# ADVANCES IN NEUROIMMUNOLOGY

ANNALS OF THE NEW YORK ACADEMY OF SCIENCES
Volume 540

# ADVANCES IN NEUROIMMUNOLOGY

*Edited by Cedric S. Raine*

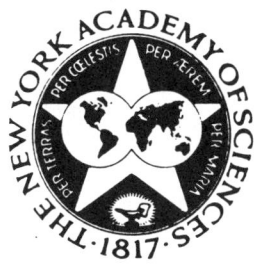

The New York Academy of Sciences
New York, New York
1988

Copyright © 1988 by the New York Academy of Sciences. All rights reserved. Under the provisions of the United States Copyright Act of 1976, individual readers of the Annals are permitted to make fair use of the material in them for teaching and research. Permission is granted to quote from the Annals provided that the customary acknowledgment is made of the source. Material in the Annals may be republished only by permission of the Academy. Address inquiries to the Executive Editor at the New York Academy of Sciences.

Copying fees: For each copy of an article made beyond the free copying permitted under Section 107 or 108 of the 1976 Copyright Act, a fee should be paid through the Copyright Clearance Center, Inc., 21 Congress St., Salem, MA 01970. For articles of more than 3 pages the copying fee is $1.75.

∞ The paper used in this publication meets the minimum requirements of American National Standard for Information Sciences—Permanence of Paper for Printed Library Materials, ANSI Z39.48-1984.

### Library of Congress Cataloging-in-Publication Data

Advances in neuroimmunology.

(Annals of the New York Academy of Sciences, ISSN 0077-8923 ; v. 540)
Based on the Second International Congress of Neuroimmunology, held by the New York Academy of Sciences in Philadelphia, Pa., Sept. 8-11, 1987.
Includes bibliographies and index.
1. Nervous system—Diseases—Immunological aspects—Congresses. 2. Neuroimmunology—Congresses. I. Raine, Cedric S., 1940- . II. International Congress of Neuroimmunology (2nd : 1987 : Philadelphia, Pa.) III. New York Academy of Sciences. IV. Series.
[DNLM: 1. Nervous System—immunology—congresses. 2. Nervous System Diseases—immunology—congresses. W1 AN626YL v.540 / WL 100 A2439 1987]
Q11.N5 vol. 540      500 s      88-32916
[RC346.5]      [616.8'0479]
ISBN 0-89766-476-0
ISBN 0-89766-477-9 (pbk.)

PCP
*Printed in the United States of America*
**ISBN 0-89766-476-0** (cloth)
**ISBN 0-89766-477-9** (paper)
**ISSN 0077-8923**

ANNOTATION OF THE NEW YORK ACADEMY OF SCIENCES

*Volume 540*
*November 28, 1988*

# ADVANCES IN NEUROIMMUNOLOGY[a]

*Editor*
CEDRIC S. RAINE

## CONTENTS

Preface. *By* CEDRIC S. RAINE ........................................ xxiii

### Part I. Basic Immunology and Immune Regulation

The T-Cell Antigen Receptor: Structure and Mechanism of Activation. *By* LAWRENCE E. SAMELSON AND RICHARD D. KLAUSNER ...................................................... 1

Immunoregulation in Rapidly Progressive Multiple Sclerosis. *By* BARRY G. W. ARNASON, AVERTANO B. C. NORONHA, AND ANTHONY T. REDER ............................................. 4

Autoimmunity in Demyelinating Diseases. *By* BYRON H. WAKSMAN ........................................................ 13

Autoimmunity in Neuromuscular Disease. *By* JOHN NEWSOM-DAVIS ........................................................... 25

### Part II. Nervous System Differentiation

Expression of Neural Cell Adhesion Molecules in Normal and Pathologic Tissues. *By* ROBERT BRACKENBURY ................. 39

Where do Different Neurons Come From? Identification and Immortalization of CNS Precursor Cells. *By* RON MCKAY ..... 47

Astrocyte Diversity. *By* A. PROCHIANTZ AND M. MALLAT .......... 52

Relevance for Neurobiology and Neurooncology of Antigens of Malignant Gliomas As Defined by Monoclonal Antibodies. *By* FOTIOS D. VRIONIS, CAROL J. WIKSTRAND, AND DARELL D. BIGNER ......................................................... 64

Diagnostic Markers in Human Neurooncology: A Progress Report. *By* LUCIEN J. RUBINSTEIN ...................................... 78

[a] This volume is the result of a conference entitled Second International Congress of Neuroimmunology, which was held by the New York Academy of Sciences on September 8-11, 1987 in Philadelphia, Pennsylvania.

Paraneoplastic Autoimmunity. *By* ANDREAS J. STECK AND E.
    NARDELLI........................................................ 91

### Part III. Clinical Neuroimmunology

Immunology of Multiple Sclerosis. *By* HENRY F. MCFARLAND ..... 99
Narcolepsy and HLA in the Japanese. *By* TAKEO JUJI, KAZUMASA
    MATSUKI, KATSUSHI TOKUNAGA, TOHRU NAOHARA, AND
    YUTAKA HONDA.................................................. 106
Neurologic Complications of Collagen Vascular Diseases. *By*
    ROBERT P. LISAK, PATRICIA M. MOORE, ARNOLD I.
    LEVINSON, AND BURTON ZWEIMAN............................. 115
Immune Mechanisms in Inflammatory Polyneuropathy. *By* H. P.
    HARTUNG, K. HEININGER, B. SCHÄFER, W. FIERZ, AND K.
    V. TOYKA ....................................................... 122
Infection of the Central Nervous System by Human
    Immunodeficiency Virus: Role of the Immune System in
    Pathogenesis. *By* RICHARD W. PRICE AND BRUCE BREW....... 162
Strategies for the Treatment of Myasthenia Gravis. *By* DANIEL B.
    DRACHMAN, KEVIN R. MCINTOSH, SHARI DE SILVA, RALPH
    W. KUNCL, AND CAROLYN KAHN............................... 176

### Part IV. Virus-Induced Disease and Autoimmunity

Autoimmune Demyelination in the Central Nervous System. *By*
    TAKESHI TABIRA................................................. 187
Autoimmune Reactions Against Myelin Basic Protein Induced by
    Corona and Measles Viruses. *By* VOLKER TER MEULEN ........ 202
Virus-Induced Autoimmunity Through Molecular Mimicry. *By*
    ROBERT S. FUJINAMI ............................................ 210
Immunobiology of Microglial Cells. *By* KARL FREI, CHRISTINE
    SIEPL, PETER GROSCURTH, STEFAN BODMER, AND ADRIANO
    FONTANA....................................................... 218
Cell-Mediated Immunity in Virus Infections of the Central Nervous
    System. *By* PETER C. DOHERTY.................................. 228
Mechanisms of Virus-Induced Demyelination and Remyelination.
    *By* MOSES RODRIGUEZ .......................................... 240

### Workshop 1. Immunogenetics and Gene Regulation

Brain Transplantation in Genetic Analysis of Experimental Allergic
    Encephalomyelitis. *By* FRED D. LUBLIN, ROBERT L.
    KNOBLER, JOSEPH MARINI, AND DAN GOLDOWITZ............ 252

Molecular Identification of Regulatory DNA Sequences for Basal and Gamma-Interferon-Induced Expression of HLA DRα in Human Multiforme Glioblastoma Cell Lines. *By* P. BASTA, P. SHERMAN, AND J. TING ......................................... 255

Generation of Antibodies to Gangliosides GM1 and GD1b: Genetic Control of Fine Antigenic Specificity. *By* HIROAKI ITO, ROBERT K. YU, AND NORMAN LATOV......................... 258

Quantitation of IgG Subclasses in Cerebrospinal Fluid of Patients with Multiple Sclerosis. *By* P. D. MEHTA........................ 261

Gene Activation During Experimental Allergic Encephalomyelitis: Cloning of New cDNAs. *By* HERMANN J. SCHLUESENER, KAI W. WUCHERPFENNIG, AND HOWARD L. WEINER............... 264

Associations of the Autoimmune Myasthenias with Genetic Markers in the Immunoglobulin Heavy Chain Region. *By* ANDY DEMAINE, NICK WILLCOX, KEN WELSH, AND JOHN NEWSOM-DAVIS................................................. 266

Determination of RFLPs Linked to Multiple Sclerosis Susceptibility. *By* VIVIAN H. COHN, DOTY SEARS, MARK HESS, RICHARD S. SPIELMAN, NORMAN ARNHEIM, AND LESLIE P. WEINER............................................. 269

Molecular Genotypes of the T-Cell Receptor Beta Chain in Families with Multiple Sclerosis. *By* T. A. CIULLA, M. A. ROBINSON, E. SEBOUN, T. H. DOOLITTLE, T. HAYASHI, T. J. KINDT, AND S. L. HAUSER....................................... 271

Antibody-Producing Cells in CSF and Peripheral Blood: A New Principle for Evaluation of B-Cell Response in Inflammatory Nervous System Diseases. *By* H. LINK, S. BAIG, T. OLSSON, AND A. ZACHAU............................................... 277

Bone Marrow Cells in Multiple Sclerosis: A Functional and Phenotypic Study. *By* S. KAM-HANSEN, S. FREDRIKSON, AND C. Z-LU ...................................................... 282

Intrathecal Antimeasles Immunity in 140 Patients with Multiple Sclerosis. *By* E. SCHULLER, E. RUZICKA, B. ALLINQUANT, P. LEBON, A. GOVAERTS, AND J. D. DEGOS ....................... 286

Autoantibodies in Serum and CSF of Patients with Multiple Sclerosis. *By* A. BLANCHER, P. MATSIOTA, B. GUILBERT, B. DOYON, M. CLANET, E. KOUVELAS, A. RASCOL, AND S. AVRAMEAS ...................................................... 290

**Workshop 2. T-Cell and Immune System Product Localization in Target Tissue**

B-Cell Compartment in the Thymus of Patients with Myasthenia Gravis and Control Subjects. *By* B. CHRISTENSSON, P. BIBERFELD, AND G. MATELL ................................... 293

Thymopoietin: A Marker of the Human Nicotinic Acetylcholine Receptor. *By* E. MOREL, B. VERNET-DER-GARABEDIAN, F. RAIMOND, T. K. AUDHYA, G. GOLDSTEIN, AND J. F. BACH... 298

Expression and Cellular Localization of Major Histocompatibility Complex Antigens in Active Multiple Sclerosis Lesions. *By* TATSUHIKO HAYASHI, JACK S. BURKS, AND STEPHEN L. HAUSER .......................................................... 301

Immunohistochemical Analysis of Suppressor-Inducer and Helper-Inducer T Cells in Multiple Sclerosis Brain Tissue. *By* RAYMOND A. SOBEL, DAVID A. HAFLER, EDUARDO E. CASTRO, CHIKAO MORIMOTO, AND HOWARD L. WEINER...... 306

Demonstration of α, β, and γ Interferon in Active Chronic Multiple Sclerosis Lesions. *By* U. TRAUGOTT AND P. LEBON... 309

Immunoglobulin G (IgG) Localization During Acute Autoimmune Demyelination. *By* G. R. WAYNE MOORE AND CEDRIC S. RAINE .......................................................... 312

Endothelial Cell Ia Increases Before Inflammatory Cell Infiltration in EAE Induced in Long-tailed Macaques. *By* LYNN M. ROSE, ROSEMARIE PETERSON, RAJ MEHRA, AND ELLSWORTH C. ALVORD, JR. ...................................................... 315

Occurrence of HLA-DR Reactive Microglia in Alzheimer's Disease. *By* P. L. MCGEER, S. ITAGAKI, H. TAGO, AND E. G. MCGEER .......................................................... 319

Interleukin-2 Blocks Oligodendrocyte Progenitor Proliferation. *By* ROBERT L. KNOBLER, RUSSELL P. SANETO, AMNON ALTMAN, HOWARD M. JOHNSON, AND JEAN DE VELLIS....... 324

Comparison of Indirect Immunofluorescence and Immunogold-Silver Staining on Cell Surface Antigens of PNS and CNS Cells. *By* CONSTANCE J. DIFIGLIA AND KAY L. FIELDS........ 327

Loss of Functional Suppression Is Linked to Decreases in Circulating Suppressor-Inducer (CD4+2H4+) T Cells in Multiple Sclerosis. *By* MICHEL CHOFFLON, HOWARD L. WEINER, AND DAVID A. HAFLER .............................. 330

A 70-Kd Polypeptide Secreted by Human Peripheral Blood Mononuclear Cells That Suppresses Proliferation of a Human Glioblastoma Cell Line. *By* TIMOTHY J. HEMESATH, DARREL TARASEWICZ, ALISON O'NEILL, JEFFREY R. GULCHER, AND KARI STEFANSSON ................................................ 333

## Workshop 3. Lymphocyte Lines and Disease

Response of Rat Encephalitogenic T Cells to Synthetic Peptides of Guinea Pig Myelin Basic Protein. *By* ARTHUR A. VANDENBARK, GEORGE HASHIM, AND HALINA OFFNER....... 337

Analysis of Helper T-Cell Specificity Involved in the Antibody Response to the Acetylcholine Receptor. *By* JOSEPH A. TAMI AND KEITH A. KROLICK ............................................. 340

Experimental Allergic Encephalomyelitis Mediated by Murine Encephalitogenic T-Cell Lines Specific for Myelin Proteolipid Apoprotein. *By* JUN-ICHI SATOH, FUMIHIKO KOIKE, AND TAKESHI TABIRA ........................................................ 343

Fine Specificities of Myelin Basic Protein-Specific Human T-Cell Clones. *By* J. R. RICHERT, C. A. REUBEN-BURNSIDE, G. E. DEIBLER, AND M. W. KIES ............................................ 345

Alterations in the Pattern of MHC Restriction of T Cells in Relapsing Murine Experimental Allergic Encephalomyelitis. *By* R. M. MCCARRON, R. FALLIS, AND D. E. MCFARLIN ......... 349

Recognition of Intracellular Measles Virus Antigens by HLA Class II Restricted Measles Virus-Specific Cytotoxic T Lymphocytes. *By* STEVEN JACOBSON, RAFICK P. SEKALY, WILLIAM J. BELLINI, CONNIE L. JOHNSON, HENRY F. MCFARLAND, AND ERIC O. LONG ................................................... 352

Blood and Thymic Lymphocyte Responses to Peptide Sequences of the Acetylcholine Receptor in Myasthenia Gravis. *By* G. HARCOURT, N. SOMMER, J. ROTHBARD, D. BEESON, N. WILLCOX, AND J. NEWSOM-DAVIS ............................ 354

T-Cell Clones Specific to Acetylcholine Receptor, Its Subunits, and Peptides. *By* YOSHITAKA FUJII AND JON LINDSTROM .......... 357

Synergism in the Pathogenesis of EAE Induced by an MBP-Specific T-Cell Line and Monoclonal Antibodies to Galactocerebroside or a Myelin Oligodendroglial Glycoprotein. *By* W. FIERZ, K. HEININGER, B. SCHAEFER, K. V. TOYKA, C. LININGTON, AND H. LASSMANN .................................................. 360

A Suppressor Cell Line That Prevents the Adoptive Transfer of EAE in Lewis Rats. *By* KAREN ELLERMAN AND STEVEN BROSTOFF ...................................................... 364

Isolation of Human Lymphocyte Cell Lines Reactive with Whole Human Myelin. *By* JAMES BURNS AND KIMBERLY LITTLEFIELD .................................................. 367

**Workshop 4. Antibodies and Complement in Autoimmunity**

Voltage-Dependent $CA^{2+}$ Channels in Small Cell Carcinomas Are Blocked by Autoantibodies from Patients with Lambert-Eaton Myasthenic Syndrome. *By* HENRY J. DE AIZPURUA, GUY E. GRIESMANN, EDWARD H. LAMBERT, AND VANDA A. LENNON ......................................................... 369

Complement Allotyping Explains MHC Associations in Multiple Sclerosis. *By* W. J. ZHANG, T. J. COBAIN, R. L. DAWKINS, G. GRIMSLEY, AND I. R. MACKAY.................................. 372

Myelin Vesicles As an *in Vitro* Model to Study Mechanisms of Myelin Damage by Immune Effectors. *By* PADMAVATHY VANGURI AND MOON L. SHIN ................................... 374

Serum Antibodies to Peripheral Nerve Antigens in Guillain-Barré Syndrome. *By* T. NEGISHI, T. YAMASHITA, K. NOMURA, T. HOSOKAWA, R. OHNO, K. HAMAGUCHI, AND K. YUEMURA... 376

Neuropathy and Monoclonal IgM M-Protein with Antibody Activity Against Gangliosides. *By* E. NARDELLI, A. J. STECK, M. SCHLUEP, K. FELGENHAUER, AND F. JERUSALEM .......... 378

Mechanism of Arachidonic Acid Release by Terminal Complement Complexes from Rat Oligodendrocyte X C6 Glioma Cell Hybrids. *By* Y. SHIRAZI, F. A. MCMORRIS, AND M. L. SHIN .. 381

Clonal Restriction of Complement-Fixing Antineural Antibodies in the Guillain-Barré Syndrome. *By* BJÖRN RYBERG ............... 384

Terminal Complement Complexes (SC5b-9) in Cerebrospinal Fluid in Autoimmune Nervous System Diseases. *By* M. E. SANDERS, E. L. ALEXANDER, C. L. KOSKI, M. L. SHIN, Y. SANO, M. M. FRANK, AND K. A. JOINER......................................... 387

**Workshop 5. Neural Cell Markers in Health and Disease**

Expression of Voltage-Gated Calcium Channels in Tumor Cell Lines of Neuroectodermal or Other Origin. *By* BETHAN LANG, NITA NAGVEKAR, JASVINDER GILL, ANGELA VINCENT, AND JOHN NEWSOM-DAVIS........................................... 389

Rat Astrocyte Proliferation by Human B-Cell Growth Factors. *By* ETTY N. BENVENISTE, JOSEPH L. BUTLER, DAVID A. GIBBS, ALICE CHEN, AND JOHN N. WHITAKER....................... 392

EAE Serum Decreases CNPase Activity in Cultures of B104 Cells. *By* R. ELKIN, W. D. LYMAN, C. F. BROSNAN, AND M. B. BORNSTEIN ..................................................... 396

Antibody for Nerve Growth Factor Detected in Patients with Alzheimer's Disease. *By* BENJAMIN F. ROY, TREY SUNDERLAND, DENNIS L. MURPHY, AND JOHN M. MORIHISA 398

Cytotoxic Response of Cultured Tumor Infiltrating Lymphocytes to Autologous Human Glioblastoma Cells. *By* M. C. KUPPNER, M. F. HAMOU, AND N. DE TRIBOLET ......................... 401

Phospholipase $A_2$ Activity in Cultured Glial Cells: Correlation with Appearance of Myelin Markers and Effects of Steroid

Hormones. *By* T. Brenner, S. Yedgar, J. Weidenfeld, and O. Abramsky ................................................. 403

Cloning of cDNA for Two Large Polypeptides Found in Myelinating Oligodendrocytes. *By* Jeffrey R. Gulcher, Linda S. Marton, and Kari Stefansson .................... 405

Neuroleukin Secretion Is Highly Regulated in T Cells But Constitutive in C6 Glioma Cells. *By* Gregory T. Spear and Mark E. Gurney ................................................ 407

A Peanut Agglutinin Binding Glycoprotein in CNS Myelin and Oligodendrocytes. *By* Daniel D. Mikol, Sara Szuchet, and Kari Stefansson ........................................... 409

Cells Proliferating *in Vitro* to Local Brain Injury Are Primarily of Hematic Origin and Differ from Those Associated with Anterograde Degeneration. *By* I. R. Katz, L. Iacovitti, and D. J. Reis ....................................................... 413

## Workshop 6.  Glia-Neuron Interactions

Interactions of Astroglia-Derived Factors with Hippocampal Neurons. *By* H. P. Matthiessen, C. Schmalenbach, and H. W. Müller .................................................. 416

Changes in Astrocyte Extracellular Matrix with Differentiation and after Contact with Neurites. *By* March D. Ard and Richard P. Bunge ............................................. 420

Antisera to an Axolemma-Enriched Fraction Have Antiaxon and Antimyelin Effects *in Vitro*. *By* Dennis N. Bourdette, Fredrick J. Seil, Charles K. Meshul, John W. Bigbee, George H. DeVries, and Harish C. Agrawal ............. 423

Substance P Stimulates Release of Arachidonic Acid Cyclooxgenation Products from Primary Culture Rat Astrocytes. *By* Hans-Peter Hartung, Kurt Heininger, Bärbel Schäfer, and Klaus V. Toyka ...................... 427

Insulin-Like Growth Factor-I Stimulates Regeneration of Oligodendrocytes *in Vitro*. *By* Robin L. Mozell and F. Arthur McMorris ............................................. 430

Intracellular Messengers: Influence of Oligodendrocyte Substratum Adhesion. *By* Timothy Vartanian, Glyn Dawson, and Sara Szuchet ................................................. 433

Glioblastoma-Cell-Derived T-Cell Suppressor Factor (G-TsF): Sequence Analysis and Biologic Mechanism of G-TsF. *By* C. Siepl, S. Bodmer, E. Hofer, M. Wrann, K. Frei, and A. Fontana ........................................................ 437

## Workshop 7. Cross-Recognition Between Nervous and Immune System Antigen

Antineuronal Autoantibodies in Neurologic Paraneoplastic
  Syndromes. *By* NEIL E. ANDERSON AND JEROME B. POSNER .. 440

Antibodies to Sulfated Glucuronic Acid Containing
  Glycosphingolipids in Neuropathy Associated with Anti-Mag
  Antibodies and in Normal Individuals. *By* SCOTT MCGINNIS,
  TATSUO KOHRIYAMA, ROBERT K. YU, MICHAEL A. PESCE,
  AND NORMAN LATOV ............................................. 442

Mammalian Reovirus Receptor Expression by Oligodendrocytes. *By*
  JEFFREY A. COHEN, ROBERT C. SERGOTT, HERBERT M.
  GELLER, MARK J. BROWN, AND MARK I. GREENE ............ 445

Isolation and Characterization of *Borrelia Burgdorferi*-Specific and
  Autoreactive T-Cell Lines from the Cerebrospinal Fluid of
  Patients with Lyme Meningoradiculomyelitis. *By* ROLAND
  MARTIN, JOHANNES ORTLAUF, VERONIKA STICHT-GROH,
  AND HANS GEORG MERTENS .................................... 449

Monoclonal Antibodies Against the P2 Protein of Peripheral
  Myelin and d18 Protein of PC Cells Bind to Antigen-
  Presenting Cells and Inhibit T-Cell Activation. *By* DONARD S.
  DWYER, F. PIERRE VANDERVEGT, JOACHIM BARTELS, AND
  GEORGE B. BROWN............................................... 452

Expression of Leukocyte Antigens on an Oligodendroglial Cell Line.
  *By* LYNN M. ROSE, SUSANNE L. JACKEVICIUS, AND EDWARD
  A. CLARK ....................................................... 455

Characterization and *in Vitro* Use of a Monoclonal Anti-Idiotypic
  Antibody Against HNK-1. *By* M. SCHLUEP, N. PAGE, G.
  PERRUISSEAU, AND A. J. STECK ................................ 459

Lesion-Induced Changes of Astrocyte Morphology and Protein
  Expression in Rat Optic Nerve. *By* GUIDO STOLL AND HANS-
  WERNER MUELLER............................................... 461

Glia Cells as Immunoregulatory Elements: Up- and Down-
  Regulatory Activities of Astrocyte Clones. *By* DEMING SUN,
  RICHARD MEYERMANN, AND HARTMUT WEKERLE ............ 463

Autoantibody Reactive Integral Membrane Antigens of Thymocytes
  and Brain. *By* A. NARENDRAN AND S. A. HOFFMAN ........... 466

A Monoclonal Antibody with Anti-Lipomodulin Activity Reverses
  a $\beta$-Adrenergic Response. *By* NINA L. PAUL, CURTIS A.
  WILLIAMS, AND NICOLE SCHUPF ................................ 467

Antibody Cross-Reactivity Between Myelin Basic Protein and CD3
  Antigen of T Cells: Implications for Autoimmunity. *By* W.
  WEBER, Z. JINGWU, J. BORST, AND W. BUURMAN.............. 470

Expression of Class II Antigens on Peripheral Nerve Allografts. *By* L. T. Yu, W. F. Hickey, W. S. Silvers, D. LaRossa, and A. M. Rostami .................................................... 472

**Workshop 8. MHC Antigens on Nervous Tissue**

Down-Regulation of Gamma-Interferon-Induced Class II Expression of Human Glioma Cells by Recombinant Beta-Interferon. *By* Jeymohan Joseph, Concetta D'Imperio, Robert L. Knobler, and Fred D. Lublin ................... 475

Neurotransmitter Modulation of the Human Class II Gene DRα on Multiforme Glioblastoma Cell Lines: A Molecular Analysis. *By* J. Ting, P. Sherman, S. Yokota, T. Moore, and P. Basta    477

Functional Implications of Class I MHC Modulation in Neural Tissue. *By* Lois A. Lampson, James P. Whelan, and Gabriela Siegel ............................................... 479

West Nile Virus Infection Modulates the Expression of Class I and Class II MHC Antigens on Astrocytes *in Vitro*. *By* Y. Liu, N. King, A. Kesson, R. V. Blanden, and A. Müllbacher.... 483

Measles Virus Infection Causes Expression of Class I and Class II MHC Antigens in Rat Brain. *By* T. Olsson, J. Maehlen, A. Löve, L. Klareskog, E. Norrby, and K. Kristensson..... 486

Tumor Necrosis Factor Induces Expression of MHC Class I Antigens on Mouse Astrocytes. *By* E. Lavi, A. Suzumura, D. M. Murasko, E. M. Murray, D. H. Silberberg, and S. R. Weiss......................................................... 488

Characterization of B Cells and IA Expression in Sindbis Virus Encephalitis. *By* W. R. Tyor, T. R. Moench, and D. E. Griffin ....................................................... 491

MHC-Dependent Neural Allograft Rejection. *By* K. Rao, H. W. Kunz, T. J. Gill, III, and R. D. Lund....................... 493

MHC Antigen Expression on Glial Cells. *By* Akio Suzumura and Donald H. Silberberg ......................................... 495

Accessory Cell Competence of Human Glial Cells in Mitogenic Activation of Resting Peripheral T Cells. *By* N. Cashman, S. Boulet, L. Cragg, L. Bambridge, and J. Antel............ 498

Microglia Express MHC Class II in Normal and Demyelinating Human White Matter. *By* G. M. Hayes, M. N. Woodroofe, and M. L. Cuzner ............................................ 501

**Workshop 9. Monoclonal Antibodies in AChR Epitopes**

Proliferative Responses to Acetylcholine Receptor Peptides in Myasthenia Gravis. *By* S. BERRIH-AKNIN, S. COHEN-KAMINSKY, D. NEUMANN, J. F. BACH, AND S. FUCHS......... 504

Responsiveness of Myasthenia Gravis Lymphocytes to Recombinant Interleukin-2. *By* S. COHEN-KAMINSKY, S. BERRIH-AKNIN, AND D. SAFAR .................................................. 506

Monoclonal Antibodies as Probes for Acetylcholine Receptor Epitopes in Thymuses and Thymic Epithelial Tumors of Patients with Myasthenia Gravis and Nonmyasthenic Controls. *By* THOMAS KIRCHNER, SOCRATES TZARTOS, FLORIAN HOPPE, BERTHOLD SCHALKE, HARTMUT WEKERLE, AND HANS KONRAD MÜLLER-HERMELINK ........................ 508

Stimulation of Autoimmune Helper T Lymphocytes from Patients with Myasthenia Gravis with Synthetic Peptides of the Acetylcholine Receptor Alpha Subunit. *By* REINHARD HOHLFELD, KLAUS V. TOYKA, LUCINDA L. MINER, AND BIANCA M. CONTI-TRONCONI................................ 511

MHC Association Between Antistriational Antibody-Negative Myasthenia Gravis in the Chinese. *By* W. GIN, B. R. HAWKINS, W. J. ZHANG, V. WONG, Y. L. YU, AND R. L. DAWKINS......................................................... 513

Synthetic Peptide of Human Acetylcholine Receptor α-Subunit Sequence 125–147 (Methionine 144), a More Potent Autoantigen Than Its Norleucine 144 Analog. *By* VANDA A. LENNON, ZHONG-XIAN HUANG, DANIEL J. MCCORMICK, GUY E. GRIESMANN, NAOKI FUJII, AND EDWARD H. LAMBERT...................................................... 516

Probing for the Main Immunogenic Region of the Human Acetylcholine Receptor. *By* H. ENG, H. JÖRNVALL, M. CARLQUIST, AND A. K. LEFVERT............................... 520

*In Vitro* Blockade of Neuromuscular Transmission by Monoclonal Anti-Acetylcholine Receptor Antibodies. *By* RICARDO A. MASELLI, BRIAN JOW, DAVID P. RICHMAN, AND DEBORAH J. NELSON ...................................................... 523

Antibodies Against the Acetylcholine Receptor also in Nonmyasthenic Autoimmune Disease. *By* ANN-CHARLOTT SUNDEWALL AND ANN KARI LEFVERT ........................ 525

Standardization of Acetylcholine Receptor Antibody Measurement. *By* E. BONIFACIO, R. L. DAWKINS, M. S. GRIFFITHS, AND T. J. COBAIN ..................................................... 528

**Workshop 10. Immunotherapy of Autoimmune Diseases**

Specific Suppression of the Antibody Response to Acetylcholine Receptor *in Vitro* and *in Vivo* by Daunomycin-Acetylcholine Receptor Conjugates. *By* DIANE SHELTON, YOSHITAKA FUJII, WOLFGANG KNOGGE, AND JON LINDSTROM .................... 530

Effect of Lymphoid Irradiation on Clinical Course, Lymphocyte Count, and T-Cell Subsets in Chronic Progressive Multiple Sclerosis. *By* S. D. COOK. C. DEVEREUX, R. TROIANO, C. ROHOWSKY-KOCHAN, G. ZITO, AND P. C. DOWLING .......... 533

Cumulative Experience with High-Dose Intravenous Cyclophosphamide and ACTH Therapy in Chronic Progressive Multiple Sclerosis. *By* JONATHAN L. CARTER, DAVID M. DAWSON, DAVID A. HAFLER, ROBERT J. FALLIS, LYNN STAZZONE, JOHN ORAV, AND HOWARD L. WEINER............ 535

Suppressor Cell Regulation of Chronic Relapsing Experimental Allergic Encephalomyelitis. *By* RUTH H. WHITHAM, DENNIS N. BOURDETTE, HALINA OFFNER, CHARLES K. MESHUL, AND ARTHUR A. VANDENBARK................................. 537

Attenuated T-Lymphocyte Lines As Vaccinating Agents Against Experimental Autoimmune Encephalomyelitis. *By* HALINA OFFNER, RICHARD JONES, AND ARTHUR A. VANDENBARK .... 540

Inhibition of Passive Allergic Encephalomyelitis by Sulfated Polysaccharides. *By* DAVID O. WILLENBORG AND CHRISTOPHER R. PARISH........................................ 543

Suppression of Experimental Allergic Neuritis by Cyclosporin A. *By* H. NAKAYASU, K. OTA, H. TANAKA, H. IRIE, AND K. TAKAHASHI..................................................... 546

Low-dose Cyclosporin A Induces Relapsing Experimental Allergic Encephalomyelitis in the Lewis Rat. *By* CHRISTINE D. DIJKSTRA, C. J. A. DE GROOT, J. C. KOETSIER, I. MATTHAEI, C. H. POLMAN, AND T. SMINIA................................... 549

Treatment of Experimental Allergic Myasthenia Gravis with a New Immunosuppressant: 15-Deoxyspergualin. *By* YASUNORI ISHIGAKI, TAKESHI SATO, SONG TONG-LIN, AND KYOZO HAYASHI ........................................................... 551

Therapeutic Immunoadsorption of Acetylcholine Receptor Antibodies in Myasthenia Gravis. *By* TAKESHI SATO, YASUNORI ISHIGAKI, TADATOSHI KOMIYA, AND HIROSHI TSUDA ................................................................ 554

## Workshop 11. Monoclonal Antibody and Lymphokine Therapy

Anti-CD4 and Anti-CD2 Monoclonal Antibody Infusions in Subjects with Multiple Sclerosis: Immunosuppressive Effects and Human Antimouse Responses. *By* DAVID A. HAFLER AND HOWARD L. WEINER ............................................. 557

Effects on Experimental Allergic Neuritis in Rats by *in Vivo* Treatment with Monoclonal Anti-T-Cell Antibodies. *By* T. OLSSON, K. STRIGÅRD, P. LARSSON, R. HOLMDAHL, AND L. KLARESKOG ..................................................... 560

Suppression of P2-T-Cell Line Mediated Experimental Autoimmune Neuritis by Interleukin-2 Receptor Blockade. *By* H. P. HARTUNG, B. SCHÄFER, T. DIAMANTSTEIN, W. FIERZ, K. HEININGER, AND K. V. TOYKA ................................. 563

Sindbis Virus Neutralization. *By* M. E. WESTARP, J. STANLEY, AND D. E. GRIFFIN ............................................. 566

Tumor Necrosis Factor Mediates Myelin Damage in Organotypic Cultures of Nervous Tissue. *By* KRZYSZTOF SELMAJ AND CEDRIC S. RAINE ....................................................... 568

Recombinant Human Lymphokines Induce Changes in Visual Evoked Potentials in the Rabbit. *By* C. F. BROSNAN, K. SELMAJ, C. E. SCHROEDER, M. LITWAK, C. S. RAINE, AND J. C. AREZZO ................................................... 571

Intracerebral Beta-Interferon in Brain Tumor Therapy: Monitoring Cerebral Function with Compressed Spectral Analysis. *By* ROBERT L. KNOBLER, FRED D. LUBLIN, LEOPOLD J. STRELETZ, MICHAEL ZIMMER, JEYMOHAN JOSEPH, CONCETTA D'IMPERIO, BRUCE NORTHRUP, GIANCARLO BAROLAT, AND STEPHEN G. MARCUS .......................................... 573

Clonal Modulation of Experimental Allergic Encephalomyelitis by a Monoclonal Antibody Directed to the T-Cell Receptor. *By* E. HEBER-KATZ, M. OWHASHI, M. P. HAPP, F. BURNS, N. SHEN, AND X. LI .............................................. 576

Inhibition of Experimental Allergic Encephalomyelitis by a New Anti-Inflammatory Compound — SK&F 86002. *By* M. J. DIMARTINO, C. E. WOLFF, G. K. CAMPBELL, JR., AND N. HANNA ................................................... 578

Anti-CD4 Monoclonal Antibody Therapy of Experimental Allergic Encephalomyelitis in Longtailed Macaques. *By* LYNN M. ROSE, ELLSWORTH C. ALVORD, JR., SARKA HRUBY, SUSANNE L. JACKEVICIUS, ROSEMARIE PETERSEN, NOEL WARNER, AND EDWARD A. CLARK ................................................. 581

**Workshop 12. Clinical Immunogenetics**

Blood Lymphocyte β-Adrenergic Receptors in Multiple Sclerosis. *By* BARRY G. W. ARNASON, MARGARET BROWN, RICARDO MASELLI, JOE KARASZEWSKI, AND ANTHONY REDER ......... 585

ACTH Production by Human Mononuclear Cells. *By* ANTHONY T. REDER, SUSMITHA PINAMANENI, WILLIAM SMYKA, AND DANIEL NUTTER.................................................. 589

Identification of Myelin Basic Protein-Specific Oligoclonal Bands in Multiple Sclerosis. *By* KEISUKE MORIMOTO, SHIN-ICHIRO IKEBE, AND TAKESHI SATO ...................................... 592

Human T-Cell Response to Human and Heterologous Myelin Basic Proteins. *By* E. TOURNIER-LASSERVE, G. HASHIM, AND M. A. BACH ............................................................ 594

Changes in Immune Function in Relapsing Multiple Sclerosis Correlate with Disease Activity as Assessed by Magnetic Resonance Imaging. *By* J. OGER, M. O'GORMAN, E. WILLOUGHBY, D. LI, AND D. W. PATY ........................ 597

Immunodiagnosis and Immunotherapy in Autistic Children. *By* V. K. SINGH, H. H. FUDENBERG, D. EMERSON, AND M. COLEMAN ...................................................... 602

Long-Term Follow-up Study of Relapse in Symptoms and Reelevation of Acetylcholine Receptor Antibody Titers in Patients with Myasthenia Gravis. *By* TADATOSHI KOMIYA AND TAKESHI SATO.................................................. 605

Lymphocyte Subsets after Stroke. *By* A. CZŁONKOWSKA, J. KORLAK, AND A. KUCZYŃSKA................................... 608

**Workshop 13. Neuroimmunology of AIDS and Slow Virus Infections**

Human Immunodeficiency Virus gp120 and p24 Oligoclonal Antibody in Acquired Immunodeficiency Syndrome Cerebrospinal Fluid and Sera. *By* LUIGI M. E. GRIMALDI, RAYMOND P. ROOS, ADRIANO LAZZARIN, MARIO MORONI, JAMES M. CASEY, AND SUSHILKUMAR G. DEVARE............ 611

Intrathecal Synthesis of Anti-HIV Oligoclonal IgG in HIV-Seropositive Patients Having No Signs of HIV-Induced Neurologic Diseases. *By* P. GALLO, A. DE ROSSI, P. CADROBBI, E. FRANCAVILLA, L. CHIECO-BIANCHI, AND B. TAVOLATO ...................................................... 615

Intrathecal Immunity in 37 Patients Seropositive for Anti-HIV-1 Antibody. *By* J. REBOUL, E. SCHULLER, G. PIALOUX, M. A. REY, P. LEBON, AND F. BRUN-VEZINET ....................... 619

Cerebrospinal Fluid Changes in HIV-1 Infection. *By* MATS ANDERSSON, TOMAS BERGSTRÖM, CHRISTIAN BLOMSTRAND, SVANTE HERMODSSON, CHARLES HÅKANSSON, AND GUN-BRITT LÖWHAGEN................................................. 624

An AIDS Virus-Associated Antigen Localized in Human Fetal Brain. *By* W. D. LYMAN, Y. KRESS, W. K. RASHBAUM, T. A. CALVELLI, E. STEINHAUER, J. M. KASHKIN, C. E. HENDERSON, AND A. RUBINSTEIN............................... 628

Pathogenesis of Human Immunodeficiency Virus (HIV)-Associated Brain Lesions: A Neuropathologic Evaluation. *By* HERBERT BUDKA ............................................................. 630

Host-Virus Interaction in Caprine Arthritis-Encephalitis. *By* M. C. ZINK AND O. NARAYAN............................................ 634

HTLV-I Myelitis: Isolation of Virus, Genomic Analysis, and Infection in Neural Cell Cultures. *By* T. SAIDA, K. SAIDA, M. FUNAUCHI, E. NISHIGUCHI, M. NAKAJIMA, S. MATSUDA, M. OHTA, K. OHTA, H. NISHITANI, AND M. HATANAKA.......... 636

Sera from Patients with Multiple Sclerosis React with Human T-Cell Lymphotropic Virus-I GAG Proteins: Western Blotting and Solid-Phase Radioimmunoassay Analyses. *By* M. OHTA, T. SAIDA, K. OHTA, F. MORI, H. NISHITANI, R. FUJINO, AND M. IKEDA ................................................................ 639

Immune Effects of Intracerebral Infection with Mouse Hepatitis Virus. *By* Robert L. Knobler, George C. Brainard, Marielle Perreault, Concetta D'Imperio, Paula Phenix, and Fred D. Lublin ....................................................................... 642

Impaired Measles-Specific Cytotoxic T-Cell Response in Subacute Sclerosing Panencephalitis. *By* SUHAYL DHIB-JALBUT, STEVEN JACOBSON, DALE E. MCFARLIN, AND HENRY F. MCFARLAND  645

**Workshop 14. Molecular Mimicry and Virus-Induced Demyelination**

Caprine Retroviral Encephalitis in Previously Infected and in Specific Pathogen-Free Goats. *By* G. C. JOHNSON, D. S. ADAMS, AND T. C. MCGUIRE..................................... 649

Sequence Comparison of a Highly Virulent and a Less Virulent Strain of Theiler's Virus. Amino Acid Differences on a Three-Dimensional Model Identify the Location of Possible Immunogenic Sites. *By* DANIEL C. PEVEAR, JOSEPH BORKOWSKI, MING LUO, AND HOWARD LIPTON ............... 652

Herpes Simplex Virus Type 1 Induced Multifocal Demyelination of the Central Nervous System in Mice. *By* L. F. KASTRUKOFF, A. S. LAU, AND S. U. KIM............................................. 654

Enumeration and Distribution of T-Cell Subsets, Macrophages, and IgG Positive Cells in the CNS of SJL/J Mice Infected with Theiler's Virus. *By* MARK D. LINDSLEY, ROGER L. THIEMANN, AND MOSES RODRIGUEZ........................... 657

Borna Disease. An Immunopathologic Response to Viral Infection in the CNS. *By* K. M. CARBONE, C. S. DUCHALA, AND O. NARAYAN ...................................................... 661

Coronavirus-JHM-Induced Demyelinating Encephalomyelitis in Rats. Analysis of the Intrathecal Immune Response. *By* R. DORRIES, S. SCHWENDER, H. WEGE, H. HARMS, R. WATANABE, AND V. TER MEULEN ............................ 663

Early Viral Proteins As Autoantigens. Evidence from JC Virus Large T Antigen. *By* G. L. STONER, C. F. RYSCHKEWITSCH, D. L. WALKER, D. SOFFER, D. G. BRAUN, H. K. HOCHKEPPEL, AND H. DEF. WEBSTER ......................... 665

Increases in the Immune Responses to Theiler's Murine Encephalomyelitis Virus after Neonatal Treatment with Anti-T-Cell Receptor Antibody. *By* MARY CRANE, STEPHEN MILLER, HOWARD LIPTON, AND BYUNG KIM .................. 669

Semliki Forest Virus (A7[74]) Infection of Adult Mice Induces an Immune-Mediated Demyelinating Encephalomyelitis. *By* J. K. FAZAKERLEY, A. KHALILI-SHIRAZI, AND H. E. WEBB ......... 672

Fine Specificity of T-Cell-Mediated Immune Responses of Susceptible and Resistant Strains in Theiler's Murine Encephalomyelitis Virus-Induced Demyelinating Disease. *By* STEPHEN D. MILLER, RICHARD J. CLATCH, AND HOWARD L. LIPTON ....................................................... 674

A Study of Persistent Viral Infections Using Nude Mice and a Temperature-Sensitive Mutant of Vesicular Stomatitis Virus. *By* SHARON C. DOLL AND TERRY C. JOHNSON ..................... 678

**Workshop 15. Neuroimmunomodulation**

Potentiation of Il-1-Induced BALB/3T3 Fibroblast Proliferation by Substance P. *By* EDWARD S. KIMBALL AND M. C. FISHER..... 681

Suppression of Anaphylactic Shock by Enkephalins. *By* DRAGAN MARIĆ AND BRANISLAV D. JANKOVIĆ......................... 684

Neurokinin-Induced Generation of Interleukin-1 in a Macrophage Cell Line. *By* EDWARD S. KIMBALL, FRANCIS J. PERSICO, AND JEFFREY L. VAUGHT ........................................ 688

Enkephalins Modulate *in Vivo* Immune Reactions Through Delta- and Mu-Opioid Receptors. *By* BRANISLAV D. JANKOVIĆ AND DRAGAN MARIĆ ................................................. 691

Opioid Receptors on Murine Splenocytes. Possible Coupling to $K^+$ Channels. *By* D. J. J. CARR, J. K. BUBIEN, W. T. WOODS, AND J. E. BLALOCK........................................... 694

Somatotropin and Prolactin Enhance Respiratory Burst Activity of Macrophages. *By* CARL K. EDWARDS, III, JEANETTE M. SCHEPPER, LIBBY M. YUNGER, AND KEITH W. KELLEY....... 698

Effect of Sound Stress on the Migration of Prethymic Stem Cells. *By* CATHERINE E. BOMBERGER AND JACK L. HAAR............ 700

Interaction of Endogenous Opioids and Developing T Lymphocytes. *By* DELANE BAILEY, LEONOR GONZALES, AND MARIE METLAY....................................................... 702

Neuroendocrine Regulation of Immune Parameters. Photoperiod Control of the Spleen in Syrian Hamsters. *By* GEORGE C. BRAINARD, MARCIA WATSON-WHITMEYER, ROBERT L. KNOBLER, AND FRED D. LUBLIN............................. 704

Sympathectomy Augments the Severity of Experimental Allergic Encephalomyelitis in Rats. *By* EWA CHELMICKA-SCHOFF, MARGARET CHECINSKI, AND BARRY G. W. ARNASON......... 707

**Workshop 16. Autoimmune Models of Demyelination**

Susceptibility of PLP-Induced EAE Is Regulated by Non-H-2 Genes. *By* VINCENT K. TUOHY, RAYMOND A. SOBEL, AND MARJORIE B. LEES............................................. 709

Oligodendrocyte Proliferation and Enhanced CNS Remyelination after Therapeutic Manipulation of Chronic Relapsing EAE. *By* C. S. RAINE, R. HINTZEN, U. TRAUGOTT, AND G. R. W. MOORE........................................................ 712

Effects of $OX8^+$ Lymphocytes on *in Vitro* Lymphocyte Reactivity During Experimental Allergic Encephalomyelitis. *By* D. M. ESSAYAN, J. A. COHEN, B. ZWEIMAN, AND R. P. LISAK....... 715

Evidence for an Immunosuppressive Autoantibody in Experimental Allergic Encephalomyelitis. *By* IAIN A. M. MACPHEE AND DONALD W. MASON............................................ 718

Changes in T-Cell Subsets in Experimental Allergic Neuritis. *By* T. YAMASHITA, T. NEGISHI, K. NOMURA, T. HOSOKAWA, R. OHNO, AND K. HAMAGUCHI...................................... 720

Presence and Distribution of Nervous System-Associated Mast Cells That May Modulate Experimental Autoimmune Encephalomyelitis. *By* EDWARD L. ORR........................ 723

Role of Mast Cells in Peripheral Nervous System Demyelination. *By* DAVID JOHNSON, HOWARD L. WEINER, AND PIERRETTE A. SEELDRAYERS.............................................. 727

Resistance to Induction of Experimental Allergic Encephalomyelitis. Role of Adjuvant Components and Antigen. *By* T. BRENNER, R. MIZRACHI, AND O. ABRAMSKY............................. 729

Demyelination of the Peripheral Nervous System Causes Neurologic Signs in Myelin Basic Protein-Induced Experimental Allergic Encephalomyelitis. Implications for the Etiology of Multiple Sclerosis. *By* MICHAEL P. PENDER............................. 732

Genetic Regulation of Susceptibility and Severity of Demyelination. *By* ROBERT L. KNOBLER, FRED D. LUBLIN, D. SCOTT LINTHICUM, MEL COHN, ROGER D. MELVOLD, HOWARD L. LIPTON, BENJAMIN A. TAYLOR, AND WESLEY G. BEAMER.... 735

Adoptive Transfer Experimental Autoimmune Encephalomyelitis. Evidence for Central Nerve and Spinal Root Dysfunction. *By* KURT HEININGER, WALTER FIERZ, BARBEL SCHAFER, HANS-PETER HARTUNG, AND KLAUS V. TOYKA...................... 738

Index of Contributors................................................ 741

**Major funding was provided by:**

- NATIONAL INSTITUTE OF NEUROLOGICAL COMMUNICATIVE DISORDERS & STROKE/NIH
- SANDOZ PHARMACEUTICALS CORPORATION

Additional funding was provided by:

- ACCURATE CHEMICAL AND SCIENTIFIC CORPORATION
- AMERICAN CYANAMID COMPANY
- AMERSHAM CORPORATION
- BOEHRINGER-MANNHEIM PHARMACEUTICALS
- CIBA-GEIGY CORPORATION
- EASTMAN KODAK COMPANY
- HOFFMANN-LA ROCHE, INC.
- IMPERIAL CHEMICAL INDUSTRIES
- LILLY RESEARCH LABORATORIES
- MARCH OF DIMES BIRTH DEFECT FOUNDATION
- MONSANTO COMPANY
- NATIONAL MULTIPLE SCLEROSIS SOCIETY
- NATIONAL INSTITUTES OF HEALTH
- PFIZER PHARMACEUTICAL CORPORATION
- STUART PHARMACEUTICALS/DIVISION OF ICI AMERICAS
- THE UPJOHN COMPANY

The New York Academy of Sciences believes it has a responsibility to provide an open forum for discussion of scientific questions. The positions taken by the participants in the reported conferences are their own and not necessarily those of the Academy. The Academy has no intent to influence legislation by providing such forums.

# Preface

CEDRIC S. RAINE

*Department of Pathology
Albert Einstein College of Medicine
Bronx, New York 10461*

This volume represents the proceedings of the Second International Congress of Neuroimmunology, which was held in Philadelphia, September 8-11, 1987 and which brought together basic researchers and clinicians involved in the application of immunologic methodologies to the elucidation of problems related to nervous system development and disease. Neuroimmunology as a discipline is still in its infancy although its roots date back more than 50 years when it was realized that certain neurologic disorders were related to allergic reactions. Since then, it has been shown that immunologic mechanisms are involved not only in a growing number of disease processes of the nervous system, but also in the development of nervous tissue. It is now widely accepted that the nervous system shares a unique relationship with the immune system, sometimes through shared receptors, and possesses a large repertoire of specific antigens. Thus, with the continuing and intensive application of immunologic techniques to the neurologic sciences, the specialty of neuroimmunology has evolved. As will become evident from the following pages, neuroimmunology involves workers in a large number of different disciplines. In addition to clinical neurologists, neuropathologists, and immunologists, there are virologists, biochemists, pharmacologists, endocrinologists, psychologists, anatomists, and biologists. The major diseases that now fall into its realm include multiple sclerosis, myasthenia gravis, peripheral neuropathy, systemic lupus erythematosus, AIDS, leprosy, narcolepsy, tumors, viral encephalitis, and their experimental counterparts. As a result of a need for neuroimmunology to be given an identity, in 1982 the First International Congress of Neuroimmunology was held in Stresa, Italy.

When the first meeting of what was to become the Program Planning Committee for the Second International Congress of Neuroimmunology was held in New York City in March 1986, there was little consensus as to what should comprise the proposed Congress format, its venue and participant list, or whether a publication on the proceedings should ensue, but one issue on which all were in agreement was that a second congress was long overdue. Because the First International Congress of Neuroimmunology was little more than a successful experiment involving about 150 investigators, mostly invited, from the inception of the Second Congress, it was the charge of all concerned to ensure that it would be an open meeting, genuinely international in flavor and truly representative of the field of neuroimmunology as of 1987. The net result of our combined efforts was an attendance of approximately 600 participants and a full program consisting of plenary lectures and simultaneous platform and poster sessions—a resounding testimony to the current interest in the field.

The Editor is exceedingly grateful to the plenary speakers for their didactic lectures, to the platform and poster presenters who showed us where the new frontiers lie, to the session chairpersons who stimulated audience participation, and to the discussants from the floor who helped elevate the Congress to an exciting event. No longer can neuroimmunology be perceived as a territory inhabited by esoteric scientists divorced from the realities of basic immunology, molecular biology, and clinical neurology. As was evident to all attendees, neuroimmunology has become a multidisciplinary field bent on the further understanding of fundamental and clinically related problems. Witness, therefore, in these proceedings the large selection of papers, the impressive number of front-line investigators, the high level of the science, and the diversity of the subjects covered. Those few speakers who found at the last moment that they would be unable to contribute a manuscript will miss the opportunity of being listed in this milestone document. It is indeed unfortunate that not all poster presentations could be accommodated because of space limitations, although the latter essential contributions did not go unnoticed, having appeared in abstract form in the *Journal of Neuroimmunology* (September 1987), an issue jointly sponsored by the World Federation of Neurology and Elsevier/North Holland Publishers Inc., to whom we are most grateful.

Let it be said that neuroimmunology came of age in Philadelphia. Not only were seminal works on all facets of the field presented (to which the pages embraced by this cover will attest), but also its very own International Society was born on September 11, 1987. The perceived success of the Congress, the laying of the Society's foundation stone, and the commitment of our Israeli colleagues to host the Third International Congress of Neuroimmunology in Jerusalem in 1991 appear firm pronouncements that neuroimmunology will continue to prosper for years to come.

At the outset, funding for the Congress appeared to be largely covered by a generous donation from Sandoz, Inc., but as is common with such ventures, with the march of time, costs escalated and additional support had to be solicited. Therefore, a few words of appreciation are in order: first, to our major sponsor, Sandoz, Inc., who donated graciously and requested nothing, and NINCDS/NIH; second, to the generosity of our secondary sponsors, the National Institutes of Health, the National Multiple Sclerosis Society, and the March of Dimes, who brought us within sight of our final target; and third, to the Pfizer Pharmaceutical Corp., Accurate Chemical & Scientific Corp., Ciba-Geigy Corp., Amersham Corp., Imperial Chemical Industries, American Cyanamid Co., Boehringer-Mannheim, Eastman Kodak Co., The Upjohn Co., Lilly Research Laboratories, Monsanto Company, Stuart Pharmaceuticals/Division of ICI Americas, and Hoffman-La Roche, Inc., for additional contributions that enabled us to meet our obligations. Accolades are also in order for the many unseen persons who provided organizational assistance. A local planning committee chaired by Dr. Lisak provided a splendid social program and information to introduce Philadelphia to its visitors. The staff of the New York Academy of Sciences is to be commended for making this a very successful meeting, particularly the Conference Department, with whom it was a pleasure to work, the Conference Committee, for their program guidance, and the Editorial Department, and particularly Mrs. Angela Fink, who conscientiously and skillfully saw this volume through the press. Without the collective administrative and knowledgeable backing of the Academy personnel, the goals of the Congress could never have been brought to fruition. Last but not least, the Editor and the Congress Planning Committee thank the participants who traveled from every corner of the world to make this Congress the highlight of the 1987 neuroimmunology calendar. Without their input, there would have been no need to pen these words and no comprehensive neuroimmunology text to serve as our bible for the next few years. Thank you one and all.

PART I. BASIC IMMUNOLOGY AND IMMUNE REGULATION

# The T-Cell Antigen Receptor

## Structure and Mechanism of Activation

LAWRENCE E. SAMELSON AND
RICHARD D. KLAUSNER

*Cell Biology and Metabolism Branch*
*National Institute of Child Health and Human Development*
*National Institutes of Health*
*Bethesda, Maryland 20892*

T lymphocytes initiate and regulate the complex immune response of the organism to foreign antigens. T cells upon activation engage immune effector cells by cell-cell interaction or production of soluble lymphokines. Subsequent events include, where appropriate, B-cell proliferation and differentiation, cytotoxic T-cell-induced target lysis, or activation of suppressor T cells. This T-cell immune response begins when antigen receptors on the surface of T cells engage antigen in the context of surface molecules encoded by the major histocompatibility complex. Over the past 5 years the structure of the antigen receptor responsible for these interactions has been very well characterized.[1] On the majority of the peripheral T cells this clonotypic structure is a heterodimer comprised of disulfide-linked $\alpha$ and $\beta$ chains, which are encoded by separate rearranging genes. Both $\alpha$ and $\beta$ are members of the immunoglobulin supergene family, and they contain both variable and constant region domains. Transfection studies have now confirmed that these two gene products confer upon the receptor both antigen and major histocompatibility complex restriction specificity.[2,3] Recently a second form of heterodimeric antigen receptor has been identified encoded by two other rearranging genes.[4] The products of these genes, $\gamma$ and $\delta$, are found on a small percentage of peripheral T cells and thymocytes. The ligand for this receptor is not yet known.

These clonotypic receptors exist as multichain receptor complexes on the T-cell surface. This conclusion was originally derived from work showing that antibodies binding the CD3 complex (T3) had functional effects on T cells.[5] Subsequently these antibodies were shown to co-immunoprecipitate the $\alpha$ and $\beta$ chains from T-cell clones.[6,7] On human T cells it thus became clear that the $\alpha$-$\beta$ heterodimer was part of a complex with the CD3 complex, the $\gamma$, $\delta$, and $\epsilon$ chains. Our initial studies in the mouse confirmed the existence of these chains and showed that they could be co-immunoprecipitated with the $\alpha$-$\beta$ heterodimer.[8] In these initial studies an additional murine subunit was observed. The $\zeta$ chain is a 16-kd nonglycosylated protein that exists as a homodimer within the complex. We generated antibodies binding this chain which immunoprecipitated the murine complex and cross-reacted on a homologous human protein.[9] Thus the $\zeta$ chain homodimer was shown to be an integral part of the human T-cell antigen receptor.

Yet another antigen receptor subunit has been demonstrated. This subunit, $\eta$, is a 22-kd protein. Recent studies (M. Baniyash, P. Garcia-Morales, L. E. S., R. D. K., submitted) prove that this subunit is disulfide linked to a ζ chain monomer. Of interest is that only 20% of receptors bear this heterodimer, leading to the conclusion that there are two classes of T-cell receptors, those with and those without the ζ-η heterodimer. The complexity of this receptor is obvious. Precedents exist for such receptor complexes including the well-characterized acetylcholine receptor. However, it is not at all certain that the antigen receptor components function similarly to form an ion channel. An alternative explanation is that these chains are involved in receptor coupling to multiple effector systems.

Signal transduction through receptors is only beginning to be understood, but in many systems receptor occupancy leads to protein kinase activation. In T cells it has been known that two activators of protein kinases, phorbol esters and calcium ionophores, in synergy can activate T cells.[11] We have looked at the receptor itself to observe whether its phosphorylation would indicate kinase activation.

We and others have found that antigen or antireceptor antibodies induce polyphosphoinositide breakdown, resulting in protein kinase C activation.[11,12] This activation results in phosphorylation of the CD3-γ chain of the receptor on a serine residue. Similar observations have been made with human T cells. More recently we observed that an additional receptor subunit, the ζ chain, serves as a substrate for a protein tyrosine kinase upon receptor activation.[12] In a murine T-cell hybridoma and in human resting peripheral blood lymphocytes, activation by antigen, lectin, or antireceptor monoclonal antibodies results in this phosphorylation (M. B., P. G.-M., L. E. S., R. D. K., submitted). Phosphorylation of other cellular substrates on tyrosine indicates that a tyrosine kinase or tyrosine kinase pathway is likely to be activated by these ligands. We have shown that activation of the protein tyrosine kinase is independent of protein kinase C activation. As yet, the identity of the kinase responsible for this phosphorylation has not been determined, and the role of this signal transduction pathway is under investigation.

Regulation of signal transduction in many systems has been shown to involve protein kinase pathways.[13] Some have speculated, for example, that T-cell antigen receptor CD3-γ chain phosphorylation induced by protein kinase C is itself responsible for receptor internalization.[14] Another example, activation of the cyclic AMP-dependent protein kinase, inhibits T-cell activation. We have shown that elevation of intracellular cAMP blocks polyphosphoinositide metabolism and thereby prevents protein kinase C activation.[12] Subsequent phosphorylation of the CD3-γ chain is blocked. Physiologically this thus represents a form of heterologous desensitization mediated through kinase activation.

The independent tyrosine kinase pathway is also modulated by elevations of cAMP. Antigen-induced phosphorylation of the ζ chain is blocked in a dose-dependent manner by cAMP. When T cells are activated by antireceptor monoclonal antibodies, elevations of cAMP also block protein kinase C activation. However, cAMP does not inhibit tyrosine kinase activation by these ligands. These data indicate further complexity in the system. Different ligands, as exemplified by antigen and antireceptor antibodies, induce differential coupling between the receptor and the kinase pathways.[15]

Receptor occupancy leads to activation of multiple kinase pathways in T cells which can be modulated by other kinases and presumably by phosphatases as well. These complex interactions are probably critical for fine regulation and control of cellular function and ultimately the immune response. Immune dysfunction might at times reflect derangement of these pathways. The mouse *lpr* and *gld* strains serve as an example. A subpopulation of T cells in these mice proliferates in an uncontrolled manner. They are unresponsive to lectin or alloantigen. We have shown that the antigen receptors on these cells are constitutively tyrosine phosphorylated on the ζ chain. Unlike antigen activation of hybridomas, receptor activation has no effect on this phosphorylation and fails to result in protein kinase C activation and CD3-γ phosphorylation. Our hypothesis is that abnormalities in the tyrosine kinase pathway could be related to both abnormalities of growth regulation and signal transduction in these cells. Understanding proximal events in T-cell activation may lead to further insights into the pathogenesis of immune dysfunction.

## REFERENCES

1. MARRACK, P. & J. W. KAPPLER, 1986. Adv. Immunol. **38:** 1-36.
2. DEMBIC, Z. et al. 1986. Nature **320:** 232-238.
3. SAITO, T., A. WEISS, J. MILLER, M. A. NORCROSS & R. N. GERMAIN. 1987. Nature **325:** 125.
4. BRENNER, M. B. et al. 1986. Nature **322:** 145-149.
5. REINHERZ, E. L., R. E. HUSSEY & S. F. SCHLOSSMAN. 1980. Eur. J. Immunol. **10:** 758-762.
6. REINHERZ, E. L. et al. 1983. Proc. Natl. Acad. Sci. USA **80:** 4104-4104.
7. OETTGEN, H. C., J. KAPPLER, W. J. M. TAX & C. TERHORST. 1984. J. Biol. Chem. **259:** 12039-12048.
8. SAMELSON, L. E., J. B. HARFORD & R. D. KLAUSNER. 1985. Cell **43:** 223-231.
9. WEISSMAN, A. M., L. E. SAMELSON & R. D. KLAUSNER. 1986. Nature **324:** 480-482.
10. SAMELSON, L. E., M. D. PATEL, A. M. WEISSMAN, J. B. HARFORD & R. D. KLAUSNER. 1986. Cell **46:** 1083-1090.
11. WEISS, A. et al. 1986. Ann. Rev. Immunol. **4:** 593-619.
12. PATEL, M. D., L. E. SAMELSON & R. K. KLAUSNER. 1987. J. Biol. Chem. **262:** 5831-5838.
13. SIBLEY, D. R., J. L. BENOVIC, M. G. CARON & R. J. LEFKOWITZ. 1987. Cell **48:** 913-922.
14. CANTRELL, D. A., A. A. DAVIES & M. J. CRUMPTON. 1985. Proc. Natl. Acad. Sci. USA **82:** 8158-8162.
15. KLAUSNER, R. D. et al. 1987. J. Biol. Chem. **262:** 12654-12659.
16. SAMELSON, L. E., W. F. DAVIDSON, H. C. MORSE & R. D. KLAUSNER. 1986. Nature **324:** 674-676.

# Immunoregulation in Rapidly Progressive Multiple Sclerosis[a]

BARRY G. W. ARNASON, AVERTANO B. C. NORONHA, AND ANTHONY T. REDER

*Department of Neurology and the Brain Research Institute*
*The University of Chicago*
*Chicago, Illinois 60637*

Numerous abnormalities of the immune system have been detected in multiple sclerosis (MS) in recent years. Changes in the activity of blood monocytes have been noted that coincide with altered activity of the disease itself.[1] Activation of B cells within the brain with production *in situ* of immunoglobulin that shows clonal restriction is characteristic of the disease. In addition, aberrancies of natural killer cells, helper T cells, and suppressor-inducer cells in terms of both cell number and function, at least as measured *in vitro*, have been noted in MS. We recently reviewed these aspects of immune function in MS.[2]

In this communication we will discuss T suppressor cell function in MS, drawing primarily on results of our own studies. In 1978 we showed that production and release of suppressor factors by blood T cells from MS patients exposed to the lectin concanavalin A *in vitro* were defective during flares of disease.[3] At the same time the capacity of concanavalin A to drive T cells from the same MS patients to proliferate was normal.

In subsequent work we were able to establish that T cells bearing the surface phenotypic marker known as CD8 were the producers of the nonspecific suppressor factor, or factors, that we were studying. More recently we developed two additional assays to measure suppressor cell function in MS. The first involves a measure of IgG production by blood-derived mononuclear cells exposed to the lectin pokeweed mitogen. IgG production in MS is increased on average in this assay system.[4] By mixing CD8 positive cells from MS patients with CD4 positive helper cells plus B cells and monocytes from controls and *vice versa*, we were able to show that augmented IgG production by B cells occurred in MS because the normal down damping effect of CD8 positive cells on IgG production failed, that is, augmented IgG production reflected reduced suppressor cell function. In the second assay we substituted OKT3 monoclonal antibody for concanavalin A as the stimulator for cell activation. Again T suppressor cell function was subnormal.[5] One additional point should be made. The defect in T suppressor function observed during attacks of disease is no longer seen once an attack has given way to a remission, indicating that the defect is reversible and that its presence correlates reasonably well with disease activity. The question of whether loss of suppressor activity permits an attack to occur or is a consequence of

---

[a] The original research reported was supported by a grant from the National Multiple Sclerosis Society and a gift from the Arthur L. Swim Foundation to Barry Arnason. Anthony J. Reder is a Harry Weaver Scholar of the National Multiple Sclerosis Society and the recipient of a clinical investigator development award from NINCDS.

the attack, that is, whether it is a first, a second, or even a third order phenomenon, remains unresolved.

Inasmuch as CD8 positive cells are responsible for suppressor function, or at least that aspect of suppressor function that we are measuring, the question quickly arose as to whether the number of cells bearing the CD8 phenotype might not be reduced when MS is active. Were this the case the absence of function might simply reflect depletion from the blood of the requisite cell population. The first reports in which T-cell phenotype in MS was evaluated did indicate significant reductions in the numbers of CD8 positive cells in the blood during flares of MS.[6,7] More recent reports, including our own, have revealed only a modest or marginal reduction in CD8 positive cell number during flares of MS, and in some studies there were none (reviewed in 2). We conclude that the defect in suppressor cell function seen during exacerbations of MS cannot be attributed to a depletion of CD8 positive cells.

It is now known that the CD8 positive cell population contains cytotoxic cells in

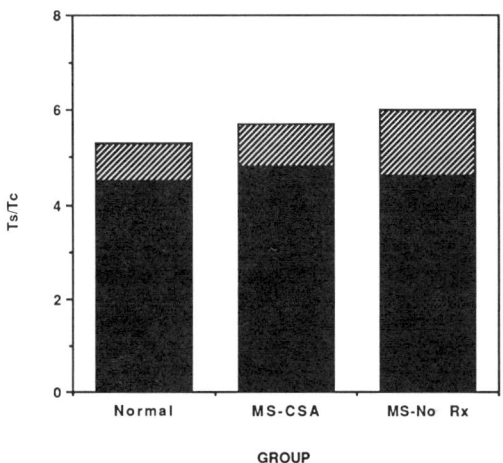

**FIGURE 1.** The ratio of Leu2+,9.3+ (cytolytic), or Tc, and Leu2+,9.3− (suppressor), or Ts, cells is equivalent between MS patients and healthy control subjects. Peripheral blood cells from patients with rapidly progressive MS, untreated (MS-no Rx) or treated with cyclosporin A (MS-CSA), and from age-matched control subjects were analyzed in this representative experiment with a fluorescence-activated cell sorter using dual fluorescence staining. The **black bars** give the Ts/Tc ratios for MS cases and control subjects; the **hatched bars** give the standard deviations.

addition to suppressor cells. The two populations can be discriminated one from the other, taking advantage of the monoclonal antibody designated as 9.3.[8] This antibody recognizes cytotoxic cells but not suppressor cells. Sorting of CD8 positive cells into 9.3 positive ones (cytotoxic) and 9.3 negative ones (suppressors) has permitted us to establish that cytotoxic to suppressor cell ratios are normal in MS (FIG. 1). The finding excludes the possibility that the CD8 positive cell number is normal in MS because a downshift in suppressor cell number is masked or counterbalanced by an upshift in cytotoxic cell number.

We have also evaluated cytotoxic cell function in MS using an *in vitro* assay in which cytotoxic cells are generated by exposure to Epstein-Barr virus-infected cell lines.[9] Cytotoxic function is normal, indicating that the defect in MS is not one of all CD8 positive cell functions but only of some (TABLE 1).

Three years ago we enrolled a group of 40 patients with rapidly progressive MS into a clinical trial of cyclosporine A as a treatment for the disease. Half the patients received cyclosporine A; the other half, a placebo. All patients accepted into the trial had rapidly progressive disease and had lost at minimum 1 point on the Kurtzke scale over the preceding year. It is well known that once patients develop progressive disease, their condition usually continues to worsen.

The number of CD8 positive cells in the blood is moderately reduced in patients with progressive disease (reviewed in Ref 2). Suppressor function in our patients with rapidly progressive disease at entry into the trial was in all instances subnormal. The magnitude of the defect could not be accounted for by the decrease in CD8 positive cell number, pointing to a defect in the cells themselves rather than to their depletion from the blood. In the placebo-treated patients suppressor function remained low in every case over the 2 years of the trial as detected by serial sampling. Cyclosporine treatment did not correct the problem. In contrast, cyclosporine treatment did depress cytotoxic function below the normal values found at entry. Interleukin-2, a lymphokine the production of which is shut off by cyclosporine A treatment, restored cytotoxic function when added to cells *in vitro,* but it had no effect on suppressor cell function.[10]

TABLE 1. Suppressor versus Cytolytic Function

| Subjects | Suppression[a] | Cytolysis[b] |
|---|---|---|
| Control | 56 ± 4% ($n = 14$)[c] | 27 ± 4% ($n = 16$) |
| MS | 17 ± 4 ($n = 17$) | 29 ± 5 ($n = 20$) |
| Significance | $p < 0.0001$ | Not significant |

[a] $\%$ suppression = $1 - \dfrac{\text{responder cells + suppressor cells (con-A-stimulated)}}{\text{responder cells + unstimulated cells}}$.

[b] MNC cytolysis of Epstein-Barr virus-transformed B cell lines, 30:1 effector to target ratio.

[c] ± SEM.

Because the placebo-treated patients had predictably abnormal suppressor function, we studied their suppressor cells in several ways, comparing them to cells of healthy age-matched controls. OKT8 is a mouse monoclonal antibody that binds to the CD8 molecule. The amount of OKT8 that binds to cells of the CD8 lineage can be quantitated by adding fluorescein-labeled goat antiserum directed against mouse IgG to cells that have bound the mouse OKT8 antibody and measuring the amount of fluorescence emitted by individual cells as they pass single file through a laser beam of light. The technique employs a fluorescence-activated cell sorter (FACS) apparatus. Using this method we found that the number of CD8 molecules per positive cell was lower in cells from progressive MS cases than in cells from control subjects or MS patients with stable disease.[11] The finding was confirmed recently.[12]

Cells exposed to OKT8 and incubated at 37°C overnight shed or internalize OKT8-CD8 complexes. The end result is a stripping of CD8 from the cell surface. Cells stripped of their CD8 had a modestly but nonetheless significantly reduced capacity to mount a suppressor response.[13] The defect hints at a role for the CD8 molecule itself in suppressor function. At the same time the deficiency seen in progressive MS is far more profound than that which we were able to induce by removal of CD8, suggesting that some additional defect was likely to be present.

Many MS patients have a relapsing-remitting course during the first years of their disease but ultimately switch to a progressive one. This clinical finding points to some change in them or in their disease during its course. What determines this switch is unknown, nor is it understood why other patients have a progressive course from the outset whereas still others never enter the progressive phase.

When we collected our 40 cases of rapidly progressive disease, we noted that all patients were spastic. This finding suggested that the sites of their lesions might be a determining factor in how they fared. We wondered whether some "strategic hit" of the disease itself might not be influencing its subsequent course.

Clearly there are abnormalities in immune function in progressive MS. Might nervous system lesions contribute in some way to these abnormalities? Although it is evident that the immune system enjoys considerable autonomy, as witnessed by most *in vitro* assays used to assess immune system function, evidence also exists that the nervous and immune systems communicate *in vivo* and that the nervous system exerts at least some level of control over the immune system. This can be shown directly in experimental animals. The approach employed by us in this regard has been to ablate the sympathetic nervous system with the drug 6-hydroxydopamine (6-OHDA) which is taken up by sympathetic nerve endings, and, once taken up, it destroys them. The lymphoid organs normally receive sympathetic innervation. Following 6-OHDA treatment the norepinephrine content of the lymphoid organs is reduced.

Immune responses are altered following sympathetic nervous system ablation with 6-OHDA. Antibody responses to immunization are increased,[14] the severity of experimentally induced myasthenia gravis is increased,[15] as is the severity of experimental allergic encephalomyelitis.[16] Experimentally induced myasthenia gravis is an antibody-mediated autoimmune disease; experimental allergic encephalomyelitis is a T-cell-mediated autoimmune disease. Thus, loss of sympathetic input seems to be followed by an up-regulation of both antibody and T-cell-mediated immune responses. It would therefore seem that one role of the sympathetic nervous system is to down-regulate immune responses. If "stress" is accompanied by increased sympathetic activity, then one consequence of "stress" might well be to increase the risk of infection by lessening the immune response.

When target cells for neurotransmitters are deprived of their innervation, they tend to up-regulate their number of surface receptors for the neurotransmitter that they are no longer receiving. The process is known as denervation hypersensitivity. Lymphocytes from sympathetic nervous system-ablated animals up-regulate their adrenergic receptors.[17] The same occurs in patients with orthostatic hypotension, a disease in which there is a failure of sympathetic function.[18] Adrenergic receptors on lymphocytes are of the $\beta 2$ type (TABLE 2). In man, T suppressor cells have three times as many $\beta 2$ adrenergic receptors as do cytotoxic T cells.[19] Helper T cells have very few. B cells have more $\beta$-adrenergic receptors than do T cells, but they are of lower affinity (FIG. 2). Because suppressor T cells have more $\beta$-adrenergic receptors than do other T cell types, one might anticipate that the sympathetic nervous system's down-damping control over the immune response would be exerted, at least in part, by suppressor cell activation.

If a "strategic hit" of MS interrupts or lessens sympathetic outflow from the nervous system to the immune system and if this loss of sympathetic "tone" lessens suppressor function, which of course is characteristic of progressive MS, then it should be possible to demonstrate that sympathetic function is defective in progressive MS. This is known to be the case,[20] and we have extended earlier work in this area by showing that pedal sweating responses to galvanic stimulation are absent in 50% of cases of progressive MS even though they are invariably present in control subjects.[21]

TABLE 2. Displacement of Specific Binding on T Cells

| Agonist | $K_D$ Controls | $K_D$ MS Patients |
|---|---|---|
| (−)-isoproterenol | 2.0 μM | 5.5 μM |
| (−)-epinephrine | 40.0 μM | 50.0 μM |
| (−)-norepinephrine | 65.0 μM | 90.0 μM |
| (+)-isoproterenol | 50.0 μM | 70.0 μM |

NOTE: Adrenergic agonists competitively and stereospecifically displace the binding of Iodo[$^{125}$]cyanopindolol ([$^{125}$]CYP) to T cells in MS patients and control subjects. $2 \times 10^5$ cells were incubated in the presence of 25 pM [$^{125}$]CYP with varying concentrations of agonists ($10^{-3} - 10^{-8}$ M) at 30°C for 90 minutes. Specific binding was determined as the difference in [$^{125}$]CYP binding in the presence of agonists and agonists plus 6 μM DL-propranolol. MS patients and control subjects responded similarly to the order of agonist potency in displacing [$^{125}$]CYP: (−)-isoproterenol >> (−)-epinephrine > (−)-norepinephrine, and (−)-isoproterenol >> (+)-isoproterenol. The displacement obtained with the three beta-adrenergic agonists suggests that the receptor sites are primarily of the beta-2 type. The experiment shown is representative of five such experiments.

Sweating responses were chosen for testing because the relay path involves a spinal cord loop.

An additional expectation would be that β-adrenergic receptors on lymphocytes might be up-regulated. They are (FIG. 2). Patients with progressive MS exhibit three times as many β-adrenergic receptors (as measured by $^{125}$I-cyanopindolol binding) on blood-derived CD8 positive cells as do age-matched controls. It will be of interest

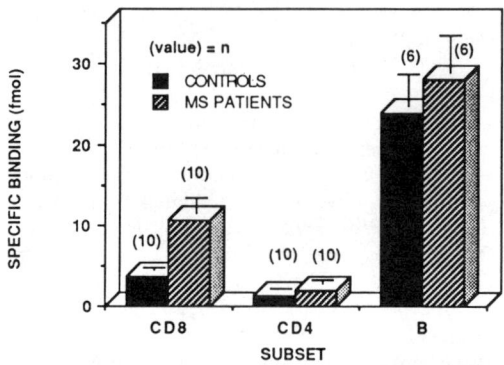

FIGURE 2. Specific Iodo[$^{125}$]cyanopindolol ([$^{125}$]CYP) binding to subsets of lymphocytes in MS patients and control subjects. $5 \times 10^5$ cells were incubated in the presence of increasing concentrations of [$^{125}$]CYP at 30°C for 90 minutes. Specific binding was determined as the difference in [$^{125}$]CYP in the absence and presence of 6 micromolar DL-propranolol. For CD8 cells, $B_{max} = 3.6 +/- 0.4$ fmol/$10^6$ cells in control subjects and $10.6 +/- 1.9$ fmol/$10^6$ in MS patients ($p < 0.01$, $n = 10$); for CD4 cells, $B_{max} = 1.3 +/- 0.1$ fmol/$10^6$ cells in control subjects and $2 +/- 0.3$ fmol/$10^6$ in MS patients ($p < 0.05$, $n = 10$); and for B cells, $B_{max} = 23.9 +/- 3.9$ fmol/$10^6$ cells in control subjects and $28.1 +/- 4.5$ fmol/$10^6$ in MS patients (n.s., $n = 6$). Note that β-adrenergic receptor density on CD8 positive cells is increased approximately 3-fold in progressive MS patients compared to control subjects. Note also that in control subjects as in those with MS, there are more β-adrenergic receptors on CD8 positive cells than on CD4 positive cells.

to determine the effects of $\beta$-adrenergic agonists and antagonists on T suppressor cell function.

We have detected an additional surface phenotype abnormality on T suppressor cells from progressive MS patients. T cells bind sheep red blood cells (SRBC). For many years the capacity to bind three or more SRBC was the operational definition of a T cell. Some T cells bind many more SRBC than do others. In 1975 we reported that MS patients in a mixed cohort of relapsing-remitting and stable cases formed fewer avid T-cell rosettes than did control subjects, an avid T cell being defined as one that bound 10 or more SRBC.[22] Recently we reexamined this question in cases of rapidly progressive disease. Avid T cells are markedly reduced in progressive MS (TABLE 3). The SRBC receptor on T cells is a protein with a molecular weight of 55,000 daltons that carries the designation of CD2. The amount of CD2 on the cell surface is greater on CD8 positive cells than on helper cells. By cell sorting techniques it can be shown that it is the CD8 positive cell that forms the avid rosette.

The finding of a change in avid T cells in MS has taken on new meaning with the realization that CD2 is an alternative cell activation pathway. Monoclonal antibodies to CD2 have been generated, and certain combinations of them will drive T cells to proliferate.[23] Activation is thought to occur via the diacylglycerol-trisphosphoinositol-protein kinase C pathway. Using fluorescein-conjugated monoclonal antibody to CD2 and the FACS method mentioned earlier, we quantitated CD2 on T cells from progressive cases of MS. The amount found was in the normal range, so

TABLE 3. Avid T Cells in Progressive Multiple Sclerosis

| Subjects | $T_A$ % | p |
|---|---|---|
| Control ($n = 5$) | 43.6 ± 2.2 | < 0.0001[a] |
| MS ($n = 7$) | 10.5 ± 2.2 | |

[a] Unpaired $t$ test.

that loss of avidity does not equate to loss of CD2 (A. Reder, unpublished observations). We also activated T cells via their CD2 pathway by pairing SRBC with a monoclonal antibody to CD2. Proliferative responses varied considerably between individuals, but no meaningful differences between progressive MS cases and control subjects were observed. We have not yet studied whether CD2 engagement by SRBC and monoclonal antibody to CD2 activates suppressor cell function. However, we have studied the ability of phorbol myristate acetate (PMA) to activate suppressor cell function. Phorbol myristate acetate can substitute for diacylglycerol (DAG) and activate the DAG-dependent component of the DAG-trisphosphoinositol-protein kinase C pathway implicated in cell activation via CD2. Phorbal myristate acetate activates suppressor cell function of T cells from control subjects but not of T cells from patients with progressive MS.

Taken together the findings just outlined suggest that $\beta$-adrenergic receptor engagement (which activates the cAMP-protein kinase A pathway) and perhaps the CD2 protein (acting via protein kinase C) may both play roles in T suppressor cell activation. The fact that suppressor cell function returns to normal when remission follows an attack of MS suggests that it may prove possible to reactivate suppressor function in progressive MS by pharmacologic intervention. Whether reactivation of suppressor cells will be accompanied by an arrest in disease progression remains to be seen.

There is a hint that this may be the case. In preliminary trials, beta-interferon has been reported to exert a beneficial effect in MS.[24] The finding should be contrasted to that observed with gamma-interferon which in a brief trial appeared to provoke attacks of MS.[25] Beta- and gamma-interferon often exhibit mutually antagonistic actions. We studied the effect of recombinant beta-interferon (Betaseron, kindly supplied by Triton Biosciences, Inc.) on T suppressor cell function. Suppressor cells were activated by concanavalin A and the adjunctive effect of beta-interferon was assessed. T suppressor cell function was augmented by the addition of beta-interferon (FIG. 3). The increase was more apparent with cells from progressive MS cases than with cells from control subjects.

The data indicate that defective T suppressor cell function, as observed in progressive MS, is correctable at least *in vitro*. It remains to be seen whether a like

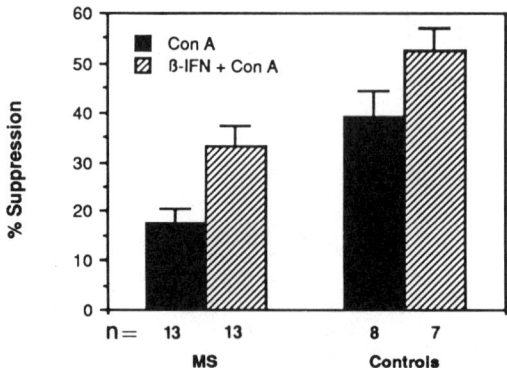

**FIGURE 3.** Suppressor cells were generated from freshly isolated peripheral blood mononuclear cells by treatment with con A or human recombinant beta-interferon (Triton BioSci) $10^3$ units/ml plus con A for 48 hours. They were then added to fresh responder cells and con A for 72 hours. $^3$H-thymidine incorporation was measured and the percentage of suppression calculated by comparing the responses of fresh responder cells to which activated suppressor cells had been added to those of responder cells to which nonactivated cells (also carried for 48 hours *in vitro* before mixing with fresh cells) had been added. Suppressor response is reduced in progressive MS. The addition of beta-interferon augments suppressor response both for cells from MS patients and for cells from control subjects. Augmentation is more marked in cells from MS patients than in cells from control subjects.

correction will occur *in vivo* during beta-interferon treatment and, if it is achieved, whether it will translate into a favorable response on the course of the disease.

## ACKNOWLEDGMENTS

We appreciate the excellent technical support of Margaret Brown, Joseph Karasewski, Mark Jensen, and Angela Toscas. We thank Madeline Murphy for typing and editing the manuscript.

## REFERENCES

1. Dore-Duffy, P., C. Siok & J. O. Donaldson. 1982. Prostaglandin E synthesis in patients with multiple sclerosis: Correlation with disease activity. Neurology **32:** 164A.
2. Reder, A. T. & B. G. W. Arnason. 1985. Immunology of multiple sclerosis. *In* Handbook of Clinical Neurology, Vol. **3.** P. J. Vinken & C. W. Bruyn, Eds. 337-395. Elsevier, New York.
3. Arnason, B. G. W. & J. P. Antel. 1978. Suppressor cell function in multiple sclerosis. Ann. Immunol. (Inst. Pasteur) **129C:** 159-170.
4. Antel, J. P., M. Rosenkoetter, A. Reder, J. J.-F. Oger & B. G. W. Arnason. 1984. Multiple sclerosis: Relation of IgG secretion to T suppressor cell number and function. Neurology **35:** 1155-1160.
5. Antel, J. P., M. B. Bania, A. Reder & N. Cashman. 1986. Activated suppressor cell dysfunction in progressive multiple sclerosis. J. Immunol. **137:** 137-141.
6. Reinherz, E. L., H. L. Weiner, S. K. Hauser, J. A. Cohen, J. A. Kistaso & S. F. Schlossman. 1980. Loss of suppressor T cells in active multiple sclerosis. N. Engl. J. Med. **303:** 125-129.
7. Bach, M.-A., E. Phan-Dinh-Tuy, E. Tournier, L. Chatenoud & J.-F. Bach. 1980. Deficit of suppressor cells in active multiple sclerosis. Lancet **2:** 1221-1223.
8. Hara, T., S. M. Fu & J. A. Hansen. 1985. Human T cell activation. II. A new activation pathway used by a major T cell population via a disulfide-bonded dimer of a 44 kilodalton polypeptide (9.3 antigen). J. Exp. Med. **161:** 1513-1524.
9. Antel, J. P., M. K. Nicholas, M. B. Bania, A. T. Reder, B. G. W. Arnason & L. Joseph. 1986. Comparison of T8+ cell-mediated suppressor and cytotoxic functions in multiple sclerosis. J. Neuroimmunol. **12:** 215-224.
10. Bania, M. B., J. P. Antel, A. T. Reder, M. K. Nicholas & B. G. W. Arnason. 1986. Suppressor and cytolytic cell function in multiple sclerosis: Effects of cyclosporine A and interleukin 2. J. Clin. Invest. **78:** 582-586.
11. Reder, A. T., J. P. Antel, J. Oger, T. A. McFarland, M. Rosenkoetter & B. G. W. Arnason. 1984. Low T8 antigen density on lymphocytes in active multiple sclerosis. Ann. Neurol. **16:** 242-249.
12. Kastrukoff, L. F. & T. N. Buican. 1987. Multiplex labeling analysis of peripheral blood lymphocytes in multiple sclerosis (abstract). Ann. Neurol. **22:** 138.
13. Antel, J. P., J. J.-F. Oger, S. Jackevicius, H. H. Kuo & B. G. W. Arnason. 1982. Modulation of T lymphocyte differentiation antigens: Potential relevance for multiple sclerosis. Proc. Natl. Acad. Sci. USA **79:** 3330-3334.
14. Miles, K., J. Quintans, E. Chelmicka-Schorr & B. G. W. Arnason. 1981. The sympathetic nervous system modulates antibody response to thymus-independent antigens. J. Neuroimmunol. **1:** 101-106.
15. Agius, M. A., M. E. Checinski, D. P. Richman & E. Chelmicka-Schorr. 1987. Sympathectomy enhances the severity of experimental autoimmune myasthenia gravis (EAMG) (abstract). J. Neuroimmunol. **16:** 11.
16. Chelmicka-Schorr, E., M. E. Checinski & B. G. W. Arnason. 1987. Sympathectomy augments the severity of experimental allergic encephalomyelitis (EAE) in rats (abstract). J. Neuroimmunol. **16:** 31.
17. Miles, K., S. Atweh, G. Otten, B. G. W. Arnason & E. Chelmicka-Schorr. 1985. $\beta$-adrenergic receptors on splenic lymphocytes from axotomized mice. J. Immunopharmacol. **6:** 171-177.
18. Bannister, R., A. W. Boulston, I. B. Davies, C. J. Mathias, P. S. Sever & D. Sudera. 1981. $\beta$-receptor numbers and thermodynamics in denervation supersensitivity. J. Physiol. **319:** 369-377.
19. Kahn, M. M., P. Sansoni, E. D. Silverman, E. G. Engleman & K. L. Melmont. 1986. Beta adrenergic receptors on human suppressor, helper and cytolytic lymphocytes. Biochem. Pharmacol. **33:** 1137-1142.
20. Senaratne, M. P. J., D. Carroll, K. G. Warren & T. Kappagoda. 1984. Evidence for cardiovascular autonomic nerve dysfunction in multiple sclerosis. J. Neurol. Neurosurg. Psychiatr. **47:** 947-952.

21. ARNASON, B. G. W., M. BROWN, A. REDER, M. CHECINSKI, E. CHELMICKA-SCHORR & R. MASELLI. 1987. Lymphocyte $\beta$-adrenergic receptors in multiple sclerosis (abstract). Ann. Neurol. **22:** 117.
22. OGER, J., B. G. W. ARNASON, S. H. WRAY & P. KISTLER. 1975. A study of B and T cells in multiple sclerosis. Neurology **25:** 444.
23. MEUER, S. C., R. E. HUSSEY, M. FABBI, D. FOX, O. ACUTO, K. A. FITZGERALD, J. C. HODGDON, J. P. PROTENTIS, S. F. SCHLOSSMAN & E. L. REINHERZ. 1984. An alternative pathway of T-cell activation: A functional role for the 50 kd T11 sheep erythrocyte receptor protein. Cell **36:** 897-906.
24. JACOBS, L., A. M. SALAZAR, R. HERNDON, P. A. REESE, A. FREEMAN, R. JOZEFOWICZ, A. CUETTER, F. HUSAIN, W. A. SMITH, R. EKES & J. A. O'MALLEY. 1987. Intrathecally administered natural human fibroblast interferon reduces exacerbations of multiple sclerosis: Results of a multicenter, double-blinded study. Arch. Neurol. **44:** 589-595.
25. PANITCH, H. S., A. S. HALEY, R. L. HIRSCH & K. P. JOHNSON. 1986. A trial of gamma interferon in multiple sclerosis: Clinical results. Neurology **36**(Suppl. 1): 285.

# Autoimmunity in Demyelinating Diseases

## BYRON H. WAKSMAN

*National Multiple Sclerosis Society
New York, New York 10017*

Immunologic research over more than half a century has defined a number of distinct immunopathologic mechanisms (TABLE 1). "Neuroimmunologic" diseases to a large extent have been firmly identified with one or another of these mechanisms. The most important distinctions to be made are:

1. The distinction between processes primarily mediated by antibody or immune (antigen-antibody) complexes (TABLE 2), those involving T cells (TABLE 3), and those in which absence of a T-cell response is the decisive pathogenetic factor (TABLE 4);

2. The distinction between processes involving microbial infection or tumor with autoimmunization against neural components (Newsom-Davis, Fujinami, this volume) and those in which there is persistent microbial infection of the nervous system with or without an immune response against the pathogen (ter Meulen, this volume);

3. The distinction between acute monophasic diseases and chronic progressive and/or exacerbating-remitting diseases.

TABLE 1. Immunologic Mechanisms in Neurologic Diseases

| Immunologic Mediator[a] | Functional Effect |
| --- | --- |
| Antibody *vs* cellular antigen | Neuronal stimulation |
|  | Blocking or accelerated degradation of membrane receptors |
|  | Neuronal death |
| Antibody *vs* myelin components | Myelinolysis (C-mediated) |
|  | Myelinolysis (ADCC) |
| Antigen-antibody complexes (exogenous or tissue antigen) | Subendothelial deposition, vascular necrosis, and inflammation |
| T-cell-mediated reactions (exogenous or tissue antigen) | Perivascular mononuclear cell infiltration and parenchymal destruction |

ABBREVIATIONS: ADCC = antibody-dependent cell-mediated cytotoxicity; C = complement.
[a] Induction by autoimmunization or by cross-reactive viral, bacterial, or tissue antigen (e.g., in tumor). Elicitation by autoantigen or by virus antigen or viral gene-encoded neoantigen.

TABLE 2. Neuroimmunologic Diseases (Primarily Antibody-Mediated)

| Disease | Target Antigens | Cross-Reacting Antigens |
|---|---|---|
| Myasthenia gravis (and EAMG) | ACHR in myoneural junction | Gram-negative rods and thymic myocytes |
| Sydenham's chorea | Caudate and subthalamic neurones | Streptococci |
| Paraneoplastic syndromes | Various: Eaton-Lambert syndrome, cerebellar degeneration, dysautonomia, etc. | Tumor cells |
| | Neuropathy with gammopathy: myelin-associated glycoprotein, myelin glycolipids | Bacterial lipids[a] |
| Systemic lupus erythematosus (and SLE in NZB mouse) | Cerebral neurones, also choroid plexus (immune complex deposits) | Bacterial cell walls, viral and tissue components |
| Polyarteritis nodosa | Vascular wall, CNS and PNS (immune complex deposits) | None |
| ALS (subset of cases) | Motor neurones | (?) |
| Schizophrenia (?) | Dopaminergic neurones (?) | (?) |

ABBREVIATIONS: ACHR = acetylcholine receptor; ALS = amyotrophic lateral sclerosis; EAMG = experimental autoimmune myasthenia gravis; NZB = New Zealand Black; SLE = systemic lupus erythematosus.
[a] Plasma-cell (or B-cell) tumors of natural antibody-forming cells produce monoclonal antibody vs myelin-associated glycoprotein or myelin glycolipid.

TABLE 3. Neuroimmunologic Diseases (Primarily T-Cell-Mediated)

| Disease | Target Antigens | Cross-Reacting Antigens |
|---|---|---|
| Post-rabies vaccination encephalomyelitis (and EAE) | PLP, MBP: other CNS myelin proteins and lipids (?) | None |
| Postinfectious encephalomyelitis (EAE with viruses) | MBP: other CNS myelin proteins and lipids (?) | Viral antigens: measles, rubella (JHM in rats) |
| Multiple sclerosis (and REAE) | CNS myelin antigens (?) MHC (?) | Common viral antigens (?) |
| Post-rabies vaccination polyneuritis (and EAN) | P2; other PNS myelin antigens (?) | None |
| Guillain-Barré syndrome (and Marek's disease) | P2; other PNS myelin antigens (?) PNS myelin antigens | Viral antigens (?) MDV antigens (?) |
| Chronic relapsing polyneuropathy | PNS myelin antigens (?) | (?) |
| Tropical spastic paraparesis, HAM (and Visna, TMEV) | Persistent viral antigens | None |
| Tertiary Lyme disease | Persistent spirochetes | None |

ABBREVIATIONS: CNS and PNS = central and peripheral nervous systems; EAE and REAE = acute and chronic relapsing experimental autoimmune encephalomyelitis; EAN = experimental autoimmune neuritis; HAM = HTLV-associated myelopathy; JHM = a strain of murine hepatitis virus; MBP = myelin basic protein; MDV = Marek's disease virus; MHC = major histocompatibility complex antigens; PLP = proteolipid protein; TMEV = Theiler's murine encephalitis virus.

In every instance, the fundamental question concerns the identity of the specific antigen that serves as the target (or local "trigger") of the pathogenetic immune response. In addition, in chronic disease there are important genetic components of the disease process affecting, to the best of our present knowledge, the level of host responsiveness to the antigen in question, possibly also faulty regulation of the response, and local vascular and tissue factors (Arnason, this volume).[1] Finally, for each case

TABLE 4. Neuroimmunologic Diseases (Absence of T-Cell Response)

| Disease | Target Cells | Virus | Mechanism of Nonreactivity |
|---|---|---|---|
| Progressive multifocal leukoencephalopathy (JHM in mice) | Oligodendrocytes, astrocytes | JC, SV40 (JHM) | Nonspecific (affecting lymphoid organs) |
| SSPE (LCMV in carrier mice?) | Neurons, glia | Measles, rubella (LCM) | Specific (tolerance) |
| AIDS dementia | Macrophages | HIV (HTVL3) | Nonspecific (affecting T4+ cells) |
| Spongiform disorders | Neurons | "Prions" (?) | (?) |

ABBREVIATIONS: AIDS = acquired immune deficiency syndrome; HIV (HTLV3) = human immunodeficiency virus; JC SV40 = well-known papovaviruses; JHM = a strain of murine hepatitis virus; LCMV = lymphocytic choriomeningitis virus; SSPE = subacute sclerosing panencephalitis.

there are many details to be worked out, such as the nature of secondary and tertiary events in the inflammatory destructive lesions initiated by T-cell recognition of specific antigen at a particular site in the nervous system. Because other participants in this conference (see Arnason, McFarland) will be addressing these questions in detail, I will only mention a few highlights here.

Of the antibody-mediated processes (TABLE 2), only the peripheral neuropathy associated with gammopathy affects myelin.[2, 3] The antibody specificity is directed to either myelin-associated glycoprotein, an adhesion molecule binding myelin to the axon, or myelin glycolipids. The pathologic autoreactive immunoglobulins are secreted by tumors of plasma cells (or B cells) producing antibody to naturally occurring glycolipids, perhaps of microorganisms in the gastrointestinal flora. The lesion is not particularly inflammatory, because the attack is directed at myelin. Because immunoglobulin passes the blood-brain barrier at very low concentrations, comparable lesions are not produced in the CNS.

Model diseases comparable to this human condition are produced by immunizing animals with myelin lipids such as galactocerebroside, gangliosides, or SGGL[4, 5] or by direct injection of such antibody into nerves.[6] The latter, however, while instructive for studies of pathogenesis, is a poor model both because of the local experimental manipulation and consequent disturbance of the blood-tissue barrier and because the condition is acute and intense rather than a slowly evolving process. Again CNS lesions are not produced unless the barriers are bypassed by direct intrathecal injection[7] or injection into the neural parenchyma.[8]

T-cell-mediated immunity is the principal mechanism of inflammatory demyelinative disease affecting either the CNS or peripheral nervous system (TABLE 3). In the acute situation, the distinction is perfectly clear between autoimmunity induced by immunization with tissue antigen, as in post-rabies vaccination encephalomyelitis and neuritis, and autoimmunity induced by viral infection, as in postinfectious encephalomyelitis and Guillain-Barré polyneuritis and their models, JHM virus infection in rats and Marek's disease in chickens. The use of purified antigens and of T-cell clones specific for these antigens has made it possible to identify MBP, PLP, P2, and Po as the effective antigens in most of the animal systems,[9-19] and T lymphocytes reactive with MBP and P2 have accordingly been found in the corresponding human diseases.[20-23] At the same time, antibodies to MBP[23] and P2[24] are also present and undoubtedly contribute to the pathologic picture in patients with these acute diseases, and antibody to protein and glycolipid antigens of myelin are prominent in some of the animal models as well.[25] Conversely, acute encephalitis produced by viral infection of the CNS and T-cell response to virus has not been regarded as a model of demyelinative disease, because the lesions have different morphologic characteristics and tend to affect gray and white matter alike (Doherty, this volume). In postinfectious demyelinative diseases, no virus can be isolated from or identified in the target tissues,[26] and it seems clear that these diseases are truly autoimmune.

In the chronic situation, the findings remain less clear-cut for diseases like multiple sclerosis (MS) and chronic relapsing inflammatory polyneuropathy. Both are thought to resemble autoimmune processes[27-31] and chronic relapsing experimental allergic encephalomyelitis (REAE), whether induced with whole myelin or with proteolipid protein or myelin basic protein, is an excellent model for MS both clinically and histopathologically.[15,16,32,33] Yet T cells specific for myelin antigens and clearly related to the disease process have not been identified unequivocally in either disease, and it must be assumed that if such cells exist, they have migrated from the blood into the target tissue (further discussion to follow). In MS, free antibody to MBP and to glycolipid antigens of myelin is found in cerebrospinal fluid and can be related to disease activity,[35,36] and similar antibody is found in the lesions.[34] That the underlying immunization results from viral infection has been inferred from epidemiologic data, which we will consider, and from the well-established viral induction of autoimmunity associated with acute demyelinative diseases.

Rapid progress has been made recently in our understanding of chronic demyelinative diseases associated with persistent infection of the CNS and the immune response to the infecting microorganism. Tropical spastic paraparesis (TSP) and its Japanese equivalent, HTLV-associated myelopathy (HAM), both of which strongly resemble chronic progressive MS,[37-39] are associated with persistent infection of the CNS with HTLV-1 or a closely related virus.[40] The model disease produced by Theiler's murine encephalitis virus (TMEV), which closely resembles chronic EAE,[41] also is associated with persistent viral infection and the T-cell-mediated immune response to virus[42] (Rodriguez, this volume). No evidence of autoimmunization is found in TMEV-infected animals.[43] Visna is a similar model in sheep infected with a retrovirus.[44] Again persistence of virus and the reaction to virus rather than autoimmunization seem to be the key elements in the disease pathogenesis.[45] In Visna, the tendency of the virus to mutate freely results in exacerbations with an uncanny resemblance to those of MS.[45] An attempt has been made to identify a similar infection as the basis of MS itself,[46] but there is much disagreement about the evidence brought to bear so far. Because HTLV-1 infection appears to be spreading among drug abusers in northern cities,[47] confusion between TSP and MS will probably occur with increasing frequency. Tertiary Lyme disease, caused by persistent infection with the spirochete, *Borrelia burgdorferi*, also can be confused with progressive MS, but it is distinguished from it by specific antibody to the spirochete.[48]

A brief comment is in order on the diseases associated with specific or nonspecific failure of the T-cell response (TABLE 4). Only progressive multifocal leukoencephalopathy (PML) is primarily demyelinative, although the causative papovaviruses infect astrocytes as well as oligodendrocytes.[49] It occurs in individuals whose T-cell responses are compromised by such diseases as sarcoidosis or Hodgkin's lymphoma. Progressive multifocal leukoencephalopathy has a good animal model in the murine demyelinative disease associated with infection by JHM virus mutants that target oligodendrocytes primarily.[50,51] In many mouse strains this disease is unaccompanied by an immunologically mediated inflammatory response, apparently because of thymic damage by the virus.

It is of interest to consider pairs of experimental situations characterized by the presence or absence of a specific T-cell response. In the case of the JHM virus just cited, mouse strains that can mount an effective T-cell response show inflammation and associated demyelination like that seen in Theiler's virus model. In AIDS produced by the retrovirus HIV (HTLV-3), there is a pure infection of CNS macrophages (microglia) without inflammation (Price, in this volume). Visna virus is very closely related to HIV,[52] and it infects the same cells. However, it also induces an ongoing T-cell and antibody response, and the lesions are inflammatory and demyelinative.[45] A comparison that suggests itself strongly is that with lepromatous and tuberculoid leprosy (in macrophages of nerve, skin), characterized respectively by the absence and presence of a specific T-cell response and the accompanying inflammation.[53]

To return to the question of MS,[27,28,54] the evidence for autoimmunity and for a relationship to viral infection in this disease remains largely circumstantial (TABLE 5).[54,55] The pattern of epidemiologic findings is strikingly reminiscent of the pattern of poliomyelitis in the earlier part of the present century.[56,57] Polio infection in early childhood, it will be recalled, induces gastrointestinal disease and immunity, usually without CNS involvement, whereas polio in adolescence or early adult life frequently induces neurologic disease as well. Thus, as domestic hygiene gradually improved in countries of the developed world, the number of children per family diminished, and the size, heating, and other features of family dwellings improved, there was a substantial diminution in the probability of viral transmission in early childhood. In fact, poliovirus infections occurred later and later in life with an abrupt increase by mid-century of cases of neurologic involvement, sometimes in "epidemic" form. This finding was especially true in countries in the temperate zone (a "latitude effect") and in higher socioeconomic groups within the affected populations.

These features are seen in MS as well: the latitude effect is well known,[58,59] and there is an increased incidence of MS among members of higher socioeconomic groups. The early migration studies of Dean[60] pinpointed early adolescence (before age 15) as the optimal period for the triggering of the MS process by environmental factors. In the Faeroe Islands epidemic, which clearly involved an infectious agent carried to the islands by British troops, the MS susceptibility "window" was defined with some precision as between ages 13 and 26.[61] In studies of twins as well, the occurrence of MS could be tentatively linked to repeated and severe viral infections in this same

TABLE 5. Infection with Common Viruses Probably Initiates Both the Primary Multiple Sclerosis (MS) Process and Most Exacerbations

Viral infection readily induces autoimmunization to components of myelin and demyelinating disease in man and animal.

MS in susceptible monozygotic twin pairs is related to frequency and severity of viral infection in late childhood, adolescence, or early adult life.

MS occurs in epidemic form in island populations.

MS in migrant populations can be related to environmental influences before age 15.

Early adolescence is a period of maximum susceptibility to MS.

Common virus infections (measles, mumps, EBV) occur at an older age in those who get MS than in matched control subjects.

MS prevalence is increased in temperate zone among Caucasians.

MS prevalence is increased in higher socioeconomic groups.

A high proportion of MS exacerbations is triggered by upper respiratory infection.

Such infection probably acts by systemic release of gamma-interferon and up-regulation of MHC.

It is possible that some relapses may be triggered by stress.

period.[62] Finally, several studies establish that individuals who get MS experience infection with common exanthematic and other viruses significantly later in life than do matched control subjects, that is, in late childhood or early adolescence.[63-65]

Why MS susceptibility is maximal during this particular phase of individual development is unknown. However, the induction of chronic relapsing EAE in guinea pigs is most readily achieved with immunization at weaning. Earlier in life the animals lack some part of the machinery required for an effective T-cell response that can produce disease. Later, EAE tends to be monophasic as a result of a strong specific suppressor T-cell response.[66] It is probable that weaning (and adolescence in man) is associated with maturation of the system of suppressor cells and immune regulation in ways that we do not yet understand.

None of this establishes the role of viral infection in MS as being the induction of autoimmunity. That relationship can only be established by actual isolation of the specific effector T cells that initiate the primary disease process and identification of their specificity for viral and/or autoantigen. The missing measles-specific T cells identified by Jacobson et al.[67] may be the long-sought effector cell. Meanwhile the alternative theory, that MS is not autoimmune but involves persistent infection, continues to spur efforts to identify a responsible pathogen comparable to HTLV-1 in tropical spastic paraparesis or JC virus in progressive multifocal leukoencephalopathy.[46]

The problem of MS exacerbations is complex. The study by Sibley et al.[68] suggests that a major proportion of such exacerbations is triggered by antecedent viral infection. However, the emphasis here is on respiratory viruses rather than exanthematic viruses, and the latent period is measured in days or weeks rather than several years (estimated by Kurtke as 6 years, in the Faeroe Islands study)[61] intervening between viral infection and the onset of a first attack of MS. Although during exacerbation the appearance of new lesions identified by neurologic examination or by imaging techniques implies a renewal of the process that triggered the first lesions (and presumably a new shower of virus or myelin-reactive T cells traveling through the bloodstream), some lesions seem simply to enlarge or reexpress themselves. The implication here is that there is somehow reactivation of the local inflammatory process. One explanation offered is that systemic gamma-interferon release is associated with each new viral infection. This up-regulates expression of major histocompatibility antigens on local auxiliary cells in the CNS (astrocytes, macrophages)[1] (Fontana, this volume) and stimulates virus or myelin-specific T cells which may remain at any lesion site to renewed activity.[69] This explanation is supported by the observation that injected gamma-interferon does indeed reactivate earlier MS lesions in association with increased MHC expression on many cells.[70]

The possibility that some MS exacerbations may be triggered by stress has had a great deal of anecdotal support, but an attempt to establish such a relationship in the cohort of patients studied by Sibley[71] was unsuccessful. New information about the sensitivity of certain lymphocyte subsets to particular neurotransmitters provides a plausible mechanism whereby emotional reactions could affect immunologic events, as discussed by Arnason elsewhere in this volume. Clearly more data are needed before this possibility can be affirmed or denied.

Since others will discuss the MS lesion, I will only comment here that the early lesion shows the main morphologic features we associate with reactions of T-cell-mediated immunity: infiltration of T cells of various phenotypes, some B cells and/or plasma cells, and a preponderance of activated macrophages associated with vascular damage and varying degrees of parenchymal destruction from loss of myelin to total tissue necrosis.[32,34] At the same time, antibody may be present and has been shown to bind macrophages to the "target" myelin, thus promoting a process of ligand-mediated endocytosis, a major element of myelin destruction in the lesion.

The key issue that remains unresolved is the identity and specificity of the effector T cells active in initiating the lesion. Studies of cerebrospinal fluid have been largely noncontributory except for the single report of Lisak and Zweiman[72] that MBP-specific T cells appear transiently in the acute phase of MS and the additional finding of T cells reactive with a variety of viruses in more advanced MS.[73] One attempt to show myelin reactivity (MBP, PLP) of T cells within fresh CNS lesions was unsuccessful.[74] However, with proper methodology, it is relatively easy to isolate MBP-reactive T-cell clones even from normal blood![75] It is important to comment again on the measles-specific cytotoxic T-cell precursor absent from the blood in over half of MS patients, whereas other virus-reactive cells of similar phenotype and MHC restriction are present in normal numbers.[67] It is tempting to think that these cells have localized in the actual lesions. They may be myelin specific as well, because there is no convincing evidence of the presence of persistent measles virus in the CNS (but see Haase et al.[76]). In EAE induced with MBP, MBP-specific T cells appear briefly in the blood and then move rapidly to the CNS.[77] However, cross-reactivity of measles-specific cells (from non-MS control subjects) with myelin antigens has not been shown (but see reference 78). McFarland will undoubtedly discuss this question further in his presentation.

The literature on MS has been dominated for the last 10 years by studies of essentially nonspecific cell changes in CSF and blood (TABLE 6). Surely one of the most interesting is the recently described diminution of T4+2H4+ suppressor/inducer T cells related to disease activity.[79] The loss of nonspecific suppressor T-cell function[80] may be directly related to this change or may instead be determined by the observed modulation of T-cell surface components such as T8[81] (by antibody? prostaglandins?). No study has yet been reported of antigen-specific suppressor T cells comparable to the MBP-specific cells shown to disappear during exacerbations of REAE in guinea pigs.[82] Even in the more readily studied guinea pig experiment, we have no clue as to what makes such cells disappear, and such information is also entirely lacking in MS patients.

The dominant finding in MS is a massive continuing nonspecific activation affecting all the cellular elements of the blood. It is difficult to interpret this activation as anything other than secondary to the ongoing disease process in the CNS and the systemic release from the lesions of a variety of lymphokines and monokines, such as gamma-interferon,[83] interleukin-1,[84] and surely others. The activation of MHC-autoreactive T cells[85] may be part of this nonspecific activation process. However, it may also depend in part on the loss of suppressor/inducer T cells.[79] These are known to function as both suppressors[85] and AMLR effectors.[86] The entry of large numbers of

TABLE 6. Cellular Abnormalities of Blood and Cerebrospinal Fluid in Multiple Sclerosis

Primary: Related to New Lesion Formation?
Transient T4+ cells (specificity?) in CSF
Absence of "measles-specific" CTL precursors (T4+) in blood
Absence of $T_{s/i}$ (AMLR suppressors) (T4+ 2H4+) in blood

Secondary: Due to Primary Events
Polyclonal activation of T cells and B cells: LK and Ig release
Entry of MHC-autoreactive T cells into CSF
Activation of monocytes: release of enzymes (myelinotoxic) and PGE2
Activation of granulocytes (enzymes) and platelets (stickiness)
Activation of endothelium, glia (MHC expression)

Tertiary: Due to Monocyte Enzymes, PGE2
Modulation of T8+ cells: loss of markers and suppressor function
Modulation of NK cells: loss of markers, killer function, IFN production
Altered adherence properties of lymphocytes and other cells

ABBREVIATIONS: AMLR = autologous mixed lymphocyte reaction; IFN = interferon; LK = lymphokines; MHC = major histocompatibility antigen; NK = natural killer; PGE2, prostaglandin E2; T4, T8, 2H4 = T-cell markers recognized with monoclonal antibodies; $T_{s/i}$ = suppressor/inducer T cells.

TABLE 7. Other Cerebrospinal Fluid (and Plasma) Abnormalities in Multiple Sclerosis

Myelin basic protein fragments
Other myelin and nonmyelin breakdown products
Antibodies reactive with above
Antibodies to pituitary (neural lobe) peptides
Immune complexes
Complement fixation: C2, C9

Elevated immunoglobulins, oligoclonal bands
Elevated antiviral (especially antimeasles) antibody
Antibodies to oligodendrocytes (?)
Myelinotoxic and neuroelectric blocking factors
Lymphocytotoxic factors

Elevated ACTH, prolactin, $\beta$-endorphin, substance P
$\gamma$-interferon, other lymphokines, prostaglandin E2
Decreased essential fatty acids
Abnormal levels of zinc, selenium (cells and/or plasma)

---

such cells into cerebrospinal fluid[87] may reflect their entry into CNS lesions and the generation there of changes characteristic of graft-vs-host lesions (local MLR), a second type of "autoimmunity."[69]

The modulation of T8+ and NK cells[81,88] and reported changes in adherence properties of lymphocytes (e.g., to myelin, to virus-infected cells in culture) may simply reflect "activation" of these cells or may be a consequence of the action of prostaglandin E2 released by activated blood monocytes.[88,89] At present we cannot estimate for the disease process itself or for the patient what the consequences may be of these "secondary" and "tertiary" cellular events.

The noncellular changes in cerebrospinal fluid and plasma (TABLE 7) fall into three groups. First are products of myelin breakdown and more generally neural tissue damage, antibodies against them, immune complexes, and fixation of complement components. MBP release shows a significant relation to disease activity,[90] as does the formation of antibody against MBP.[35] Proteolipid and myelin glycolipids and the corresponding antibodies behave similarly, but their relationship to disease activity appears less sharp. However, release of some neural components, notably S100, may reflect astroglial activation.[91]

Much of the immunoglobulin in the cerebrospinal fluid (including that in the famous oligoclonal bands) cannot be related in any meaningful way to the MS disease process, other than as reflecting nonspecific B-cell activation (TABLE 6) and recruitment of these cells into the CNS and CSF compartments, where they produce Arnason's "nonsense antibodies."[28] The immunoglobulin includes antibodies to a wide variety of viruses[92] as well as neuroelectric blocking factor[93] and lymphocytotoxic factor. The myelinotoxic factor may simply reflect the sum of proteolytic and other enzymes released from activated monocytes (macrophages) and blood granulocytes. It does not appear to be antibody.[95]

Of the other nonantibody products found at abnormal levels in blood and CSF, some like gamma-interferon and prostaglandin E2 can be directly traced to the activated lymphocytes and macrophages in the CNS lesions (and in the periphery).[83] These cells may also be the source of hormones like ACTH and prolactin and of neuropeptides such as beta-endorphin and substance P,[96] but this possibility is less certain. Both lymphokines and hormones may exert significant effects on the clinical state of the MS patient, but this is also conjectural at present. Even more conjectural is the meaning of changes in certain metals, such as zinc, in red cell membranes.[97] Particular fatty acid levels may simply reflect inactivity and altered dietary habits.[98]

## SUMMARY

Demyelinative diseases of the CNS and peripheral nervous system can be distinguished on the basis of primary mediation by antibody or T lymphocytes (or failure of the T-cell-mediated response) and on the basis of chronicity. The principal mechanisms are autoimmunization to myelin antigens after actual immunization with tissue or infection with cross-reactive viruses or, alternatively, persistent infection of the nervous system (viral or spirochetal) with an associated immune response to the pathogen.

## REFERENCES

1. GONATAS, N. K., M. I. GREENE & B. H. WAKSMAN. 1986. Immunology Today **7:** 121-126.
2. LATOV, N., W. H. SHERMAN, R. NEMNI et al. 1980. N. Engl. J. Med. **303:** 618-621.
3. MURRAY, N., & A. J. STECK. 1984. Lancet **1:** 711-713.
4. SAIDA, T., K. SAIDA, S. H. DORFMAN et al. 1979. Science **204:** 1103-1106.
5. ARIGA, T., KOHRIYAMA, L. FREDDA et al. 1987. J. Biol. Chem. **262:** 848-853.
6. SAIDA, T., K. SAIDA, M. J. BROWN & D. H. SILBERBERG. 1979. J. Neuropathol. Exp. Neurol. **38:** 498-518.
7. LASSMANN, H., B. SCHWERER, K. KITZ et al. 1983. Progr. Brain Res. **59:** 305-315.
8. SERGOTT, R. C., M. J. BROWN, D. H. SILBERBERG & R. P. LISAK. 1984. J. Neurol. Sci. **64:** 297-303.
9. BEN-NUN, A., H. WEKERLE & I. R. COHEN. 1981. Eur. J. Immunol. **11:** 195-199.
10. PEPOSE, J. S., J. G. STEVENS, M. L. COOK & P. W. LAMPERT. 1981. Am. J. Pathol. **103:** 309-320.
11. WANTANABE, R., H. WEGE & V. TER MEULEN. 1983. Nature **305:** 150-153.
12. MOKHTARIAN, F., D. E. McFARLIN & C. S. RAINE. 1984. Nature **309:** 354-358.
13. LININGTON, C., S. IZUMO, M. SUZUKI et al. 1984. J. Immunol. **133:** 1946-1950.
14. WEGE, H., R. WATANABE & V. TER MEULEN. 1984. J. Neuroimmunol. **6:** 325-336.
15. YOSHIMURA, T., T. KUNISHITA, K. SAKAI et al. 1985. J. Neurol. **69:** 47-58.
16. ROSTAMI, A., J. B. BURNS, M. J. BROWN et al. 1985. Cell Immunol. **91:** 354-361.
17. HEININGER, C., G. STOLL, C. LININGTON et al. 1986. Ann. Neurol. **19:** 44-49.
18. TROTTER, J. L., H. B. CLARK, K. G. COLLINS et al. 1987. J. Neurol. Sci. **79:** 173-188.
19. SATOH, J., K. SAKAI, M. ENDOH et al. 1987. J. Immunol. **138:** 179-184.
20. LISAK, R. P., P. O. BEHAN, B. ZWEIMAN & T. SHETTY. 1974. Neurology **24:** 560-564.
21. JOHNSON, R. T., D. E. GRIFFIN, R. L. HIRSCH et al. 1984. N. Engl. J. Med. **310:** 137-141.
22. GECZY, C., R. RAPER, I. M. ROBERTS, P. MEYER & C. C. A. BERNARD. 1985. J. Neuroimmunol. **9:** 179-191.
23. HEMACHUDHA, T., D. E. GRIFFIN, J. J. GIFFELS et al. 1987. N. Engl. J. Med. **316:** 369-374.
24. KOSKI, C. L., R. HUMPHREY & M. L. SHIN. 1985. Proc. Natl. Acad. Sci. USA **82:** 905-909.
25. WEBB, H. E., S. MEHTA, S. LIEBOWITZ & N. A. GREGSON. 1984. Neuropathol. Appl. Neurobiol. **10:** 77-84.
26. GENDELMAN, H., J. S. WOLINSKY, R. T. JOHNSON et al. 1984. Ann. Neurol. **15:** 353-360.

27. WAKSMAN, B. H. & W. E. REYNOLDS. 1984. Proc. Soc. Exp. Biol. Med. **175:** 282-294.
28. REDER, A. T. & B. G. W. ARNASON. 1985. *In* Handbook of Clinical Neurology: Demyelinating Diseases. J. C. Koetsier, Ed. Vol. **3**(47): 337-395.
29. MCFARLIN, D. E. & H. F. MCFARLAND. 1982. N. Engl. J. Med. **307:** 1183-1188, 1246-1251.
30. WEINER, H. L. & D. A. HAFLER. 1986. *In* Current Neurology. S. Appel, Ed. : 123-151. Year Book Medical Publishers, Chicago, IL.
31. DALAKAS, M. C. & W. K. ENGEL. 1981. Ann. Neurol. **9**(Suppl.): 134-145.
32. RAINE, C. S. 1984. Lab. Invest. **50:** 608-635.
33. LASSMANN, H. 1983. Comparative Neuropathology of Chronic Experimental Allergic Encephalomyelitis and Multiple Sclerosis. Springer-Verlag, Berlin.
34. PRINEAS, J. W. 1985. *In* Handbook of Clinical Neurology: Demyelinating Diseases. J. C. Koetsier, Ed. Vol. **3**(47): 213-257.
35. WARREN, K. G. & I. CATZ. 1986. Ann. Neurol. **20:** 20-25.
36. HUKKANEN, V., A. SALMI & H. FREY. 1982. J. Neuroimmunol. **3:** 295-305.
37. ROMAN, G., P. S. SPENCER & B. SCHOENBERG. 1985. Neurology **35:** 1158-1170.
38. OSAME, M., M. MATSUMOTO, K. USUKU *et al.* 1987. Ann. Neurol. **21:** 117-122.
39. JOHNSON, R. T. & J. C. MCARTHUR. 1987. Ann. Neurol. **21:** 113-116.
40. HIROSE, S., Y. UEMURA, M. FUJISHITA *et al.* 1986. Lancet ii: 397-398.
41. DAL CANTO, M. C. & H. L. LIPTON. 1975. Lab. Invest.**33:** 626-637.
42. CLATCH, R. J., R. W. MELVOLD, S. D. MILLER & H. L. LIPTON. 1985. J. Immunol. **135:** 1408-1414.
43. MILLER, S. D., R. J. CLATCH, D. C. PEVEAR *et al.* In press.
44. GEORGSSON, G., J. R. MARTIN, J. KLEIN, P. A. PALSSON *et al.* 1982. Acta Neuropathol. **57:** 171-178.
45. CLEMENTS, J. E. 1985. Rev. Infect. Dis. **7:** 68-74.
46. KOPROWSKI, H., E. C. DEFREITAS, M. E. HARPER *et al.* 1985. Nature **318:** 154-160.
47. ROBERT-GUROFF, M., S. H. WEISS, J. A. GIRON *et al.* 1986. JAMA **255:** 3133-3137.
48. PACHNER, A. R. & A. C. STEERE. 1986. (Abstract) Neurology **36**(Suppl.): 286.
49. JOHNSON, R. T. 1982. Viral Infections of the Nervous System :255-263. Raven Press, New York, NY.
50. STOHLMAN, S. A. & L. P. WEINER. 1981. Neurology **31:** 38-44.
51. KNOBLER, R. L. & M. B. A. OLDSTONE. 1983. *In* Viruses & Demyelinating Diseases. C. A. Mims, M. L. Cuzner & R. E. Kelly, Eds. :53-65. Academic Press, London.
52. GONDA, M. A., F. WONG-STAAL, R. C. GALLO *et al.* 1985. Science **227:** 173-177.
53. KAPLAN, G. & Z. A. COHN. 1986. Int. Rev. Exp. Pathol. **28:** 45-78.
54. JOHNSON, R. T. 1985. *In* Handbook of Clinical Neurology: Demyelinating Diseases. J. C. Koetsier, Ed. Vol. **3**(47): 319-336.
55. WAKSMAN, B. H. & S. C. REINGOLD. 1986. Trends in Neuroscience **9:** 388-390.
56. POSKANZER, D. C., J. L. SHERIDAN, L. B. PRENNEY & A. M. WALKER. 1980. J. Epidemiol. Community Health **34:** 240-252.
57. NATHANSON, N. & J. R. MARTIN. 1979. Am. J. Epidemiol. **110:** 672-692.
58. HALLPIKE, J. F., C. W. M. ADAMS & W. W. TOURTELLOTTE. 1983. Multiple Sclerosis: Pathology, Diagnosis & Management. Williams & Wilkins. Baltimore, MD.
59. KURTZKE, J. F. 1977. *In* Multiple Sclerosis. A Critical Conspectus. E. J. Field, Ed. :83-142. MTP Press Ltd, Lancaster, England.
60. DEAN, G. & J. F. KURTZKE. 1971. Br. Med. J. **3:** 725-729.
61. KURTZKE, J. F. & K. HYLLESTED. 1986. Neurology **36:** 307-328.
62. CURRIER, R. D. & R. ELDRIDGE. 1982. Arch. Neurol. **39:** 140-144.
63. SULLIVAN, C. B., B. R. VISSCHER & R. DETELS. 1984. Neurology **34:** 1144-1148.
64. ANDERSON, O., M. DALTON, A. VAHLNE & C. LINDBERG. 1985. J. Neurol. **232**(Suppl.): 104.
65. COMPSTON, D. A. S., B. N. VAKARELIS, E. PAUL *et al.* Brain **109:** 325-344.
66. ARNON, R. 1981. Immunol. Rev. **55:** 5-30.
67. JACOBSON, S., M. L. FLERLAGE & H. F. MCFARLAND. 1985. J. Exp. Med. **162:** 839-850.
68. SIBLEY, W. A., C. R. BAMFORD & K. CLARK. 1985. Lancet **1:** 1313-1315.
69. WAKSMAN, B. H. 1985. Nature **318:** 104-105.
70. PANITCH, H. S., R. L. HIRSCH, A. S. HALEY & K. P. JOHNSON. 1987. Lancet i: 893-895.

71. SIBLEY, W. A. 1987. *In* A Multidisciplinary Approach to Myelin Diseases. G. Serlupi Crescenzi, Ed. In press. Plenum Press, New York.
72. LISAK, R. P. & B. ZWEIMAN. 1977. N. Engl. J. Med. **297:** 850-853.
73. REUNANEN, M., J. ILONEN, T. ARNADOTTIR *et al.* 1983. J. Neurol. Sci. **58:** 211-221.
74. HAFLER, D. A., D. S. BENJAMIN, J. BURKS & H. L. WEINER. 1987. J. Immunol. **139:** 68-72.
75. BURNS, J., A. ROSENZWEIG, B. ZWEIMAN & R. P. LISAK. 1983. Cell. Immunol. **81:** 435-440.
76. HAASE, A. T., P. VENTURA, C. J. GIBBS, JR., & W. W. TOURTELLOTTE. 1981. Science **212:** 672-674.
77. BURNS, J., A. ROSENZWEIG, B. ZWEIMAN *et al.* 1984. J. Immunol. **132:** 2690-2692.
78. RICHERT, J. R., H. F. MCFARLAND & D. E. MCFARLIN. 1983. Proc. Natl. Acad. Sci. USA **80:** 555-559.
79. MORIMOTO, C., D. A. HAFLER, H. L. WEINER *et al.* 1987. N. Engl. J. Med. **316:** 67-72.
80. ANTEL, J. P., B. G. W. ARNASON & M. E. MEDOF. Ann. Neurol. **5:** 338-342.
81. REDER, A. T., J. P. ANTEL, J. J.-F. OGER *et al.* 1984. Ann. Neurol. **16:** 242-249.
82. LYMAN, W. D., C. F. BROSNAN & C. S. RAINE. 1985. J. Neuroimmunol. **7:** 345-353.
83. HIRSCH, R. L., H. S. PANITCH & K. P. JOHNSON. 1985. J. Clin. Immunol. **5:** 386-389.
84. HOFMAN, F. M., R. I. VON HANWEHR, C. A. DINARELLO *et al.* 1986. J. Immunol. **136:** 3239-3245.
85. GREENSTEIN, J. I. & D. T. CRISP. 1987. Fed. Proc. **46:** 1378.
86. TAKEUCHI, T., C. E. RUDD, S. F. SCHOLSSMAN & C. MORIMOTO. 1987. Eur. J. Immunol. **17:** 97-103.
87. BIRNBAUM, G., L. KOTILINEK, M. STERNAD & M. SCHWARTZ. 1984. J. Clin. Invest. **74:** 1307-1317.
88. MERRILL, J. E., R. H. GERNER, L. W. MYERS & G. W. ELLISON. 1983. J. Neuroimmunol. **4:** 223-237, 239-251.
89. DORE-DUFFY, P. & R. B. ZURIER. 1981. Clin. Immunol. Immunopathol. **19:** 303-313.
90. WHITAKER, J. N. & D. S. SNYDER. 1984. CRC Crit. Rev. Clin. Neurol. **1:** 45-82.
91. MASSARO, A. R., F. MICHETTI, A. LAUDISIO & P. BERGONZI. 1985. Ital. J. Neurol. Sci. **6:** 53-56.
92. CREMER, N. E., K. P. JOHNSON, G. FEIN & W. H. LIKOSKY. 1980. Arch. Neurol. **37:** 610-615.
93. SCHAUF, C. L. & F. A. DAVIS. 1978. Neurology **28:** 34-39.
94. SCHOCKET, A., H. L. WEINER, J. WALKER *et al.* 1977. Clin. Immunol. Immunopathol. **7:** 15-23.
95. GRUNDKE-IQBAL, I. & M. B. BORNSTEIN. 1979. Brain Res. **160:** 489-503.
96. SMITH, E. M. & J. E. BLALOCK. 1981. Proc. Natl. Acad. Sci. USA **78:** 7530-7534.
97. DORE-DUFFY, P., F. CATALANOTTO, J. O. DONALDSON *et al.* 1983. Ann. Neurol. **14:** 450-454.
98. UTERMOHLEN, V., J. CONIGLIO, D. MAO *et al.* 1981. Prog. Lipid. Res. **20:** 739-741.

# Autoimmunity in Neuromuscular Disease

### JOHN NEWSOM-DAVIS

*University of Oxford*
*Department of Clinical Neurology*
*Radcliffe Infirmary*
*Oxford, England*

Autoimmune mechanisms are increasingly being implicated in the pathology of neuromuscular disease. They appear to be the principal cause of neuromuscular disorders presenting acutely such as myasthenia gravis (MG) and acute inflammatory polyneuritis, and contribute significantly to chronic conditions such as the neuropathies associated with plasma cell dyscrasias, and chronic inflammatory neuropathies. Autoimmunity also was recently shown to underlie neuromuscular disorders that are associated with cancer, notably the Lambert-Eaton myasthenic syndrome (LEMS) and perhaps also subacute sensory neuropathy (SSN).

There are several clinical features that point to the possibility of an autoimmune causation. The symptoms may fluctuate in severity and be made worse by infection, although these changes will depend on the capacity of the target organ to recover from attack and thus to reflect variations in the severity of the autoimmune process. The disease may be associated with other disorders of known autoimmune origin, and the incidence of autoantibodies to irrelevant antigens may be increased. There may be immunogenetic associations, notably an increased frequency of particular HLA antigens and Ig heavy chain markers. In addition, clinical improvement following plasma exchange (PE) or in response to immunosuppressive drug (ISD) treatment may be seen. However, none of these features establishes unequivocally an autoimmune causation. For this, certain postulates, similar to those proposed by Koch for establishing an infective process, need to be fulfilled.[1] First, an immune response, either antibody-mediated or cell-mediated, should be demonstrable. Second, active immunization with the purified antigen and/or passive immunization with the patient's immunoglobulin (Ig) should induce the disorder in experimental animals. Finally, the disease should be capable of propagation from affected animals, in which the disease was experimentally induced, to normal syngeneic animals by transfer of antibody in serum and/or immunologically competent cells.

This paper reviews how far the current clinical and experimental data support an autoimmune causation in neuromuscular disorders, focusing on antibody-mediated mechanisms for which, currently at least, much more evidence is available.

## MYASTHENIA GRAVIS

Myasthenia gravis is unquestionably the best model of autoimmunity in human neurologic disease, and indeed it is arguably so for any system, making it an appropriate starting point in this review. Clinical clues that led Simpson[2] to propose an autoimmune mechanism in MG included its association with thyroid disease and other autoimmune disorders, and the occurrence of neonatal myasthenia, in which about 1 in 8 babies born to mothers with MG have a transient myasthenic disorder. Moreover, MG illustrates some of the difficulties in establishing an autoimmune process, in particular the initial failure of the immunohistologic approach because of the lack of sensitivity of the techniques available at that time, and the role that apparently unrelated advances in another field can play, notably the purification and characterization of a component of a snake venom (alpha-Bungarotoxin, a-BuTx) that proved to be a specific ligand for the acetylcholine receptor (AChR).[3] The use of a-BuTx in MG[4,5] established that the primary abnormality was a reduced number of functional acetylcholine receptors, and that this reduction was adequate to account for the primary physiologic abnormality, namely, a reduced amplitude of the miniature end plate potentials (mepps) and end plate potentials discovered about 10 years earlier.[6]

The availability of a-BuTx also lay behind the study by Patrick and Lindstrom[7] who used the toxin to purify AChR from the electric organ of electric eel and then immunized rabbits further to characterize the receptor. As is now well known, this induced experimental autoimmune MG (EAMG), a finding that has been confirmed by similar experiments in other species including primates in whom the disease bears a striking resemblance to human MG.[8] Autologous AChR was also effective in inducing EAMG.[9] It was shown that EAMG could be propagated by passive transfer of serum[10] and by adoptive transfer of spleen cells.[11]

In parallel with these studies, it was found that serum anti-AChR antibody was detectable in the majority (85-90%) of MG patients.[12,13] The antibody was of IgG class and was heterogeneous in its fine specificity, as demonstrated in competition studies using experimentally raised monoclonal anti-AChR antibodies.[14] Most antibody binds to a restricted site (the main immunogenic region) of the alpha subunit of the receptor.

The role of the IgG antibody in MG was at first in doubt, but the successful passive transfer of the electrophysiologic features of MG to mice by intraperitoneal injection of MG IgG established its pathogenic characteristics.[15] Transplacental transfer of maternal anti-AChR antibody similarly appeared to account for neonatal MG. Consistent with this role of anti-AChR antibody, PE was shown to induce a short-term improvement in MG[16] that was associated with the decline of specific antibody in serum,[17,18] and many studies have shown improvement following ISD treatment. The principal mechanisms inducing AChR loss appear to be complement-mediated lysis and down-regulation of AChR secondary to cross-linking of receptors.[19]

Further analysis of the clinical and immunologic features of MG patients suggested a degree of heterogeneity in the AChR-antibody-positive population of patients, as shown by differences in sex incidence, onset age, thymic pathology, and HLA and Ig heavy chain marker associations, possibly implying diversity in the factors initiating the disease[20] (TABLE 1). There exists, in addition, a group of MG patients in whom serum anti-AChR antibodies are persistently undetectable, but who otherwise appear to have typical clinical features of MG. These patients respond to PE and ISD treatment (TABLE 1), suggesting that pathogenic antibodies of a different specificity may be present. Ig or IgG from these patients injected into mice transferred a defect in neuromuscular transmission without a concomitant reduction in AChRs or significant amounts of antibody bound to AChRs, suggesting the presence of antibodies directed to determinants at the neuromuscular junction other than the AChR.[21] Recent passive transfer studies using plasma from one of these cases confirmed a striking reduction in mepp amplitudes in the injected mice, but there was no evidence of antibody bound to AChR or of a decrease in postsynaptic acetylcholine sensitivity.[22]

TABLE 1. Myasthenia Gravis

|  | Serum Anti-AChR | | | |
|---|---|---|---|---|
|  | Positive | | Negative | |
| Thymus | Hyperplasia[a] | Atrophy[a] | Thymoma | Normal[a] |
| Age (yr.) at onset | <40 | >40 | Any | Any |
| Sex (M:F) | 1:3 | 2:1 | 1:1 | 2:1 |
| HLA association | A1, B8, DR3 | A3, B7, DR2 | None | n.a.[b] |
| Ig heavy chain (Gm) (Japanese) | 1,2,21 | 1,2,21 | 1,2,21 | n.a. |
| Associated autoantibodies | 63% | 46% | 62% | 53% |
| Treatment response Plasmapheresis | + | + | + | + |
| Immunosuppression | + | + | + | + |

[a] Typical pathology.
[b] Not available.

These findings raised the possibility that the plasma factor, presumably an antibody, is acting in some way to reduce the size of the ACh packet. A recent report also showed that Ig from MG patients who had no detectable serum anti-AChR antibody neither accelerated degradation nor blocked AChRs, an effect that is in contrast to those of MG Ig.[23] It is conceivable that such antibodies might also be present in some MG patients who have detectable anti-AChR antibody.

## LAMBERT-EATON MYASTHENIC SYNDROME

The primary physiologic abnormality in LEMS is a reduced quantal content of the end plate potential, that is, a reduction in the number of packets of transmitter released by each nerve impulse.[24] The disorder was first recognized in association with bronchial carcinoma.[25] It is now clear that this association is specifically with small cell lung cancer (SCLC), but it occurs in only about 60% of LEMS cases.[26] Guttmann et al.[27] first drew attention to the association with other autoimmune diseases. Other features suggestive of autoimmunity are also present (TABLE 2) and include an increase in autoantibodies[28] and association with HLA and Ig heavy chain markers[29] (see also Demaine et al., page 266, this volume). Patients also respond to PE[30] and, in non-SCLC cases, to ISD treatment. Interestingly, as TABLE 2 indicates, there are no clear clinical or immunologic distinguishing features between those with SCLC and those with no detectable cancer.

Evidence of an autoimmune etiology was first provided by the finding that LEMS IgG injected into mice transferred the principal physiologic abnormalities[31,32] and that the time course closely followed that of the titer of human IgG in the mouse serum.[33] Furthermore, the primary morphologic abnormality in LEMS—paucity and disorganization of active zone particles of the nerve terminal[34]—was also transferred to mice by LEMS IgG.[35] Immunolocalization of LEMS IgG has proved to be technically difficult, but it was recently demonstrated in the region of the presynaptic active

TABLE 2. Lambert-Eaton Myasthenic Syndrome

|  | Small Cell Lung Carcinoma | No Cancer Detected |
|---|---|---|
| Incidence ratio | 3 | 2 |
| Sex (M:F) | 14:11 | 18:7 |
| Age (yr.) at onset | >30 | Any |
| Associated |  |  |
| Autoantibodies | 24% | 44% |
| Autoimmune disease | 24% | 28% |
| HLA-B8 (13%)[a] | 39%[b] | 48%[b] |
| -DR3 (30%) | 20% | 52% |
| Ig heavy chain |  |  |
| Glm[2] (17%)[a] | 45%[b] | 50%[b] |
| Response to treatment |  |  |
| Plasma exchange | + | + |
| Immunosuppression | +/− | + |

[a] Control frequency.
[b] All cases: $p < 0.001$.

zones.[36] Active zone particles are thought to represent voltage-gated $Ca^{2+}$ channels (VGCCs), and the physiologic abnormalities in LEMS-IgG-injected mice are also consistent with a decrease in the number of functional VGCCs.[37] Thus, the pathogenic antibody in LEMS may be directed to VGCCs or structures closely associated with them.

The role of the SCLC in triggering the autoimmune process was recently investigated. Small cell lung cancer is thought possibly to be of neuroectodermal origin. The cells express VGCCs, and $K^+$-stimulated (voltage-dependent) $^{45}Ca^{2+}$ flux can be detected in cultured human SCLC cell lines using $^{45}Ca^{2+}$.[38] Cells cultured in LEMS IgG showed a significant decrease in $K^+$-stimulated $Ca^{2+}$ flux compared with cells grown in control human IgG.[38] This finding was consistent with the view that LEMS IgG contained antibodies that bound SCLC VGCCs; cross-reactivity of these antibodies with similar determinants at the nerve terminal could lead to the neurologic syndrome. Thus, in SCLC-associated LEMS, tumor VGCCs may initiate the autoimmune process; the stimulus in those without detectable SCLC is unknown.

## INFLAMMATORY POLYNEUROPATHIES

Acute inflammatory polyneuritis, by definition, is a monophasic illness that does not progress beyond 5−6 weeks from its onset. Characteristically, the neuropathy is demyelinating in type (acute inflammatory demyelinating polyneuropathy, AIDP); however, a less common form of AIDP can be distinguished in which the pathology is primarily axonal in type,[39] as summarized in TABLE 3. This distinction needs to be kept in mind in the search for autoimmune mechanisms which, in view of this, are likely to be heterogeneous. In chronic inflammatory polyneuropathy the clinical course may be progressive or relapsing and the pathology is demyelinating in type (chronic inflammatory demyelinating polyneuropathy, CIDP[40,41]). These cases are occasionally associated with multifocal CNS demyelination.[42] Evidence suggesting underlying autoimmune mechanisms in the demyelinating neuropathies includes the inflammatory cell infiltrate of peripheral nerve[40,41,43] and, in CIDP only, an association with HLA antigens A1, B8, and DR3.[44] Association with other autoimmune disorders has not been a prominent feature in either AIDP or CIDP.

Several groups have reported clinical improvement following PE in CIDP,[45,46] and three results have now been substantiated in a double-blind trial using sham exchange,[47] clearly pointing to a humoral factor. The CIDP patient also typically responds to ISD treatment.[48]

In AIDP, a response to PE has been more difficult to show, in part owing to the monophasic nature of the disorder and a wide variation in outcome in untreated cases. A control study of 30 patients failed to show a significant difference,[49] but the large multicenter U.S. trial demonstrated a benefit for those receiving PE particularly within the first week of the illness.[50] However, the control group did not receive sham exchange. Response of AIDP to ISD treatment has not been shown convincingly. A control trial of prednisolone failed to demonstrate benefit in the treatment group.[51]

There is growing experimental evidence of a humoral demyelinating factor in AIDP. Sera from 26 of 31 patients produced primary demyelination of cultured fetal muscle dorsal root ganglion cells and was complement dependent.[52] However, the effect was not specific for AIDP. It occurred with sera of 1 of 11 healthy control subjects and 14 of 41 of those with other neurologic diseases. Intraneural injection of AIDP sera into rat nerve induced the morphologic changes of demyelination in many cases[53,54] that correlated with the severity of the disease, whereas less than 10% of control sera caused demyelination usually of less severity.[54] Some of the sera produced mild weakness. The morphologic effects of the sera were lost after heating to 56°C[53] and were not restored by adding a source of fresh complement. Electrophysiologic findings using a similar experimental approach were consistent with morphologic data,[55,56] producing a significant degree of conduction block compared with that in the controls. This effect depended upon sera being fresh and obtained early in the course of the illness; serum stored even at $-70°C$ does not retain the activity. Such factors may account for the failure of some studies to confirm the effects of intraneural injection.

TABLE 3. Inflammatory Polyneuropathies

|  | Acute Axonal | Acute Demyelinating | Chronic Demyelinating |
|---|---|---|---|
| Sex (M:F) | n.a.[a] | 2:1 | 2:1 |
| Peak severity | Day 7 | Day 14 | Progressive or relapsing |
| Mononuclear cell infiltration | Absent or minimal | Present | Present |
| Associated autoimmunity | Absent | Absent | Absent? |
| HLA association | n.a. | Absent | A1,B8,DR3 |
| Response to treatment |  |  |  |
| Plasmapheresis | n.a. | + | + |
| Immunosuppression | n.a. | ? | + |

[a] Not available.

This work has established that AIDP sera are more likely to be myelinotoxic than are control sera, and it points to a disease-specific factor. The decline of myelinotoxic activity during storage argues against the view that an antibody alone underlies the effect. If an antibody is involved, then its action seems to require a further heat-labile factor(s) that may not simply be complement. A protease may be implicated. However, the question has not yet been resolved of how the blood-nerve barrier is breached. Systemic (intraperitoneal) injection of AIDP sera failed to transfer the disorder to mice.[57] By contrast, systemic injection of crude Ig fractions or a purified IgG from 5 of 6 CIDP patients caused a significant decrease in nerve conduction velocity in primates, although no clear morphologic changes were observed.[58]

Early immunofluorescence studies suggested that IgM and complement were bound to peripheral nerve myelin sheaths in 4 of 6 AIDP patients, but not in a (small) number of control subjects.[59] Recently IgM antibody against peripheral myelin has been detected in AIDP sera, using an assay based on the fixation of the C1 component of complement.[60] Eleven of eleven acute phase sera showed a 6- to 56-fold increase in titer compared with that of controls. Serum titers were highest when first sampled and declined rapidly over the first 2 weeks of the illness, being scarcely detectable thereafter. Depletion studies (by precipitation with anti-class-specific anti-serum) confirmed that the antibody was an IgM. Serial measurements of antibody titer and muscle strength showed a clear inverse relationship consistent with a role for the antibody in the demyelinating process, but low levels of antibody could persist for several months.[61] Significantly raised titers of this antibody were also found in patients with CIDP and neuropathy and in those with neuropathy associated with paraproteins.[60] Low titers of the antibody were also present in some healthy individuals and those with other neurologic diseases.

Does demyelination in AIDP and CIDP depend on complement activation by antibody? For this to be the case there would need to be a breakdown in the blood-brain barrier, particularly because low levels of the antibody are present in some healthy individuals. That blood-brain permeability is enhanced is suggested by the preliminary finding of late complement components in the CSF of AIDP patients but not of control subjects.[62] In CIDP, however, the studies of Heininger et al.[58] suggest that IgG alone appears able to induce a defect in nerve conduction. Those studies were undertaken in marmosets, and the possibility that relevant antibody specificities may have been missed in the earlier transfer studies in AIDP because of lack of species cross-reactivity needs to be kept in mind.

The experimental animal diseases induced by immunizing with components of peripheral nerve with or without Freund's adjuvant have proved of great interest,[63] but the extent to which any one of them may be a true model of AIDP or CIDP is not yet clear and may depend on first identifying the antigen(s) relevant to the human disease.

## PLASMA CELL DYSCRASIAS

Neuropathies can occur with paraproteins that are benign in type or that associate with osteoclastic myeloma or Waldenström's macroglobulinemia (TABLE 4). Most cases of neuropathy that associate with benign gammopathy are demyelinating in type,[64] although some are axonal,[65] and males are much more frequently affected. The paraprotein is typically an IgMκ, directed against carbohydrate determinants shared

TABLE 4. Polyneuropathy in Plasma Cell Dyscrasias

| | Benign Gammopathies | | Waldenström's Macroglobulinemia | Osteoclastic Myeloma |
|---|---|---|---|---|
| | Demyelinating | Axonal | | |
| Age | 40–70 | — | Elderly | 40–70 |
| Sex (M:F) | 6:1 | — | 2:1 | 1:1 |
| Clinical features | Sensory/motor Tremor | Sensory/motor | Sensory/motor Systemic features | Severe weakness Systemic features |
| MCV[b] | Slow | Normal | Variable | Slow |
| Ig heavy chain (Gm) | +/− | n.a.[a] | n.a. | n.a. |
| M-protein | IgMκ | IgM | IgM | IgGλ, IgAλ |
| Target | Carbohydrate determinant MAG/glycoproteins/ glycolipids | Chondroitin sulfate | ? | ? |
| Histology | IgM on myelin Segmental demyelination Mononuclear cell infiltration | IgM on endoneurium | IgM on myelin/ endoneurium Mononuclear cell infiltration | Axonal/demyelinating |

[a] Not available.
[b] Motor conduction velocity.

by myelin-associated glycoprotein (MAG), other glycoproteins, and glycolipids.[66-69] In studies using mouse anti-idiotype monoclonal antibodies to IgM reacting with MAG, there appeared to be no idiotypic cross-reactivity between the IgM anti-MAG paraproteins in a group of 34 patients.[70] A study of a small group of patients suggested differences in the Gm phenotype compared with that in the controls.[71] In the axonal neuropathy found with some benign gammopathies the target appears to be chondroitin sulfate.[72] In osteoclastic myeloma, by contrast, motor rather than sensory signs predominate, the pathology is mixed axonal and demyelinating, and the associated paraprotein is usually IgG or IgAλ. The association of gammopathy and neuropathy provides circumstantial evidence of a causative role for the paraprotein. The improvement following PE and ISD treatment in a proportion of cases is also supportive.[73] Strong experimental evidence in the case of IgG-myeloma-associated neuropathies was provided by passive transfer of physiologic changes from man to mice by intraperitoneal injection of the purified monoclonal IgG.[74] In IgM anti-MAG paraprotein, intraneural injection in cats induces demyelination,[75] but how the IgM crosses the blood-nerve barrier in human disease is not known.

## SUBACUTE SENSORY NEUROPATHY

It has been suggested that autoimmune mechanisms may underlie the painful SSN that occurs in association with SCLC. The principal pathologic changes involve the dorsal root ganglia (DRG) in which there is cellular infiltration and neuronal degeneration. These patients do not seem to show any clear-cut improvement following PE. Such a finding does not exclude a circulating pathologic autoantibody because DRG cells may well lack the ability to regenerate. Serum antibodies in SSN patients that bind to neuronal (e.g., DRG or trigeminal) nuclei but not to other non-neuronal nuclei to any substantial degree have been described.[76] These antibodies appear to cross-react with a SCLC antigen.[77] Although these antibodies may be implicated in SSN, it is not clear how an antibody to an intracellular antigen leads to cell lysis, unless similar determinants are also on the cell surface, perhaps at too low a density to be detected. Successful passive transfer studies have not yet been reported, possibly because the putative autoantibody failed to cross the blood-nerve barrier.

## SUMMARY AND CONCLUSIONS

A number of confounding factors can be identified from the search for autoimmune mechanisms over the last 2 decades that may be relevant for future studies. (1) An apparently homogeneous clinical disorder may represent more than one disease process and thereby imply antibody/antigen heterogeneity as, for example, in MG with and without detectable anti-AChR antibodies. In some cases, physiologic studies allow the different forms of the disease to be distinguished as in AIDP and acute inflammatory axonal polyneuropathy. (2) A homogeneous disorder (e.g., LEMS) may have at least two different triggering mechanisms (SCLC and an unknown stimulus). (3) Antigen density may be too low to be detected by the immunohistologic techniques available, as initially occurred in MG and LEMS. (4) Autoantibodies may be detected that are

TABLE 5. Autoimmune Mechanisms in Neuromuscular Disorders

| | Antigen | Ig | Passive Transfer | Animal Models Active Immunization | Propagation |
|---|---|---|---|---|---|
| MG: anti-AChR positive | AChR | IgG | Systemic + | EAMG | + |
| Lambert-Eaton | Voltage-gated $Ca^{2+}$ channel | IgG | Systemic + | — | — |
| Benign demyelinating gammopathy | Carbohydrate determinant on MAG, glycoproteins, glycolipids | IgMκ | Intraneural + | — | — |
| Osteoclastic myeloma | ? | IgGλ IgAλ | Systemic + | — | — |
| AIDP | ? | IgM? | Intraneural + | EAN? | — |
| CIDP | ? | IgG | Systemic + | EAN? | — |
| MG: anti-AChR undetectable | ? | Ig IgG | + | — | — |

ABBREVIATIONS: AChR = acetylcholine receptor; AIDP = acute demyelinating polyneuropathy; CIDP = chronic inflammatory demyelinating polyneuropathy; EAMG = experimental autoimmune myasthenia gravis; EAN = experimental allergic neuritis; MG = myasthenia gravis.

irrelevant to the primary disease, such as anti-striated muscle antibodies in MG. (5) Poor antibody cross-reactivity between species may mean that the pathogenic antibody is undetected in binding assays or in experimental passive transfer studies. For example, anti-AChR antibody in MG shows less than 5% reactivity with Torpedo AChR. (6) A poor regenerative capacity of the target antigen may mean that reduction of circulating autoantibodies by either plasma exchange or ISD treatment is not associated with detectable clinical improvement, as may be the case in SSN in which DRG cells appear to be the target.

TABLE 5 summarizes the extent to which the data reviewed have established a role for pathogenic antibodies in the light of the postulates for autoimmunity set out earlier and ranks the disorders accordingly. Only in MG with detectable anti-AChR antibody are all the postulates met, including definition of the antigen, experimental passive transfer by the IgG fraction of MG sera, active immunization of experimental animals, and propagation. In both LEMS and the IgMκ anti-MAG demyelinating neuropathy the antigen is known, although better characterized in LEMS; the epitopes are not yet defined in either. Data relating to passive transfer are more extensive in LEMS, however; systemic passive transfer of anti-MAG has not yet been reported. In neither condition is an animal model available. In the demyelinating neuropathies, the case for autoimmunity is less complete. Neither in AIDP nor in CIDP is the antigen known, and thus the relevance of the different EAN disorders is uncertain. Current evidence thus rests on the demonstration of serum IgM antibodies that react with peripheral nerve myelin and fix complement and on the intraneural passive transfer studies. In some cases of MG without detectable anti-AChR antibody, the passive transfer data are strongly suggestive of autoantibodies that are directed against determinants of the neuromuscular junction other than the AChR, and that may themselves be heterogeneous. Finally, in SSN there is currently no experimental evidence that the antineural nuclear antibody is directly implicated in the pathogenesis of DRG cell destruction.

## REFERENCES

1. HUMPHREY, J. H. & R. G. WHITE. 1970. Immunology for Students of Medicine. Autoimmunity (Auto-allergy) and Its Relation to Human Disease, 3rd ed., Chap. 15, pp 600-670. Blackwell, Oxford.
2. SIMPSON, J. A. 1960. Myasthenia gravis. A new hypothesis. Scot. Med. J. **5:** 419-439.
3. CHANG, C. E. & C. Y. LEE. 1962. Isolation of neurotoxins from the venom of Bungarus multicinctus and their modes of neuromuscular blocking action. Arch. Int. Pharmacodyn. Ther. **144:** 241-257.
4. FAMBROUGH, D., D. B. DRACHMAN & S. SATYAMURTI. 1973. Neuromuscular junction in myasthenia gravis. Decreased acetylcholine receptors. Science **182:** 293-295.
5. ITO, Y., R. MILEDI, A. VINCENT & J. NEWSOM-DAVIS. 1978. Acetylcholine receptors and endplate electrophysiology in myasthenia gravis. Brain **101:** 345-368.
6. ELMQVIST, D., W. M. HOFMANN, J. KUGELBERG & D. M. J. QUASTEL. 1964. An electrophysiological investigation of neuromuscular transmission in myasthenia gravis. J. Physiol. (Lond) **174:** 417-434.
7. PATRICK, J. & J. M. LINDSTROM. 1973. Autoimmune response to acetylcholine receptor. Science **180:** 871-872.
8. TARRAB-HAZDAI, R., A. AHARANOV, I. SILMAN & S. FUCHS. 1975. Experimental autoimmune myasthenia induced in monkeys by purified acetylcholine receptor. Nature **256:** 128-130.
9. LENNON, V. A., J. M. LINDSTROM & M. E. SEYBOLD. 1975. Experimental autoimmune myasthenia: A model of myasthenia gravis in rats and guinea-pigs. J. Exp. Med. **141:** 1365-1375.

10. LINDSTROM, J. M., A. G. ENGEL, M. SEYBOLD, V. A. LENNON & E. H. LAMBERT. 1976. Pathological mechanisms in experimental autoimmune myasthenia gravis. II. Passive transfer of experimental autoimmune myasthenia gravis in rats with anti-acetylcholine receptor antibody. J. Exp. Med. **144:** 739-753.
11. TARRAB-HAZDAI, R., A. AHARANOV, O. ABRAMSKY, I. YAAR & S. FUCHS. 1975. Passive transfer of experimental autoimmune myasthenia by lymph node cells in inbred guinea-pigs. J. Exp. Med. **142:** 785-789.
12. LINDSTROM, J. M., M. E. SEYBOLD, V. A. LENNON, S. WHITTINGHAM & D. D. DUANE. 1976. Antibody to acetylcholine receptor in myasthenia gravis. Prevalence, clinical correlates, and diagnostic value. Neurology **26:** 1054-1059.
13. VINCENT, A. & J. NEWSOM-DAVIS. 1980. Anti-acetylcholine receptor antibodies. J. Neurol. Neurosurg. & Psychiatr. **43:** 590-600.
14. TZARTOS, S. J., M. E. SEYBOLD & J. M. LINDSTROM. 1982. Specificities of antibodies to acetylcholine receptors in sera from myasthenia gravis patients measured by monoclonal antibodies. Proc. Natl. Acad. Sci. USA **79:** 188-192.
15. TOYKA, K. V., D. B. DRACHMAN, D. E. GRIFFEN, A. PESTRONK, J. A. WINKELSTEIN, K. H. FISCHBECK & I. KAO. 1977. Myasthenia gravis. Study of humoral immune mechanism by passive transfer to mice. N. Engl. J. Med. **296:** 125-131.
16. PINCHING, A. J., D. K. PETERS & J. NEWSOM-DAVIS. 1976. Remission of myasthenia gravis following plasma exchange. Lancet **11:** 1373-1376.
17. DAU, P. C., J. M. LINDSTROM, J. K. CASSEL, E. H. DENYS, E. E. SHEV & L. E. SPITTER. 1977. Plasmapheresis and immunosuppressive drug therapy in myasthenia gravis. N. Engl. J. Med. **297:** 1134-1140.
18. NEWSOM-DAVIS, J., A. J. PINCHING, A. VINCENT & S. G. WILSON. 1978. Function of circulating antibody to acetylcholine receptor in myasthenia gravis: Investigation by plasma exchange. Neurology (NY) **28:** 266-272.
19. ENGEL, A. G. 1980. Morphological and immunopathologic findings in myasthenia gravis and in congenital myasthenic syndromes. J. Neurol. Neurosurg. Psychiatr. **43:** 577-589.
20. COMPSTON, D. A. S., A. VINCENT, J. NEWSOM-DAVIS & J. R. BATCHELOR. 1980. Clinical, pathological, HLA antigen and immunological evidence for disease heterogeneity in myasthenia gravis. Brain **103:** 579-601.
21. MOSSMAN, S., A. VINCENT & J. NEWSOM-DAVIS. 1986. Myasthenia gravis without acetylcholine receptor antibody: A distinct disease entity. Lancet **i:** 116-118.
22. BURGES, J., J. NEWSOM-DAVIS, A. VINCENT & D. W-WRAY. 1987. Plasma factors from a myasthenia gravis patient without detectable anti-acetylcholine receptor antibody: Effect on mouse neuromuscular transmission. J. Physiol. in press.
23. DRACHMAN, D. B., S. DESILVA, D. RAMSAY & A. PESTRONK. 1987. 'Seronegative' myasthenia gravis: A humorally mediated variant of myasthenia. Neurology **37:** 214A.
24. LAMBERT, E. H. & D. ELMQVIST. 1971. Quantal components of endplate potentials in the myasthenic syndrome. Ann. N.Y. Acad. Sci. **183:** 183-199.
25. LAMBERT, E. H., E. D. ROOKE, L. M. EATON & C. H. HODGSON. 1961. Myasthenic syndrome occasionally associated with bronchial neoplasm: neurophysiologic studies. In Myasthenia Gravis. H. R. Viets, Ed.: 362-410. Charles C Thomas, Springfield.
26. O'NEILL, J. H., N. M. F. MURRAY & J. NEWSOM-DAVIS. The Lambert-Eaton myasthenic syndrome: A review of 50 cases. Brain, in press.
27. GUTTMANN, L., T. W. CROSBY, M. TAKAMORI & J. D. MARTIN. 1972. The Eaton-Lambert syndrome and autoimmune disorders. Am. J. Med. **53:** 354-356.
28. LENNON, V. A., E. H. LAMBERT, S. WHITTINGHAM & V. FAIRBANKS. 1982. Autoimmunit; in the Lambert-Eaton myasthenic syndrome. Muscle & Nerve **5:** S21-S25.
29. WILLCOX, N., J. NEWSOM-DAVIS, A. G. DEMAINE & K. I. WELSH. 1985. Increased frequency of IgG heavy chain marker Glm(2) and of HLA-B8 in Lambert-Eaton myasthenic syndrome with and without associated lung carcinoma. Human Immunology **14:** 29-36.
30. NEWSOM-DAVIS, J. & N. M. F. MURRAY. 1984. Plasma exchange and immunosuppressive drug treatment in the Lambert-Eaton myasthenic syndrome. Neurology (NY) **34:** 480-485.
31. LANG, B., J. NEWSOM-DAVIS, D. WRAY, A. VINCENT & N. MURRAY. 1981. Autoimmune aetiology for myasthenic (Eaton-Lambert) syndrome. Lancet **ii:** 224-226.

32. LANG, B., J. NEWSOM-DAVIS, C. PRIOR & D. WRAY. 1983. Antibodies to motor nerve terminals: An electrophysiological study of a human myasthenic syndrome transferred to mouse. J. Physiol. (Lond) **344:** 335-345.
33. PRIOR, C., B. LANG, D. WRAY & J. NEWSOM-DAVIS. 1985. Action of Lambert-Eaton myasthenic syndrome IgG at mouse motor nerve terminals. Ann. Neurol. **17:** 587-592.
34. FUKUNAGA, H., A. ENGEL, M. OSAME & E. H. LAMBERT. 1982. Paucity and disorganisation of presynaptic membrane active zones in the Lambert-Eaton myasthenic syndrome. Muscle & Nerve **5:** 686-697.
35. FUKUNAGA, H., A. G. ENGEL, B. LANG, J. NEWSOM-DAVIS & A. VINCENT. 1983. Passive transfer of Lambert-Eaton myasthenic syndrome with IgG from man to mouse depletes the presynaptic membrane active zones. Proc. Natl. Acad. Sci. USA **80:** 7636-7640.
36. FUKUOKA, T., A. G. ENGEL, B. LANG, J. NEWSOM-DAVIS & A. VINCENT. 1987. Lambert-Eaton Myasthenic Syndrome: II. Immunoelectron microscopy localisation of IgG at the mouse motor endplate. Ann. Neurol. **22:** 200-211.
37. LANG, B., J. NEWSOM-DAVIS, C. PEERS, C. PRIOR & D. W-WRAY. 1987. The effect of myasthenic syndrome antibody on presynaptic calcium channels in the mouse. J. Physiol. **390:** 257-270.
38. ROBERTS, A., S. PERERA, B. LANG, A. VINCENT & J. NEWSOM-DAVIS. 1985. Paraneoplastic myasthenic syndrome IgG inhibits $^{45}Ca^{2+}$ flux in a human small cell carcinoma line. Nature **317:** 737-739.
39. FEASBY, T. E., J. J. GILBERT, W. F. BROWN, C. F. BOLTON, A. F. HAHN, W. F. KOOPMAN & D. W. ZOCHODNE. 1986. An acute axonal form of Guillain-Barre polyneuropathy. Brain **109:** 1115-1126.
40. THOMAS, P. K., R. G. LASCELLES, J. F. HALLPIKE & R. L. HEWER. 1969. Recurrent and chronic relapsing Guillain-Barre polyneuritis. Brain **92:** 589-606.
41. DYCK, P. J., A. C. LAIS, M. OHTA, J. A. BASTRON, H. OKAZAKI & R. V. GROOVER. 1978. Chronic inflammatory polyradiculoneuropathy. Mayo Clin. Proc. **50:** 621-637.
42. THOMAS, P. K., R. W. H. WALKER, P. RUDGE, J. A. MORGAN-HUGHES, R. H. M. KING, J. M. JACOBS, K. R. MILLS, I. E. C. ORMEROD, N. M. F. MURRAY & W. I. MCDONALD. 1987. Chronic demyelinating peripheral neuropathy associated with multifocal central nervous system demyelination. Brain **110:** 53-76.
43. ASBURY, A. K., B. G. ARNASON & R. D. ADAMS. 1969. The inflammatory lesion in idiopathic polyneuritis: Its role in pathogenesis. Medicine (Baltimore) **48:** 173-215.
44. ADAMS, D., H. FESTENSTEIN, J. D. GIBSON, R. A. C. HUGHES, J. JARAQUEMADA, C. PAPASTERIADIS, J. SACHS & P. K. THOMAS. 1979. HLA antigens in chronic relapsing idiopathic inflammatory neuropathy. J. Neurol. Neurosurg. & Psychiatr. **42:** 184-186.
45. GROSS, M. L. P. & P. K. THOMAS. 1981. The treatment of chronic relapsing and chronic progressive inflammatory polyneuropathy by plasma exchange. J. Neurol. Sci. **52:** 69-78.
46. TOYKA, K. V., R. AUGSPACH, H. WIETHOLTER, U. A. BESINGER, F. HANEVELD, U. G. LEIBERT, K. HEININGER, G. SCHWENDEMANN, K. REINERS & B. GRADENSEE. 1982. Plasma exchange in chronic inflammatory polyneuropathy: Evidence suggestive of a pathogenic humoral factor. Muscle & Nerve **5:** 479-484.
47. DYCK, P. J., J. DAUBE, P. O'BRIEN, A. PINEDA, P. A. LOW, A. J. WINDEBANK & C. SWANSON. 1986. Plasma exchange in chronic inflammatory emyelinating polyradiculoneuropathy. N. Engl. J. Med. **314:** 461-465.
48. DYCK, P. J., P. C. O'BRIEN, K. F. OVIATT, R. P. DINAPOLI, J. R. DAUBE, J. D. BARTLESON, B. MOKRI, T. SWIFE, P. A. LOW & A. J. WINDEBANK. 1982. Prednisone improves chronic inflammatory demyelinating polyradiculoneuropathy more than no treatment. Ann. Neurol. **11:** 136-141.
49. GREENWOOD, R. J., J. NEWSOM-DAVIS, R. A. C. HUGHES, S. ASLAN, A. N. BOWDEN, D. W. CHADWICK, N. S. GORDON, D. L. MCLELLAN, P. MILLAC, R. B. STOTT & P. ARMITAGE. 1984. Controlled trial of plasma exchange in acute inflammatory polyradiculoneuropathy. Lancet **i:** 877-879.
50. GUILLAIN-BARRE SYNDROME STUDY GROUP. 1985. Plasmapheresis and acute Guillain-Barre syndrome. Neurology **35:** 1096-1107.
51. HUGHES, R. A. C., J. NEWSOM-DAVIS, G. D. PERKIN & J. M. PIERCE. 1978. Controlled trial of Prenisolone in acute polyneuropathy. Lancet **ii:** 750-753.

52. COOK, S. D., P. C. DOWLING, M. R. MURRAY & J. N. WHITAKER. 1971. Circulating demyelinating factors in acute idiopathic polyneuropathy. Arch. Neurol. **24:** 136-144.
53. FEASBY, T. E., A. F. HAHN & J. J. GILBERT. 1982. Passive transfer studies in Guillain-Barre polyneuropathy. Neurology **32:** 1159-1167.
54. SAIDA, T., K. SAIDA, R. P. LISAK, M. J. BROWN, D. H. SILBERBERG & A. K. ASBURY. 1982. In vivo demyelinating activity of sera from patients with Guillain-Barre syndrome. Ann. Neurol. **11:** 69-75.
55. SUMNER, A. H., R. P. LISAK, M. J. BROWN & A. K. ASBURY. 1983. Demyelinative activity of Guillain-Barre (GBS) serum. Neurology **33:** 81A.
56. HARRISON, B. M., L. A. HANSEN, J. D. POLLARD & J. G. MCLEOD. 1984. Demyelination induced by serum from patients with Guillain-Barre syndrome. Ann. Neurol. **15:** 163-170.
57. TANDON, D. S., J. W. GRIFFIN, D. B. DRACHMAN, D. L. PRICE & P. L. COYLE. 1980. Studies on the humoral mechanisms of inflammatory demyelinating neuropathies. Neurology **30:** 362A.
58. HEININGER, K., U. G. LIEBERT, K. V. TOYKA, F. T. HANEVELD, G. SCHWENDEMANN, V. KOLB-BACHOFEN, H.-G. ROSS, S. CLEVELAND, U. A. BESINGER, E. GIBBELS & W. WECHSLER. 1984. Chronic inflammatory polyneuropathy: Reduction of nerve conduction velocities in monkeys by systemic passive transfer of immunoglobulin G. J. Neurol. Sci. **66:** 1-14.
59. LUIJTEN, J. A. F. M. & E. H. BAART DE LA FAILLE-KUYPER. 1972. The occurrence of IgM and complement factors along myelin sheaths of peripheral nerves. An immunohistochemical study of the Guillain-Barre syndrome. Preliminary communication. J. Neurol. Sci. **15:** 219-224.
60. KOSKI, C. L., R. HUMPHREY & M. L. SHIN. 1985. Anti-peripheral myelin antibody in patients with demyelinating neuropathy: Quantitative and kinetic determination of serum antibody by complement component 1 fixation. Proc. Natl. Acad. Sci. USA **82:** 905-909.
61. KOSKI, C. L., E. GRATZ, J. SUTHERLAND & R. F. MAYER. 1986. Clinical correlation with anti-peripheral-nerve myelin antibodies in Guillain-Barre syndrome. Ann. Neurol. **19:** 573-577.
62. KOSKI, C. L., P. VANGURI & M. L. SHIN. 1985. Activation of the alternative pathway of complement by human peripheral nerve myelin. J. Immunol. **134:** 1810-1814.
63. WAKSMAN, B. H. & R. D. ADAMS. 1955. Allergic neuritis: An experimental disease of rabbits induced by the injection of peripheral nervous tissue and adjuvants. J. Exp. Med. **102:** 213-236.
64. SMITH, I. S., S. N. KAHN, B. W. LACEY, R. H. M. KING, R. A. EAMES, D. J. WHYBREW & P. K. THOMAS. 1983. Chronic demyelinating neuropathy associated with benign IgM paraproteinaemia. Brain. **106:** 169-195.
65. NEMNI, R., G. GALASSI, N. LAROV, W. H. SHERMAN, M. R. OLARTE & A. P. HAYS. 1983. Polyneuropathy in nonmalignant IgM plasma cell dyscrasia: A morphological study. Ann. Neurol. **14:** 43-54.
66. ILYAS, A. A., R. H. QUARLES, T. D. MACINTOSH, M. J. DOBERSEN, B. D. TRAPP, M. C. DALAKAS & R. O. BRADY. 1984. IgM in a human neuropathy related to paraproteinaemia binds to a carbohydrate determinant in the myelin-associated glycoprotein and to a ganglioside. Proc. Natl. Acad. Sci. USA **81:** 1225-1229.
67. NOBILE-ORAZIO, E., N. LATOV, A. P. HAYS, M. TAKATSU, M., G. M. ABRAMS, W. H. SHERMAN, J. R. MILLER, M.-J. M. T. SAITO, A. TAHMOUSH, R. E. LOVELACE & L. P. ROWLAND. 1984. Neuropathy and anti-MAG antibodies without detectable serum M-protein. Neurology (Cleveland) **34:** 218-221.
68. FREDDO, L., T. ARIGA, M. SAITO, L. C. MECALS, R. K. YU & N. LATOV. 1985. The neuropathy of plasma cell dyscrasia: Binding of IgM M-proteins to peripheral nerve glycolipids. Neurology **35:** 1420-1424.
69. HAFLER, D. A., D. JOHNSON, J. J. KELLY, H. PANITCH, R. KYLE & H. L. WEINER. 1986. Monoclonal gammopathy and neuropathy: Myelin-associated glycoprotein reactivity and clinical characteristics. Neurology **36:** 75-78.
70. MURRAY, N., N. PAGE & A. J. STECK. 1986. The human anti-myelin-associated glycoprotein IgM system. Ann. Neurol. **19:** 473-478.
71. KAHN, S. N. & J. P. PANDEY. 1987. IgG heavy-chain (Gm) allotypes in demyelinating

polyneuropathy associated with MAG-binding monoclonal IgM autoantibodies. Ann. Neurol. **21:** 507-509.
72. SHERMAN, W. H., N. LATOV, A. P. HAYS, M. TAKATSU, R. NEMNI, G. GALASSI & E. F. OSSERMAN. 1983. Monoclonal IgM antibody precipitating with chondroitin sulfate C from patients with axonal polyneuropathy and epidermolysis. Neurology **33:** 192-201.
73. SHERMAN, W. H., M. R. OLARTE, G. MCKIERNAN, K. SWEENEY, N. LATOV & A. P. HAYS. 1984. Plasma exchange treatment of peripheral neuropathy associated with plasma cell dyscrasia. J. Neurol. Neurosurg. Psychiatry **47:** 813-819.
74. BESINGER, U. A., K. V. TOYKA, A. P. ANZIL, A. FATEH-MOGHADAM, D. NEUMEIER, R. RAUSCHER & K. HEININGER. 1981. Myeloma neuropathy: Passive transfer from man to mouse. Science **213:** 1027-1030.
75. HAYS, A. P., N. LATOV, M. TAKATSU & W. H. SHERMAN. 1987. Experimental demyelination of nerve induced by serum of patients with neuropathy and an anti-MAG IgM M-protein. Neurology **37:** 242-256.
76. GRAUS, F., C. CORDON-CARDO & J. B. POSNER. 1985. Neuronal antinuclear antibody in sensory neuronopathy from lung cancer. Neurology **35:** 538-543.
77. GRAUS, F., K. B. ELKON, C. CORDON-CARDO & J. B. POSNER. 1986. Sensory neuronopathy and small cell lung cancer. Antineuronal antibody that also reacts with the tumor. Am. J. Med. **80:** 45-52.

PART II. NERVOUS SYSTEM DIFFERENTIATION

# Expression of Neural Cell Adhesion Molecules in Normal and Pathologic Tissues

ROBERT BRACKENBURY

*University of Cincinnati Medical Center
Department of Anatomy and Cell Biology
Cincinnati, Ohio 45267-0521*

Specific cell-cell interactions have long been recognized as a key factor guiding the differentiation and morphogenesis of higher organisms. These interactions are a hallmark of the developing nervous system, presumably playing important roles in events such as primary induction of the neural plate, closure of the neural tube, the precise migration and differentiation of neural crest cells, and formation of the elaborate and specific connections of the mature nervous system. The desire to understand these processes at a fundamental level led to intense efforts over the last 20 years to identify and characterize molecules that mediated cell-cell adhesion or "recognition."

The first of these molecules to be defined, the neural cell adhesion molecule, or "N-CAM,"[1,2] was detected by an indirect immunologic assay, but eventually was shown to have binding activity,[3] as would be expected of a ligand. A second major adhesion molecule on epithelial cells, L-CAM (also called E-cadherin, Cell-CAM 120/80, or uvomorulin), was subsequently identified in a similar manner.[4-7] As will be discussed, these molecules are representative of two major families of adhesion molecules.

## THE N-CAM FAMILY OF ADHESION MOLECULES

N-CAM mediates the calcium-independent adhesion of nerve cells[8] and the binding between neurons and myotubes.[9] The molecule is a large and abundant cell-surface glycoprotein[10] encoded by a single gene[11] located on human chromosome 11.[12] Alternative splicing of the N-CAM transcript gives rise to three major polypeptides in neural tissue[13-15] (FIG. 1). Recently, two smaller variations that do not appreciably alter the electrophoretic mobility of these polypeptides were also shown to result from alternative patterns of splicing.[16,17] Except for these minor changes, the extracellular portion of the three polypeptides is identical. Strikingly, there are major differences between the three forms in their attachment to the membrane and in the extent of their cytoplasmic domains.[15,17-21]

The binding region of N-CAM is located within the amino-terminal portion of the molecule.[15,18] Interestingly, this region consists of five segments that are homologous to each other and to members of the immunoglobulin gene superfamily[15,17,19,21] (FIG.

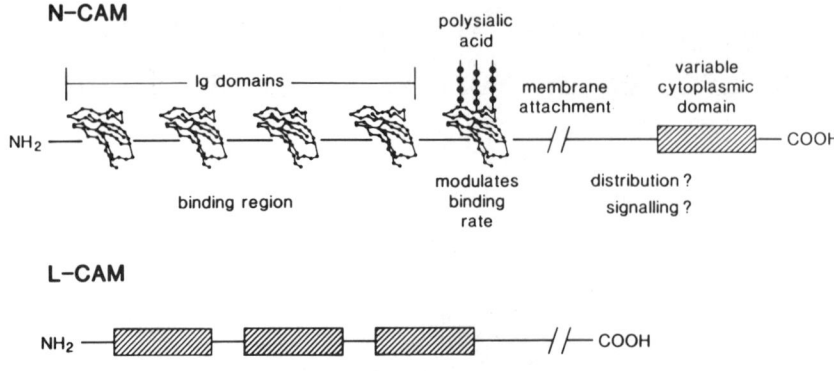

**FIGURE 1.** Structure of N-CAM and L-CAM. *Upper panel:* N-CAM polypeptides contain immunoglobulin-like domains that extend away from the cell surface. This common extracellular portion contains the binding region. Carbohydrate constitutes about one third of the mass of N-CAM and includes an exceptionally large amount of sialic acid attached (*filled circles*) as long, unbranched polymeric chains. The three major N-CAM polypeptides differ in their form of membrane attachment: Both the Mr 180,000 and Mr 140,000 polypeptides contain identical hydrophobic segments that span the cell membrane but differ in the extent of their cytoplasmic domains. The largest chain, which is found only in neural tissue, contains a unique region (*crosshatched*) coded by a single large exon that is included via a tissue-specific splicing event. The smallest chain does not contain the membrane-spanning domain, but instead incorporates a different hydrophobic-rich segment that is attached to the membrane by a phosphotidylinositol linkage. *Lower panel:* Thus far, only a single polypeptide form of the calcium-dependent adhesion molecule L-CAM has been detected. The large extracellular domain consists of three repeated homology units that are unrelated to the immunoglobulin domains of N-CAM. The polypeptide spans the membrane and contains a cytoplasmic domain of approximately 150 amino acids. This model is drawn from recent studies of cDNA clones of mouse and chicken L-CAM.[34-36] Other studies show that the calcium-dependent adhesion molecules N-cadherin and P-cadherin are structurally similar to L-CAM.[41,43]

1). Because N-CAM binding is homophilic, that is, N-CAM on one cell binds to another N-CAM on an adjacent cell, the binding mechanism apparently involves interactions among immunoglobulin-like domains. Inhibition studies with different monoclonal antibodies[15,22] suggest that domains 1 and 3 may directly participate in binding.

In contrast to the immunoglobulin genes, there is no evidence for any heterogeneity in the sequence at the amino-terminal portion of N-CAM that might change the specificity of its binding. However, several posttranslational modifications may serve to regulate N-CAM's expression or activity. N-CAM is glycosylated,[10] phosphorylated, sulfated, and acylated,[23] but little is presently known about the effect of these modifications on binding activity. One change, in the carbohydrate component of N-CAM, *is* known to affect its binding: N-CAM isolated from adult brains has only about one third the amount of sialic acid of N-CAM from embryos,[24,25] and the low-sialic acid forms of N-CAM mediate binding at four times the rate of the high-sialic acid form.[26] The decrease in sialic acid during development might serve to strengthen or finalize transient connections, although there is no direct evidence for this view.

The functional significance of the major variations at the carboxyl end of N-CAM is unknown. The different structures could be involved in directing different forms of N-CAM to various locations on an individual cell. For example, it is known that the

$M_r$ = 180,000 form is preferentially expressed on axon processes,[14,27] and recent evidence suggests that spectrin binds specifically to this form.[28] Such an association could provide a mechanism for selective localization. A second possibility is that N-CAM plays a role in transmembrane signaling. In this case, the variations in structure at the carboxyl terminus could lead to different cellular responses to binding.

Several other neural cell surface components that may function as adhesion molecules were found to be structurally related to N-CAM (TABLE 1). The most striking example is the myelin-associated glycoprotein (MAG), which may play a role in the interactions between Schwann cell membranes and neural axons. Like N-CAM, MAG has an extracellular portion composed of immunoglobulin-like domains, and a variable cytoplasmic domain that arises by alternative splicing.[29-31] In addition, Thy-1 and the myelin protein $P_0$, which are suggested to have adhesive functions, also consist of immunoglobulin-like domains.[31,32] Comparison of these sequences with other members of the immunoglobulin gene superfamily suggests that N-CAM is closely related to the primitive immunoglobulin domain gene precursor.[15,32] These observations suggest that the compact immunoglobulin domain structure, consisting of back-to-back β-pleated sheets, serves as an excellent scaffolding for constructing a variety of adhesive molecules. They support the idea[33] that immune recognition evolved from an early cell-cell recognition system.

## THE L-CAM FAMILY OF ADHESIVE MOLECULES

A second family of CAMs is represented by the epithelial cell adhesion molecule L-CAM. Like N-CAM, L-CAM is a large and relatively abundant glycoprotein that spans the plasma membrane and has a moderate cytoplasmic domain (FIG. 1). However, the complete sequence of L-CAM, deduced from cDNA clones,[34-36] indicates that the two molecules are not related structurally. L-CAM has no homology to immunoglobulin domains, but rather consists of three internally repeated homology units.[34-36] L-CAM has little or no associated sialic acid, but is phosphorylated and acylated.[37]

Both the binding activity and the structure of L-CAM depend on calcium.[4-7] Takeichi[38,39] first suggested that this property was diagnostic of a class of calcium-dependent adhesion molecules, termed "cadherins," that are expressed on a variety of cells. Together with co-workers, Takeichi has characterized several of these molecules, including E-cadherin[35] (the mouse form of L-CAM), P-cadherin[40,41] (enriched in placenta), and N-cadherin,[42] the neural calcium-dependent adhesion molecule. The

TABLE 1. Neural Cell Surface Molecules Composed of Immunoglobulin Domains[15,31,32]

| Molecule | Number of Ig Domains | Function |
|---|---|---|
| N-CAM | 5 | Neuron-neuron and neuron-myotube adhesion |
| MAG | 5 | Schwann cell-axon interactions |
| $P_0$ | 1 | Myelin compaction (?) |
| Thy-1 | 1 | Concentrated at synapses |

structures of these molecules are closely related,[35,40-43] indicating that they form a family of evolutionarily related adhesion molecules that is distinct from the N-CAM family.

## THE FUNCTION OF CAMs

Generally speaking, what do CAMs do and how many are required? As a specific example, most neural cells simultaneously express both N-CAM and N-cadherin, and the detailed tissue distributions of these two molecules are similar, but not identical. Why do neural cells employ two virtually ubiquitous adhesion systems, and how are the activities of these molecules coordinated? Are there perhaps additional, as yet undiscovered, CAMs expressed on these cells?

It is likely that many different functions may fall under the rubric of "CAM." In this connection, it is important to note that CAMs are defined operationally. The assays that have been used so far have limited the molecules that could be identified to those that are present on most cells, are immunogenic, and are able to withstand appreciable shear. Any CAMs that are specific to small subsets of cells would not have been detected, nor would secondary adhesion molecules that merely strengthen or modulate primary binding events. New classes of CAMs will be detected only through the development of assays that focus on different aspects of cell-cell interactions.

Many kinds of roles can be imagined for cell surface adhesive molecules. During early embryogenesis, differential expression of CAMs may guide morphogenetic rearrangements. For example, cell-cell adhesions mediated by N-CAM or N-cadherin might be essential for neural tube closure. The differentiation of neural crest cells provides another intriguing example. Crest cells initially express N-CAM, then lose it during their period of active migration, and finally re-express N-CAM at the same time as they aggregate to form dorsal root ganglia.[44] It is tempting to infer that adhesion mediated by N-CAM plays a key role in regulating the decision to migrate or adhere. Another possibility is that cell-contact mediated by CAMs could trigger specific differentiation events. In other situations, the degree of cell contact might affect the rate at which nutrients, hormones, or "morphogens" pass through a tissue. In this case CAM function could indirectly modulate the pattern or rate of differentiation. A striking example illustrating this role is the finding that the pattern of feather bud differentiation is disrupted by antibodies to L-CAM.[45]

The most familiar example of specific cell adhesion is the precise connectivity of the visual system of vertebrates. The chemoaffinity model of Sperry[46] accounted for this precise mapping by postulating a large number of complementary pairs of adhesive molecules distributed on individual cells. This view has been superseded to some extent by evidence emphasizing that the initial pattern of connectivity is sharpened or regulated by subsequent activity.[47] Nevertheless, many workers, encouraged by results from arthropod embryos, continue to search for recognition molecules specific to small subsets of neurons. It is clear that molecules such as N-CAM or N-cadherin are too widely distributed to determine point-to-point mapping, although Edelman[48] has argued persuasively that a substantial degree of ordered pattern can emerge from the dynamic interaction of several basic processes.

In all of these situations, CAMs might have passive, mechanical roles, or active, "signaling" functions. A passive role implies that CAMs are "simply" cell-surface glue, serving to ligate cells. In this view, adjacent cells would adhere or not according to the developmental program of expression for specific CAMs and CAM receptors. As already discussed, a "passive" role could nevertheless be a major determinant in morphogenetic processes. In the contrasting view, CAMs would not only mediate cell ligation but would also actively transmit information on the state of cell association across the cell membrane. In many developing systems it is known that cell contact triggers specific differentiation events. Thus, the binding of N-CAM on one cell to N-CAM on an adjacent cell might alter the conformation of the molecule, thereby changing its association with the cytoskeleton or activating an enzymatic activity associated with its cytoplasmic domain. Such changes could be directly translated into altered differentiation signals inside the cell. Thus far, however, all assays for CAM function have focused on binding events rather than intracellular consequences of binding.

Both of these views suggest that mechanisms that control CAM expression or activity would be central regulatory systems of development and prime targets for evolutionary changes.[49] Although mutations that changed the primary structure of CAMs would ordinarily lead to embryonic lethality, mutations that altered the timing of CAM expression or altered the posttranslational modifications of CAMs might have less devastating consequences.

## CHANGES IN CAM EXPRESSION ASSOCIATED WITH PATHOLOGIC STATES

Recent studies suggest that a variety of pathologic changes may be accompanied by alterations in CAM expression. Three examples, including the effects of malignant transformation, a neurologic mutation, and response to peripheral nerve injury will be briefly discussed.

It is widely believed that a key alteration in malignant cells is changes in their cell surfaces that cause disruption of normal cell-cell interactions. The correlation between N-CAM expression and migration of neural crest cells already discussed also supports this idea. To test this possibility, we determined the effect of transformation by Rous sarcoma virus (RSV) on N-CAM expression. In one study,[50] using established cell lines containing a temperature-sensitive mutant of RSV, the expression of N-CAM was temperature sensitive. When grown at the permissive temperature, the cells became morphologically transformed, lost N-CAM, and adhered poorly. N-CAM expression was also decreased to about one tenth the normal level in primary chick neuroepithelial cells transformed by RSV.[51] We also found that the transformed cells had become highly motile, migrating rapidly over the culture dish and under or through aggregates of cells. The increase in motility may result from or be augmented by the reduction in cell-cell adhesiveness. We are currently testing the possibility that these changes significantly enhance the invasiveness of the transformed cells.

A particularly interesting alteration in CAM expression occurs in the mouse neurologic mutant *staggerer*. Mice that are homozygous for this recessive mutation have abnormal posture and gait, and die at about 3 weeks, in part because of an inability to feed. The cerebellum of *sg*/*sg* mice is substantially reduced in size because of massive death of granule cells and Purkinje neurons. Cytologic studies suggest that granule cell survival depends on successful synapse formation between the parallel fibers of the granule cells and the Purkinje dendritic tree. Edelman and Chuong[52] found that the normal conversion of the high sialic acid form of N-CAM to the low sialic acid form is greatly delayed in $sg/sg$ mice. Although this alteration in N-CAM is certainly an indirect effect of the primary mutation, the failure to reduce the sialic acid content could prevent a strengthening of N-CAM mediated connections, leading to extensive granule cell death.

Finally, changes in CAM expression may play important roles in nerve regeneration. N-CAM is normally concentrated at neuromuscular junctions, but its expression in extrajunctional regions increases after nerve crush or transection.[53,54] In addition, Schwann cells that proliferate after nerve damage express increased amounts of N-CAM and Ng-CAM.[55,56] The possibility that these increased levels of CAMs serve to guide nerve fiber regeneration is being actively explored by several laboratories, with a view toward creating CAM-coated substrates that could serve as useful prostheses.

These examples suggest the wide variety of possible effects that result from altered expression of CAMs, and raise the hope that new information about the structure and expression of CAMs may prove useful in ameliorating these effects.

## SUMMARY

Because cell-cell and cell-matrix interactions directly affect the growth, differentiation, and morphogenesis of neural tissue, abnormal changes in these processes could have severe pathologic consequences. Over the last few years, it has become possible to investigate these interactions at the molecular level due to advances in the identification and characterization of matrix components and receptors and cell adhesion molecules (CAMs). Emerging evidence suggests that two broad classes of CAMs are represented by the neural CAM, N-CAM, and the epithelial CAM, L-CAM. N-CAM and several other neural adhesion molecules contain immunoglobulin-like domains and do not require calcium for binding. In contrast, L-CAM, N-cadherin, and P-cadherin depend on calcium for activity and share structural features that differ from those of the N-CAM family. All of these CAMs are expressed in early embryos and in a variety of tissues throughout development, although each has a characteristic pattern. Initial studies suggest that injury, oncogenic transformation, and some genetic neurologic disorders are accompanied by changes in CAM expression that alter the adhesive or migratory behavior of cells.

## REFERENCES

1. BRACKENBURY, R., J.-P. THIERY, U. RUTISHAUSER & G. M. EDELMAN. 1977. J. Biol. Chem. **252:** 6835-6840.
2. THIERY, J.-P., R. BRACKENBURY, U. RUTISHAUSER & G. M. EDELMAN. 1977. J. Biol. Chem. **252:** 6841-6845.
3. RUTISHAUSER, U., S. HOFFMAN & G. M. EDELMAN. 1982. Proc. Natl. Acad. Sci. USA **79:** 685-689.
4. GALLIN, W. J., G. M. EDELMAN & B. A. CUNNINGHAM. 1983. Proc. Natl. Acad. Sci. USA **80:** 1038-1042.
5. HYAFIL, F., D. MORELLO, C. BABINET & F. JACOB. 1980. Cell **21:** 927-934.
6. DAMSKY, C. H., J. RICHA, D. SOLTER, K. KNUDSEN & C. A. BUCK. 1983. Cell **34:** 455-466.

7. YOSHIDA-NORO, C., N. SUZUKI & M. TAKEICHI. 1984. Dev. Biol. **101:** 19-27.
8. BRACKENBURY, R., U. RUTISHAUSER & G. M. EDELMAN. 1981. Proc. Natl. Acad. Sci. USA **78:** 387-391.
9. GRUMET, M., U. RUTISHAUSER & G. M. EDELMAN. 1982. Nature (Lond.) **295:** 693-695.
10. HOFFMAN, S., B. C. SORKIN, P. C. WHITE, R. BRACKENBURY, R. MAILHAMMER, U. RUTISHAUSER, B. A. CUNNINGHAM & G. M. EDELMAN. 1982. J. Biol. Chem. **257:** 7720-7729.
11. OWENS, G. C., G. M. EDELMAN & B. A. CUNNINGHAM. 1987. Proc. Natl. Acad. Sci. USA **84:** 294-298.
12. NGUYEN, C., M.-G. MATTEI, J.-F. MATTEI, M.-J. SANTONI, C. GORIDIS & B. R. JORDAN. 1986. J. Cell Biol. **102:** 711-715.
13. MURRAY, B. A., J. J. HEMPERLY, E. A. PREDIGER, G. M. EDELMAN & B. A. CUNNINGHAM. 1986. J. Cell Biol. **102:** 189-193.
14. MURRAY, B. A., G. OWENS, K. L. CROSSIN, G. M. EDELMAN & B. A. CUNNINGHAM. 1986. J. Cell Biol. **103:** 1431-1439.
15. CUNNINGHAM, B. A., J. J. HEMPERLY, B. A. MURRAY, E. A. PREDIGER, R. BRACKENBURY & G. M. EDELMAN. 1987. Science **236:** 799-806.
16. DICKSON, G., H. J. GOWER, C. H. BARTON, H. M. PRENTICE, V. L. ELSOM, S. E. MOORE, R. D. COX, C. QUINN, W. PUTT & F. S. WALSH. 1987. Cell **50:** 1119-1130.
17. SMALL, S. J., G. E. SHULL, M.-J. SANTONI & R. AKESON. 1987. J. Cell Biol. **105:** 2335-2343.
18. CUNNINGHAM, B. A., S. HOFFMAN, U. RUTISHAUSER, J. J. HEMPERLY & G. M. EDELMAN. 1983. Proc. Natl. Acad. Sci. USA **80:** 3116-3120.
19. HEMPERLY, J. J., B. A. MURRAY, G. M. EDELMAN & B. A. CUNNINGHAM. 1986. Proc. Natl. Acad. Sci. USA **83:** 3037-3041.
20. HEMPERLY, J. J., G. M. EDELMAN & B. A. CUNNINGHAM. 1986. Proc. Natl. Acad. Sci. USA **83:** 9822-9826.
21. BARTHELS, D., M.-J. SANTONI, W. WILLE, C. RUPPERT, J.-C. CHAIX, M.-R. HIRSCH, J. C. FONTECILLA-CAMPS & C. GORIDIS. 1987. EMBO J. **6:** 907-914.
22. COLE, G. J., A. LOEWY, N. V. CROSS, R. AKESON & L. GLASER. 1984. J. Cell Biol. **103:** 1739-1744.
23. SORKIN, B. C., S. HOFFMAN, G. M. EDELMAN & B. A. CUNNINGHAM. 1984. Science **225:**
24. ROTHBARD, J. B., R. W. BRACKENBURY, B. A. CUNNINGHAM & G. M. EDELMAN. 1982. J. Biol. Chem. **257:** 7720-7729.
25. ROUGON, G., H. DEAGOSTINI-BAZIN, M. HIRN & C. GORIDIS. 1982. EMBO J. **1:** 1239-1244.
26. HOFFMAN, S. & G. M. EDELMAN. 1983. Proc. Natl. Acad. Sci. USA **80:** 5762-5766.
27. POLLERBERG, E. G., R. SADOUL, C. GORIDIS & M. SCHACHNER. 1985. J. Cell Biol. **101:** 1921-1929.
28. POLLERBERG, E. G., M. SCHACHNER & J. DAVOUST. 1986. Nature **324:** 462-465.
29. ARQUINT, M., J. RODER, L.-S. CHIA, J. DOWN, D. WILKINSON, H. BAYLEY, P. BRAUN & R. DUNN. 1987. Proc. Natl. Acad. Sci. USA **84:** 600-604.
30. SALZER, J. L., W. P. HOLMES & D. R. COLMAN. 1987. J. Cell Biol. **104:** 957-965.
31. LAI, C., M. A. BROW, K.-A. NAVE, A. B. NORONHA, R. H. QUARLES, F. E. BLOOM, R. J. MILNER & J. G. SUTCLIFFE. 1987. Proc. Natl. Acad. Sci. USA **84:** 4337-4341.
32. WILLIAMS, A. F. 1987. Immunol. Today **8**(10): 298-303.
33. WILLIAMS, A. F. 1982. J. Theoret. Biol. **98:** 221-234.
34. GALLIN, W. J., B. C. SORKIN, G. M. EDELMAN & B. A. CUNNINGHAM. 1987. Proc. Natl. Acad. Sci. USA **84:** 2808-2812.
35. NAGAFUCHI, A., Y. SHIRAYOSHI, K. OKAZAKI, K. YASUDA & M. TAKEICHI. 1987. Nature **329:** 341-343.
36. RINGWALD, M., R. SCHUH, D. VESTWEBER, H. EISTATTER, F. LOTTSPEICH, J. ENGEL, R. DOLZ, F. JAHNIG, J. EPPLEN, S. MAYER, C. MULLER & R. KEMLER. 1987. EMBO J. **6:** 3647-3653.
37. CUNNINGHAM, B. A., Y. LEUTZINGER, W. J. GALLIN, B. C. SORKIN & G. M. EDELMAN. 1984. Proc. Natl. Acad. Sci. USA **81:** 5787-5791.
38. TAKEICHI, M. 1977. J. Cell Biol. **75:** 464-474.
39. URUSHIHARA, H., H. S. OZAKI & M. TAKEICHI. 1979. Dev. Biol. **70:** 201-216.

40. NOSE, A. & M. TAKEICHI. 1986. J. Cell Biol. **103:** 2649-2658.
41. NOSE, A., A. NAGAFUCHI & M. TAKEICHI. 1987. EMBO J. **6**(12): 3655-3661.
42. HATTA, K. & M. TAKEICHI. 1986. Nature **320:** 447-449.
43. SHIRAYOSHI, Y., K. HATTA, M. HOSODA, S. TSUNASAWA, F. SAKIYAMA & M. TAKEICHI. 1986. EMBO J. **5**(10): 2485-2488.
44. THIERY, J.-P., J.-L. DUBAND, U. RUTISHAUSER & G. M. EDELMAN. 1982. Proc. Natl. Acad. Sci. USA **79:** 6737-6741.
45. GALLIN, W. J., C.-M. CHUONG, L. H. FINKEL & G. M. EDELMAN. 1986. Proc. Natl. Acad. Sci. USA **83:** 8235-8239.
46. SPERRY, R. W. 1963. Proc. Natl. Acad. Sci. USA **50:** 703-710.
47. EASTER, S. S., D. PURVES, P. RAKIC & N. C. SPITZER. 1985. Science **230:** 507-511.
48. EDELMAN, G. M. 1984. Trends Neurosci. **7:** 78-84.
49. EDELMAN, G. M. 1984. Proc. Natl. Acad. Sci. USA **81:** 1460-1464.
50. GREENBERG, M. E., R. BRACKENBURY & G. M. EDELMAN. 1984. Proc. Natl. Acad. Sci. USA **81:** 969-973.
51. BRACKENBURY, R., M. E. GREENBERG & G. M. EDELMAN. 1984. J. Cell Biol. **99:** 1944-1954.
52. EDELMAN, G. M. & C.-M. CHUONG. 1982. Proc. Natl. Acad. Sci. USA **79:** 7036-7040.
53. RIEGER, F., M. GRUMET & G. M. EDELMAN. 1985. J. Cell Biol. **101:** 285-293.
54. COVAULT, J. & J. SANES. 1985. Proc. Natl. Acad. Sci. USA **82:** 4544-4548.
55. DANILOFF, J. K., G. LEVI, M. GRUMET, F. RIEGER & G. M. EDELMAN. 1986. J. Cell Biol. **103:** 929-945.
56. NIEKE, J. & M. SCHACHNER. 1985. Differentiation **30:** 141-151.

# Where Do Different Neurons Come From?

## Identification and Immortalization of CNS Precursor Cells

RON McKAY

*Massachusetts Institute of Technology
Cambridge, Massachusetts 02139*

Early events in neural development establish functionally important features of the adult nervous system. The *number* of neurons in the adult brain is derived from two independent processes, an early proliferative process operating on neuronal precursor cells and a later process of selective cell death.[1] Transplantation experiments show that the *types* of neuron found in the adult brain are also importantly influenced by events that occur at early stages in embryogenesis.[2-4] In *Drosophila*, genetic methods of cell lineage analysis show that cell-cell interaction plays an important role in defining neuronal type at the time neurons are first generated.[5,6] These experiments suggest that early in development, as neurons differentiate from neuroepithelial precursor cells, they interact with cells in their environment, and this interaction leads to the choice of a specific cellular fate.

As this early time in the embryo is important in making neurons different, it has been carefully studied with available methods. During neurogenesis, cell proliferation, migration, and axon navigation are three major steps in the life of a developing neuron. Neuroepithelial cells proliferate under an extraordinarily precise set of controls so that neurons become postmitotic in precise numbers on specific days of development.[7] Postmitotic neurons then migrate from the specialized proliferative zone to the location occupied by the adult neuron.[8-10] Once the neuronal cell body reaches this location, an axon is extended which grows along defined cellular cues.[11-18] In spite of what is known about these early processes, we still do not have a detailed picture of the way a neuron differentiates.

What cell types are present in the neuroepithelium at the time of neurogenesis? In the vertebrate neural tube there are three major morphologically defined cell types during the restricted period when neurons differentiate. A columnar epithelial cell is the only cell found in the neuroepithelium before neurogenesis. During neurogenesis the two additional cell types, postmitotic neurons and radial glial cells, appear at the same time. As we know that cell interactions are important in controlling the number and types of neuron found in the adult brain, our group has concentrated on identifying the cell types in the early mammalian CNS and studying their functions and fates. We have particularly focused on the precursor cells from the rat CNS. We have identified a major precursor population and established a tissue culture system in which these precursors differentiate.

## IDENTIFYING NEURONAL PRECURSORS

We have made monoclonal antibodies that recognize the major cell types in the embryonic rat CNS at the time of neurogenesis.[19] In this experiment we immunized mice with the E 15 (15th day of gestation) CNS of the rat and screened the resulting hybridomas by immunohistochemistry on cross-sections of rat embryos. By choosing this strategy we could readily identify antibodies that were specific for neurons and radial glial cells. The monoclonal antibody Rat 401 was shown to bind radial glial cells by an extensive survey at the light and electron microscopic levels of rat embryos from E 9 to adult. These experiments showed that the cell population recognized by the Rat 401 antibody stained columnar epithelial cells before neurons differentiate, and the expression of the antigen was lost from the brain at the end of the period when neurons are born. The early and transient expression of the Rat 401 antigen around the time when neurons are born suggested that Rat 401 might recognize a precursor population.

To determine directly if the Rat 401 positive population was a precursor population we developed methods for dissociating, counting, and characterizing Rat 401 cells through embryonic development.[20] The Rat 401 positive cell population has properties expected of neuronal precursors:

1. Almost all (98%) the cells of the CNS are Rat 401 positive immediately before neurons differentiate.
2. The proportion of Rat 401 cells decreases during neurogenesis.
3. During neurogenesis Rat 401 positive cells form the major proliferating cell type.
4. The total number of positive cells is large enough to account for the number of neurons born.

These results provide very strong evidence that Rat 401 positive cells are neuronal precursors in the animal. However, it is difficult to use population studies to prove lineage relationships.

## GENERATING PRECURSOR CELL LINES

The next stage in our studies was designed to obtain direct evidence of lineage relationships in the developing brain. We set out to establish clonal cell lines that expressed the precursor marker Rat 401. If these cells were still capable of differentiation, then precursor-product relationships between cells expressing particular marker antigens could be proved.

To obtain Rat 401 positive cell lines we used retroviruses to transduce immortalizing oncogenes into primary brain cells. We chose to put particular emphasis on the use of the large T antigen oncogene from SV40 virus. Recent work shows that the large T antigen immortalizes (or establishes) fibroblasts from the rat.[21] These immortal cell lines differ from fully transformed cells as they do not form tumors. The lack of tumors was important to our strategy, because we planned to transplant immortal cells into the developing brain where we hoped the cells would differentiate. (See Ref. 22 for further discussion of the use of immortal cell lines in transplantation studies.) SV40 large T antigen appeared to be suitable for our studies for two other reasons.

Firstly, others had shown that SV40 virus could be used to generate transformed cells with characteristics of neurons and glia.[23,24] This finding indicates that expression of large T antigen is compatible with expression of CNS-differentiated properties. This conclusion has been strengthened by recent work with transgenic mice in which T antigen expression can be found in postmitotic neurons (Erfrat and Hanahan, personal communication).

Secondly, T antigen is available in a temperature-sensitive form, so that when cells are grown at 33°C, the gene is active but at 39°C the gene product is rapidly degraded. Previous work with muscle cells suggested that the reduction of oncogene function might promote differentiation.[25,26] We constructed a retrovirus carrying the temperature-sensitive form of SV40 T antigen tsA58. This retrovirus was based on a previous construct carrying a wild type large T antigen pZipNeoSV40.[27] The retrovirus carrying the tsA58 gene also carries a gene that confers on the infected cells resistance to the cytotoxic drug neomycin or G418. The presence of the neo® allows selection against uninfected cells that would obscure immortal cells carrying T antigen. (See reference 28 for further details of this strategy and the construction of the pZipneoSv(X)1 shuttle vector.)

Cells lines were generated from the postnatal cerebellum because neurons are formed in the cerebellum in large numbers in the first 2 weeks of life. Nine of the 10 cell lines we obtained with tsA58 were Rat 401 positive. The expression of Rat 401 antigen encouraged us to believe that the cells were capable of differentiating, and we have used three different conditions to differentiate these cells.

1. We have grown the cells at 39°C where the amount of T antigen decreases, the cells lose Rat 401 expression, and, in the presence of particular batches of fetal calf serum, they gain the intermediate filament protein characteristic of astrocytes, GFAP.

2. We have grown the cells in serum-free medium where we have obtained cells that are morphologically similar to neurons and express the intermediate filaments characteristic of neurons.

3. We have grown the immortal cells in the presence of primary cerebellar cells, and this method is the most reproducible one for obtaining both neuronal and glial differentiation.

These results suggest that the cell lines we obtained are derived from brain precursor cells and are capable of generating both neurons and astrocytes. The third major class of cells found in the adult brain are oligodendroglia, and the expression of the galactocerebroside (galC) glycolipid is characteristic of this cell type. A small proportion of the immortal cells express a surface antigen recognized by a monoclonal anti-galC antibody. We must extend our characterization of these differentiated states, but our early data suggest that large T antigen of SV40 is capable of immortalizing multipotential brain precursor cells.

## A MODEL OF CELL LINEAGE IN THE EARLY CNS

A diagram showing a representation of precursor-product relationships in the brain is shown in FIGURE 1.

Our data show that a cloned Rat 401 positive cell line can induce gene products that are restricted *in vivo* to three major differentiated cell types of the adult brain. A further feature of this model is the classification of the radial glial cell as being

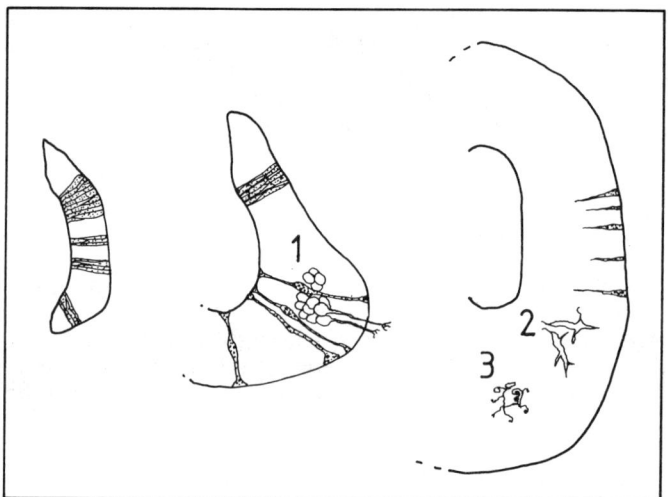

**FIGURE 1.** Diagram showing a representation of precursor-product relationships in the brain. Rat 401 positive cells are *stippled*. Three different times in development are shown from *left* to *right*. At early times the Rat 401 positive cells are columnar. At later times neurons (marked **1**) are the first products of the Rat 401 positive multipotent precursor to differentiate. At later times the two major glial cell types, astrocytes (**2**) and oligodendroglia (**3**), differentiate.

closely related to the neuronal precursor cell. This assignment is based on our cell lineage studies *in vivo* and *in vitro*,[20,29] which suggest that Rat 401 positive cells are major sources of neurons and glia; however, our morphologic studies show that Rat 401 positive cells are radial glial cells.[19] This way of looking at radial glial cell function is new, and it has an attractive feature. If neuronal number and type are a consequence of cell-cell interaction, then the direct presence of the precursor cell in the peripheral regions where postmitotic neurons are differentiating allows a simple mechanism for events in this region to influence subsequent rounds of neuron production.

## SUMMARY

The ability to make functionally competent brain precursor cell lines may have important consequences for a number of outstanding questions in mammalian CNS development. The diversity of neurons is one of the most striking conclusions of recent molecular studies of the nervous system. In our work we provided some of the earliest data to support this conclusion.[30–32] Our preliminary data with precursor cell lines suggest that these cells give neurons with highly differentiated characteristics. If further work continues to support this conclusion, then immortal cell lines will be useful in analyzing the mechanisms that make neurons different. The methods that can be applied to these cell lines include manipulation in tissue culture, transplantation into the developing CNS, and application of the methods of mammalian cell genetics to link gene function to neuronal specificity.

## REFERENCES

1. COWAN, W. M. 1979. Selection and control in neurogenesis. *In* The Neurosciences: A Fourth Study Program. F. O. Schmitt & F. G. Worden, Eds.: 59-79. M.I.T. Press, Cambridge, MA.
2. SPEMANN, H. 1938. Embryonic Development and Induction. Yale University Press, New Haven.
3. CHUNG, S. H. & J. COOKE. 1975. Nature 258: 126-132.
4. JACOBSON, M. 1978. Developmental Neurobiology. Plenum Press, NY.
5. READY, D. F., D. E. HANSEN & S. BENZER. 1976. Dev. Biol. 53: 217-240.
6. LAWRENCE, P. A. & S. M. GREEN. 1979. Dev. Biol. 71: 142-152.
7. SIDMAN, R. L., I. L. MIALE & N. FEDER. 1959. Exp. Neurol. 1: 322-333.
8. RAKIC, P. 1971. Brain Res. 33: 471-476.
9. RAKIC, P. 1971. J. Comp. Neurol. 141: 283-312.
10. RAKIC, P. 1981. Trends in Neurosci. 4: 184-187.
11. CONSTANTINE-PATON, M. & M. I. LAW. 1978. Science 202: 639-641.
12. ANDERSON, H. 1978. J. Embryol. Exp. Morphol. 46: 147-159.
13. MACAGNO, E. 1978. Nature 275: 318-320.
14. GHYSEN, A. 1978. Nature 274: 869-872.
15. KATZ, M. J. & R. J. LASEK. 1979. J. Comp. Neurol. 183: 817-832.
16. LANCE-JONES, C. & L. LANDMESSER. 1980. J. Physiol. 302: 581-602.
17. GOODMAN, C. S., M. J. BASTIANI, C. Q. DOE, S. DU LAC, S. L. HELFAND, J. Y. KUWADA & J. B. THOMAS. 1984. Science 225: 1271-1279.
18. KUWADA, J. Y. 1986. Science 233: 740-746.
19. HOCKFIELD, S. & R. MCKAY. 1985. J. Neurosci. 5: 3310-3328.
20. FREDERIKSEN, K. & R. MCKAY. 1987. J. Neurosci. in press.
21. JAT, P. S. & P. A. SHARP. 1986. J. Virol. 59: 746-750.
22. MCKAY, R. 1987. Prog. Brain Res. in press.
23. DE VITRY, F., M. CAMIER, P. CZERNICHOW & A. TIXIER-VIDAL. 1974. Proc. Natl. Acad. Sci. 71: 3575-3579.
24. NETO, V. M., M. MALLAT, H. CHNEIWEISS, J. PREMONT, F. GROS & A. PROCHIANTZ. 1986. Dev. Brain Res. 26: 11-22.
25. FISZMAN, M. & P. FUCHS. 1975. Nature 254: 429-431.
26. HOLTZER, H., J. BRIEHL, G. YEOH, R. MEGANATHAN & A. KAJI. 1975. Proc. Natl. Acad. Sci. 72: 4051-4055.
27. JAT, P. S., C. L. CEPKO, R. C. MULLIGAN & P. A. SHARP. 1986. Mol. Cell Biol. 6: 1204-1217.
28. CEPKO, C. L., B. E. ROBERTS & R. C. MULLIGAN. 1984. Cell 37: 1053-1062.
29. FREDERIKSEN, K., P. S. JAT, N. VALTZ, D. LEVY & R. MCKAY. Submitted.
30. ZIPSER, B. & R. MCKAY. 1981. Nature. 289: 549-554.
31. MCKAY, R., S. HOCKFIELD, J. JOHANSEN & K. FREDERIKSEN. 1983. Cold Spring Harbor Symp. XLVIII: 599-610.
32. HOCKFIELD, S., R. MCKAY, S. H. C. HENDRY & E. G. JONES. 1983. Cold Spring Harbor Symp. XLVIII: 877-890.

# Astrocyte Diversity

A. PROCHIANTZ AND M. MALLAT

*Collège de France, INSERM U 114*
*Chaire de Neuropharmacologie*
*11, place Marcelin Berthelot*
*75231 Paris cedex 05, France*

If the paucity of different cell types involved in its construction is considered, the brain appears like a rather simple organ. It is not simple enough, however, for most of us who until recently had thought that astrocytes were simple accessory cells only able to foster the neurons during development and to stick them together in adulthood.

It is becoming more and more obvious that this view of the so-called satellite cells was oversimplified. In the following pages the various and important functions fulfilled by the astrocytes will be reviewed. We shall see that in addition to maintenance of brain homeostasis these cells play a key role in all phenomena involving neuronal plasticity. Moreover, astrocytes may be the key to the protection of the brain through "immune-like" mechanisms and to the establishment of the blood-brain barrier (BBB). The existence of so many different functions explains why the astrocytic family has to be subdivided into specialized subpopulations.

In addition to the functional heterogeneity of the astrocyte, one has to consider structural and even regional variation contributing, to a degree not yet clearly understood, to the overall complexity of the brain.

## FUNCTIONAL HETEROGENEITY OF THE ASTROCYTE

The definition of the astrocyte is not any more morphological. An astrocyte is defined by the presence of the glial fibrillary acidic protein (GFAP) in the intermediate filaments.[1] TABLE 1 summarizes the different astrocytic functions presently known and attempts to relate molecular properties to possible functions.

### *Extracellular Buffering*

Astrocytes share with the neurons the capacity to capture and to bind several neuromediators. In addition, they possess several ionophores including $NA^+$, $K^+$, and $Ca^+$ channels.[2] High affinity uptake has been demonstrated for serotonin, dopamine, norepinephrine, and several inhibitory or excitatory amino acids.[3-8] It is generally believed that astrocytic uptake participates in the clearing of the neurotransmitter from the synaptic cleft.

TABLE 1. Astrocyte-Derived Molecules and Associated Functions

| Structure | Function |
|---|---|
| Potassium channel | Extracellular buffering |
| Sodium channel | ? |
| Receptors to neuromediators | ? |
| Neuromediator carriers | ? |
| Major histocompatibility complex class II antigens | Antigen presentation |
| Interleukin 1 | Autocrin factor ? |
| Interleukin 3 | Paracrin factor |
| Complement 3 | ? |
| Factor B | ? |
| Neural cell adhesion molecule | Neuronal development |
| Laminin | ID |
| Fibronectin | ID |
| Cytotactin-J1 | ID |
| Matrix protein receptors | ID |
| Growth factors | ID |

Astrocytes are also able to capture glutamine.[9,10] It is likely that glutamine is transformed into glutamate and transported under that form into the neurons where it participates in the newly synthesized pool of neurotransmitters. The presence of several neuromediator receptors has been reported repeatedly. Among these can be quoted the amine, the amino acid, and the peptide receptors.[11-25] Their role has not been elucidated. They could intervene in the metabolic and trophic responses of the astrocytes to the neuronal release of neurotransmitters.[22,26]

In addition to receptors and carrier molecules the astrocytic membrane contains different ionophores. The sodium channel is activated in the presence of veratridine and therefore resembles its neuronal equivalent.[27,28] The potassium channel has been studied by several authors. Its function seems to be homeostatic in that it can remove the potassium accumulating in the synaptic cleft in the course of neuronal depolarization and repolarization.[29,30] In a series of experiments on the Müller cell in the retina, Newman has shown that potassium channels are exclusively located at the end feet of the cell.[31,32] In addition, he could demonstrate the existence of $CA^{++}$-activated, fast inactivating, and inward rectifying $K^+$ channels. This list of channels must be completed with the existence on the Müller cell of a $Ca^{++}$ channel.[33]

It can therefore be concluded that astrocytes express several "neuronal-specific" molecules. The main difference with the neurons resides in the density of these molecules and in the fact that the presence of synapses involving an astrocytic partner has so far not been demonstrated.

### *Astrocytes and Brain Immunity*

*Blood-Brain Barrier*

The BBB is the separation between the CNS and the blood compartments. This separation prevents cells and macromolecules from the two compartments from mingling. This phenomenon may contribute to the "immune-privileged" status of the CNS.

It is this property of the CNS that explains why immunosuppressive treatment is not absolutely necessary for the survival and development of embryonic neuron xenografts into adult brains. In fact, the BBB is not perfect and plenty of leakage seems to be allowed.[34] This leakage may explain why the "immune privilege" of the brain is far from being absolute.

The BBB is constituted by the formation of tight junctions between the endothelial cells of the brain vessels. Janzer and Raff[35] recently demonstrated that astrocytes induce the *in vitro* formation of tight functions by epithelial cells and proposed that it could also be the case *in vivo*.

If we may soon know how the BBB is built, the need for its existence remains obscure. It has been speculated by Fierz and Fontana[34] that this separation prevents the occurrence of tissue destruction by cytolytic processes. However, these authors proposed that when an immune reaction is necessary, the astrocytes could regulate the infiltration of T cells. Another nonexclusive explanation could be based on the fact that similar and even identical molecules (neuromediators, lymphokines, complement molecules, and matrix protein receptors) are used for different functions in the nervous and immune systems. In the absence of BBB a complete confusion of signals would be created. Therefore, the BBB allows two separate cellular systems of comparable complexity to communicate in two different languages by means of identical or closely related molecules.

*Secretion of Interleukins*

The presence of interleukins in the brain has been reported by several authors. Whereas the production and secretion of IL-3 by astrocytes are a well-accepted fact, the origin of IL-1 is still controversial. Fontana and collaborators and also other investigators have demonstrated the synthesis of IL-1 by the C6 glioma and by pure astrocyte primary cultures.[34,36] Giulian and Lachman[37] challenged this hypothesis and proposed that IL-1 synthesis in astrocyte cultures is due to contaminating microglial cells.

In fact, when the microglia is eliminated by L-leucine methyl ester treatment, IL-1 cannot be detected in the astrocyte cultures.[38] Moreover, purified microglial cells characterized by the presence of nonspecific esterase and Mac-1 antigen synthesize high amounts of IL-1 on lipopolysaccharide treatment.[39] Similar results were also obtained in our laboratory (Hetier *et al.,* unpublished results).

Another problem with IL-1 concerns its mode of secretion. Following genetic cloning of the molecule it appears that no signal peptide could possibly be coded by the sequences present in the 5' regions of the mRNA.[40,41] Therefore, how does IL-1 get across the membrane? It has been proposed that IL-1 leaks through cell membranes damaged during tissue injury and inflammation.[41]

This hypothesis is of interest to the neurobiologist, because bFGF, a neurotrophic and gliotrophic molecule, presents sequence homologies with IL-1 and also seems to be lacking a signal peptide.[42-44] The fact that in the CNS bFGF is synthesized by the neurons allows speculation that neuronal death, which occurs at high levels during normal CNS ontogeny, results in the release of bFGF and stimulates both astrocytic division and neuronal maturation.

The role of interleukins in the CNS appears to be the modulation of cell growth. Interleukin-1 stimulates astroglial divisions, IL-3 induces microglial proliferation, and IL-2 modulates the proliferation of oligodendrocytes and oligodendrocyte precursors.[34,45] Because IL-3 is synthesized by the astrocytes, it is possible that a strong positive cooperation exists between the microglial and astrocytic populations.[34,46] For example, it could be proposed that in injury or neuronal death, IL-1 would leak out from dying microglia and provide a mitotic signal to the astrocytes. Conversely, IL-3-secreting astrocytes would contribute to maintenance of the normal number of microglial cells.

*Antigen Presentation*

The problem of brain immunity is indeed linked to the presence not only of T cells but also of antigen-presenting cells (APC). Several possible APCs exist in the CNS: peripheral macrophages (in disruption of the BBB), microglial cells, and astrocytes. In fact, good evidence exists that astrocytes are also APCs.[34] Most convincing is the fact that a subpopulation of astrocytes expresses MHC II antigens (Ia in the mouse) and that this expression is stimulated in the presence of interferon (IFN) and murine hepatitis virus antigens.[47–51]

The ability of some astrocytes to act as APCs suggests that these cells may have an important function in autoimmune diseases, and particularly encephalomyelitis. In this disease astrocytes can present the myelin basic protein in an MHC II context.[52] In addition, Massa and collaborators have demonstrated that a strong correlation exists between the genetic fragility towards experimentally induced encephalomyelitis and astrocytic Ia inducibility.[52] Even more intriguing is that the increased IFN-induced Ia expression seen in sensitive strains is restricted to the astrocytic population and is not shared by the peritoneal macrophages.[53]

*Other Macrophage-Like Properties of the Astrocyte*

It is not in the scope of this short review to enumerate all the similarities between astrocytes and macrophages. In addition to Ia presentation, we would like to stress two points of interest. One is the capacity of the astrocytes to synthesize and release apolipoprotein E (ApoE). This property might be important during neuritogenesis (developmental or post-traumatic) because it is taken up by neuronal growth cones *in vitro* and *in vivo*.[54,55] In fact, the neuritogenic action of ApoE was first proposed by Shooter and his collaborators following studies on the regenerating sciatic nerve.[56] A possible role of ApoE is the recycling of the cholesterol necessary for the synthesis of neuronal membranes.

A second important point is the synthesis of the complement molecule C3. The role of C3 could indeed be classical, a possibility reinforced by the property of astrocytes to synthesize factor B.[57] In this case aggressive microorganisms might get coupled to iC3bH (one product of the cleavage of C3 by factor B) and phagocytosed by either astrocytes or microglial cells. However, it cannot be precluded that C3 serves more neurobiologic functions. In support of the latter point is that the C3 receptor (CR3) belongs to a super family of molecules among which several (particularly the receptor to laminin and fibronectin) are implicated in the mechanism of neuroastroglial adhesion.[58-61] Moreover, iC3b itself contains the Arg-Gly-Asp sequence present in fibronectin and necessary for its morphogenetic activity. In fact, the homologies between iC3b and fibronectin (and also vitronectin) extend to a segment of 50 residues surrounding the tripeptide.[62]

## ASTROCYTE HETEROGENEITY AND DEVELOPMENT

### *Lineage*

*Astrocyte Lineage*

Astrocytic heterogeneity has clearly been demonstrated in the optic nerve by immunostaining *in vitro*. Fibrous astrocytes (type 2) are decorated by a monoclonal antibody (A2B5) which recognizes a tetrasialoganglioside normally present on neurons only.[63] Velamentous astrocytes (type 1) do not carry the antigen. Interestingly enough the A2B5 epitope is also neuronal and is responsible for tetanus toxin binding. Therefore, type 2 astrocytes can also be recognized by their property to bind tetanus toxin.

Raff and collaborators[64,65] have demonstrated that astrocytes type 1 and 2 do not belong to the same lineage. In fact, it is well established that astrocyte type 2 and oligodendrocytes have a common progenitor. This progenitor replicates a limited number of time (supposedly under an astrocyte type 1-derived mitotic signal) and is then committed to establish itself as an astrocyte type 2 or an oligodendrocyte.

The optic nerve is not the only region of the CNS where astrocytes exhibit different morphologic and biochemical traits. In fact, the division between fibrous and velamentous can be extended to the entire CNS. However, a precise lineage study has only been achieved in the optic nerve, and the results obtained with this structure cannot yet be generalized to the rest of the brain. It could be that the fibrous astrocytes with their stellate shape derive from the radial glia.[66] If this is the case, what about the developmental status of the velate astrocyte? Does it belong to a separate lineage? Is it the *in vitro* equivalent of the *in vivo* radial astrocyte? Further lineage studies will be necessary to clarify these points.

From a functional point of view, radial glia appears responsible for the oriented migration of neurons leaving the germinative zone, whereas the stellate astrocytes are associated with postmigratory neurons. Good evidence of these separate functions has been demonstrated by the elegant *in vitro* experiments of Hatten *et al.*[67]

*Microglial Lineage*

The origin of the brain macrophage (ameboid and ramified microglia) is still a controversial issue.[68-73] Two hypotheses at least coexist. One is that brain macrophages are derived from astrocytic progenitors. In support of this hypothesis are the numerous similarities found between macrophages and astrocytes, as just described.

The second hypothesis is based on lineage studies using tracers such as carbon particles injected into the circulation and found in the brain macrophages.[74] It was demonstrated (in the rat) that no monocyte precursor could enter the brain before postnatal day 5. Although these lineage experiments are rather convincing, there is no doubt that the use of artificial and stable genetic markers should soon help to resolve this question.[75]

## Neurotrophic Functions of Astrocytes

### Diffusible Trophic Factors

The influence of astrocytes on the survival and biochemical maturation of neurons has been reported several times.[76-81] However, so far few astrocyte-derived diffusible neurotrophic molecules have been truly characterized. It seems that astrocytes can synthesize nerve growth factor (NGF) *in vitro*, but the physiologic role of this phenomenon is not clearly defined.[82,83] It might be a property restricted to astrocytes in culture or to reactive astrocytes that begin to divide following neuronal damage. However, it cannot be precluded that astrocytes from regions innervated by the terminals of NGF-sensitive cholinergic neurons synthesize the neurotrophic factor. It would constitute an interesting case of regional astrocytic specialization.[84-86]

Another astrocytic diffusible molecule is the S100 protein which has been shown by Kligman and Marshak[87] to act as a neurite-elongating factor. It is likely that several brain-derived factors recently purified are synthesized by astrocytes *in vivo* and *in vitro*.[88-91] However, this still awaits direct confirmation.

### Peripheral and Matrix Molecules

TABLE 1 lists the matrix molecules that are synthesized by developing astrocytes. Laminin and fibronectin are important for neuritic extension as demonstrated in several experiments *in vitro*.[92-100] Interestingly enough, although these molecules certainly participate in the induction of neurite elongation, the inhibition of neurite growth on astrocyte monolayers requires the presence not only of anti-matrix molecule antibodies but also of antibodies directed against the receptors to these molecules.[101-103]

These receptors belong to a superfamily of receptors that also includes the receptor to C3, the *Drosophila* position-specific antigens, and the very late lymphocytic antigens (VLA).[58-62] Each of these receptors is composed of a unique $\alpha$ subunit and a ubiquitous $\beta$ subunit. (The extent of the similarities between these $\beta$ subunits is not completely clarified yet.)

Cytotactin (also called J1) is another astroglial matrix glycoprotein involved in neuroastroglial adhesion and migration.[104-105] It seems to be endowed with a high degree of biochemical heterogeneity possibly generated by differential splicing and stage- and region-specific glycosylations.

*Adhesion Molecules*

The only true adhesion molecule known to be synthesized by astrocytes is N-CAM.[106] Several forms of N-CAM are present in the brain and are generated by differential splicing.[107] The astrocytes only synthesize the 120-kd isoform.[107] The isoform is attached to the membrane by a glycophospholipid anchor and can be released into the medium on treatment with phosphatidyl inositol-phospholipase C (PI-PLC). The function of astrocytic N-CAM might be to promote neuroastroglial attachment. After its release into the extracellular space, it could also participate in the formation of extracellular adherons.[108,109]

*Regional Heterogeneity of the Astrocytes*

Recent experiments have led to speculation on a segmental organization of the vertebrate nervous system.[110-113] It is conceivable that astroglial cells from different segments can be distinguished on a physiologic and biochemical basis.

A way to test this hypothesis is to look for some regional specificity of the neuroastroglial interactions during development. In our laboratory we compared the morphologic traits of mesencephalic and striatal neurons cultured for 2 days with mesencephalic and striatal astrocytes in the four possible combinations. The neuronal polarity (dendrite growth) established itself faster in homotopic (neurons and astrocytes from the same region) than in heterotopic neuroastroglial co-cultures.[114,115]

We then began to characterize the surface molecules synthesized by mesencephalic and striatal astrocytes, which led us to demonstrate a very important degree of heterogeneity between forebrain and midbrain astrocytes. In particular, mesencephalic and cerebellar astrocytes synthesize a 190-kd fucosylated glycoprotein that is not present in the striatum and is only slightly expressed in the cortex.[116] Experiments are underway to examine the possible role of gp190 in region-specific neuroastroglial interactions.

## REFERENCES

1. BIGNAMI, A., L. F. ENG, D. DAHL & C. T. UYEDO. 1972. Localization of the glial fibrillary acidic protein in astrocytes in immunofluorescence. Brain Res. **43**: 429-435.
2. ABBOT, N. J. 1985. Are glial cells excitable after all? TINS **8**: 141-142.
3. CURRIE, D. N. & G. R. DUTTON. 1970. $^3$H-GABA uptake as a marker for cell type in primary cultures of cerebellum and olfactory bulb. Brain Res. **199**: 473-481.
4. SCHOUSBOE, A., G. SVENNEBY & L. HERTZ. 1977. Uptake and metabolism of glutamate in astrocytes cultured from dissociated mouse brain hemispheres. J. Neurochem. **29**: 999-1005.
5. CURRIE, D. N. & J. S. KELLY. 1981. Glial versus neuronal uptake of glutamate. J. Exp. Biol. **95**: 181-193.
6. KIMELBERG, H. K. & E. W. PELTON, II. 1983. High-affinity uptake of ($^3$H)norepinephrin by primary astrocyte cultures and its inhibition by tricyclic antidepressant. J. Neurochem. **40**: 1265-1270.
7. WILKIN, G. P., G. LEVI, S. R. JOHNSTONE & P. N. RIDDLE. 1983. Cerebellar astroglial cells in primary culture. Expression of different morphological appearances and different ability to take up $^3$H-D-aspartate and $^3$H-GABA. Dev. Brain Res. **10**: 265-277.

8. KATZ, D. M. & H. K. KIMELBERG. 1985. Kinetics and autoradiography of high affinity uptake of serotonin by primary astrocyte cultures. J. Neurosci. **5:** 1901-1908.
9. RAMAHAROBANDRO, N., J. BORG, P. MANDEL & J. MARK. 1982. Glutamine and glutamate transport in cultured neuronal and glial cells. Brain Res. **244:** 113-121.
10. LINSER, P. & A. A. MOSCONA. 1983. Hormonal induction of glutamine synthetase in cultures of embryonic retina cells: Requirement for neuron-glia contact interactions. Dev. Biol. **96:** 529-534.
11. HÖSLI, L., P. F. ANDRES & E. HÖSLI. 1979. Depolarization of cultured astrocytes by glutamate and aspartate. Neuroscience **4:** 1593-1598.
12. EBERSOLT, C., M. PEREZ & J. BOCKAERT. 1981. Neuronal, glial and meningeal localization of neurotransmitter-sensitive adenylate cyclase in cerebral cortex of mice. Brain Res. **213:** 139-150.
13. TARDY, M., M. F. COSTA, B. ROLLAND, C. FAGES & P. GONNARD. 1981. Benzodiazepine receptors on primary cultures of mouse astrocytes. J. Neurochem. **36:** 1587-1589.
14. REPKE, H. & K. MADERSPACH. 1982. Muscarinic acetylcholine receptors on cultured glial cells. Brain Res. **232:** 206-211.
15. MAGISTRETTI, P. J., M. MANTHORPE, F. E. BLOOM & S. VARON. 1983. Functional receptors for vasoactive intestinal polypeptide in cultured astroglia from neonatal rat brain. Regulatory Peptide **6:** 71-80.
16. KETTENMANN, H., K. H. BACKUS & M. SCHACHNER. 1984. Aspartate, glutamate and GABA depolarize cultured astrocytes. Neurosci. Lett. **52:** 25-29.
17. TRIMMER, P. A., T. EVANS, M. M. SMITH, T. K. HARDEN & K. D. MCCARTHY. 1984. Combination of immunocytochemistry and radioligand receptor assay to identify adrenergic receptor subtypes on astroglia in vitro. J. Neurosci. **4:** 1598-1606.
18. BUNN, S. J., M. R. HANLEY & G. WILKIN. 1985. Evidence for a kappa-opioid receptor on pituitary astrocytes: An autoradiographic study. Neurosci. Lett. **55:** 317-323.
19. CHNEIWEISS, H., J. GLOWINSKI & J. PREMONT. 1985. Modulation by monoamines of somatostatin-sensitive adenylate cyclase on neuronal and glial cells from the mouse brain in primary cultures. J. Neurochem. **44:** 1825-1831.
20. BAKER, S. P., C. SUMMERS, J. PITHA & M. K. RAIZADA. 1986. Characteristics of the $\beta$-adrenoreceptor from neuronal and glial cells in primary cultures of the rat brain. J. Neurochem. **47:** 1318-1326.
21. TORRENS, Y., J. C. BEAUJOUAN, M. SAFFROY, M. C. DAGUET DE MONTETY, L. BERGSTROM & J. GLOWINSKI. 1986. Substance P receptors in primary cultures of cortical astrocytes from the mouse. Proc. Natl. Acad. Sci. USA **83:** 9216-9220.
22. WHITAKER-AZMITIA, P. M. & E. C. AZMITIA. 1986. ($^3$H)-hydroxy-tryptamine binding to brain astroglial cells: Differences between intact and homogenized preparations and mature and immature cultures. J. Neurochem. **46:** 1186-1189.
23. BRIDGES, R. J., J. P. KESSLAK, M. NIETO-SAMPEDRO, J. T. BRODERCK, J. YU & C. W. COTMAN. 1987. A L-($^3$H)glutamate binding site on glia: An autoradiographic study on implanted astrocytes. Brain Res. **415:** 163-168.
24. HAN, V. K. M., J. M. LAUDER & A. J. D'ERCOLE. 1987. Characterization of somatomedine/Insuline-like growth factor receptors and correlation with biologic action in cultured neonatal rat astroglial cells. J. Neurosci. **7:** 501-511.
25. RAIZADA, M. K., M. I. PHILLIPS, F. T. CREWS & C. SUMNERS. 1987. Distinct angiotensin II receptor in primary cultures of glial cells from rat brain. Proc. Natl. Acad. Sci. USA **84:** 4655-4659.
26. BRENNEMAN, D. E., E. A. NEALE, B. A. FOSTER, S. W. D'AUTREMONT & G. L. WESTBROOK. 1987. Non neuronal cells mediate neurotrophic action of vasoactive intestinal peptide. J. Cell Biol. **104:** 1603-1610.
27. BOWMAN, C. L., H. K. KIMELBERG, M. V. FRANGAKIS, Y. BERWALD-NETTER & C. EDWARDS. 1984. Astrocytes in primary culture have chemically activated sodium channels. J. Neurosci. **4:** 1527-1534.
28. NOWAK, L., P. ASCHER & Y. BERWALD-NETTER. 1987. Ionic channels in mouse astrocytes in culture. J. Neurosci. **7:** 101-109.
29. PENTREATH, V. W. & M. A. KAI-KAI. 1982. Significance of the potassium signal from neurons to glial cells. Nature **295:** 58-61.

30. WALZ, W., W. WUTTKE & L. HERTZ. 1984. Astrocytes in primary cultures: Membrane potential characteristics reveal exclusive potassium conductance and potassium accumulator properties. Brain Res. **292:** 367-374.
31. NEWMAN, E. A. 1984. Regional specialization of retinal glial membrane. Nature **309:** 155-157.
32. NEWMAN, E. A., D. A. FRAMBACH & L. L. ODETTE. 1984. Control of extracellular potassium levels by retinal glial cell $K^+$ siphoning. Science **225:** 1174-1175.
33. NEWMAN, E. A. 1985. Voltage-dependent calcium and potassium channels in retinal glial cells. Nature **317:** 809-811.
34. FIERZ, W. & A. FONTANA. 1986. The role of astrocytes in the interaction between the immune and nervous system. In Astrocytes, Vol. 3. F. Fedoroff & A. Vernadakis, Eds.: 203-229. Academic Press. New York.
35. JANZER, R. C. & M. C. RAFF. 1987. Astrocytes induce blood-brain barrier properties in endothelial cells. Nature **325:** 253-255.
36. NIETO-SAMPEDRO, M. & M. A. BERMAN. 1987. Interleukin-1-like activity in rat brain: Sources, targets, and effect of injury. J. Neurosci. Res. **17:** 214-219.
37. GIULIAN, D. & L. B. LACHMAN. 1985. Interleukin-1 stimulation of astroglial proliferation after brain injury. Science **228:** 497-498.
38. GIULIAN, D., T. J. BAKER, L.-C. N. SHI & L. B. LACHMAN. 1986. Interleukin-1 of the central nervous system is produced by ameboid microglia. J. Exp. Med. **164:** 594-604.
39. GIULIAN, D. & T. J. BAKER. 1986. Characterization of ameboid microglia isolated from developing mammalian brain. J. Neurosci. **6:** 2163-2178.
40. AURON, P. E., A. C. WEBB, L. J. ROSEBWASSER, S. F. MUCCI, A. RICH, S. M. WOLFF & C. A. DINARELLO. 1984. Nucleotide sequence of human monocyte interleukin-1 precursor cDNA. Proc. Natl. Acad. Sci. **81:** 7907-7911.
41. LOMEDICO, P. T., U. GUBLER, C. P. HELLMANN, P. DUKOVICH, J. G. GIRI, Y.-C. E. PAN, C. COLLIER, R. SEMIONOW, A. O. CHUA & S. B. MIZEL. 1984. Cloning and expression of murine interleukine-1 cDNA in *Escherichia coli.* Nature **312:** 458-462.
42. GIMENEZ-GALLEGO, G., J. RODKEY, C. BENNETT, M. RIOS-CANDELORE, J. DISALVO & K. THOMAS. 1985. Brain-derived acidic fibroblast growth factor: Complete aminoacid sequence and homologies. Science **230:** 1385-1388.
43. MORRISON, R. S., A. SHARMA, J. DE VELLIS & R. A. BRADSHAW. 1986. Basic fibroblast growth factor supports the survival of cerebral cortical neurons in primary culture. Proc. Natl. Acad. Sci. USA **83:** 7537-7541.
44. WALICKE, P., W. M. COWAN, N. VENO, A. BAIRD & R. GUILLEMIN. 1986. Fibroblast growth factor promotes survival of dissociated hippocampal neurons and enhances neurite extension. Proc. Natl. Acad. Sci. USA **83:** 3012-3016.
45. SANETO, R. P., A. ALTMAN, R. L. KNOBLER, H. M. JOHNSON & J. DE VELLIS. 1986. Interleukin 2 mediates the inhibition of oligodendrocyte progenitor cell proliferation in vitro. Proc. Natl. Acad. Sci. USA **83:** 9221-9225.
46. FREI, K., S. BODMER, C. SCHWERDEL & A. FONTANA. 1986. Astrocyte-derived interleukin 3 as a growth factor for microglial cells and peritoneal macrophages. J. Immunol. **137:** 3521-3527.
47. HIRSCH, M.-R., J. WIETZERBIN, M. PIERRES & C. GORIDIS. 1983. Expression of Ia antigens by cultured astrocytes treated with interferon. Neurosci. Lett **41:** 199-204.
48. WONG, G. H. W., P. F. BARTLETT, I. CLARK-LEWIS, F. BATTYE & J. W. SCHRADER. 1984. Inducible expression of H-2 and Ia antigens on brain cells. Nature **310:** 688-691.
49. MASSA, P. T., R. DÖRRIES & V. TER MEULEN. 1986. Viral particles induce Ia antigen expression on astrocytes. Nature **320:** 543-546.
50. TEDESCHI, B., J. N. BARRETT & R. W. KEANE. 1986. Astrocytes produce interferon that enhances the expression of H-2 antigens on a subpopulation of brain cells. J. Cell Biol. **102:** 2244-2253.
51. MASSA, P. T. & V. TER MEULEN. 1987. Analysis of Ia induction on Lewis rat astrocytes in vitro by virus particles and bacterial adjuvants. J. Neuroimmunol. **13:** 259-271.
52. SUN, D. & H. WEKERLE. 1986. Ia-restricted encephalitogenic T lymphocytes mediating EAE lyse autoantigen-presenting astrocytes. Nature **320:** 70-72.
53. MASSA, P. T., V. TER MEULEN & A. FONTANA. 1987. Hyperinducibility of Ia antigen

on astrocytes correlates with strain-specific susceptibility to experimental autimmune encephalomyelitis. Proc. Natl. Acad. Sci. USA **84:** 4219-4223.
54. STOLL, G. & H. W. MULLER, 1986. Macrophages in the peripheral nervous system and astroglia in the central nervous system of rat commonly express apolipoprotein E during development but differ in their response to injury. Neurosci. Lett. **72:** 233-238.
55. IGNATIUS, M. J., E. M. SHOOTER, R. E. PITAS & R. W. MAHLEY. 1987. Lipoprotein uptake by mouse brain astrocytes and its modulation by interferon. Brain Res. **410:** 45-51.
56. MULLER, H. W., P. J. GEBICKE, D. H. HANGEN & E. M. SHOOTER. 1985. A specific 37,000-dalton protein that accumulates in regenerating but not in non regenerating mammalian nerves. Science **228:** 499-501.
57. LEVI-STRAUSS, M. & M. MALLAT. 1987. Primary cultures of murine astrocytes produce C3 and factor B, two components of the alternative pathway of complement activation. J. Immunol. **139:** 2361-2366.
58. LAW, S. K., J. GAGNON, J. E. K. HILDRETH, C. E. WELLS, A. C. WILLIS & A. J. WONG. 1987. The primary structure of the $\beta$-subunit of the cell structure adhesion glycoprotein LFA-1, CR3 and P150,95 and its relationship to the fibronectin receptor. EMBO. J. **6:** 915-919.
59. LEPTIN, M. P., AEBERSOLD, R. & M. WILCOX. 1987. Drosophila position-specific antigens resemble the vertebrate fibronectin-receptor family. EMBO. J. **6:** 1037-1043.
60. TAKADA, Y., C. HUANG & M. E. HEMLER. 1987. Fibronectin receptor structures in the VLA family of heterodimers. Nature **326:** 607-609.
61. TAKADA, Y., J. L. STROMINGER & M. E. HEMLER. 1987. The very late antigen family of heterodimers is part of a superfamily of molecules in adhesion and embryogenesis. Proc. Natl. Acad. Sci. USA **84:** 1965-1968.
62. WRIGHT, S. D., P. A. REDDY, M. T. C. JONG & B. W. ERICKSON. 1987. C3bi receptor (complement receptor type 3) recognizes a region of complement protein C3 containing the sequence Arg-Gly-Asp. Proc. Natl. Acad. Sci. USA **84:** 1965-1968.
63. ABNEY, E. R., B. P. WILLIAMS & M. C. RAFF. 1983. Tracing the development of oligodendrocytes from precursor cells using monoclonal antibodies fluorescence-activated cell sorting and cell culture. Dev. Biol. **100:** 166-171.
64. RAFF, M. C., R. H. MILLER & M. NOBLE. 1983. A glial progenitor cell that develops in vitro into an astrocyte or an oligodendrocyte depending on culture medium. Nature **303:** 390-396.
65. FFRENCH-CONSTANT, C. & M. C. RAFF. 1986. The oligodendrocyte-type-2 astrocyte cell lineage is specialised for myelination. Nature **323:** 335-338.
66. LEVITT, P. & P. RAKIC. 1980. Immunoperoxydase localization of glial fibrillary acidic protein in radial glial cells and astrocytes of the developing rhesus monkey brain. J. Comp. Neurol. **193:** 815-840.
67. HATTEN, M. E., R. K. LIEM & C. A. MASON. 1984. Two forms of cerebellar glial cells interact differently in vitro. J. Cell Biol. **98:** 193-204.
68. MURABE, Y., Y. IBATA & Y. SANO. 1982. Morphological studies on neuroglia. IV. Proliferative response of non-neuronal elements in the hippocampus of the rat to kainic acid-induced lesions. Cell Tissue Res. **222:** 223-226.
69. PERRY, V. H., D. A. HUME & S. GORDON. 1985. Immunocytochemical localization of macrophages and microglia in the adult and developing mouse brain. Neuroscience **15:** 313-326.
70. VAUGHN, J. E., P. L. HINDS & R. P. SKAFF. 1970. Electron microscopic studies of Wallerian degeneration in the rat optic nerve. I. The multi-potential glia. J. Comp. Neurol. **140:** 175-206.
71. KITAMURA, T., T. MIYAKE & S. FUJITA. 1984. Genesis of resting microglia in the gray matter of mouse hippocampus. J. Comp. Neurol. **226:** 421-433.
72. KUSAKA, H., A. HIRANO, M. B. BORNSTEIN, G. R. W. MOORE & C. S. RAINE. 1986. Transformation of cells of astrocyte lineage into macrophage-like cells in organotypic cultures of mouse spinal cord tissue. J. Neurol. Sci. **72:** 77-89.
73. SMINIA, T., J. A. DE GROOT, C. D. DIJKSTRA, J. C. KOETSIER & C. H. POLMAN. 1987. Macrophages in the central nervous system of the rat. Immunobiology **174:** 43-50.

74. LING, E. A., D. PENNEY & C. P. LEBLOND. 1980. Use of carbon labeling to demonstrate the role of blood monocytes as precursors of the ameboid cells present in the corpus callosum of postnatal rat. J. Comp. Neurol. **193**: 631-657.
75. TURNER, D. L. & C. L. CEPKO. 1987. A common progenitor for neurons and glia persists in rat retina late in development. Nature **328**: 131-136.
76. BANKER, G. A. 1980. Trophic interactions between astroglial cells and hippocampal neurons in culture. Science **209**: 809-810.
77. FOUCAUD, B., R. REEB., M. SENSENBRENNER & G. COMBOS. 1982. Kinetics and morphological analysis of the preferential adhesion of chick embryo neuronal cells to astroglial cells in culture. Exp. Cell Res. **137**: 285-294.
78. RAKIC, P., 1982. The role of neuronal glia interaction during brain development. Life Sci. Res. Rep. **20**: 25-38.
79. NOBLE, M., J. FOK-SEANG & J. COHEN. 1984. Glia are a unique substrate for the in vitro growth of central nervous system neurons. J. Neurosci. **4**: 1892-1903.
80. FALLON, J. R. 1985. Preferential outgrowth of central nervous system neurites on astrocytes and schwann cells as compared to non glial cells in vitro. J. Cell Biol. **100**: 198-207.
81. MALLAT, M., V. MOURA NETO, F. GROS, J. GLOWINSKI & A. PROCHIANTZ. 1986. Two simian virus 40 (SV40)-transformed cell lines from the mouse striatum and mesencephalon presenting astrocytic characters. II. Interactions with mesencephalic neurons. Dev. Brain Res. **26**: 23-31.
82. LINDSAY, R. M. 1979. Adult rat brain astrocytes support survival of both NGF-dependent and NGF-insensitive neurons. Nature **282**: 80-82.
83. LINDSAY, R. M., P. C. BARBER, M. R. C. SHERWOOD, J. ZIMMER & G. RAISMAN. 1982. Astrocyte cultures from adult rat brain. Characterization and neurotrophic properties of pure astroglial cells for corpus callosum. Brain Res. **243**: 329-343.
84. KORSHING, S., G. AUBURGER, R. HEUMANN, J. SCOTT & H. THOENEN. 1985. Levels of nerve growth factor and its mRNA in the central nervous system of the rat correlate with cholinergic innervation. EMBO. J. **4**: 1389-1393.
85. SHELTON, D. L. & L. F. REICHARDT. 1986. Studies on the expression of the $\beta$ nerve growth factor (NGF) gene in the central nervous system: Level and regional distribution of NGF mRNA suggest that NGF functions as a trophic factor for several distinct populations of neurons. Proc. Natl. Acad. Sci. USA **83**: 2714-2718.
86. WITHMORE, S. R., T. EBENDAL, L. LÄRKFORS, L. OLSON, A. SEIGER, I. STRÖMBERG & H. PERSSON. 1986. Developmental and regional expression of $\beta$ nerve growth factor in the rat central nervous system. Proc. Natl. Acad. Sci. USA **83**: 817-821.
87. KLIGMAN, D. & D. R. MARSHAK. 1985. Purification and characterization of a neurite extension factor from bovine brain. Proc. Natl. Acad. Sci. USA **82**: 7136-7139.
88. BARDE, Y.-A., D. EDGAR & H. THOENEN. 1982. Purification of a new neurotrophic factor from mammalian brain. EMBO J. **1**: 549-553.
89. GUENTER, J., H. NICK & D. MONARD. 1985. A glia-derived neurite-promoting factor with protease inhibitory activity. EMBO. J. **4**: 1963-1966.
90. PATTERSON, P. H. 1985. On the role of proteases, their inhibitors and the extracellular matrix in promoting neurite outgrowth. J. Physiol. (Paris) **80**: 207-211.
91. GLOOR, S., K. ODINK, J. GUENTER, H. NICK & D. MONARD. 1986. A glia-derived neurite promoting factor with protease inhibitory activity belongs to the protease nexins. Cell **47**: 687-693.
92. AKERS, R. M., D. F. MOSHER & J. E. LILIEN. 1981. Promotion of retinal neurite outgrowth by substratum-bound fibronectin. Dev. Biol. **86**: 179-188.
93. LIESI, P., D. DAHLAND & A. VAHERI. 1983. Laminin is produced by early rat astrocytes in primary culture. J. Cell Biol. **96**: 920-924.
94. MANTHORPE, M., E. ENGVALL, E. RUOSLATTI, F. M. LONGO, G. E. DAVIS & S. VARON. 1983. Laminin promotes neuritic regeneration from cultured peripheral and central neurons. J. Cell Biol. **97**: 1882-1890.
95. ROGERS, S. L., P. C. LETOURNEAU, S. L. PALM, J. MCCARTHY & L. T. FURCHT. 1983. Neurite extension by peripheral and central nervous system neurons in response to substratum-bound fibronectin and laminin. Dev. Biol. **98**: 212-220.

96. EDGAR, D., R. TIMPLE & H. THOENEN. 1984. The heparin-binding domain of laminin is responsible for its effect on neurite outgrowth and neuronal survival. EMBO. J. **3**: 1463-1468.
97. LIESI, P., S. KAAKKOLA, D. DAHL & A. VAHERI. 1984. Laminin is induced in astrocytes of adult brain by injury. EMBO. J. **3**: 683-686.
98. SMALHEISER, N. R., S. M. CRAIN & L. M. REID. 1984. Laminin as a substrate for retinal axons in vitro. Dev. Brain Res. **12**: 136-140.
99. LANDER, A. D., D. K. FUJII & L. F. REICHARDT. 1985. Laminin is associated with the "neurite outgrowth promoting factor" found in conditioned media. Proc. Natl. Acad. Sci. USA **82**: 2183-2187.
100. PRICE, J. & R. O. HYNES. 1985. Astrocytes in culture synthesize and secrete a variant form of fibronectin. J. Neurosci. **5**: 2205-2211.
101. BOZYCZKO, D. & A. F. HORWITZ. 1986. The participation of a putative cell surface receptor for laminin and fibronectin in peripheral neurite extension. J. Neurosci. **6**: 1241-1251.
102. BIXBY, J. L., R. S. PRATT, J. LILIEN & L. F. REICHARDT. 1987. Neurite outgrowth on muscle cell surfaces involves extracellular matrix receptors as well as $Ca^{++}$-dependent and -independent cell adhesion molecules. Proc. Natl. Acad. Sci. USA **84**: 2555-2559.
103. HALL, D. E., K. M. NEUGEBAUER & L. F. REICHARDT. 1987. Embryonic neural retina cell response to extracellular matrix proteins: Developmental changes and effects of the cell substratum attachment antibody (CSAT). J. Cell Biol. **104**: 623-634.
104. GRUMET, M., S. HOFFMANN, L. L. CROSSIN & G. E. EDELMAN. 1985. Cytotactin, an extracellular matrix protein of neural and non-neural tissues that mediates glia-neuron interaction. Proc. Natl. Acad. Sci. USA **82**: 8075-8079.
105. KRUSE, J., G. KEILHAUER, A. FAISSNER, R. TIMPL & M. SCHACHNER. 1985. The J1 glycoprotein—a novel nervous system cell adhesion molecule of the L2/HNK-1 family. Nature **316**: 146-148.
106. NOBLE, M., M. ALBRECHTSEN, C. MOLLER, J. LYLES, E. BOCK, C. GORIDIS, M. WATANABE & U. RUTISHAUSER. 1985. Glial cells express N-CAM D2-CAM-like polypeptides in vitro. Nature **316**: 725-728.
107. GENNARINI, G., M.-R. HIRSCH, H.-T. HE, M. HIRN, J. FINNE & C. GORIDIS. 1986. Differential expression of mouse neural cell-adhesion molecule (N-CAM) mRNA species during brain development and in neural cell lines. J. Neurosci. **6**: 1983-1990.
108. HE, H.-T., J. BARBET, J.-C. CHAIX & C. GORIDIS. 1986. Phosphatidylinositol is involved in the membrane attachment of NCAM-120, the smallest component of the neural cell adhesion molecule. EMBO J. **5**: 2489-2494.
109. HE, H.-T., J. FINNE & C. GORIDIS. In press. Biosynthesis, membrane-association and release of NCAM-120, a phosphatidylinositol-linked form of the neural cell adhesion molecule. J. Cell. Biol.
110. GEHRING, W. J. 1987. Homeo boxes in the study of development. Science **236**: 1245-1252.
111. MORI, K., S. C. FUJITA, Y. WATANABE, K. OBATA & O. HAYAISHI. 1987. Telencephalon-antigen identified by monoclonal antibody. Proc. Natl. Acad. Sci. USA **84**: 3921-3925.
112. SHEARD, P. & M. JACOBSON. 1987. Clonal restriction boundaries in xenopus embryos demonstrated with two intracellular lineage tracers. Science **236**: 851-854.
113. TAGUCHI, T., M. HUCHET, M. ROA, J.-P. CHANGEUX & C. E. HENDERSON. In press. A sub-population of embryonic telencephalic neurons survive and develop in vitro in response to factors derived from the periphery. Dev. Brain Res. **465**: 125-132.
114. DENIS-DONINI, S., J. GLOWINSKI & A. PROCHIANTZ. 1984. Glial heterogeneity may define the three-dimensional shape of mouse mesencephalic dopaminergic neurons. Nature **307**: 641-643.
115. CHAMAK, B., A. FELLOWS, J. GLOWINSKI & A. PROCHIANTZ. 1987. MAP2 expression and neurite outgrowth and branching are co-regulated through region-specific neuro-astroglial interactions. J. Neurosci. **7**: 3163-3170.
116. BARBIN, G., D. M. KATZ, B. CHAMAK, J. GLOWINSKI & A. PROCHIANTZ. 1988. Brain astrocytes express region-specific surface glycoproteins in culture. Glia **1**: 96-103.

# Relevance for Neurobiology and Neurooncology of Antigens of Malignant Gliomas As Defined by Monoclonal Antibodies[a]

FOTIOS D. VRIONIS,[b] CAROL J. WIKSTRAND,[b] AND
DARELL D. BIGNER [b,c]

[b] *Department of Pathology, and the*
[c] *Preuss Laboratory for Brain Tumor Research*
*Duke University Medical Center*
*Durham, North Carolina*

Glioblastoma multiforme (GBM) is the most common primary brain tumor, accounting for 15 to 20% of all intracranial neoplasms in adults.[1] Brain tumors are only second to leukemia as the most frequent form of cancer in childhood. Approximately 11,000 to 15,000 new brain tumor cases per annum are predicted in the United States, making malignant brain tumors more common than Hodgkin's disease.[1] Despite significant progress in the treatment of some types of cancer, there currently is no truly effective therapy for human GBM. Even with the best multimodality treatment, that is, surgical resection, external radiation, and BCNU chemotherapy, the prognosis for patients with malignant glioma remains extremely poor, with a median survival of less than a year.[2]

In gliomas, tumor heterogeneity at several levels is one of the most important determinants of resistance to treatment.[3] Cellular heterogeneity has traditionally being considered to consist of two aspects: genotypic and phenotypic heterogeneity. Genotypically, individual malignant gliomas are composed of multiple, related subpopulations of cells that differ in modal chromosome number and DNA content but retain a common set of numerical deviations and structural rearrangements.[4] This pattern suggests that the tumors have undergone clonal evolution in a genotypic sense,[5] but there is no evidence that gliomas initiate other than as uniclonal neoplasms. To date, a consistent chromosomal rearrangement or karyotypic pattern such as those found in chronic myelogenous leukemia or Burkitt's lymphoma has not been detected in gliomas, although a few chromosomal deviations occur more frequently than expected by chance and have been associated with oncogene(s) activation (i.e., gains of chromosome number 7, losses of chromosome number 10, and the presence of double minute chromosomes).[6] Phenotypically, both within and between cell lines, cultured glioma cells differ in antigen expression, growth properties, response to chemotherapy, and tumorigenicity in nude mice.[3,7,8] Heterogeneity of gliomas has two important implications with regard to immunotherapy. First, antigens uniformly expressed on

---

[a]This work was supported by NIH Grants RO1-CA 42324, RO1-CA 43638, RO1-CA 11898, NIH-CA 32672, and NS-20023.

all cells of any individual glioma or among different gliomas from different individuals are unlikely to exist. Second, the concept of heterogeneity suggests that for any given antigen a null cell exists. Therefore, monoclonal antibody cocktails to different antigens may be more preferable than single ones. Furthermore, Mabs may be labeled with a particle and gamma ray emitting radioisotope (such as $^{131}$I), so that both antigen-positive cells and any neighboring antigen-negative tumor cells can be killed, at least within the effective cell kill radius of the radiolabeled antibody.[9]

The existence of the blood-brain barrier (BBB) is also of crucial importance in immunotherapy and drug delivery in intracerebral tumors. Although spontaneous BBB disruption has been demonstrated in glioblastomas, there is considerable variability in BBB permeability within different areas of the same tumor.[10] Regional variations in BBB permeability may be circumvented by temporary, reversible hyperosmotic BBB disruption in normal brain.[11] Studies in rats showed increased antibody delivery to normal brain after hyperosmotic BBB disruption, but whether such BBB disruption can increase antibody localization to brain tumors rather than merely increase antibody levels in normal brain is still moot.[12]

## GLIOMA-ASSOCIATED ANTIGEN DETECTION WITH MONOCLONAL ANTIBODIES VERSUS POLYCLONAL ANTISERA

Earlier studies with polyclonal antisera demonstrated that the autologous and allogenic response to gliomas could be separated into three major categories: (1) response to glioma-restricted antigens; (2) response to idiotypic tumor antigens; and (3) response to antigens expressed by neuroectodermal tumors and fetal brain.[1] None of the extensively absorbed heteroantisera was specific enough to allow the identification of a well-defined tumor-associated antigen. Batch-to-batch variation, limitations in producing large amounts of antiserum, cross-reactivity with normal brain and other organs, interspecies reactivity, and the need for extensive absorption to achieve specificity with consequently very low antibody titers compromised the use of polyclonal antisera in studies of brain tumors.[1] The hybridoma technology, introduced by Köhler and Milstein[13] in 1975, revolutionized the serologic and biochemical analysis of human cancer by reducing the problems of specificity, reproducibility, and limited supply encountered with heterologous antisera. The exquisite specificity of Mab technology has, nevertheless, created new problems in that epitopes recognized by Mabs may be present on more than one molecular species, such as the shared epitopes reported among the intermediate filament proteins of nervous system cells, that is, neurofilament protein, glial fibrillary acidic protein (GFAP), and vimentin.[14] It is essential for basic research applications in neurobiology, for diagnosis, and especially for therapy, that molecular monospecificity of Mabs be documented, especially with protein, carbohydrate, and glycolipid antigens.[14]

## HUMAN GLIOMA-ASSOCIATED ANTIGENS DEFINED BY MONOCLONAL ANTIBODIES

### *Normal CNS-Associated Antigens*

Most normal brain-associated antigens were characterized by means of heterologous sera and were found to be intracellular in location. Examples of such well-characterized markers are: GFAP for astrocytes, 14-3-2 or neuron-specific enolase for neurons, and galactocerebroside for oligodendrocytes.[1] Many antigens or "markers" of normal cell types become more broadly expressed in neoplasia, and their value as "markers" of differentiation and diagnostic reagents is decreased.[15,16]

Three specific anti-GFAP Mabs reacting with an interspecies determinant on GFAP were used as a monoclonal "cocktail" in the diagnostic evaluation of formalin-fixed, paraffin-embedded surgical brain biopsy specimen.[17] This "cocktail" preparation was shown to be equally sensitive in detecting GFAP as the reference polyvalent anti-GFAP antiserum and superior with regard to specificity, continuous supply, and defined titer.[17] Similarly, monospecific antibodies against NFP protein have been useful in diagnosing neuronal tumors, and determining neuronal differentiation of medulloblastoma cells.[18-20]

*Extracellular Matrix Antigens*

The extracellular matrix (ECM) plays an important role in cell adhesion, motility, migration, and differentiation of both normal and neoplastic cell.[21] Its importance in the biology of gliomas became more apparent with the discovery of the glioma-mesenchymal extracellular matrix antigen (GMEM), a human ECM protein specifically recognized by Mab 81C6 which was derived following immunization with the GFAP-positive glioma cell line U-251 MG.[22] The same antigen in other species (i.e., chicken, rat, and mouse) was simultaneously or later identified by other groups and was assigned several names: myotendinous antigen,[23] hexabrachion,[24] cytotactin,[25] and tenascin[26] (the latter to be used in the rest of this review). Immunochemically these proteins have identical cross-reactivities.[27]

Tenascin is a high molecular weight macromolecule composed of 250 kd disulfide-bonded glycoprotein subunits[28] and appearing as a six-armed structure under electron microscopy.[24] It is predominantly expressed around the newly formed blood vessels in gliomas, which suggests a role in tumor angiogenesis.[22,29] Moreover, the tenascin epitope detected by Mab 81C6 is not restricted to tumors of neuroectodermal origin and is present in normal adult liver and kidney but not in human adult brain.[22] Similarly, in rats it is expressed in the fetal but not the adult mammary gland, and it reappears in chemically induced mammary tumors.[26] Studies in chicken embryos show a changing pattern of tenascin expression during neural development and suggest a role for tenascin similar to the one for fibronectin in neuronal crest cell migration.[30] Finally, a role of tenascin in limb morphogenesis has been postulated.[23] These observations demonstrate that a glioma-associated antigen, as originally identified by a Mab, can also be a molecule of particular importance in developmental neurobiology and in normal tissue differentiation and morphogenesis.

The 81C6 Mab is the most well-studied Mab for antibody localization and therapy in gliomas. Initial paired label studies showed specific localization of radiolabeled 81C6 in subcutaneous and intracranial human glioma xenografts as indicated by localization indices of up to 15 and persistence up to 7 days after administration.[31] Xenografts in both subcutaneous and intracranial sites were readily radioimaged. Imaging of intracranial xenografts was successful with tumor sizes as small as 20 mg, whereas control radiolabeled Mab localized nonspecifically only in tumors greater in size than 300 mg.[32]

Furthermore, the therapeutic efficacy of radiolabeled 81C6 was assessed in both subcutaneous and intracranial human glioma tumors transplanted into immunocompromised animals. The estimated dose delivered to subcutaneous mouse D54 MG human glioma xenografts was 9,719 rads for 1 mCi/100 μg of $^{131}$I-81C6 administered, and 1,585 rads from a dose of 1.25 mCi/100 μg of $^{131}$I-81C6 administered to rats with intracranial xenografts. In both animal models significant growth delay, increased survival, or tumor regression was noted.[33,34] A lack of toxicity to normal organs in these xenograft studies and in nonhuman primates, along with promising imaging and therapeutic results, have led to series of imaging and biodistribution results in patients with malignant gliomas, in collaboration with Hugh Coakham in England.[35] In this study, specific tumor localization, as indicated by localization indices ranging from 1.4 to 12.6, was observed in three patients with intracranial gliomas following intracarotid injection of $^{131}$I-81C6. Moreover, serial imaging showed relatively little binding of labeled 81C6 in normal tissues with the exception of liver and spleen, justifying further imaging and biodistribution studies in patients with malignant gliomas.[35]

Another well-characterized antigen with a pericellular distribution is the melanoma-associated chondroitin sulfate proteoglycan (MPG). This antigen was defined with the Mab 9.2.27, originally derived following immunization with urea extracts of human melanoma cells.[36] Immunohistochemical studies showed a high MPG expression in 8 of 10 glioma biopsies in addition to all primary and metastatic melanomas that were tested.[37] The MPG is a well-defined target for immunotherapy as indicated by the fact that simultaneous injection of Mab 9.2.27 and immunologic effector cells eradicated established melanoma tumors in nude mice.[36] Furthermore, radioiodinated Me 1-14 Mab, which like 9.2.27 Mab reacts with MPG, was demonstrated to localize specifically in human glioma xenografted in nude mice.[38] The potential of Me 1-14 in human glioma imaging is presently being evaluated in a Phase I trial with $^{123}$I-labeled Me 1-14 F(ab')$_2$ fragments. Preliminary results in patients with malignant glioma studied to date show diagnostic quality image and specificity ratios similar to those obtained with Mab 81C6 (de Tribolet, personal communication, 1987).

*Brain-Lymphoid Antigens*

Since evaluation of the cross-reactivity of rabbit polyclonal antihuman brain antiserum with human T cells, it has been appreciated that there is extensive shared antigenicity between the brain and the lymphoid system.[39] Delineation of these shared antigens has proceeded with the introduction of Mab technology. Thy-1, a thymocyte differentiation marker recognized by Mab 390, was found in gliomas, in neuroblastomas, as well as in normal brain.[40] Further studies established that Thy-1 is a highly conserved antigen in gliomas as indicated by its expression in 16 of 17 human glioma cell lines and within 8 subclones of the parent cell line D-54MG.[41] Also of great interest was the finding that some normal and malignant glioma cells express high levels of HLA-DR (Ia) and several lymphoid-tumor-associated markers, such as common acute lymphoblastic leukemia antigen (CALLA), "T-L," and DU-ALL-1.[41-43] Furthermore, gamma interferon (IFN-γ) was shown to superinduce MHC class II antigen expression and enhance the mixed lymphocyte response of two human glioma cell lines with constitutive levels of Ia,[44,45] suggesting a prospect for adoptive immunotherapy in patients with gliomas.

## Gangliosides

*Antiganglioside Monoclonal Antibodies*

Gangliosides are important cell surface molecules that have been implicated in cell growth, transformation, and metastasis, in cell attachment, in recognition of toxins from infectious agents, and also in differentiation and development. Certain gangliosides, namely, GM2, GD2, 3'-iso-LM1, and 3',6'-iso-LD1, may be "differentiation" antigens as indicated by their quantitative increased expression in fetal in contrast to adult brain and their association largely with neoplasms of neuroectodermal origin. Glioma biopsies and cell lines show an increased concentration of GM3, GM2, GD2, and GD3 compared with that of the normal brain, which is concordant with earlier reports that showed a marked shift of ganglioside expression in gliomas, namely, that from the more complicated, polysialylated gangliosides towards the simpler, less polar ones.[45–48] Two glioma-associated gangliosides, 3'-iso-LM1 and 3'6'-iso-LD1, have been isolated from the D-54MG human cell line.[49] The 3'-iso-LM1 ganglioside was first isolated from human meconium and has been detected in small cell lung carcinomas,[50] the teratoma cell line Tera-1,[51] and the embryonal carcinoma cell line PA-1.[52,53] Similarly 3',6'-iso-LD1 has been detected in the human PA-1 cell line[52] and extracted from human colonic cancer.[54] The significant observations relevant to glioma expression were that these moieties comprised the major mono- and disialoglioses of the extensively characterized human glioma cell line D-54MG[49] and subsequently that 3'-iso-LM1 was broadly expressed in human glioma tissue.[55] Although 3'-iso-LM1 can be isolated from normal human infant brain, only trace amounts can be detected in normal adult brain,[56] thus allowing its potential use as a glioma cell marker within the adult CNS.

Several Mabs have been raised against neuroectodermal-tumor-associated gangliosides (presented in detail in TABLE 1). Mab R24, directed against GD3, showed that GD3 is the major ganglioside component of melanomas; R24 also reacted with two of five astrocytoma cell lines.[57] An antineuroblastoma Mab 14.18, which reacts with GD2, also cross-reacted with gliomas and fetal brain.[58] Finally, a human Mab OFA I-1[59] and a murine 5-3[60] recognizing the GM2 ganglioside reacted with eight of eight astrocytoma cell lines, glioma and melanoma tissues, and fetal brain. A significant humoral and cellular response against GM2 was also observed in patients with OFA-I-1-positive tumors, making GM2 a candidate molecule for active immunization.[61] Results from the foregoing studies suggest that tumors of neuroectodermal origin may express exploitable levels of GM2, GD2, and GD3, indicating that panels of Mabs might be more useful than single ones in immunotherapy. The necessity for a thorough analysis of the structural specificity of antiganglioside Mabs has been demonstrated on at least two occasions.[62,63] Such an analysis showed that three described anti-GD3 Mabs cross-react with 3',8'-LD1, or disialylparagloboside, and with lesser affinities to GT1a and GQ1b; all of these gangliosides share the NeuAc $\alpha$2-8NeuAc $\alpha$2-3Gal$\beta$1-4 sequence.

*Applications of Antiganglioside Monoclonal Antibodies*

One of the most important implications of hybridoma technology is that a laboratory-generated Mab can quickly be applied in the clinical setting. The anti-GD$_3$ Mab R$_{24}$ was used in a phase I clinical trial in patients with metastatic melanoma and achieved marked tumor regression in 5 of 12 patients with only mild side effects.[64] Furthermore, regression of cutaneous metastatic melanoma was observed in six of eight patients treated with intratumoral injections of the human anti-$GD_2$ Mab L72 (OFA-I-2).[65] An anti-idiotype Mab with the internal image of $GD_2$ was raised against Mab L72 to be used for active immunization of melanoma patients.[66] In another study, 12 patients with neuroblastoma, malignant melanoma, and osteogenic sarcoma were treated with the anti-$GD_2$ Mab 3F8. Complete and partial remission of the tumors was noted, and 10 of 12 patients had positive *in vivo* localization using $^{131}$I-3F8 radioimaging.[67] The same group used an anti-$GD_2$ IgM Mab together with complement to purge tumor cells from autologous bone marrow of patients with neuroblastoma and proposed that Mabs can be used for removal of residual tumor cells before autologous bone marrow transplantation not only in leukemia, but also in neuroblastomas with osseous involvement.[68]

TABLE 1. Summary of Representative Antiganglioside Mabs Reactive with Tumors of Neuroectodermal Origin

| Ganglioside | Mab | Ref. |
|---|---|---|
| GD3 | R24 | 57 |
| | 4.2 | 97 |
| | 3.6, 11C 64 | 98 |
| | 2B2, 1F4, MG21 | 99 |
| 9-0-acetyl GD3 | D1.1 | 100 |
| GD2 | OFA I.2 (L72) | 101 |
| | 3F8, 2F7, 3G6, 3A7 | 68 |
| | 14.18, 12G | 58 |
| GM2 | OFA I.1 | 59 |
| | 5.3 | 60 |
| (3'-iso) LM1 | $C_{50}$ | 102 |
| | $K_4$ | 51 |
| (3',6'-iso)LD1 | FH9 | 54 |
| GM3 | $M_{2590}$ | 103 |

Although antiganglioside Mabs have not been used specifically in studies with gliomas, the significance of the findings in other neuroectodermal tumors and the documented increased expression of these target gangliosides in gliomas indicate their substantial potential in brain tumor oncology.

*"Neuroectodermal-Oncofetal" Antigens*

The descriptive phrase, "neuroectodermal-oncofetal" antigens, was used previously[69] as an operational framework to include antigens with a pattern of reactivity best described in that manner. At that time, antibodies such as OFA-I-1, OFA I-2, and Me 1-14 would have fallen into this category. Now these Mabs have been demonstrated to detect defined moieties, such as $GM_2$ and $GD_2$ in the case of OFA I-1 and OFA I-2, respectively, and MPG in the case of Me 1-14. It is apparent then that as technology evolves and we move from an operational definition to a biochemical one, operational terms such as neuroectodermal-oncofetal will be shown to include a variety of defined moieties.

Mabs of limited biochemical characterization that fall into this category, including 2F3, 4C7, and 5B7, were raised against the human glioma cell line D-54MG and show a more restricted oncofetal-neuroectodermal tissue distribution.[69] A similar distribution pattern was demonstrated by Mabs BF7, GE2, and CG12, but the latter was also present in normal adult brain.[43] Furthermore, two Mabs, C12 and D12, recognizing proteins of 180 and 88 kd, respectively, specifically localized to human glioma xenografts in athymic mice.[38,70] Finally, UJ13A, a "pan-neuroectodermal" monoclonal antibody raised against a 16-week fetal homogenate,[71] recognizes a cell-surface antigen widely expressed on most normal and tumor tissues of neuroectodermal origin with the exception of melanomas.[71] Radiolabeled UJ13A was initially shown to localize to gliomas and neuroblastomas in patients with advanced disease;[72] when both UJ13A and a nonspecific immunoglobulin were used, however, specific localization was not observed, indicating that nonspecific antibody uptake by the tumor had occurred.[72] However, UJ13A has shown promising clinical use as one of a panel of Mabs to remove tumor cells from the bone marrow of patients with neuroblastoma before autologous bone marrow transplantation.[71]

## INTRATHECAL THERAPY AND CONCEPT

Various methods have been proposed to increase Mab delivery to malignant gliomas in intracranial xenograft rodent models once specificity has been demonstrated. These include the use of Fab[73] or F(ab')2[74] fragments, the disruption of the BBB,[12] and the exploitation of alternative routes of administration, that is, intracarotid[75] and intrathecal injection.

The intrathecal approach offers the theoretic advantage of allowing the injected Mab contact with brain tumor cells and normal brain before contact with other normal tissues. Mabs selectively chosen for their reactivity with brain tumor cells, but not with normal brain, thus may have enhanced tumor cell binding compared to antibodies administered by vascular routes. Because of limited Mab diffusion into normal brain and intraparenchymal brain tumors, intrathecal therapy is most feasible with tumors with ventricular projection or leptomeningeal seeding with tumor cells in contact with the CSF. In this respect, radiolabeled monoclonal antibody (UJ181.4, F8.111, or Me 1-14, depending on the immunophenotype of the particular tumor) was intrathecally administered in a phase I clinical trial to five patients with carcinomatous meningitis. Striking therapeutic responses with remissions of up to 22 months and only minimal side effects were observed, suggesting that intrathecal antibody administration may find a place in the treatment of malignancies that involve leptomeninges (Coakham, H. & Kemshead, J., personal communication).

## HUMAN HYBRIDOMAS

Mouse monoclonal antibodies, when administered to immunocompetent patients, provoke an immune response that can greatly compromise the efficacy of the monoclonal antibody treatment. This response was demonstrated in 50% of patients with cutaneous T-cell leukemia treated with the T101 Mab.[76] To date there are little available data on the immune response of glioma patients to mouse IgG. Because glioma patients are often immunosuppressed even before radiation and chemotherapy,[77] it is possible that repeated doses of mouse immunoglobulins, and especially Fab or F(ab')2 fragments, may be administered without eliciting or boosting an immune response. Indeed, Courteney-Luck et al.[78] found no increase in anti-mouse immunoglobulin levels in one of two glioma patients treated with radiolabeled anti-EGF receptor Mab 9A whereas the second patient developed only a moderate response.

Human-human hybridomas may limit the anti-mouse immunoglobulin immune response further to only anti-idiotype problems; moreover, it is likely that human-human hybridoma specificity will be different from that of murine hybridoma. To date there has been little success in producing human-human hybridomas of sufficient specificity and affinity to consider large scale human trial[79] within the glioma patient population; however, the reported regression of cutaneous melanoma metastases following intralesional injection of the human anti-GD2 monoclonal antibody L72[65] is a positive indication of further progress in this area.

## GROWTH FACTORS AND ONCOGENES IN GLIOMAS

Growth factors and oncogenes may play a major role in human glioma growth. Several mechanisms of oncogene activation operate in different types of tumors; of these, amplification is the process more frequently documented in human gliomas, although laborious searches for point mutation have not been extensively carried out with tissue from patients with malignant glioma. Double minute chromosomes, a cytogenetic abnormality associated with gene amplification, are found in approximately 50% of malignant gliomas, and their presence correlates with epidermal growth factor receptor (EGFR) gene amplification.[80] In biopsy tissue, approximately 40% of gliomas showed EGFR gene amplification and increased levels of EGFR gene transcript.[81,82]

Furthermore, rearrangements of the EGFR gene resulting in abnormal protein products were shown in five of six glioma xenografts with EGFR gene amplification.[83] Of particular interest was the finding of an aberrant EGFR lacking the external EGF-binding domain and structurally resembling the V-erB transforming protein. This amino-truncated, predominantly intracytoplasmic EGFR possesses intrinsic tyrosine kinase activity and may fire constitutively, leading to uncontrolled cell growth.[83] Because EGFR is highly expressed in a large percentage of malignant gliomas, it may become a useful target for immunotherapy. *In vitro*, anti-EGFR Mabs show a direct cytostatic effect on the growth of A431 cells (an epidermoid carcinoma cell line expressing very high numbers of EGFR) and also suppress a tumorigenic growth of the same cells in nude mice.[84] Radiolabeled F(ab')2 fragments of the anti-EGFR Mab 425 showed specific localization in U-87MG human glioma xenografts.[74] Furthermore, Epenetos et al.[85] claimed that one patient with glioma experienced transient improvement following treatment with a radiolabeled Mab, recognizing a carbohydrate determinant of the EGFR identical to that of blood group A. However, the ubiquitous nature of EGFR and the proposed requirement of EGF for normal growth and development may set a limit on immunotherapy with anti-EGFR Mabs.

Apart from EGF and its receptor, other growth factors and oncogenes implicated in gliomas include: platelet-derived growth factor (PDGF), the cellular homologue of the v-sis viral oncogene, which was detected in three of five glioblastomas,[86] and the nuclear protooncogenes N-myc and c-myc, which were amplified in three glioma biopsies[82] and one medulloblastoma cell line,[87] respectively. Platelet-derived growth factor, like EGF, has been implicated in glioma growth by its autocrine or paracrine action. Mabs against either the growth factor or its receptor may interrupt such circuits. In mouse cells transformed by v-sis, for example, proliferation of the transformed cells can be inhibited by adding antibodies to PDGF.[88] Finally, a highly amplified, overexpressed gene, called gli, was recently identified in two human gliomas. It is distinct from other previously described oncogenes.[89] DNA sequencing analysis of this putative oncogene will allow construction of synthetic peptides that can be used as immunogens in raising Mabs potentially reactive with the transformed cell gene product. In this respect, the gli gene product, like the EGFR, may also become a target for immunotherapy if its cellular location is suitable and its normal tissue distribution not prohibitive.

Gene amplification is only one mechanism of oncogene activation in gliomas. Another possible mechanism is a point mutation that can alter the structure of the oncogene protein. This mechanism is well documented in the case of the neu oncogene that was first identified from ethyl-nitrosourea-induced neuroectodermal tumors in rats. A simple point mutation converts the neu oncogene into a potent one by changing a single amino acid in the transmembrane domain of the neu-encoded protein.[90] The biologic significance of the neu oncogene is exemplified by the fact that the Mab 7.16.4, which recognizes the neu gene protein, inhibits the anchorage independent growth of neu-transformed cells in soft agar. Furthermore, treatment with the same Mab results in inhibition of the tumorigenic growth of the rat cell line (B104) from which neu was initially derived in nude mice and in syngeneic rats.[91] It is worth mentioning that a simple point mutation converts the normal ras gene, like the neu gene, to its oncogenic, active counterpart. It was recently shown that about 40% of colon cancers contain activated ras oncogenes,[92] suggesting that a mutation-activated neu oncogene can be similarly operating in gliomas.

## USE OF PANELS OF MONOCLONAL ANTIBODIES IN DIAGNOSIS AND PHENOTYPIC CHARACTERIZATION OF BRAIN TUMORS

Virtually all leukemias and lymphomas express some lineage-specific surface antigens that allow us not only to differentiate between B- and T-cell leukemias but also to identify the stage during B- or T-cell ontogeny at which the leukemic clone arose. The specific immunophenotype of a leukemia or lymphoma is of particular prognostic and therapeutic significance. Although such a classification has not been demonstrated in brain tumors, considerable progress has been made in defining distinct phenotypic patterns of human medulloblastoma and glioma cell lines. In a recent study, an extensive panel of Mabs reactive against neuroectodermal, glial, neuronal, and HLA and lymphoid-associated antigens was used to characterize the phenotype of four distinct medulloblastoma cell lines.[19] Two readily distinguishable phenotypic patterns, one more "glial" and the other more "neuronal," were found, suggesting that there may be subtypes of medulloblastoma with differences in biologic behavior, chemotherapy, and prognosis.

Panels of Mabs have been used successfully to demonstrate the phenotypic heterogeneity of gliomas. A panel comprised of 10 Mabs with restricted but not absolute specificity for gliomas was used to demonstrate the antigenic heterogeneity of the established glioma line D-54 MG and its eight single-cell derived clones.[93]

The use of Mabs as immunodiagnostic agents in surgical pathology and cytopathology has great potential. It is known that the identification of malignant cells in CSF is an accurate indicator of CNS involvement by tumor. In many of these cases, the distinction among a primary brain tumor, a primary cerebral lymphoma, or a metastasis from an occult primary tumor elsewhere in the body is difficult.[94] A carefully designed panel of Mabs can pinpoint the different origins of neoplastic cells and substantially help in making the correct diagnosis. Such a panel of four Mabs was immunohistochemically applied in a series of 53 CNS cases (consisting of specimens of CSF, needle aspirates, and imprints) and accurately classified the encountered malignant cells to one of the three broad categories of neoplasms already mentioned (presented in detail in TABLE 2).[94] A similar panel of Mabs was applied to CSF specimens from patients with suspected neoplastic meningitis and accurately identified

TABLE 2. A Representative Proposed Monoclonal Antibody Panel For the Evaluation of Cytologic Specimens from the Central Nervous System (reproduced from Vick et al., 1987)

|  | UJ13a Neuroectodermal Associated Antigen | Anti-GFAP (A Mab "cocktail") | B72.3 Carcinoma-Associated Antigen | $2D_1$ Common Leukocyte Antigen |
|---|---|---|---|---|
| Gliomas | + | + | − | ± |
| Nonglial primary brain tumors | + | − | − | − |
| Oat cell carcinoma Rhabdomyosarcoma | + | − | − | − |
| Metastatic adenocarcinoma (non-oat cell carcinomas) | − | − | + | − |
| Melanoma | − | − | − | − |
| Lymphoma leukemia | − | − | − | + |

neoplastic cells of epithelial, lymphoid, or neuroectodermal origin in 16 of 17 cases.[95] In addition, such panels of Mabs can be of value in assessing the efficacy of therapy (radiation, chemotherapy, etc.) in patients with CSF cytology previously positive for malignant cells, because many of these cells revert to normal during the course of treatment.

## SUMMARY AND PROSPECTS

There is little doubt that monoclonal antibodies directed to human glioma-associated antigens have had a substantial impact on our understanding of the biologic aspects of glioma. Unique extracellular matrix antigens, abnormally expressed gangliosides, brain lymphoid antigens, and other cross-reactive neuroectodermal moieties have all been identified during continuing investigations of brain tumor cell biology. Furthermore, the combined approaches of hybridoma technology and molecular biology have delineated the presence of activated growth factors and oncogenes in gliomas, a finding of considerable therapeutic significance.

Despite the limited use of Mabs in patients with glioma, their clinical potential is remarkable. They can be applied, either alone or in panels, as immunodiagnostic agents in neuropathology, cytopathology and neuroradiology and, finally, in antitumor therapy, as originally proposed by Ehrlich[96] in 1906. As reagents in neurobiology, they are helping to unravel problems of developmental neurobiology, glial and neuronal mobility, attachment, and cell-cell communication.

## REFERENCES

1. WIKSTRAND, C. J. & D. D. BIGNER. 1980. Am. J. Pathol. **98:** 515-568.
2. GREEN, S. B., D. P. BYAR, M. D. WALKER, et al. 1983. Cancer Treat. Rep. **67:** 121-132.
3. BIGNER, D. D. 1982. Neurosurgery **9:** 320-326.
4. BIGNER, S. H., R. BJERKVIG & O. D. LAERUM. 1985. Neurolog. Clin. **3:** 769-784.
5. BIGNER, S. H., J. MARK, P. C. BURGER, M. S. MAHALEY, JR., D. E. BULLARD, L. H. MUHLBAIER & D. D. BIGNER. 1987. Submitted for publication.
6. BIGNER, S. H., J. MARK, D. E. BULLARD, M. S. MAHALEY, JR., & D. D. BIGNER. 1986b. Cancer Genet. Cytogenet. **22:** 121-135.
7. BIGNER, D. D., S. H. BIGNER, J. PONTEN, B. WESTERMARK, M. S. MAHALEY, E. RUOSLAHTI, H. HERSMAN, L. F. ENG & C. J. WIKSTRAND. 1981. J. Neuropathol. Exp. Neurol. **40:** 201-229.
8. BULLARD, D. E., S. C. SCHOLD, S. H. BIGNER & D. D. BIGNER. 1981. J. Neuropathol. Exp. Neurol. **40:** 410-427.
9. BOURDON, M. A., R. E. COLEMAN & D. D. BIGNER. 1984a. Prog. Exp. Tumor Res. **28:** 79-101.
10. GROOTHUIS, D. R., J. M. FISHER, N. A. VICK & D. D. BIGNER. 1981. Cancer Treat. Rep. **65:** 13-18.
11. NEUWELT, E. A., E. P. FRENKEL, J. T. DIEHL, L. H. VU, S. RAPAPAPORT & S. HILL. 1980. Neurosurgery **7:** 44-53.
12. BULLARD, D. E., M. BOURDON & D. D. BIGNER. 1984. J. Neurosurg. **61:** 901-911.
13. KOHLER, G. & C. MILSTEIN. 1975. Nature **256:** 495-497.
14. PEGRAM, C. N., L. F. ENG, C. J. WIKSTRAND, R. D. McCOMB, Y.-L. LEE & D. D. BIGNER. 1985. Neurochem. Pathol. **3:** 119-138.
15. DRANOFF, G. & D. D. BIGNER. 1984. Arch. Pathol. Lab. Med. **108:** 535.
16. VINORES, S. A., J. M. BONNIN, L. J. RUBINSTEIN & P. J. MARANGOS. 1984. Arch. Pathol. Lab. Med. **108:** 536-540.
17. McLENDON, R. E., P. C. BURGER, C. N. PEGRAM, L. F. ENG & D. D. BIGNER. 1986. J. Neuropathol. Exp. Neurol. **45:** 692-703.
18. TROJANOWSKI, J. Q., H. S. FRIEDMAN, P. C. BURGER & D. D. BIGNER. 1987. Am. J. Pathol. **126:** 358-363.
19. HE, X.-M., S. X. SKAPEK, C. J. WIKSTRAND, H. S. FRIEDMAN, J. T. KEMSHEAD, H. B. COAKHAM, S. H. BIGNER & D. D. BIGNER. 1987. Submitted for publication.
20. FRIEDMAN, H. S., P. C. BURGER, S. H. BIGNER, J. Q. TROJANOWSKI, C. J. WIKSTRAND, E. C. HALPERIN & D. D. BIGNER. 1985. J. Neuropathol. Exp. Neurol. **44:** 592-605.
21. HAY, E. D. 1981. J. Cell Biol. **91:** 205-223.
22. BOURDON, M. A., C. J. WIKSTRAND, H. FURTHMAYR & D. D. BIGNER. 1983. Cancer Res. **43:** 2796-2806.
23. CHIQUET, M. & D. M. FAMBROUGH. 1984. J. Cell Biol. **98:** 1926-1936.
24. ERICKSON, H. P. & J. L. IGLESIAS. 1984. Nature **311:** 267-269.

25. GRUMET, M., S. HOFFMAN, K. L. CROSSIN & G. M. EDELMAN. 1985. PNAS **82:** 8075-8079.
26. EHRISMANN, R. C., E. J. MACKIE, C. A. PEARSON & T. SAKAKURA. 1986. Cell **47:** 131-139.
27. ERICKSON, H. P. & H. C. TAYLOR. 1987. J. Cell Biol. in press.
28. BOURDON, M. A., T. J. MATTHEWS, S. V. PIZZO & D. D. BIGNER. 1985. J. Cell Biol. **28:** 183-195.
29. MCCOMB, R. D., J. M. MOUL, J. P. DAVID & D. D. BIGNER. 1987. J. Neuropathol. Exp. Pathol. in press.
30. CROSSIN, K. L., S. HOFFMAN, M. GRUMET, J.-P. THIERY & G. M. EDELMAN. 1986. J. Cell. Biol. **102:** 1917-1930.
31. BOURDON, M. A., R. E. COLEMAN, R. G. BLASBERG, D. R. GROOTHUIS & D. D. BIGNER. 1984b. Antican. Res. **4:** 133-140.
32. BULLARD, D. E., C. J. WIKSTRAND, P. A. HUMPHREY, Y. S. LEE, R. E. COLEMAN, M. ZALUTSKY & D. D. BIGNER. 1986. Nucl. Med. **25:** 210-215.
33. BULLARD, D. E., Y. S. LEE, M. R. ZALUTSKY, R. E. COLEMAN, H. S. FRIEDMAN, E. V. COLAPINTO & D. D. BIGNER. 1987. Can. Res. in press.
34. LEE, Y. S., D. E. BULLARD, P. A. HUMPHREY, E. V. COLAPINTO, H. S. FRIEDMAN, M. R. ZALUTSKY, R. E. COLEMAN & D. D. BIGNER. 1987a. Submitted for publication.
35. MOSELEY, R., M. R. ZALUTSKY, H. B. COAKHAM, R. E. COLEMAN & D. D. BIGNER. 1987. J. Nucl. Med. **28:** 603.
36. REISFELD, R. A. 1986. Sem. Oncol. **13:** 153-164.
37. SCHREYER, M., M.-F. HAMOU, S. CARREL, J.-P. MACH, N. DE TRIBOLET. 1985. *In* Markers of Human Neuroectodermal Tumors, Chap 4. Staal and Van Veelan, Eds. CRC Press, USA.
38. WIKSTRAND, C. J., R. E. MCLENDON, S. CAVREL, J. T. KEMSHEAD, J. MACH, H. B. COAKHAM, N. DE TRIBOLET, D. E. BULLARD, M. R. ZALUTSKY & D. D. BIGNER. 1987. J. Neuroimmunol. **15:** 37-56.
39. WHITESIDE, T. L. 1977. Am. J. Pathol. **86:** 1-16.
40. SEEGER, R. C., Y. L. DANON, S. A. RAYNER & F. HOOVER. 1981. J. Immunol. **128:** 983-987.
41. WIKSTRAND, C. J., F. C. GRAHMANN, R. D. MCCOMB & D. D. BIGNER. 1985. J. Neuropathol. Exp. Neurol. **44:** 229-241.
42. CARREL, S., A. SCHMIDT-KESSEN, J.-P. MACH, D. HEUMANN & C. ZIRARDET. 1983. J. Immunol. **130:** 2456-2460.
43. PIQUET, V., A.-C. DISERENS, S. CARREL, J.-P. MACH & N. DE TRIBOLET. 1985. Springer Sem. Immunopathol. **8:** 111-127.
44. TAKIGUCHI, M., J. P. TING, S. C. BUERSOW, C. BOYER, Y. GILLESPIE & J. A. FRELINGER. 1985. Eur. J. Immunol. **15:** 809-814.
45. BASTA, P. V., P. A. SHERMAN & J. P.-Y. TING. 1987. J. Immunol. **138:** 1275-1280.
46. FREDMAN, P., H. VAN HOLST, V. P. COLLING, A. AMMAR, B. DELLHEDEN, B. WAHREN, L. GRANHOLM & L. SVENNERHOLM. 1986. Neurol Res. **8:** 123-126.
47. YATES, A. J., D. K. THOMPSON, C. P. BOESEL, C. ALBRIGHTSON & R. W. HART. 1979. J. Lipid Res. **20:** 428-436.
48. TAYLOR, D. T. & E. L. HOGAN. 1980. J. Neurochem. **34:** 126-131.
49. MÄNSSON, J.-E., P. FREDMAN, D. D. BIGNER, K. MOLIN, B. ROSENGREN, H. S. FRIEDMAN & L. SVENNERHOLM. 1986. FEBS Lett. **201:** 109-113.
50. NILSSON, O., J.-E. MANSSON, L. LINDHOLM, J. HOLMGREN & L. SVENNERHOLM. 1985. FEBS Lett. **182:** 398-401.
51. RETTIG, W. J., C. E. CARDO, S. C. JENNIFER, H. F. OETTGEN, L. J. OLD & K. O. LLOYD. 1985. Cancer Res. **45:** 815-821.
52. FUKUDA, M. N., K. BOTHNER, K. O. LLOYD, W. J. RETTIG, P. R. TILLER & A. DELL. 1986. J. Biol. Chem. **261:** 5141-5153.
53. SVENNERHOLM, L. 1987. New Trends in Ganglioside Research. In press.
54. FUKUSHI, Y., E. NUDELMAN, S. B. LEVERY, T. HIGUSHI & J. HAKOMORI. 1986. Biochemistry **25:** 2859-2866.
55. FREDMAN, P. 1987. New Trends in Ganglioside Research. In press.

56. SVENNERHOLM, L., P. FREDMAN, B. JUNGBJER, J.-E. MANSSON, B.-M. RYNMARK, K. BOSTROM, B. HAGBERG, L. NOREN & P. SANTAVOURI. 1987. J. Neurochem. in press.
57. PUKEL, C. S., K. O. LLOYD, L. R. TRAVASSOS, W. G. DIPPOLD, H. F. OETTGEN & L. J. OLD. 1982. J. Exp. Med. **155:** 1133-1147.
58. MUJOO, K., D. A. CHERESH, M.-Y. HSIN, R. A. REISFELD. 1987. Cancer Res. **47:** 1098-1104.
59. TAI, T., J. C. PAULSON, L. D. CAHAH & R. F. IRIE. 1983. PNAS **80:** 5392-5396.
60. NATOLI, E. J., JR., P. O. LIVINGSTON, C. S. PUKEL, K. O. LLOYD, H. WIENGANT, J. SZALAY, H. F. OETTGEN & L. J. OLD. 1986. Cancer Res. **46:** 4116-4120.
61. LIVINGSTON, P. O., E. J. NATOLI, M. J. CALVES, E. STOCKERT, H. F. OETTGEN & L. J. OLD. 1987. PNAS **84:** 2911-2915.
62. FREDMAN, P., J. L. MAGNAMI, M. NIRENBERG & V. GINSBURG. 1984. Arch. Biochem. Biophys. **233:** 661-666.
63. BRODIN, T., S. HELLSTROM, K. E. HELLSTROM, K. A. KARLSSON, H.-O. SJOGREN, N. STOMBERG & J. THURIN. 1985. Biochem. Biophys. Acta **837:** 349-353.
64. HOUGHTON, A. N., D. MINTZER, C. C. CARDO, S. WELT, B. FLIEGEL, S. VADHAN, E. CARSWELL, M. R. MELAMED, H. F. OETTGEN & L. J. OLD. 1985. PNAS **82:** 1242-1246.
65. IRIE, R. F. & D. L. MORTON. 1986. PNAS **83:** 8694-8698.
66. SAXTON, R. E., K. KONO & R. F. IRIE. 1987. Proc. AACR **28:** 389.
67. CHEUNG, N.-K., N. BERGER, P. COCCIA, S. KALLICK, H. LAZARUS, F. MIRALDI, U. SAARINEN & S. STRANDJORD. 1986. Proc. AACR **27:** 318.
68. CHEUNG, N. V., V. M. SAARINEN, J. E. NEELY, B. LANDMEYER, D. DONOVAN & P. T. COCCIA. 1985. Cancer Res. **45:** 2642-2649.
69. GRAHMANN, F. C., C. J. WIKSTRAND & D. D. BIGNER. 1984. *In* Neuroimmunology. Ed: P. Behan & F. Spreatico, Eds.: 311-323. Raven Press, New York.
70. WIKSTRAND, C. J., R. E. MCLENDON, D. E. BULLARD, P. FREDMAN, L. SVENNERHOLM & D. D. BIGNER. 1986. Cancer Res. **46:** 5933-5940.
71. ALLEN, P. M., J. A. GARSON, E. I. HARPER, V. ASSER, H. B. COAKHAM, B. BROWNELL & J. T. KEMSHEAD. 1983. Int. J. Cancer, **31:** 591-598.
72. DAVIES, A. G., R. B. RICHARDSON, S. P. BOURNE, J. T. KEMSHEAD & H. B. COAKHAM. 1986. *In* Tumors of the Brain. N. M. Bleehan, Ed.: 83-99. Springer Verlag, New York.
73. COLAPINTO, E. V., Y. S. LEE, P. A. HUMPHREY, D. E. BULLARD & D. D. BIGNER. 1987. Manuscript in preparation.
74. TAKAHASHI, H., D. HERLYN, B. ATKINSON, J. POWE, V. RODECK, A. ALAVI, D. A. BRUCE & H. KOPROWSKI. 1987. Cancer Res. **47:** 3847-3850.
75. LEE, Y. S., D. E. BULLARD, C. J. WIKSTRAND, M. R. ZALUTSKY, L. H. MUHLBAIER & D. D. BIGNER. 1987b. Cancer Res. **47:** 1931-1946.
76. DILLMAN, R. O., J. B. DILLMAN & M. CLUTTER. 1985. Proc. Am. Soc. Clin. Oncol. **4:** 230.
77. MAHALEY, M. S., JR., W. H. BROOKS, T. L. ROSZMAN, D. D. BIGNER, L. DUKA & S. RICHARDSON. 1977. J. Neurosurg. **46:** 467-476.
78. COURTENEY-LUCK, N.S., A. A. EPENETOS, R. MOORE, M. LARCHE, D. PECTASIDES, B. DHOKIA & M. A. RITTER. 1986. Cancer Res. **46:** 6489-6493.
79. SIKORA, K. 1984. Exp. Cell Biol. **52:** 189-195.
80. BIGNER, S. H., A. J. WONG, J. MARK, L. H. MUHLBAIER, K. W. KINZLER, B. VOGELSTEIN & D. D. BIGNER. 1986a. Cancer Genet. Cytogenet. **22:** 121-135.
81. LIBERMANN, T. A., H. R. NUSBAUM, N. RAUCOM, R. KRIS, I. LAX, H. SOREG, N. WHITTLE, M. D. WETERFIELD, A. ULLRICH & J. SCHLESSINGER. 1985. Nature **313:** 144-147.
82. WONG, A. J., S. H. BIGNER, D. D. BIGNER, K. W. KINZLER, J. R. HAMILTON & B. VOGELSTEIN. 1987. PNAS in press.
83. HUMPHREY, P. A., A. J. WONG, P. BOGELSTEIN, S. H. BIGNER, H. S. FRIEDMAN, M. W. WERNER & D. D. BIGNER. 1987. Submitted for publication.
84. MASUI, H., T. KAWAMOTO, J. D. SATO, B. WOLF, G. SATO & J. MENDELSON. 1984. Cancer Res. **44:** 1002-1007.
85. EPENETOS, A. A., L. N. COURTENAU, D. PICKERING, G. HOOKER, H. DURBIN, J. P. LAVENDER & C. G. MCKENZIE. 1985. Br. Med. J. **290:** 1463-1466.

86. EVA, A., K. C. ROBBINS, P. R. ANDERSON, A. SRINIVASSAN, S. R. TRONICK, E. P. REDDY, N. W. ELLMORE, A. T. GALEN, J. A. LAUTENBERGER, T. S. PAPAS, E. H. WESTIN, F. WONG-STALL, R. C. GALLO & S. A. AARONSON. 1982. 295: 116-119.
87. FRIEDMAN, H. S., P. C. BURGER, J. H. BIGNER, J. Q. TROJANOWSKI, G. M. BRODEUR, C. J. WIKSTRAND, J. KURTZBERG, M. BERENS, E. C. HALPERIN & D. D. BIGNER. 1987. Submitted for publication.
88. JOHNSSON, A., C. BETSHOLTE & C.-H. HELDON. 1985. Nature **317**: 438-440.
89. KINZLER, K. W., S. H. BIGNER, D. D. BIGNER, J. M. TRENT, M. L. LAW, S. J. O'BRIEN, A. J. WONG & B. VOGELSTEIN. 1987. Science **236**: 70-73.
90. BARGMANN, C., M. HUNG & R. WEINBER. 1986. Cell **45**: 649-657.
91. DREBIN, J., V. LINK, R. WEINBER & M. GREEN. 1986. 1985 PNAS **83**: 9129-9133.
92. BOS, J. L., E. R. FEARON, S. R. HAMILTON, M. V. DE VRIES, J. H. VAN BOOM, A. J. VANDEREB & B. VOGELSTEIN. 1987. Nature **327**: 293-297.
93. WIKSTRAND, C. J., S. H. BIGNER & D. D. BIGNER. 1983. Cancer Res. **43**: 3327-3334.
94. VICK, W. W., S. H. BIGNER, C. J. WIKSTRAND, D. E. BULLARD, J. KEMSHEAD, H. B. COAKHAM, J. SCHLOM, W. W. JOHNSTON & D. D. BIGNER. 1987. Acta Cytol. in press.
95. COAKHAM, H. B., B. BROWNELL, E. HARPER, J. A. GARSON, P. M. ALLAN, E. B. LANE & J. T. KEMSHEAD. 1984. Lancet **1**: 1095-1097.
96. EHRLICH, P. 1906. Collected Studies on Immunity, pp. 442-447. John Wiley & Sons, New York.
97. NUDELMAN, E., S. HAKOMORI, R. KANNAGI, S. LEVERY, M.-Y. YEH, K. E. HELSTROM & I. HELLSTROM. 1982. J. Biol. Chem. **257**: 12752-12756.
98. CHERESH, D. A., J. R. HARPER, G. SCHULZ & R. A. REISFELD. 1984a. PNAS **81**: 5767-5771.
99. HELLSTRÖM, I., V. BRANKORA & K. E. HELLSTROM. 1985. PNAS **82**: 1499-1502.
100. CHERESH, D. A., A. P. VARKI, N. M. VARK, W. B. STALLCUP, J. LEVINE & R. A. REISFELD. 1984b. J. Biol. Chem. **259**: 7453-7459.
101. CAHAL, L. D., R. I. IRIE, R. SINGH, A. CASSIDENTI & J. C. PAULSEN. 1982. PNAS **79**: 7629-7633.
102. MÄNSSON, J.-E., P. FREDMAN, O. NILSSON, L. LINHOLM, J. HOLMGREN & L. SVENNERHOLM. 1985. Biochem. Biophys. Acta **834**: 110-117.
103. HIRABAYASHI, Y., A. HAMAOKA, A. MASTUMOTO, T. MATSUBARA, M. TAGAWA, S. WABABAYASHI & M. TANAGUCHI. 1985. J. Biol. Chem. **260**: 13328-13333.

# Diagnostic Markers in Human Neurooncology

## A Progress Report[a]

LUCIEN J. RUBINSTEIN

*Division of Neuropathology*
*Department of Pathology*
*University of Virginia School of Medicine*
*Charlottesville, Virginia 22908*

The development of immunohistochemistry in the past 10 years has led to considerable advances in the diagnostic demonstration of morphologic differentiation markers. The potential of this approach in the resolution of difficult problems in surgical oncology is so great that its use in the histology laboratory has now become routine. Its many applications in the demonstration of cytoplasmic and cell surface antigenic determinants that play a role as glial, neuronal, or other markers of differentiation in cerebral tumors were recently reviewed in detail from this and other laboratories.[1-5] Many of these applications are well known, but the scope of this field is still widening, and regular reviews at relatively short intervals are needed to define the state of the art. A progress report is given here on the antigenic determinants being used today for the diagnosis of nervous system neoplasms, with emphasis on those most frequently relied on. References to the individual determinants will be found in the aforementioned reviews and will in a number of instances be supplemented here by the citation of work that has appeared after those reviews were written.

Although the differentiation markers to be considered are generally regarded as playing a significant role in nervous system function, their neural specificity is, with a few exceptions, only relative. These markers may either involve cytoskeletal structures or other particular organelles, or be related to the cell membranes; they are therefore generally known as structural proteins. Other markers function as enzymes, as systemic or local endocrine carriers, or as neurotransmitter substances; they usually are soluble proteins. Insofar as the diagnosis of tumors is concerned, there is increasing recognition that these markers, rather than being indicators of neoplastic cytogenesis, are more likely to function as signposts of tumor cell differentiation or metaplasia.[2,6] Their potential utility extends beyond their current diagnostic use in the morphologic identification of tumors. Future applications are likely to include the identification of events that precede the phenotypic manifestations of neoplasia and the recognition of emerging cellular subpopulations based on the expression of single or multiple discriminating markers. Thus, we can anticipate in the future that early diagnosis, improved prognostic assessment, and even prediction of response to various modes of therapy may result from further advances in morphologic immunohistochemistry.

[a] This work was supported by Research Grant CA 31271 from the National Cancer Institute, US Department of Health and Human Services.

# DIFFERENTIATION MARKERS

## *Intermediate Filaments*

Intermediate filaments constitute a form of insoluble cytoplasmic organelles that measure 7 to 11 nm in diameter, being intermediate in size between microtubules (22-25 nm in diameter) and microfilaments (5-7 nm). They are absent from germ cells and early embryonal cells before the stage of implantation, but they are otherwise ubiquitous. The major polypeptides forming these filaments have molecular weights that range from 40 to 70 kd, save for those of neurons, in which the polypeptides have higher molecular weights. The distribution of intermediate filaments is, to some extent, tissue specific. Five groups are well recognized: (1) the cytokeratins, which include numerous types of biochemically distinct polypeptides and are characteristic of epithelial cells; (2) neurofilaments, which are found in most neurons and their processes, with the notable exception of the sensory neurons of the olfactory mucosa; (3) glial fibrillary acidic (GFA) protein, which forms a major constituent of normal and abnormal astrocytes; (4) desmin, which is found in cardiac, skeletal, and smooth muscle cells; and (5) vimentin, which is found in normal and neoplastic cells of mesenchymal origin, including endothelial cells, fibroblasts, macrophages, and lymphocytes, and which is also expressed in the early phase of development of most other cell types.

There is increasing awareness that two or even three different intermediate filament proteins may be found in the same neoplasm and that in several cases there may be colocalization of different proteins in the same tumor cell. Until relatively recently, it was generally thought that one member of the pair was always vimentin. However, the dual expression of cytokeratin and neurofilament protein has been demonstrated in neuroendocrine tumors, and that of GFA protein and cytokeratin in normal and neoplastic salivary gland cells, whereas, in the context of nervous system growths, coexpression of cytokeratin, GFA protein, and vimentin has been found in tumors of the choroid plexus.[7]

## *Glial Fibrillary Acidic (GFA) Protein*

This marker is still the most relied on today and the most often employed for the immunomorphologic diagnosis of cerebral tumors. This is partly due to the considerable morphologic heterogeneity of tumors of the glioma group which can in some cases result in serious problems of diagnostic recognition and classification. It must also be recognized that GFA protein is a highly sensitive marker and furthermore that it may demonstrate cell specificities that extend beyond those of central neuraxial (i.e., glial) origin. Thus, its uncritical use sometimes increases the complexity of diagnostic problems that its application may initially attempt to resolve.

Although its utilization in the identification of tumors of astrocytic origin is therefore well accepted, GFA protein can be expressed in cells that not only are not astrocytic, but also may not even be of neuroepithelial origin. Within the group of central nervous system (CNS) neoplasms, such nonastrocytic tumors include oligodendrogliomas, ependymomas, and choroid plexus papillomas. In the first two types of tumor, it is generally thought that its presence recalls the transient expression of GFA protein in fetal, normally developing oligodendroglial, or ependymal cells. In choroid plexus papillomas, its expression presumably recalls the ontogenesis of the choroid plexus epithelium from primitive neuroepithelial ventricular cells. GFA protein is also sometimes found in the stromal cells of capillary hemangioblastomas. We interpret this finding as due to its uptake by cells of angiogenic origin when conspicuous reactive gliosis is present in and around the tumor. We have also seen GFA protein within reactive macrophages in foci of severe CNS damage resulting from radiation necrosis.

Outside the central neuraxis, GFA protein has been found in nonmyelinating Schwann cells. Thus, both schwannomas and neurofibromas may include tumor cells, variable in number and distribution, that are GFA protein positive.[8] The hypothesis has been stated that the protein consists of different heterogeneous polypeptides that share common antigenic determinants, but other explanations are also possible, such as chemical alteration of epitopes after fixation or even the selective expression of GFA protein by cells that contain different classes of intermediate filaments. We should also note that GFA protein has been demonstrated in the folliculostellate cells of the anterior pituitary gland, in cells forming Rathke's cleft or its remnants, in crystalline lens epithelium, in hepatic Kupffer cells, in epiglottal cartilage cells, in epithelial salivary gland cells, and in tumors of Müllerian derivation. Nonetheless, its immunohistochemical demonstration continues to play a crucial role in the differential diagnosis of glial and nonglial cerebral tumors, particularly when the traditional special histologic stains are incapable of doing so. It has also considerably increased our awareness of the frequency with which astrocytic differentiation is visualized in either poorly differentiated embryonal tumors, such as medulloblastomas, or in anaplastic tumors, such as glioblastomas and gliosarcomas. It has also permitted the identification of new tumor entities, such as pleomorphic xanthoastrocytoma and desmoplastic infantile ganglioglioma,[9] and of newly recognized variations in the appearances of malignant astrocytic gliomas.[6,10] Both glial and nonglial cell specificities shown by polyvalent antisera have been confirmed with monoclonal antibodies.

*Neurofilament Proteins*

These proteins comprise three biochemically and immunochemically distinct subunits, which possess respective molecular weights in the regions of 65-70, 145-160, and 200-220 kd. In normal adult mammalian tissues, they are generally restricted to ganglion cells. However, they are unevenly distributed in the neuronal cell soma and its processes. The 200-220-kd subunit makes its appearance later than the other two subunits in the course of neuronal development, and it constitutes the major determinant in defining the diameter of the axon. The biochemical characteristics, immunogenicity, and topographic distribution of the neurofilament (NF) protein subunits differ according to their state of phosphorylation. It is highly likely that, as defined with monoclonal antibodies, variations in the distribution of phosphorylated NF epitopes may play a significant role in human neuropathology.

In central and peripheral nervous system tumors, the expression of NF proteins raises some intriguing questions because they may be present in the neoplastic equivalents of cells that normally do not contain them. Thus, their relation to the phenotypic manifestations of neoplasia needs to be further explored.[11] In general, NF protein subunits are readily demonstrable in differentiated neoplastic nerve cells of both the central and peripheral nervous systems as well as in numerous neuroendocrine tumors such as paragangliomas, carcinoid tumors, oat cell lung carcinomas, and parathyroid adenomas. They may also be seen in Flexner-Wintersteiner rosettes of retinoblastomas.[12] In embryonal tumors of neuroepithelial origin, the demonstration of NF protein serves to indicate ganglionic differentiation in cerebellar medulloblastomas, in sympathetic, olfactory and cerebral neuroblastomas, and in desmoplastic infantile gangliogliomas.

### *Other Structure-Related Neural Proteins*

These neural proteins include in particular the microtubule-associated proteins MAP-1 and MAP-2, and synaptophysin.

MAP-1 and MAP-2 copurify with tubulin and are generally thought to favor microtubular assembly by helping the microtubules to interact with intermediate filaments and with actin. Whereas MAP-1 is widely found in axonal processes and in nonneuronal cells, MAP-2 is generally regarded as being more specific and restricted to ganglion cells, in particular the dendrites. Both MAP-1 and MAP-2 are expressed in both the less and the more mature cells of adrenal neuroblastomas.

Synaptophysin is an important glycoprotein that has a molecular weight of 38 kd and is expressed in the presynaptic vesicles of neurons. It has been demonstrated in peripheral nerve cell tumors exhibiting various degrees of differentiation, in paragangliomas, and in various types of neuroendocrine tumor, where it may be coexpressed with either NF protein or cytokeratin.[13] It is frequently expressed in cerebellar medulloblastomas,[14,15] as we have confirmed.[16] Its scope and potential as a marker currently are being actively explored; evidence indicates that it will prove to be a highly reliable and relatively specific marker for the identification of neuroblastic and neuroendocrine tumors.[4,17,18]

### *Nervous System-Related Enzymes*

Those enzymes implicated in catecholamine synthesis include in particular tyrosine hydroxylase, dopamine-$\beta$-hydroxylase, and phenylethanolamine N-methyltransferase. In the peripheral nervous system (PNS), these enzymes were demonstrated immunohistochemically in neuroblastomas and in a variety of paragangliomas. In the CNS, tyrosine hydroxylase has been visualized in a ganglioglioma.[19]

Other neural-related enzymes comprise glutamine synthetase, aldolase C, carbonic anhydrase C, neuron-specific enolase, calcineurin, glycerol-3-phosphate dehydrogenase, and 2',3' cyclic nucleotide 3'-phosphohydrolase. The last two, which have been employed as markers for normal developing and mature glia, have not so far been applied immunomorphologically in the diagnosis of human cerebral tumors.

Glutamine synthetase is a cytoplasmic astrocyte-specific marker that appears to play a significant role in the detoxification of ammonia and the metabolism of glutamate. It is positive in astrocytomas and in areas of medulloblastomas that show astrocytic differentiation. It may be useful in confirming the astrocytic nature of anaplastic gliomas in which glial fibrils are lacking.

Aldolase C is a glycolytic enzyme that is present immunomorphologically in normal and neoplastic astrocytes, especially in the more differentiated cells.

Carbonic anhydrase C is a metalloprotein enzyme that catalyzes the hydration of carbon dioxide and is generally considered to play a role in the regulation of ionic and acid-base balance. The isozyme C has been found by some workers to be a marker for normal oligodendroglia in the rodent and human brain, as well as for the Müller cells of the human retina. About 25% of oligodendrogliomas show a relatively small number of immunopositive tumor cells, but a wide variety of other neoplasms, both within and outside the CNS, are also immunopositive, as are reactive astrocytes, oligodendroglia, and neurons included in or adjacent to brain tumors.[20] Our conclusion is that anticarbonic anhydrase C antisera cannot be used as specific markers for any human cerebral tumor.

## Neuron-Specific Enolase

The $\gamma\gamma$ homodimer of enolase, a glycolytic enzyme that catalyzes the interconversion of 2-phosphoglycerate into phosphoenolpyruvate, was previously known as the 14-3-2 protein and currently bears the name of neuron-specific enolase (NSE). It is generally regarded as characteristic of, but not specific for, ganglion cells and their axons, as well as of normal endocrine and neuroendocrine cells. Its appearance correlates with the development of ganglionic maturation. There is extensive evidence,[3,4] however, that it is expressed in cells of nonneuronal origin, including reactive astrocytes (where it may in some instances be colocalized with GFA protein). It nevertheless continues to function as a useful marker to identify neoplastic cells of peripheral neuronal derivation, neuroendocrine tumor cells, and melanomas. In central neuroepithelial neoplasms, it is easily demonstrable in cerebellar medulloblastomas[21] and retinoblastomas.[12] It is present in normal pinealocytes and therefore readily visualized in tumors of the pineal parenchyma.

Its interpretation as hard evidence of ganglionic cytogenesis or as expressing early neuronal differentiation, however, must be contested in view of its frequent expression in brain tumors such as glioblastomas, astrocytomas, oligodendrogliomas, meningiomas, choroid plexus papillomas, and schwannomas. In cerebellar hemangioblastomas, stromal cells, but not endothelial cells, are also positive.[22] It has also been shown at the electron immunocytochemical level that in neoplasms the enzyme is often localized to the cytoplasmic cell membrane. More recently the $\gamma\gamma$ enolase was visualized in both neoplastic and nonneoplastic proliferating Schwann cells.[23] All this suggests that increased glycolytic activity occurs on the surface of proliferating cells irrespective of the nature of the proliferation and that it represents either an increase in the total content of enolase or a shift in the isoenzyme to a more stable form, presumably to meet the increased rate of glycolysis needed for cellular proliferation. In any event, the same loss of neuronal specificity in neoplasms was noted when a monoclonal antibody against the $\gamma\gamma$ enolase was substituted for the polyvalent antiserum.[24]

Whereas NSE may continue, therefore, to be a useful adjunct in the diagnosis of peripheral neuronal and neuroendocrine tumors, its significance in ganglionic cytogenesis remains limited, especially in anaplastic or embryonal CNS tumors. However, it may be regarded as supporting the neuronal nature of neoplasms in the light of other confirmatory evidence. Its role as a reliable, primary neuronal and neuroendocrine marker is likely to be superseded by that of synaptophysin.

Calcineurin is a calcium-dependent phosphoprotein phosphatase that is stimulated by calmodulin and whose physiologic role in the brain, where it is found in high concentrations, is unknown. It was demonstrated immunohistochemically in the neoplastic ganglion cells of CNS and PNS tumors, including medulloblastomas and retinoblastomas.[25]

*Other Nonstructural Neural-Related Proteins*

Those proteins with which we are chiefly concerned include the S-100 protein, myelin basic protein (MBP), myelin-associated glycoprotein (MAG), and the retinal S-antigen.

The S-100 protein is a calcium-binding soluble protein whose molecular weight is about 21 kd and which has been extensively investigated in the nervous system. Its role is uncertain, but it may possibly assist in the regulation of microtubular assembly and stability.[26] The S-100 protein is synthesized in both the nuclei and the cytoplasm of glia, but it has also been found in the nuclei, cytoplasm, and membranes of ganglion cells. In the PNS, it is localized in Schwann cells, but it has been expressed by numerous other cell types such as the folliculostellate cells of the anterior pituitary gland, chondrocytes, adipocytes, melanocytes, Langerhans cells, T lymphocytes, interdigitating reticulum cells of lymph nodes, as well a wide variety of tumors of epithelial and cartilaginous origin.

Its distribution in the CNS is closely similar to that of GFA protein, but it is considerably less specific. It is valuable in the demonstration of amelanotic melanomas, whereas in PNS tumors it is positive in the more differentiated nerve sheath growths. It permits Schwann cells to be distinguished from perineurial cells, because it is characteristically absent in the latter. Its use in conjunction with the monoclonal antibodies against the Leu 7 epitope and against the human epithelial membrane antigen has recently increased its value as a differential marker.[27]

The limitations of its specificities are presumably due to the fact that it consists of several antigenically distinct polypeptides.[28] With some of the monoclonal antibodies that have been raised against the different determinants, the same heterogeneity was found.[29,30] However, in a study with a monoclonal antibody raised against the $\beta$ component of the protein, differential immunoreactivity was demonstrated in astrocytomas, glioblastomas, schwannomas, ependymomas, and craniopharyngiomas and was absent in oligodendrogliomas, meningiomas, neuroblastomas, and medulloblastomas.[31]

Myelin basic protein (MBP), while demonstrable immunomorphologically in normal immature oligodendrocytes in man and in mature oligodendrocytes in the rat, is in our experience found only in the residual myelin sheath fragments scattered in human oligodendrogliomas and not in tumor cells. Likewise, its demonstration in peripheral nerve sheath tumors is open to question.

Myelin-associated glycoprotein, like MBP, has been demonstrated immunomorphologically in immature oligodendrocytes and Schwann cells. It is also found in the Müller cells of the human adult retina. With a human monoclonal antibody against MAG, we found that only a very small number of oligodendrogliomas are immunopositive and in a few cells only. Some of these were oligodendroglial, others astrocytic. Most of the cells positive for MAG were also positive for GFA protein. All the 19 peripheral nerve sheath tumors (14 schwannomas and 5 neurofibromas) that we tested for the presence of MAG were found to be negative (Perentes, unpublished observations).

The retinal S-antigen is a highly significant protein with a molecular weight of 50 kd and closely implicated in the phototransduction of vision. It is expressed in retinal photoreceptor cells and in the pinealocytes of different vertebrates, including man. Both pineal parenchymal tumors and retinoblastomas are immunopositive.[12] In our experience it is negative in cerebral neuroblastomas and central neurocytomas, but immunopositive in a number of tumor cells in medulloblastomas.[32,33] This intriguing observation suggests a morphogenetic link between medulloblastomas and pineoblastomas.

## Neurotransmitters and Neuropeptides

These include a growing number of substances, among which should first be listed epinephrine and norepinephrine, which have been demonstrated in both adrenal and extraadrenal paragangliomas. An increasing number of neuropeptides are currently being demonstrated, particularly in neuroendocrine tumors, including pheochromocytomas and paragangliomas originating in the cauda equina or duodenum. Vasoactive intestinal peptide is expressed in a number of well-differentiated peripheral and central neuronal tumors, and $\beta$-endorphin was reported in intrasellar gangliocytomas. This area of investigation is expanding rapidly, and important results in the next few years are anticipated.

## Shared Lymphoid and Neuronal Markers

A large number of antigenic determinants displaying cross-reactivity between lymphoid and neuronal cells are currently being studied with panels of monoclonal antibodies raised against hemopoietic cells. Their contribution to tumor diagnosis is uncertain at this time, with one major exception, the HNK-1-defined antigen, which is recognized by the Leu 7 monoclonal antibody.

## Leu 7 Monoclonal Antibody

The Leu 7 monoclonal antibody was originally raised against cells of a human T-lymphoblastoid cell line. It was initially regarded as a specific marker of human cells with natural killer activity. However, it soon became evident that it recognizes myelin sheath cells in both the CNS and the PNS, that is, oligodendrocytes and Schwann cells, as well as a number of normal tissue cells such as prostatic epithelium. Generally, immunoreactivity is seen on the cytoplasmic cell membranes and myelin sheaths, although it may occasionally be diffuse throughout the cytoplasm. The antibody is generally thought to recognize a carbohydrate epitope on MAG.

Tumors composed of Schwann cells (schwannomas and neurofibromas, including their anaplastic equivalents) are recognized by the Leu 7 antibody, but perineurial cells are characteristically negative.[27] In conjunction with the S-100 protein, it may therefore help in the differential diagnosis of nerve sheath tumors from other soft tissue neoplasms; however, divergent results have been reported, presumably due to technical differences. The antibody also recognizes pheochromocytomas.

In CNS tumors, the antibody recognizes most types of neoplastic cells, but shows a preference for oligodendrogliomas, in which the number of immunoreactive cells is often very large. We have the impression that the cell membranes recognized by the antibody are usually those of well-differentiated tumors, whereas those of the more anaplastic or embryonal neoplasms tend to be immunonegative. Meningiomas are also negative, a feature that may assist in the differential diagnosis of meningioma from oligodendroglioma invading the meninges. It also helps in differentiating an anaplastic glioblastoma with desmoplasia from a meningeal sarcoma. A number of carcinomas, including those originating from the lung, kidney, ovary, endometrium, breast, and especially the prostate, show various degrees of immunoreactivity. Despite these various cross-reactions, the Leu 7 antibody has in practice been useful in the elucidation of diagnostic problems that could not be resolved with traditional special stains.

## *Human Neuroectodermal Tumor-Associated Antigens*

According to Bullard and Bigner,[34] those currently defined by monoclonal antibodies can be divided into four groups: (1) biochemically defined markers, which have already been discussed with the group of intermediate filament proteins and of soluble proteins such as the S-100 protein and NSE; (2) markers shared by neural and lymphoid cells, which include the HNK-1 antigen (noted above) and the murine Thy-1 antigen; (3) shared neuroectodermal-oncofetal markers, which include antigens that have been demonstrated on human neuroectodermal tumors, human fetal neural tissues, and glioma- or neuroblastoma-derived cell lines, and which have been reported to result in patterns of restricted reactivity that may possibly help in the recognition of some of the less differentiated tumor cell types when panels of monoclonal antibodies are used; and (4) putative tumor-restricted markers, which so far have not been recognized as specific for any particular type of human neural tumor, but have been claimed to be useful in animal tumor models.

## *Neuroectodermal-Oncofetal Markers*

Various antisera and monoclonal antibodies have been raised against such antigens shared by human fetal brain, human neuroectodermal tumors, and glioma, neuroblastoma, and melanoma cell lines.[34] Their pattern of recognition is usually complex and indicates considerable antigenic heterogeneity on the part of human gliomas and their cell lines. The use of different panels of monoclonal antibodies may be useful in permitting the differential diagnosis of highly anaplastic small round-cell tumors, especially in distinguishing poorly differentiated metastatic carcinoma, neuroblastoma, and malignant lymphoma.

### Nonneural-Associated Markers

In the present context, we are especially concerned with two such determinants: the cytokeratins and the epithelial membrane antigen.

The cytokeratins are extensively used as markers to classify epithelial neoplasms and, in cerebral tumors, to help recognize poorly differentiated metastatic carcinoma and to confirm the diagnosis of chordoma. The expression of cytokeratin in meningiomas, in which it may be coexpressed with vimentin, emphasizes the dual nature and function of arachnoid cells and their neoplasms. Concomitant expression of vimentin and cytokeratin is also found in chordomas.

We recently noted that cytokeratin may be expressed in the epithelial-like areas of glioblastomas and gliosarcomas, thus representing a rare but extreme form of cellular metaplasia.[6] It may also constitute an early expression of differentiation in immature germ cell tumors in the CNS, including germinomas and yolk sac carcinomas.[35]

The epithelial membrane antigen (EMA) is a glycoprotein originally demonstrated in human milk fat globule membranes and which has turned out to be an important marker for most normal and neoplastic epithelial cells, especially in distinguishing between anaplastic carcinoma and malignant lymphoma. In some cases it is superior to cytokeratin. Positivity for EMA, however, extends beyond cells of epithelial origin and includes the fetal notochord, chordomas, mesotheliomas, synovial and epithelial sarcomas as well as a large number of meningiomas. We also found that the luminal lining surface of normal ependymal cells as well as scattered normal epithelial cells of the choroid plexus are immunopositive and that occasionally the cells of malignant astrocytomas and ependymomas are reactive (Perentes, unpublished observations). Twenty-five oligodendrogliomas tested for EMA in our laboratory were negative. Neoplastic glial cells were also reported to be immunopositive by others.[36] The foci exhibiting squamous differentiation in the epithelial-like formations of glioblastomas and gliosarcomas[6] are immunopositive. Intracranial germinomas are also frequently positive.[3,35]

In our material, 19 schwannomas tested for EMA were immunonegative (Perentes, unpublished observation). The antigen is important in helping to distinguish perineurial cells from Schwann cells, because the former and their derivatives are consistently immunopositive.[27]

In differential diagnosis, EMA may help to distinguish a metastatic renal cell carcinoma (positive) from a cerebellar hemangioblastoma (negative), a meningioma (positive) from an oligodendroglioma invading the leptomeninges (negative), and a fibroblastic meningioma (positive) from a schwannoma (negative).

## KINETIC MARKERS

### Monoclonal Antibodies to Demonstrate the Proliferative Compartment in Brain Tumors

This approach may provide important information on the kinetics of human brain tumors. Thus, monoclonal antibodies have been raised against bromodeoxyuridine (BrdU), an analog of thymidine that is incorporated into the nuclear DNA in the S phase. The latter can therefore be estimated, especially in the more rapidly growing tumors such as anaplastic astrocytomas, glioblastomas, medulloblastomas, and malignant meningiomas.[37-39]

A human nuclear antigen, known as Ki67, is expressed on proliferating and dividing cells, and a monoclonal antibody raised against it was used to recognize the growth fraction of surgical specimens of human tumors, including those arising in the CNS.[40,41] The labeling indices of the nuclei obtained with this antibody reflect the grade of malignancy of the tumor. They range from 40 to 60% in medulloblastomas and carcinomas and from 10 to 40% in anaplastic astrocytomas and glioblastomas. The technique requires fresh or frozen tissue, and therefore paraffin-embedded material cannot be studied retrospectively. We have found it applicable, however, to smear preparations of neurosurgical material,[3] but consistent immunoreactivity is not always obtained.

## CONCLUSION

Immunohistochemistry has proved to be a powerful tool in the histopathologic diagnosis of brain tumors. It should be emphasized, however, that the technique is not devoid of pitfalls and that the identification of neoplastic cell types must therefore remain based on information obtainable by all the morphologic methods available. Thus, absence of immunopositivity does not necessarily mean absence of the antigen, whereas an unexpected immunoreaction may be caused by contaminating antibodies, cross-reactivity, or nonspecific binding to immunoglobulins. Therefore, appropriate positive and negative controls remain essential for accurate evaluation. Such controls include preabsorption of the primary antibody by saturation with the corresponding antigen when the latter is available or incubation with class-specific immunoglobulins instead of the primary antibody, particularly when monoclonal antibodies are employed, or both. Long incubation at 4°C with high dilutions of primary antibodies is important to ensure both consistency and high sensitivity. With mouse monoclonal antibodies, we have found the use of a rabbit instead of a mouse immunoperoxidase complex (resulting in a four-step reaction) to be invaluable.[3]

## SUMMARY

In this progress report, some of the most commonly used antibodies are discussed in regard to their immunohistochemical application to human neurooncology. The importance of determining the spectrum of antibody immunoreactivity in a wide panel of normal, reactive, and neoplastic tissues is stressed. In atypical and aberrant cases, immunopositivity needs to be interpreted with caution and in the context of all other available data. The demonstration of a well-characterized, cell type-specific marker in a tumor reflects not so much its cytogenesis as its differentiation potential and its capacity for metaplasia. The relation of an abnormal or aberrant expression of antigenic determinants to the process of neoplasia raises a number of intriguing questions to which research in the next few years will likely provide answers.

## REFERENCES

1. BONNIN, J. M. & L. J. RUBINSTEIN. 1984. Immunohistochemistry of central nervous system tumors. Its contributions to neurosurgical diagnosis. J. Neurosurg. **60:** 1121-1133.
2. RUBINSTEIN, L. J. 1986. Immunohistochemical signposts—not markers—in neural tumour differentiation. Neuropathol. Appl. Neurobiol. **12:** 523-537.
3. PERENTES, E. & L. J. RUBINSTEIN. 1987. Recent applications of immunoperoxidase histochemistry in human neuro-oncology. An update. Arch. Pathol. Lab. Med. **111:** 796-812.
4. KLEIHUES, P., M. KIESSLING & R. C. JANZER. 1987. Morphological markers in neuro-oncology. In Current Topics in Pathology, vol. 77: Morphological Tumor Markers. G. Seifert, Ed.: 307-338. Springer-Verlag, Berlin, Germany.
5. REIFENBERGER, G., J. SZYMAS & W. WECHSLER. 1987. Differential expression of glial- and neuronal-associated antigens in human tumors of the central and peripheral nervous system. Acta Neuropathol. **74:** 105-123.
6. MØRK, S. J., L. J. RUBINSTEIN, J. J. KEPES, E. PERENTES & D. F. UPHOFF. 1988. Patterns of epithelial metaplasia in malignant gliomas. II. Squamous differentiation of epithelial-like formations in gliosarcomas and glioblastomas. J. Neuropathol. Exp. Neurol. **47:** 101-118.
7. DOGLIONI, C., P. DELL'ORTO, G. COGGI, P. IUZZOLINO, L. BONTEMPINI & G. VIALE. 1987. Choroid plexus tumors. An immunocytochemical study with particular reference to the coexpression of intermediate filament proteins. Am. J. Pathol. **127:** 519-529.
8. STANTON, C., E. PERENTES, V. P. COLLINS & L. J. RUBINSTEIN. 1987. GFA protein reactivity in nerve sheath tumors: A polyvalent and monoclonal antibody study. J. Neuropathol. Exp. Neurol. **46:** 634-643.
9. VANDENBERG, S. R., E. E. MAY, L. J. RUBINSTEIN, M. M. HERMAN, E. PERENTES, S. A. VINORES, V. P. COLLINS & T. S. PARK. 1987. Desmoplastic supratentorial neuro-epithelial tumors of infancy with divergent differentiation potential ("desmoplastic infantile gangliogliomas"). Report on 11 cases of a distinctive embryonal tumor with favorable prognosis. J. Neurosurg. **66:** 58-71.
10. MØRK, S. J., L. J. RUBINSTEIN & J. J. KEPES. 1988. Patterns of epithelial metaplasia in malignant gliomas. I. Papillary formations mimicking medulloepithelioma. J. Neuropathol. Exp. Neurol. **47:** 93-100.
11. TROJANOWSKI, J. Q. 1987. Neurofilament proteins and human nervous system tumors. J. Histochem. Cytochem. **35:** 999-1003.
12. PERENTES, E., C. P. HERBORT, L. J. RUBINSTEIN, M. M. HERMAN, S. UFFER, L. A. DONOSO & V. P. COLLINS. 1987. Immunohistochemical characterization of human retinoblastomas in situ with multiple markers. Am. J. Ophthalmol. **103:** 647-658.
13. GOULD, V. E., B. WIEDENMANN, I. LEE, K. SCHWECHHEIMER, B. DOCKHORN-DWORNICZAK, J. A. RADOSEVICH, R. MOLL & W. W. FRANKE. 1987. Synaptophysin expression in neuroendocrine neoplasms as determined by immunocytochemistry. Am. J. Pathol. **126:** 243-257.
14. GOULD, V. E., I. LEE, B. WIEDENMANN, R. MOLL, G. CHEJFEC & W. W. FRANKE. 1986. Synaptophysin: A novel marker for neurons, certain neuroendocrine cells, and their neoplasms. Human Pathol. **17:** 979-983.
15. SCHWECHHEIMER, K., B. WIEDENMANN & W. W. FRANKE. 1987. Synaptophysin: A reliable marker for medulloblastomas. Virchows Arch. A **411:** 53-59.
16. KATSETOS, C. D., M. M. HERMAN, A. FRANKFURTER, V. P. COLLINS, C. C. WALKER, R. O. BARNARD & L. J. RUBINSTEIN. 1988. Dual neuronal and astroglial differentiation in cerebellar desmoplastic medulloblastomas: A further immunohistochemical characterization of the "pale islands" (abstract). J. Neuropathol. Exp. Neurol., **47:** 349.
17. GOULD, V. E. 1987. Synaptophysin. A new and promising pan-neuroendocrine marker. Arch. Pathol. Lab. Med. **111:** 791-794.
18. MIETTINEN, M. 1987. Synaptophysin and neurofilament proteins as markers for neuroendocrine tumors. Arch. Pathol. Lab. Med. **111:** 813-818.
19. KAWAI, K., H. TAKAHASHI, F. IKUTA, K. TANIMURA, Y. HONDA & H. YAMAZAKI. 1987. The occurrence of catecholamine neurons in a parietal lobe ganglioglioma. Cancer **60:** 1532-1536.

20. NAKAGAWA, Y., E. PERENTES & L. J. RUBINSTEIN. 1987. Non-specificity of anti-carbonic anhydrase C antibody as a marker in human neurooncology. J. Neuropathol. Exp. Neurol. **46:** 451-460.
21. BURGER, P. C., F. C. GRAHMANN, A. BLIESTLE & P. KLEIHUES. 1987. Differentiation in the medulloblastoma. A histological and immunohistochemical study. Acta Neuropathol. **73:** 115-123.
22. FELDENZER, J. A. & P. E. MCKEEVER. 1987. Selective localization of γ-enolase in stromal cells of cerebellar hemangioblastomas. Acta Neuropathol. **72:** 281-285.
23. VINORES, S. A., M. M. HERMAN & L. J. RUBINSTEIN. 1987. Localization of neuron-specific (γγ) enolase in proliferating (supportive and neoplastic) Schwann cells. An immunohisto- and electron-immunocytochemical study of ganglioneuroblastoma and schwannomas. Histochem. J. **19:** 439-448.
24. CRAS, P., J. J. MARTIN & J. GHEUENS. 1988. γ-enolase and glial fibrillary acidic protein in nervous system tumors. An immunohistochemical study using specific monoclonal antibodies. Acta Neuropathol. **75:** 377-384.
25. GOTO, S., Y. MATSUKADO, Y. MIHARA, N. INOUE & E. MIYAMOTO. 1987. An immunocytochemical demonstration of calcineurin in human nerve cell tumors. A comparison with neuron-specific enolase and glial fibrillary acidic protein. Cancer **60:** 2948-2957.
26. HESKETH, J. & J. BAUDIER. 1986. Evidence that S100 proteins regulate microtubule assembly and stability in rat brain extracts. Int. J. Biochem. **18:** 691-695.
27. PERENTES, E., Y. NAKAGAWA, G. W. ROSS, C. STANTON & L. J. RUBINSTEIN. 1987. Expression of epithelial membrane antigen in perineurial cells and their derivatives. An immunohistochemical study with multiple markers. Acta Neuropathol. **75:** 160-165.
28. HAIMOTO, H., S. HOSODA & K. KATO. 1987. Differential distribution of immunoreactive S100- α and S100-β proteins in normal nonnervous human tissues. Lab. Invest. **57:** 489-498.
29. LOEFFEL, S. C., G. Y. GILLESPIE, S. A. MIRMIRAN, E. W. MILLER, P. GOLDEN, F. B. ASKIN & G. P. SIEGAL. 1985. Cellular immunolocalization of S100 protein within fixed tissue sections by monoclonal antibodies. Arch. Pathol. Lab. Med. **109:** 117-122.
30. VANSTAPEL, M.-J., K. C. GATTER, C. DE WOLF-PEETERS, D. Y. MASON & V. D. DESMET. 1986. New sites of human S-100 immunoreactivity detected with monoclonal antibodies. Am. J. Clin. Pathol. **85:** 160-168.
31. VAN ELDIK, L. J., R. A. JENSEN, B. A. EHRENFRIED & W. O. WHETSELL, JR. 1986. Immunohistochemical localization of S100β in human nervous system tumors by using monoclonal antibodies with specificity for the S100β polypeptide. J. Histochem. Cytochem. **34:** 977-982.
32. KORF, H.-W., M. CZERWIONKA, J. REINER, W. SCHACHENMAYR, J. J. SCHALKEN, W. DE GRIP & I. GERY. 1987. Immunocytochemical evidence of molecular photoreceptor markers in cerebellar medulloblastomas. Cancer **60:** 1763-1766.
33. BONNIN, J. M. & E. PERENTES. 1988. Retinal S-antigen immunoreactivity in medulloblastomas. Acta Neuropathol., in press.
34. BULLARD, D. E. & D. D. BIGNER. 1985. Applications of monoclonal antibodies in the diagnosis and treatment of primary brain tumors. J. Neurosurg. **63:** 2-16.
35. NAKAGAWA, Y., E. PERENTES, G. W. ROSS, A. N. ROSS & L. J. RUBINSTEIN. 1988. Immunohistochemical differences between intracranial germinomas and their gonadal equivalents. An immunoperoxidase study of germ cell tumours with epithelial membrane antigen, cytokeratin and vimentin. J. Pathol., in press.
36. HITCHCOCK, E. & C. S. MORRIS. 1987. Cross reactivity of anti-epithelial membrane antigen monoclonal for reactive and neoplastic glial cells. J. Neuro-Oncol. **4:** 345-352.
37. HOSHINO, T., T. NAGASHIMA, J. A. MUROVIC, C. B. WILSON, M. S. B. EDWARDS, P. H. GUTIN, R. L. DAVIS & S. J. DEARMOND. 1986. In situ cell kinetics studies on human neuroectodermal tumors with bromodeoxyuridine labeling. J. Neurosurg. **64:** 453-459.
38. HOSHINO, T., T. NAGASHIMA, J. A. MUROVIC, C. B. WILSON & R. L. DAVIS. 1986. Proliferative potential of human meningiomas of the brain. A cell kinetics study with bromodeoxyuridine. Cancer **58:** 1466-1472.
39. NAGASHIMA, T., T. HOSHINO, K. G. CHO, M. SENEGOR, F. WALDMAN & K. NOMURA. 1988. Comparison of bromodeoxyuridine labeling indices obtained from tissue sections and flow cytometry of brain tumors. J. Neurosurg. **68:** 388-392.

40. BURGER, P. C., T. SHIBATA & P. KLEIHUES. 1986. The use of the monoclonal antibody Ki-67 in the identification of proliferating cells: Application to surgical neuropathology. Am. J. Surg. Pathol. **10:** 611-617.
41. GIANGASPERO, F., C. DOGLIONI, M. T. RIVANO, S. PILERI, J. GERDES & H. STEIN. 1987. Growth fraction in human brain tumors defined by the monoclonal antibody Ki-67. Acta Neuropathol. **74:** 179-182.

# Paraneoplastic Autoimmunity[a]

ANDREAS J. STECK AND E. NARDELLI

*Laboratory of Neurobiology*
*Department of Neurology*
*CHUV, 1011 Lausanne*
*Switzerland*

Paraneoplastic neurologic disorders are well known to neurologists and can affect both the central and the peripheral nervous systems. A major interest in these syndromes, besides the fact that the neurologic signs may precede the diagnosis of the neoplasm, resides in the interesting problems of pathogenesis that they present. New developments have implicated an autoimmune reaction in some of these disorders. In the last few years, a large amount of data have accumulated, showing that a high proportion of monoclonal Ig (usually belonging to the IgM class) of patients with peripheral neuropathy have antibody activity against various nervous tissue antigens. The demonstration of specific antibody activity of monoclonal proteins has provided useful leads in understanding the underlying pathogenic mechanism. Among the many types of autoantigens involved are structural lipids and membrane glycoproteins. Our laboratory has been involved in a comprehensive investigation of antibody activity of monoclonal proteins in patients with peripheral nerve disorders, and the present study attempts to define the major developments in this area.

## AUTOANTIBODY ACTIVITIES OF MONOCLONAL IgM IN PATIENTS WITH PERIPHERAL NERVE DISORDERS

Biochemical and immunologic analyses show that the usual target antigens in these patients are carbohydrate structures of glycoproteins or glycolipids[1] TABLE 1 summarizes the major antibody activities of human monoclonal IgM reported in patients with peripheral nerve disorders. Taking all the available data into account, it appears that more than 70% of monoclonal IgM from patients with peripheral neuropathy belongs to one or another of the aforedefined subgroups and that about half of all these IgMs are anti-myelin-associated glycoprotein (MAG) antibodies.[2] There appears to be a good correlation between nerve pathology and antibody activity. Patients with monoclonal IgM reacting with MAG have a demyelinating sensory-motor neuropathy,[3] whereas patients with monoclonal IgM binding to gangliosides GM1 and GD1b present a motor neuropathy simulating a motor neuron disorder.[4] Thus, as new antibody specificities are described, it may be possible to account for the large spectrum of disorders affecting patients with neuropathy in association with a monoclonal protein. A vexing problem concerns the specificity of monoclonal IgG or IgA in patients with

---

[a] This work was supported in part by grants from the Swiss National Science Foundation and the Swiss MS Society.

TABLE 1. Antibody Activities of Human Monoclonal IgM in Patients with Peripheral Nerve Disorders

| Antibody Activity | Clinical Syndrome | Chief Type of Nerve Injury |
|---|---|---|
| MAG | Sensory-motor NP | Demyelination |
| Acidic glycolipids | NP | ? |
| Gangliosides with disialosyl configuration | Sensory NP | Demyelination |
| Gangliosides $GM_1$ and $GD_1b$ | MND | Axonal |
| Chrondroitin sulfate C | Sensory-motor NP | Axonal |
| Phosphatidic acid and gangliosides | NP | ? |

ABBREVIATIONS: MND = motor neuron disorder; NP = neuropathy.

neuropathy. An autoantibody activity of these classes of immunoglobulins has yet to be defined.

## MONOCLONAL IgM WITH ANTI-MAG ACTIVITY

The major and best characterized group consists of patients whose IgM is an anti-MAG antibody. A sensory-motor neuropathy is usually the presenting symptom, an overt lymphoid proliferation is detectable in less than 40% of the patients, and many of these patients present a benign monoclonal gammopathy. Screening of anti-MAG activity is usually performed by an ELISA test (FIG. 1) or an immunoblotting assay. It is now well established that this antibody activity is associated with a progressive demyelinating neuropathy.[5] A constant finding on nerve biopsy is a splitting of the myelin lamellae, resulting in a widening that affects the external leaflets of the myelin sheaths. In some cases, a hypermyelination that can be as marked as that in a typical case of tomaculous neuropathy is observed. The monoclonal IgM reacts with the carbohydrate moiety of MAG and not with the polypeptide backbone.[6] Proteolytic degradation of MAG yields a number of immunoreactive peptides, the smallest with a molecular weight of 20,000 daltons. Whether only one or several glycosyl side chains carry the antigenic determinant is presently unclear. Species specificity was observed, suggesting differences in glycosylation, because these monoclonal antibodies react with myelin sheaths from humans, primates, calves, rabbits, and guinea pigs but not with myelin from rats or mice.[7]

Biochemical and immunologic data indicate that the carbohydrate epitope of MAG is shared with other glycolipids and glycoproteins in peripheral nerve and in the brain. Studies have identified the major glycolipid antigen in peripheral nerve as a sulfated glucuronic acid-containing paragloboside.[8] The carbohydrate moiety of MAG is also recognized by the HNK-1 mouse monoclonal antibody, which recognizes a surface antigen on natural killer cells.[9] In addition, the MAG/HNK-1 carbohydrate determinant is shared with several other molecules that are implicated in cell-cell interactions in the developing nervous system, including the adhesive macromolecules N-CAM, L1, and J1.[10,11] The intricacy of these cross-reactions may be related to the

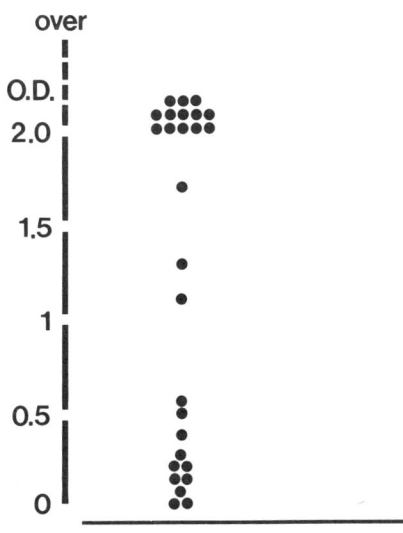

FIGURE 1. Detection of serum anti-MAG IgM antibodies by ELISA. Wells were coated with a LIS extract of MAG and sera reacted at a dilution of 1:1000. ELISA may provide a quantitative assessment of antibody, but it should be followed by the immunoblot procedure because the antigen preparation used is not pure.

recently reported homology between MAG and several neural cell adhesion molecules that are members of the immunoglobulin gene superfamily.[12]

A pathogenic role of these autoantibodies in the mechanism underlying the neuropathy is likely. Several studies have shown deposits of the appropriate class of heavy and light chain types in the affected nerves, with the IgM sometimes localized precisely to areas of myelin splitting.[13] Recently it was shown that intraneural injection of anti-MAG IgM in the rabbit causes focal demyelination[14] similar but somewhat less marked than that observed using rabbit antiserum to galactocerebroside, a major glycolipid of peripheral and central myelin. In this experimental situation, demyelination occurs acutely, which is very different from that observed in patients who present a human disease in there is chronic progressive demyelinating neuropathy. In humans, other mechanisms of antibody-mediated injury to myelin may be important, such as antigenic modulation or inhibition of remyelination. An explanation of the exact mechanism by which the anti-MAG antibodies cause demyelination in humans might result from a better understanding of the precise role of MAG in the formation and maintenance of myelin. In this context, it is interesting to note that studies of the quaking mutant, the primary defect of which is not known, but which has marked reduced levels of MAG, have revealed an abnormally widened space between the axon and the innermost myelin lamellae.[15]

## OTHER AUTOANTIBODY ACTIVITIES

A high proportion of patients with neuropathy and IgM monoclonal protein are found to react with glycolipids.[16] When the reactivity of these monoclonal antibodies is determined by ELISA with different glycosphyngolipids, they show a high degree of cross-reactivity as well as different patterns of specificity (FIG. 2). Such a degree of heterogeneity may reflect differences in reactivity between one monoclonal IgM and another as well as the presence of shared epitopes among these closely related molecules.

There have been reports of the identification and isolation of a new monoclonal IgM antibody with a distinct anti-GM1 and anti-GD1b reactivity.[4,17] This autoantibody activity is of interest for the following reasons: (1) it is associated with a motor neuron disease-like syndrome; and (2) GM1 and GD1b are major nervous tissue gangliosides. This paraneoplastic motor neuron disease syndrome may occasionally be difficult to distinguish from ALS, but uncommon pyramidal signs, electrodiagnostic studies with slowing of nerve conduction, as well as appropriate immunologic investigations may identify this subgroup of patients who have a better prognosis and may benefit from specific therapy.

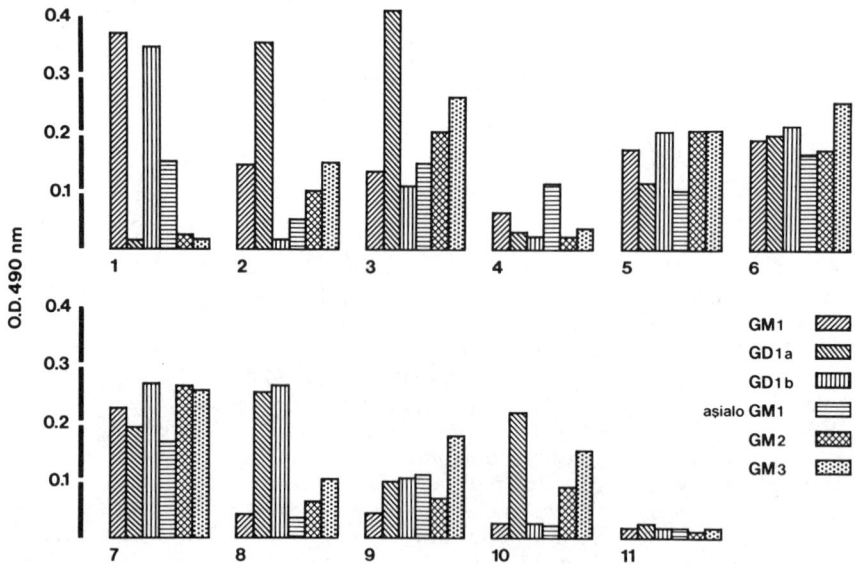

**FIGURE 2.** ELISA reactivity patterns of nine sera selected from patients with neuropathy and M-IgM binding to a crude preparation of gangliosides. Wells were coated with 5 µg of each glycolipid in methanol. Case 11 is a patient with Waldenström's disease and no neuropathy. Case 4 is a patient with a lymphoma and an IgG monoclonal protein. The anti-GM1 and asialo-GM1 activity was associated with IgM antibodies.

The pathogenesis of motor neuron disease is still obscure, and association with serum paraprotein has been reported.[18] Paraproteins of the IgG, IgM, and IgE classes have been identified in the sera of several patients presenting with a neurologic illness typical of ALS. The precise association between motor neuron disorder and paraproteinemia is unknown and could be purely coincidental. Conversely, a possible autoimmune mechanism of motor neuron disease associated with paraprotein is likely in those cases in which the M-protein has an antibody activity against a nervous tissue antigen. Thus, the few cases of motor neuron disease associated with an IgM M-protein with an antibody activity directed to gangliosides are of particular interest. In these patients, the IgM M-protein reacts with gangliosides GM1 and GD1b (FIG. 3) and cross-reacts with asialo-GM1. It has been suggested that the epitope is the

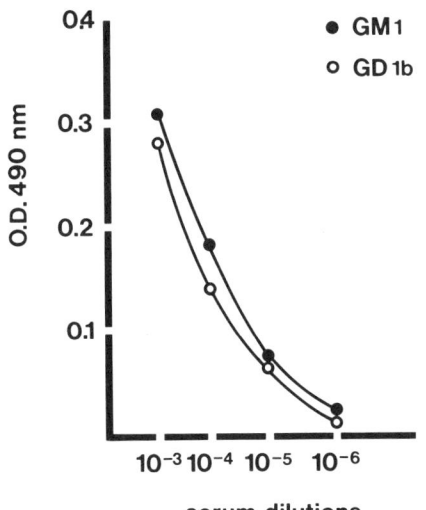

FIGURE 3. Binding curve of patient's serum (case 1) to GM1 and GD1b by ELISA at various serum dilutions.

Gal $\beta$ (1-3) GAL-NAc moiety shared by the three glycolipids (4). However, our own studies with different lectins, including peanut agglutinin, a lectin binding to the GAL $\beta$ (1-3) GAL-NAc disaccharide, suggest that the reactive epitope may be slightly different. Thus, peanut lectin inhibits the binding of IgM H.A. to GM1 and asialo-GM1 but not to GD1b (FIG. 4). Therefore, peanut agglutinin and the human M-IgM share a common binding site, but they must differ slightly in their sugar binding specificity. Helix pomatia, a lectin binding to $\alpha$-linked GAL-NAc is noninhibitory. Recently, we observed an M-IgM from a patient (A.W.) with neuropathy with an apparent specificity towards gangliosides GM1 and GD1a.[17] Here it appears that the epitope involves neuraminic acid because *Limulus polyphemus*, a lectin binding to terminal neuraminic acid, blocks the binding of the patient's M-IgM to GM1 and GD1a (FIG. 4).

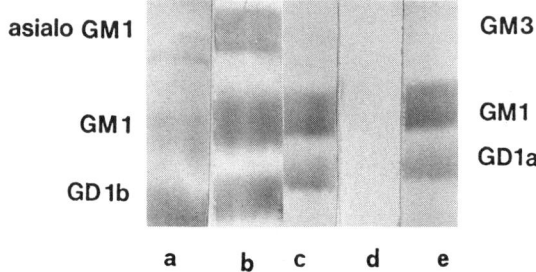

FIGURE 4. Gangliosides separated on TLC plates were immunostained with the sera of patients by an antihuman IgM peroxidase-labeled antibody. (b) Binding of patient's H.A. M-IgM (patient 1 in FIG. 2) to GM1, GD1b, and asialo-GM1; (a) inhibition of binding to GM1 and asialo-GM1 but not to GD1b by preincubation with peanut agglutinin; (c) binding of patient's A.W. M-IgM (patient 2 in FIG. 2) to GM1 and GD1a; (d) complete inhibition of binding by preincubation with *Limulus polyphemus*; (e) absence of inhibition by peanut lectin.

The presently available biochemical data suggest that human M-IgM reacting with ganglioside appears to display a degree of heterogeneity but may recognize a few immunodominant oligosaccharides. This finding correlates well with previously reported results showing a variety of patterns of reactivity among mouse monoclonal antibodies to the ganglioside GM1.[19] With respect to immunocytochemical staining, human M-IgMs with specificity for GM1 have been shown to react with granular cells in cerebellum and white matter as well as with axons in peripheral nerves. Such a distribution is in keeping with the widespread localization of ganglioside GM1 in both neuronal membrane and myelin. In patients with M-IgM with antibody activity for GM1 and GD1b, the mechanism of nerve injury is not known, nor is the reason for the predominant involvement of motor neurons. These neurons could be especially susceptible to antibodies reacting with cell surface receptors, such as gangliosides, because of the possibility that binding at the nerve terminal may result in internalization and retrograde transport of the antibody to the cell soma.[20]

Other autoantibody activities against phospholipids or phosphorylated epitopes should prove to be relatively frequent among M-IgMs. Recent studies report that an M-IgM from a patient with a slowly progressive sensory-motor neuropathy binding to myelin and to DNA appear to have a specificity for a conformational epitope formed by phosphatidic acid and gangliosides.[21] The identity of the reactive epitope in myelin is unknown, but it could involve a myelin phosphoprotein. This finding suggests that antibodies to DNA cross-reacting with phosphorylated epitopes in neural tissue may possibly cause neurologic dysfunction.

## THE ORIGIN OF MONOCLONAL AUTOANTIBODIES

Some of these monoclonal autoantibodies show a wide spectrum of cross-reactivity, and the autoreactive antigen(s) does not necessarily represent the immunogen. Whether these autoreactive proliferating B-cell clones result from stimulation by internal or external antigens is debatable. One may recall, for instance, that monoclonal antibodies to DNA may cross-react, on one hand, with various autoantigens[21] and, on the other, with bacterial polysaccharides.[22] In the human anti-MAG IgM system, the existence of a cross-reactive epitope between MAG and NK-cells may have consequences for immune regulation.[23] With IgM antibodies to gangliosides GM1 and GD1b, there is evidence that the reactive disaccharide GAL $\beta$ (1-3) GAL-NAc may represent a cross-reactive epitope with sialomucins in normal as well as neoplastic breast tissue[24] (FIG. 5). Circumstantial evidence supporting the idea that a tumor cell determinant could trigger autoimmunity is provided by the clinical history of breast cancer in one of our patients. However, the absence of underlying neoplasia in most of the dysglobulinemic neuropathies suggests that other factors are involved. In fact, the extraordinary high frequency of some autoantibody activity of monoclonal IgM, such as the anti-MAG activity, may reflect triggering by other signals. A variety of factors including viruses, oncogenes, or growth factors could activate autoantibody, producing B-cell clones.

There are some similarities between the specificities of many human monoclonal Igs and the so-called natural autoantibodies found in significant number in the normal human B-cell repertoire.[25] Recently, it was shown that a fraction of B-lymphocytes that have the Leu-1 marker are capable of making autoantibodies similar to those found in systemic lupus erythematosus and rheumatoid arthritis.[26] However, there is

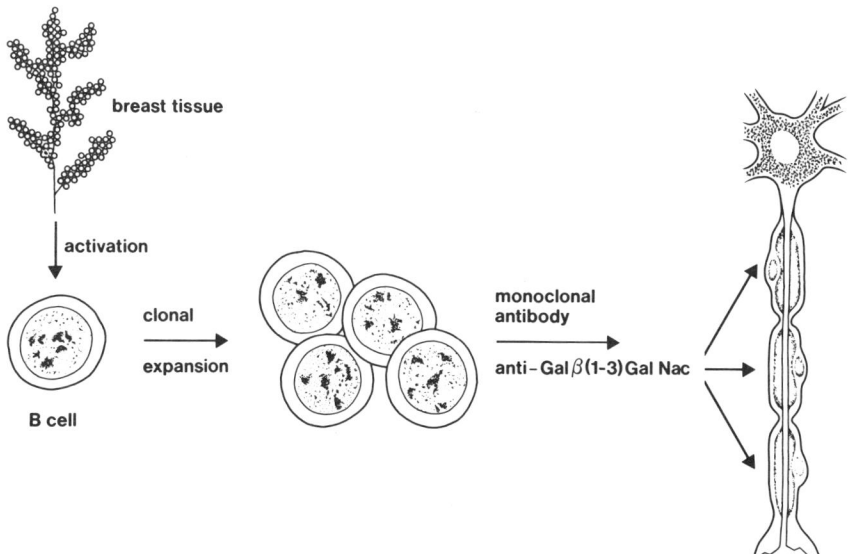

FIGURE 5. Pathogenetic significance of cross-reactions in motor neuropathy associated with IgM monoclonal antibodies to GM1 and GD1b. The shared antigen between breast tissue and motor neuron is postulated to be the Gal $\beta$ (1-3) Gal NAc sugar epitope.

so far no evidence that the anti-MAG IgM or other monoclonal IgM autoantibodies originate from such a separate lineage of B cells.[27] It should also be pointed out that a close relationship between the natural IgM autoantibodies and some pathogenic IgG antibodies of autoimmune diseases is far from proven.

The study of patients with monoclonal autoantibodies, therefore, certainly remains a fertile field for future research on antibody-mediated neurologic diseases as well as immunoproliferative disorder of B cells and autoimmunity in general.

## REFERENCES

1. STECK, A. J., N. MURRAY, K. DELLAGI, J. C. BROUET & M. SELIGMANN. 1987. Ann. Neurol. 22: 764-767.
2. MURRAY, N., N. PAGE & A. J. STECK. 1985. Ann. Neurol. 19: 473-478.
3. STECK, A. J., N. MURRAY, C. MEIER, N. PAGE & G. PERRUISSEAU. 1983. Neurology. 33: 19-23.
4. FREDDO, L., R. K. YU, N. LATOV, P. D. DONOFRIO, A. P. HAYS, H. S. GREENBERG, J. W. ALBERS, A. G. ALLESSI & D. KEREN. 1986. 36: 454-458.
5. HAFLER, D. A., D. JOHNSON, J. J. KELLY, M. PANITCH, R. KYLE & H. L. WEINER. 1986. Neurology 36: 75-77.
6. ILYAS, A. A., R. H. QUARLES, T. D. MACINTOSH, M. J. DOBERSEN, B. D. TRAPP, M. C. DALAKAS & R. D. BRADY. 1984. Proc. Natl. Acad. Sci. USA 81: 1225-1229.
7. STECK, A. J., N. MURRAY, M. VANDEVELDE & A. J. ZURBRIGGEN. 1983. J. Neuroimmunol. 5: 145-156.

8. ARIGA, T., T. KOHRIYAMA, L. FREDDO, N. LATOV, M. SAITO, K. KON, S. ANDO, M. SUSUKI, M. E. HEMLING, K. L. RINEHART, S. KUSUNOKI & R. K. YU. 1987. J. Biol. Chem. **262:** 848-853.
9. MCGARRY, K. C., S. L. HEFLAND, H. QUARLES & J. C. RODER. 1983. Nature **306:** 376-378.
10. POLTORAK, M., A. J. STECK & M. SCHACHNER. 1986. Neurosci. Lett. **65:** 199-203.
11. TUCKER, G. C., K. DELLAGI, C. SCHMITT, J. C. BROUET & J. P. THIERY. 1987. Clin. Exp. Immunol. **67:** 358-361.
12. SALZER, J. L., W. P. HOLMES & D. R. COLMAN. 1987. J. Cell Biol. **104:** 957-965.
13. MENDELL, J. R., Z. SAHENK, J. N. WHITAKER, B. D. TRAPP, A. J. YATES, R. C. GRIGGS & R. H. QUARLES. 1985. Ann. Neurol. **17:** 243-254.
14. HAYS, A. P., N. LATOV, M. TAKATSU & W. H. SHERMAN. 1987. Neurology **37:** 242-256.
15. TRAPP, B. D., R. H. QUARLES & K. SUZUKI. 1984. J. Cell Biol. **99:** 594-606.
16. ILYAS, A. A., R. H. QUARLES, C. DALAKAS & R. O. BRADY. 1985. Proc. Natl. Acad. Sci. USA **82:** 6697-6700.
17. NARDELLI, E., A. J. STECK, T. BARKAS, M. SCHLUEP, & F. JERUSALEM. Ann. Neurol. in press.
18. SHY, M. E., L. P. ROWLAND, T. SMITH, W. TROJABORG, N. LATOV, W. SHERMAN, M. A. PESCE, R. E. LOVELACE & E. F. OSSERMAN. 1986. Neurology. **36:** 1429-1436.
19. MAHADIK, P. S., H. LAEV & M. M. RAPOPORT. 1986. J. Neurochem. **47:** 1172-1175.
20. YAMAMOTO, T., Y. IWASAKI, H. KONNO & H. IIZUKA. 1987. Neurology **37:** 843-846.
21. FREDDO, L., A. P. HAYS, K. G. NICKERSON, L. SPATZ, S. MCGINNIS, R. LIEBERSON, C. A. VEDELER, M. E. SHY, L. AUTILIO-GAMBETTI, F. C. GRAUS, F. PETITO, L. CHESS & N. LATOV. 1987. J. Immunol. **131:** 3821-3825.
22. NEPARSTEK, Y., D. DUGGAN, A. SCHATTNER, M. P. MADAIO, F. GONI, B. FRANGIONE, B. D. STOLLAR, E. A. KABAT & R. S. SCHWARTZ. 1985. J. Exp. Med. **161:** 1525-1538.
23. MURRAY, N. & A. J. STECK. 1985. Lancet **I:** 321-322.
24. WALKER, R. A. 1982. Histopathology **6:** 571-579.
25. DIGHIERO, G., B. GUILBERT, J. P. FERMAND, P. LYMBERY, F. DANON & S. AVRAMEAS. 1983. Blood **62:** 264-270.
26. CASALI, P., S. E. BURASTERO, M. NAKAMURA, G. INGHIRAMI & A. L. NOTKINS. 1987. Science **236:** 77-81.
27. SPATZ, L., B. LIEBERSON, J. ABRAHAM, O. J. MILLER, D. A. MILLER & N. LATOV. 1987. Ann. Neurol **21:** 207-211.

PART III. CLINICAL NEUROIMMUNOLOGY

# Immunology of Multiple Sclerosis

### HENRY F. McFARLAND

*Neuroimmunology Branch*
*National Institute of Neurological and Communicative*
*Disorders and Stroke*
*National Institutes of Health*
*Bethesda, Maryland 20892*

Although the cause of multiple sclerosis (MS) is not known, an immunologic process is generally considered to be an important element in the pathogenesis of the disease.[1] Evidence of an immunologic mechanism is however circumstantial. The perivenular inflammatory response comprised of lymphocytes and monocytes is certainly consistent with an immunologically mediated disease and resembles the pathologic changes seen in postvaccinal encephalomyelitis, a disease of certain immunologic cause. The similarities between MS and a model of immunopathologic disease of the central nervous system (CNS), experimental allergic encephalomyelitis (EAE), also supports a similar mechanism in MS. The objections to the appropriateness of EAE as a model for MS have been partially overcome by the demonstration of an experimentally produced relapsing remitting disease with close pathologic similarities to MS.[2] The relationship between MS and EAE remains uncertain, but it is clear that the induction of MS is considerably more complex.

Further support for an immunologic mechanism in MS comes from the demonstration of abnormalities of immunoglobulin (Ig) and lymphocyte populations and function in the disease. Alterations in cerebrospinal fluid (CSF) Ig represent the most consistent immunologic changes described in MS, which reflects their diagnostic importance. The increased levels of Ig, largely synthesized locally in the CSF,[3] and the oligoclonal nature of this Ig[4] have led to the contention that MS may be directly related to antibody reactivity with components of myelin. Despite extensive investigations, a clear association between CSF Ig reactivity and the disease has not been established. Increased antibody levels to numerous viruses have been found, and in each case they represent a small fraction of the Ig present. Small amounts of antibody to myelin components have been described, but again it is unlikely that these antibodies are directly or singularly responsible for the demyelination.[5]

An alternative explanation for the increased Ig with multiple specificities is that it merely reflects the specificities of B cells or plasma cells that have migrated into the inflammatory sites within the CNS. The antibody specificities found in the CSF in MS are generally those found in high titers in the serum. This finding suggests that B cells with these specificities have a relatively high precursor frequency and, if circulating, would have a greater chance of migrating into an inflammatory site by chance. Although their accumulation may be random, the conditions permitting their differentiation into Ig-producing cells must be present within the CNS. Because the oligoclonal Ig pattern found in the CSF is often relatively constant over time, it seems likely that some B-cell populations or clones are maintained and undergo continued differentiation within the CNS. Generally, differentiation and Ig production require two signals, one of which is the perturbation of the Ig antigen receptor. If the antigens to which these antibodies react are not in the CNS, the continued differentiation of B cells must be due to factors in the CNS milieu that are capable of overriding the need for antigen binding to the Ig receptor. These factors could include lymphokines produced by an ongoing immune response or the presence of neurotransmitters with immunostimulatory activity.

With the exception of CSF Ig abnormalities, evidence of an immunologic process in the pathogenesis of MS points to a cellular immune mechanism. However, there remain fundamental unanswered questions concerning the nature of this process including: What is the mechanism of demyelination? What is the antigen responsible for stimulating this response and where is the antigen presented to T cells? Finally, what accounts for the fluctuating nature of the disease? Although there are no unequivocal answers to these questions, recent studies have begun to provide some insight.

## DEMYELINATION

Several immunologic mechanisms have been considered or suggested as the effector mechanism producing demyelination. These mechanisms include antibody or other serum factors, lymphocytes, particularly cytotoxic T cells, and macrophages. The eloquent ultrastructural studies of Prineas et al.[6] support the supposition that demyelination results from an interaction between myelin and macrophages. This finding is consistent with the observations that macrophages are the predominant cell population in regions of active demyelination. Importantly, macrophages that appear to be stripping myelin were shown to have coated pits. Similar associations between myelin and macrophages with coated pits were described in a relapsing form of EAE in the mouse.[2] These coated pits most likely represent the migration of receptors within the macrophage membrane. Included among the receptors expressed on macrophages are those of both the Fc portion of Ig and complement. Both groups of receptors are up-regulated with activation of macrophages in sites of inflammation, particularly those associated with delayed hypersensitivity (DTH) reactions.

Either type of receptor could contribute to myelin-macrophage interactions. Antibody to various components of myelin may occur in MS, and antibody bound to myelin could subsequently be bound to Fc receptors on activated macrophages. Antibody to galactocerebroside was shown to contribute to the induction of EAE in the guinea pig,[7] but it does not seem to be involved in disease production in the mouse or rat. Alternatively, complement may serve as the ligand between myelin and macrophages. Complement could certainly be fixed to antibody attached to myelin, and myelin can bind or fix complement in the absence of antibody. Macrophages express two types of complement receptors: CR 3 and CR 1.[8] In addition to being up-regulated on activated macrophages, the CR 1 complement receptor becomes mobile in the macrophage membrane and becomes associated with clathin-coated endocytic pits. Consequently, complement could form a bridge between macrophages and myelin by first binding to antibody-coated myelin or directly to myelin.

## T-CELL ACTIVATION

If activated macrophages serve as the final effector arm in demyelination, then what is the mechanism for activation of macrophages and why is not every inflammatory response in the CNS associated with demyelination? Activation may require lymphokines such as gamma interferon produced by activated T cells, and it would occur as part of a local DTH response. Still to be identified are the antigen(s) recognized by the DTH-initiating T cells and the site where antigen presentation takes place.

Either neural or viral antigens are reasonable possibilities. It was clearly demonstrated in studies of EAE that sensitization with MBP can produce an autoimmune disease often characterized by inflammation and demyelination. Recent studies showing that a relapsing form of EAE can be induced in mice by the transfer of T cells sensitized to MBP bring this experimental model closer to MS.[2] Furthermore, even the pathologic condition of these mice closely resembles that of MS. That MBP can be the relevant antigen in relapsing EAE is confirmed by the induction of the disease following transfer of T-cell clones specific for the amino terminal portion of the molecule.[9]

Evidence of an enhanced cellular immune response to MBP in patients with MS is meager. One recent study of a large number of patients in which lymphoproliferation was used to measure reactivity to MBP indicated that the response was only slightly greater than that of a control group.[10] The response to two other immunogenic components of myelin, myelin-associated glycoprotein and proteolipid protein, was not significantly different from that of the controls. In a separate study using T-cell clones generated from the CSF and blood of MS patients, none of the clones showed reactivity to MBP, whereas MBP-reactive clones were obtained from the CSF of patients with postinfectious encephalomyelitis.[11] In the same study T-cell clones were also generated from the brain of one MS patient who had died, and again, none of the clones reacted to MBP. These findings suggest that even at the site of demyelination, MBP-reactive T cells cannot be demonstrated. However, there are always questions regarding the age of the lesions sampled and the extent to which the clones reflect the repertoire of T cells in the lesions. Even the small response of lymphocytes from the blood to MBP noted in some studies may not be specific for MS because similar responses have been observed in patients with other neurologic disorders.

A relationship between a virus and MS is supported by epidemiologic studies of MS and the elevated CSF antibody levels to many viruses. Additional support for this relationship comes from studies of Theiler's murine encephalomyelitis virus (TMEV) infection in mice.[12] Neurologic signs related to demyelination occur one to several months following infection. The disease seems to be immunologically mediated, and susceptibility is influenced by the genetic makeup of the host. Genetic factors include genes in the MHC and at least one other set of genes outside the MHC and possibly coding for the beta-chain of the T-cell receptor.[13] Susceptibility to disease correlates closely with the ability to generate a DTH response to TMEV. On the basis of these observations it was proposed that T-cell recognition of virus still present within the CNS produces a DTH response that results in macrophage activation and subsequent demyelination. A process of this nature would not require persistence of infectious virus. Persistence of the viral genome and production of a single, even incomplete polypeptide that contains an epitope recognized by T cells and not antibody would be sufficient to elicit a T-cell-mediated DTH response.

Many studies have examined the reactivity of lymphocytes from MS patients to various viral antigens. Most of these investigations used lymphoproliferation to measure reactivity, and the results were inconsistent. Recently, the generation of cytotoxic T cells (CTL) was examined in patients with MS and in appropriate control groups.[14] A substantial number of patients had a significant reduction in their ability to generate measles-virus-specific CTL. In contrast, their ability to generate influenza-virus-specific CTL was the same as that of the control groups. Previous studies of measles-virus-specific CTL showed that they are CD4+ and that cytolysis is restricted by HLA class II antigens. These findings are distinct from those of CTL specific for many other viruses which are predominantly CD8+ and HLA class I restricted. The reduction in measles-virus-specific CTL is due to an approximately 5- to 10-fold reduction in their precursor frequency in peripheral blood and not their total absence.[15] The explanation for this finding remains uncertain. It could reflect a general reduction in a subset of CD4+, although preliminary evidence indicates that other CD4+ HLA class II restricted CTL are not reduced. Therefore, the alteration probably reflects a difference in the initial infection or in the mechanisms responsible for maintaining long-term immunity. It is also possible that if this population of cells was directly involved in disease production, the reduced frequency in the peripheral blood could be due to migration and sequestration of these cells within the CNS. Presently, however, there does not appear to be a correlation between the reduced measles-virus-specific CTL and the clinical course. Thus, the possibility of T-cell recognition of viral antigens in the CNS, triggering an immune response with subsequent demyelination, has remained an attractive hypothesis, but proof for it is lacking.

A final possibility is that a viral infection produces sensitization to a neural antigen either by increasing the immunogenicity of that antigen or through cross-reactivity or mimicry. A subacute demyelinating disease was produced with a coronavirus, the JHM virus, and this EAE-like disease can be transferred with lymphocytes boosted *in vitro* with MBP in a manner similar to that used in the adoptive transfer studies of EAE.[16] These findings indicate that infection with the JHM virus produces T-cell sensitization to MBP sufficient for subsequent transfer of an EAE-like disease. Sensitization to MBP following viral infections in humans was also reported. Studies of children with complicated or uncomplicated measles virus infections demonstrated that many children with measles encephalitis acquire a lymphoproliferative response to MBP.[17] It is unknown if this sensitization is produced by the release of MBP or is due to a possible cross-reactivity. Some minor degrees of sequence homology were reported between several human viruses and MBP.[18] The significance of these findings to MS is uncertain, but they do demonstrate that viral infections apparently can produce sensitization to neural antigens such as MBP.

## ANTIGEN PRESENTATION

To produce a DTH type of response within the CNS the relevant antigen(s) needs to be presented to T cells in the local environment. Cells that can function as antigen-presenting cells (APC) must be able to express MHC class II antigens on their membranes and to process antigens for presentation. Investigations over the last few years showed that two cell populations, endothelial cells and astrocytes, have the capability to express MHC class II antigens and can present MBP to sensitized T cells.[19,20] Although neither cell population normally expresses significant quantities of Ia antigens, both can be induced to do so when factors such as gamma interferon are used. When endothelial cells are obtained from animals with EAE, they express MHC class II antigens, indicating that this expression has been induced *in vivo*.[19] Studies of rats or mice susceptible or nonsusceptible to EAE showed that the ability to induce Ia antigens in cultured astrocytes from these animals correlates with susceptibility.[21] Similar differences in the ability to induce HLA class II antigens in humans could represent one of the genetic factors operating in MS.

MHC class II antigens can also be induced in rat astrocytes by viral infection. Even inactivated virus seems to be capable of inducing these MHC antigens on astrocytes, especially on those derived from strains susceptible to EAE.[22] Therefore, a persistent infection could contribute to expression of class II antigens and, in turn, could lead to presentation of either viral or neural antigens. Importantly, this possibility suggests that a persistent infection could be instrumental to disease production triggered by T-cell reactivity to nonviral antigens. These events are more likely to occur in association with a diminished cellular immune response to the virus because the ability to eliminate the virus would be reduced.

## REGULATION

One characteristic of MS is that it frequently follows a relapsing-remitting course, leading to the speculation that the disease may be related to an abnormality of suppressor cell function. In fact, deficiencies of suppressor cells were demonstrated on several experimental systems.[23,24] The finding that the number of CD8+ T cells, which includes suppressor cells, is reduced during periods of worsening has been inconsistent.[25,26] However, functional studies showed that suppression is reduced during progression or exacerbation. These studies measured suppression as generated by mitogens such as concanavalin A or OKT3 which binds to the T-cell receptor.[23] Similarly, the ability of CD8+ T cells to suppress Ig production following PWM stimulation is reduced, whereas other functional parameters of the CD8+ T cells such as CTL activity are normal.[24] A subset of CD4+ T cells, the 2H4 cells, which act to induce suppression through the CD8+ T cell, is reduced in MS patients with active disease.[27]

The autologous mixed lymphocyte reaction (AMLR) is considered an important technique in studying immunoregulatory processes, and several investigators examined the AMLR in patients with MS.[28-30] Generally, the response was increased during worsening. It has now been demonstrated that the greater response is due to a reduction in the generation of suppression which normally occurs in the AMLR.[29]

The significance of the various abnormalities of suppressor cell function is uncertain. Multiple sclerosis is not associated with multiple immunologic abnormalities, which casts some doubt on generalized suppressor cell deficiency, but episodic fluctuations in regulatory mechanisms could be involved in exacerbation. Alternatively, these changes in immunoregulation could result from the same process that triggers the immune response within the CNS. For example, up-regulation in HLA class II antigen expression could lead to increased reactivity in all of these *in vitro* tests and account for the apparent reduction in suppression. The significance of these findings is important to an understanding of the immune process in MS, and future studies hopefully will establish if these changes represent reduced suppression or enhanced reactivity secondary to the disease process.

## CONCLUSION

Evidence linking the pathogenesis of MS to an immunologic process remains indirect and tentative. It is increasingly certain that the actual destruction of myelin is caused by activated macrophages. What is uncertain is the mechanism for activation of these macrophages. Although an immunologic mechanism seems most likely, it is still possible that activation could be a direct result of a viral infection. Extrapolation from observations made in various experiment models indicates that the most likely immunologic process is the induction of a DTH response with subsequent macrophage activation. Either a neural or viral antigen could trigger this response, and the genetic influence on susceptibility may reflect the genes coding for the HLA class II and T-cell receptor makeup necessary for recognition of the relevant antigen. Failure to demonstrate unique or enhanced T-cell reactivity is disturbing, but it could be due to the techniques used or to sequestration of this population within the CNS. Sequestration seems the least likely and has little support for experimental models.

It is now clear that both astrocytes and endothelial cells can function as antigen-presenting cells. The nonspecific induction of HLA class II antigens on either population, but especially endothelial cells by lymphokines such as gamma interferon, provides an attractive mechanism for presenting antigen to circulating cells and triggering a local immune response that leads to demyelination. Periodic increases in HLA class II expression caused by nonspecific processes such as viral infections could provide a reasonable explanation for the fluctuating course of the disease. With continued disease progression the local production of lymphokines may become sufficient to maintain an ongoing immune response.

Demyelination may be enhanced by local production of antibody capable of binding myelin. B cells with appropriate specificities migrating into the inflammatory site would find both antigen and lymphokines necessary for B-cell differentiation. The continued differentiation of B cells with production of antimyelin antibody could contribute to the conversion of the disease from a relapsing-remitting course to one of continued progression.

The major unanswered questions concern the antigen and the role of the genetic influence on the response. The ability of T cells to recognize epitopes that consist of only several amino acids and that are not recognized by antibody may contribute to the difficulty in answering this question. Hopefully, techniques that allow manipulation of HLA genes and identification of characteristics of the T-cell receptor makeup, along with more specific immunologic methods, will contribute a greater understanding to these questions.

## REFERENCES

1. REDER, A. T. & B. G. W. ARNASON. 1985. Immunology of multiple sclerosis. *In* Handbook of Clinical Neurology, Vol. 47. P. J. Vinken, G. W. Bruyn, & H. C. Klawans, Eds.: 337-396. Elsevier, Amsterdam.
2. RAINE, C. S., F. MOHKTARIAN & D. E. MCFARLIN. 1984. Adoptively transferred chronic relapsing experimental autoimmune encephalomyelitis in the mouse. Lab. Invest. **51:** 534-546.
3. TOURTELLOTTE, W. W., M. J. WALSH, R. W. BAUMHEFNER *et al.* 1984. The current status of multiple sclerosis intra-blood-brain-barrier /Ig/g synthesis. Ann. N.Y. Acad. Sci. **436:** 52-67.
4. EBERS, C. G. 1984. Oligoclonal banding in MS. Ann. N.Y. Acad. Sci. **436:** 206-212.
5. LISAK, R. P., B. ZWEIMAN, J. B. BURNS *et al.* 1984. Immune response to myelin antigen in multiple sclerosis. Ann. N.Y. Acad. Sci. **436:** 221-230.
6. PRINEAS, J. W., E. E. KWON, E. CHO & L. R. SHARER. 1984. Continual breakdown and regeneration of myelin in progressive multiple sclerosis plaques. Ann. N.Y. Acad. Sci. **436:** 11-32.

7. RAINE, C. S., U. TRAUGOTT, F. MOHKTARIAN et al. 1981. Augmentation of immune-mediated demyelination by lipid haptens. Lab. Invest. **45:** 174-182.
8. ADAMS, D. O. & T. A. HAMILTON. 1984. The cell biology of macrophage activation. Ann. Rev. Immunol. **2:** 283-318.
9. ZAMVIL, S. S., P. A. NELSON, D. J. MITCHELL et al. 1985. Encephalitogenic T cell clones specific for myelin basic protein. J. Exp. Med. **162:** 2107-2124.
10. JOHNSON, D., D. A. HAFLER, R. J. FALLIS et al. 1986. Cell-mediated immunity to myelin associated glycoprotein, proteolipid protein, and myelin basic protein in multiple sclerosis. J. Neuroimmunol. **13:** 99-108.
11. HAFLER, D. A., D. S. BENJAMIN, J. BURKS, H. L. WEINER et al. 1987. Myelin basic protein and proteolipid reactivity of brain and cerebrospinal fluid-derived T cell clones in multiple sclerosis and postinfectious encephalomyelitis. J. Immunol. **139:** 68-72.
12. CLATCH, R. J., H. L. LIPTON & S. D. MILLER. 1986. Characterization of Theiler's murine encephalomyelitis virus (TMEV)-specific delayed type hypersensitivity. J. Immunol. **136:** 920-927.
13. MELVOLD, R. W., D. M. JOKINEN, R. KNOBLER & H. L. LIPTON. 1987. Variations in genetic control of susceptibility to Theiler's murine encephalomyelitis virus(TMEV)-induced demyelinating disease. J. Immunol. **138:** 1429-1436.
14. JACOBSON, S. J., M. L. FLERLAGE & H. F. MCFARLAND. 1985. Impaired measles virus-specific cytotoxic T cell responses in multiple sclerosis. J. Exp. Med. **162:** 839-850.
15. MCFARLAND, H. F., A. GOODMAN & S. J. JACOBSON. 1987. Virus specific cytotoxic T cells. Ann. N.Y. Acad. Sci. in press.
16. WATANABE, R., H. WAGE & V. TER MEULEN. 1983. Adoptive transfer of EAE-like lesions from rats with coronavirus-induced demyelinating encephalomyelitis. Nature **305:** 150-152.
17. JOHNSON, R. T., D. E. GRIFFIN, R. L. HIRSCH et al. 1984. Measles encephalomyelitis—clinical and immunological studies. N. Engl. J. Med. **310:** 137-141.
18. JAHNKE, U., E. H. FISHER & E. C. ALVORD. 1985. Sequence homology between certain viral proteins and proteins related to encephalomyelitis and neuritis. Science **229:** 282-284.
19. MCCARRON, R. M., M. SPATZ, O. KEMPSKI et al. 1986. Interaction between myelin basic protein-sensitized T lymphocytes and murine cerebral vascular endothelial cells. J. Immunol. **137:** 3428-3435.
20. FONTANA, A., W. FIENZ & H. WEKERLE. 1984. Astrocytes present myelin basic protein to encephalitogenic T cell lines. Nature **307:** 273-276.
21. MASSA, P. T., V. TER MEULEN & A. FONTANA. 1987. Hyperinductibility of Ia antigen on astrocytes correlates with strain specific susceptibility to experimental autoimmune encephalomyelitis. Proc. Natl. Acad. Sci. USA **84:** 4219-4223.
22. MASSA, P. T., R. DORRIES & V. TER MEULEN. 1986. Viral particles induce Ia antigen expression on astrocytes. Nature **320:** 543-544.
23. ANTEL, J. P., M. B. BANIA, A. REYDA & N. CASHMAN. 1986. Activated suppressor cell dysfunction in progressive multiple sclerosis. J. Immunol. **137:** 137-141.
24. ANTEL, J. P., M. K. NICKOLAS, M. B. BANIA et al. 1986. Comparison of T8+ cell-mediated suppressor and cytotoxic functions in multiple sclerosis. J. Neuroimmunol. **12:** 215-224.
25. WEINER, H. L., D. A. HAFLER & R. J. FALLIS. 1984. T cell subsets in patients with multiple sclerosis. Ann. N.Y. Acad. Sci. **436:** 281-290.
26. RICE, G. P., J. C. SIPE, S. L. BRAHERY et al. 1984. The failure of monoclonal antibody-defined lymphocyte subsets to monitor disease activity in multiple sclerosis. Ann. N.Y. Acad. Sci. **436:** 271-280.
27. MORIMOTO, C., D. A. HAFLER, H. L. WEINER et al. 1987. Selective loss of the suppressor inducer T cell subset in progressive multiple sclerosis. N. Engl. J. Med. **316:** 67-72.
28. BIRNBAUM, G. & L. KOTILINEK. 1981. Autologous lymphocyte proliferation in multiple sclerosis and the effect of intravenous ACTH. Ann. Neurol. **9:** 439-446.
29. CRISP, D. T., J. I. GREENSTEIN & J. E. KLEINER. 1985. Regulation of the autologous mixed lymphocyte response in multiple sclerosis. Ann. Neurol. **18:** 129.
30. HAFLER, D. A., M. BUCHSBAUM & H. L. WEINER. 1985. Decreased autologous mixed lymphocyte reaction in multiple sclerosis. J. Neuroimmunol. **9:** 339-347.

# Narcolepsy and HLA in the Japanese

TAKEO JUJI,[a] KAZUMASA MATSUKI,[a] KATSUSHI
TOKUNAGA,[b] TOHRU NAOHARA,[c]
AND YUTAKA HONDA[d]

[a]Blood Transfusion Service
Tokyo University Hospital
Tokyo, Japan

[b]Department of Anthropology
Faculty of Science
University of Tokyo
Tokyo, Japan

[c]Department of Research
Japanese Red Cross Central Blood Center
Tokyo, Japan

[d]Seiwa Hospital
Neuropsychiatric Research Institute
Tokyo, Japan

Many diseases have been associated with particular HLA antigens. Among these is the extremely strong association reported in 1973 between ankylosing spondylitis and HLA-B27.[1,2] Because the relative risk of ankylosing spondylitis is as high as 70% in HLA-B27 carriers, HLA typing has been valuable for diagnosis. For example, HLA-B27 is positive in about 80% of patients with ankylosing spondylitis, whereas this antigen is as rare as 0.3% in normal Japanese.

Ten years later, an exciting relationship was found between another disease and HLA antigens. HLA-DR2 has been identified in all narcoleptic patients so far tested in Japan,[3,4] England,[5] France,[6] and elsewhere, although some cases of narcolepsy without HLA-DR2 have been reported recently as rare exceptions.[7-10]

## MATERIALS AND METHODS

At the Department of Neuropsychiatry, Tokyo University Hospital, and Seiwa Hospital, Neuropsychiatric Research Institute, a total of 197 Japanese patients with narcolepsy were studied and 310 normal Japanese served as the controls.

The diagnostic criteria of narcolepsy are as follows: (1) recurrent daytime naps and/or lapses into sleep occurring almost every day for a period of at least 6 months; and (2) clinical confirmation in a patient's history of concurrent cataplexy for at least

3 months. The characteristic features of daytime sleep episodes and cataplexy were investigated by questionnaire and personal interview in 131 narcoleptic patients. HLA class I and II (DR and DQ) antigens were typed by a standard method using qualified local and exchanged antisera. Some narcoleptic patients were typed for HLA-D antigens using several homozygous typing cells (HTCs) including Dw2 and Dw12. Agarose gel electrophoresis followed by immunofixation with monospecific anti-BF antiserum was employed for typing of BF allotypes.[11] C2 allotypes were typed by thin layer, horizontal slab, polyacrylamide gel isoelectric focusing followed by a specific hemolytic overlay method.[12] Neuraminidase-pretreated EDTA plasma was typed for C4 allotypes by high-voltage agarose gel electrophoresis followed by immunofixation and C4-dependent hemolytic overlay.[13]

Haplotype frequencies in the patient population were calculated, and those in normal control subjects were obtained from family data presented at the eighth Japanese HLA workshop.[14] Seventeen families with at least one narcoleptic patient were examined to determine HLA haplotypes with narcoleptic genes.

Genomic DNA was isolated from peripheral blood leukocytes of narcoleptic patients and normal control subjects. The extracted DNA preparations were digested with restriction endonucleases. After electrophoresis and transfer to nylon membrane filters, the restriction fragments were probed with a $^{32}$P-labeled cDNA DQα probe. After washing, the filters were exposed to Kodak XAR-5 films. The patterns of bands obtained were examined to determine the HLA haplotypes of the samples.

## RESULTS

The features of recurrent daytime sleepiness were revealed in the responses of 131 narcoleptic patients to the questionnaire. In almost all patients the sleep episode did not last long, usually less than 1 hour. Daytime sleep episodes can be terminated easily by calling. In 79% of patients, sleepiness is irresistible. Three quarters of the patients feel refreshed after a nap as long as their nocturnal sleep is sufficient. Central nervous system stimulants, such as methylpheniclate, pemoline, and methamphetamine, are effective for daytime sleepiness in 100% of the patients.

Our definition of cataplexy is the sudden bilateral loss of skeletal muscle tone caused by strong emotional stimulation. All of the patients stated that their consciousness and memory are not impaired and respiration is not affected during episodes of cataplexy. Cataplexy lasts less than 5 minutes in 97% of the patients. In 99% of the patients, triggering emotional stimuli, such as roaring with laughter or experiencing feelings of pride, are pleasant. The administration of clomipramine or imipramine is effective in preventing cataplexy in 100% of the patients.

The frequencies of HLA class I antigens in 190 Japanese patients with narcolepsy and in 310 healthy Japanese are shown in TABLE 1. For HLA-A locus antigens, the increased frequency of A2 and the decreased frequencies of A24 and Aw33 were observed in the patients; however, the differences were not statistically significant. The increased frequencies of B35 and Bw67 in the patient were statistically significant. Conversely, the frequencies of B7 and Bw52 decreased significantly. A significant increase in Cw3 was also observed.

As shown in TABLE 2, all 190 patients with narcolepsy were typed DR2 and DQw1 positive, whereas the frequencies of these phenotypes in normal subjects were

TABLE 1. HLA Class I Frequencies in Japanese with Narcolepsy

| Ag | Patient ($n = 190$) No. | % | Control[a] ($n = 310$) No. | % | $X^2$ | Relative Risk | $\log_{10} p$ |
|---|---|---|---|---|---|---|---|
| A1   | 1   | 0.5  | 3   | 1.0  |        |      |       |
| A2   | 104 | 54.7 | 127 | 41.0 | 8.99   | 1.74 | −2.57 |
| A3   | 0   | 0.0  | 5   | 1.6  |        |      |       |
| A11  | 41  | 21.6 | 56  | 18.1 |        |      |       |
| A24  | 95  | 50.0 | 185 | 59.7 | −4.48  | 0.68 | −1.46 |
| A26  | 52  | 27.4 | 65  | 21.0 |        |      |       |
| A31  | 30  | 15.8 | 50  | 16.1 |        |      |       |
| Aw33 | 18  | 9.5  | 50  | 16.1 | −4.44  | 0.54 | −1.46 |
| B7   | 5   | 2.6  | 35  | 11.3 | −12.00 | 0.21 | −3.27 |
| B13  | 1   | 0.5  | 11  | 3.5  |        |      |       |
| B27  | 2   | 1.1  | 1   | 0.3  |        |      |       |
| B35  | 64  | 33.7 | 55  | 17.7 | 16.51  | 2.35 | −4.32 |
| B37  | 2   | 1.1  | 3   | 1.0  |        |      |       |
| B39  | 24  | 12.6 | 23  | 7.4  |        |      |       |
| B44  | 12  | 6.3  | 39  | 12.6 | −5.05  | 0.47 | −1.61 |
| Bw46 | 8   | 4.2  | 26  | 8.4  |        |      |       |
| Bw48 | 9   | 4.7  | 14  | 4.5  |        |      |       |
| B51  | 41  | 21.6 | 53  | 17.1 |        |      |       |
| Bw52 | 13  | 6.8  | 72  | 23.2 | −22.41 | 0.24 | −5.66 |
| Bw54 | 27  | 14.2 | 45  | 14.5 |        |      |       |
| Bw55 | 6   | 3.2  | 21  | 6.8  |        |      |       |
| Bw56 | 5   | 2.6  | 3   | 1.0  |        |      |       |
| Bw59 | 1   | 0.5  | 13  | 4.2  | −4.55  | 0.12 | −1.48 |
| Bw60 | 20  | 10.5 | 41  | 13.2 |        |      |       |
| Bw61 | 34  | 17.9 | 56  | 18.1 |        |      |       |
| Bw62 | 46  | 24.2 | 65  | 21.0 |        |      |       |
| Bw67 | 17  | 8.9  | 5   | 1.6  | 15.07  | 5.99 | −3.98 |
| Bw4  | 66  | 34.7 | 170 | 54.8 | −19.10 | 0.44 | −4.91 |
| Bw6  | 173 | 91.1 | 274 | 88.4 |        |      |       |
| Cw1  | 42  | 22.1 | 85  | 27.4 |        |      |       |
| Cw3  | 118 | 62.1 | 142 | 45.8 | 12.54  | 1.94 | −3.40 |
| Cw4  | 12  | 6.3  | 33  | 10.6 |        |      |       |
| Cw5  | 0   | 0.0  | 3   | 1.0  |        |      |       |
| Cw7  | 53  | 27.9 | 60  | 19.4 | 4.91   | 1.61 | −1.57 |

[a] Controls were randomly selected healthy Japanese subjects.

TABLE 2. HLA Class II Frequencies in Japanese with Narcolepsy

| Ag | Patient ($n = 190$) No. | % | Control[a] ($n = 310$) No. | % | $\chi^2$ | Relative Risk | $\log_{10} p$ |
|---|---|---|---|---|---|---|---|
| DR1 | 4 | 2.1 | 45 | 14.5 | −19.15 | 0.13 | −4.92 |
| DR2 | 190 | 100.0 | 104 | 33.5 | 211.99 | 752.89 | −35.0 |
| DR4 | 63 | 33.2 | 125 | 40.3 | | | |
| DRw8 | 17 | 8.9 | 84 | 27.1 | −24.07 | 0.26 | −6.03 |
| DRw9 | 20 | 10.5 | 85 | 27.4 | −20.26 | 0.31 | −5.17 |
| DRw10 | 1 | 0.5 | 2 | 0.6 | | | |
| DRw11 | 8 | 4.2 | 20 | 6.5 | | | |
| DRw12 | 17 | 8.9 | 41 | 13.2 | | | |
| DRw13 | 10 | 5.3 | 51 | 16.5 | −13.77 | 0.28 | −3.68 |
| DRw14 | 5 | 2.6 | 8 | 2.6 | | | |
| DRw52 | 57 | 30.0 | 178 | 57.4 | −35.55 | 0.32 | −8.61 |
| DRw53 | 83 | 43.7 | 189 | 61.0 | −14.19 | 0.50 | −3.78 |
| DQw1 | 190 | 100.0 | 213 | 68.7 | 71.77 | 173.99 | −16.6 |
| DQw3 | 70 | 36.8 | 157 | 50.6 | −9.05 | 0.57 | −2.58 |

[a]Controls were randomly selected healthy Japanese subjects.

33.5 and 68.7%, respectively. The relative risk of DR2 for narcolepsy was calculated to be as high as 752.89, and the relative risk of DQw1 was 173.99. Conversely, the frequencies of the remaining DR alleles, such as DR1, DRw8, DRw9, and DRw13, were significantly decreased as were the frequencies of DRw52 and DRw53.

Allotypes of HLA-linked complement markers (HLA class III antigens) of the patients and the controls were typed (TABLE 3). In C2 alleles in the patient group,

TABLE 3. Complement Alleles or Haplotype Frequencies (%) in Japanese Patients with Narcolepsy and Control Subjects

| Alleles or Haplotypes | Narcoleptic Patients | Control Subjects | p |
|---|---|---|---|
| | ($n = 46$) | ($n = 521$) | |
| C2*C | 87.8 | 93.9 | <0.05 |
| AT | 8.9 | 3.4 | <0.01 |
| B | 2.2 | 2.2 | |
| BH | 1.1 | 0.6 | |
| | ($n = 45$) | ($n = 487$) | |
| BF*S | 62.0 | 80.1 | <0.0001 |
| F | 38.0 | 19.8 | <0.0001 |
| F0.75 | 0.0 | 0.1 | |
| C4 | ($n = 43$) | ($n = 169$) | |
| A*3 B*1 | 46.3 | 53.0 | |
| A*4 B*2 | 15.3 | 12.0 | |
| A*3 B*2 | 13.1 | 3.9 | |
| A*3 B*5 | 6.1 | 5.7 | |
| A*4 B*1 | 5.9 | 1.5 | |
| A*2 B*Q0 | 3.6 | 10.8 | <0.005 |
| A*Q0 B*1 | 1.1 | 6.0 | |

TABLE 4. Estimated Haplotype Frequencies (per 10,000)

| Haplotypes | Narcoleptic Patients ($n = 190$) | | Control Subjects ($n = 414$) | | p |
|---|---|---|---|---|---|
| | Mean | SD | Mean | SD | |
| B35-DR2 | 186 | 55 | 11 | 2 | <0.001 |
| Bw62-DR2 | 129 | 54 | 16 | 3 | <0.25 |
| B51-DR2 | 114 | 54 | 9 | 2 | <0.05 |
| Bw61-DR1 | 94 | 53 | 6 | 2 | <0.05 |
| Bw54-DR2 | 74 | 53 | 3 | 2 | ... |
| Bw52-DR2 | 35 | 52 | 110 | 7 | ... |

the decreased frequency of C2*C and the increased frequency of C*AT were significant. The increase in BF*F and the decrease in BF*S were also significant in the patients. The frequency of A*2-B*QO C4 haplotype was significantly decreased in the patients.

It is known that there are two alleles of HLA-D antigens that associate with HLA-DR2, namely, HLA-Dw2 and HLA-Dw12,[15] and an estimated one third of DR2 associates with Dw2 and the remaining two thirds of DR2 associate with Dw12 in normal Japanese.[16] The aforementioned data suggest that an HLA marker primarily associated with narcolepsy might not be HLA-DR2 itself, but one of these two HLA-D alleles. This finding is also supported by the extremely different frequencies of HLA-B antigens on DR2 haplotypes between the patients and the controls (TABLE 4). This speculation was confirmed by MLC testing using HTCs including three Dw2 HTCs and a Dw12 HTC. HLA-Dw2 was positive in all seven narcoleptic patients tested, whereas HLA-Dw12 was defined in only one HLA-DR2 homozygous patient (Dw2/Dw12 heterozygote).

When genomic DNA from narcoleptic patients and controls was digested with Taq I and hybridized with a DQα cDNA probe, the patterns of bands obtained were distinct for each haplotype. As shown in TABLE 5, each of the five different sized bands was observed to associate with particular DR or D specificities. The 6.0-kb band was observed in all 11 patients with narcolepsy and also in some of DR2-, DRw6-, and DRw8-positive normal individuals. The frequency of this band was 54% in HLA-DR2-positive normal controls. On the other hand, the 6.6-kb band was observed in only one patient; however, the patient was a Dw2/Dw12 heterozygote. This band was also identified in some of DR-2, DRw6-, and DRw8-positive normal individuals. As for the HLA-D typed normal panel, the Dw12 homozygotes were positive for the 6.6-kb band and negative for the 6.0-kb band. Both 6.6- and 6.0-kb bands were observed in two Dw2/Dw12 heterozygotes. The 5.5-kb band was found in DR4-, DR7-, and DR9-positive and some of the DRw8-, DRw12-, and DR2-positive individuals. The 4.6-kb band was observed in the DRw11-positive subjects

TABLE 5. Association between DQα RFLP and HLA-DR or D Specificities

| Band | Specificity |
|---|---|
| 2.4 kb | DR1, DRw10, DR214, DR2S |
| 4.6 kb | DRw11, DRw12 |
| 5.5 kb | DR4, DR7, DRw8, DRw9, DRw12, DR2S |
| 6.0 kb | Dw2, DRw8, Dw19 |
| 6.6 kb | Dw12, DRw8, Dw18 |

and in some of the DRw12-positive subjects. The 2.4-kb band was identified in DR1-, DRw10-, and DRw14-positive individuals and in some of DR2-positive individuals.

Of the 111 patients with narcolepsy, 29 were positive for only DR2 (DR2 homozygotes and DR2/DR blank heterozygotes), and 82 patients were DR2/other DR alleles heterozygotes. As shown in TABLE 6, observed phenotypic frequencies were shown to fit with expected phenotypic frequencies calculated in a dominant model, and a recessive model was ruled out at $p < 10^{-28}$.

## DISCUSSION

The meaning of the word "narcolepsy" and the diagnostic criteria for narcolepsy differ among investigators. In our diagnostic criteria for narcolepsy, the clinical con-

TABLE 6. Observed and Expected Phenotype Frequencies in Patients with Narcolepsy

| Phenotype | Observed Number | Expected Number | |
|---|---|---|---|
| | | Dominant | Recessive |
| DR2/DR-[a] | 29 | 22.31 | 111 |
| DR2/DRx | 82 | 88.69 | 0 |
| DRx/DRx | 0 | 0 | 0 |
| Chi-square value | | 1.13 | 126 |
| $p$ | | 0.29 | $<10^{-28}$ |

[a] DR2 DR- = DR2/DR2, DR2/DR blank; DRx = DR alleles other than DR2; DRx/DRx = DRx/DRx, DRx/DR blank, DR blank/DR blank.

firmation of cataplexy in a patient's history is essential. As shown in TABLE 7, 202 patients with excessive daytime sleepiness were classified into 16 groups according to the combinations of symptoms related to narcolepsy, such as cataplexy, hypnagogic hallucinations, sleep paralysis, and sleep-onset rapid eye movement. For each group, the frequencies of HLA-DR2 were calculated. It was obvious that 100% of patients with cataplexy were HLA-DR2 positive, even though the frequency of HLA-DR2 in patients with excessive daytime sleepiness without cataplexy was high (58.5%) compared with that of normal Japanese (33.5%). If the other symptoms were used as criteria, HLA-DR2-negative cases would be included among cases of narcolepsy. If it is difficult to get a consensus for the common diagnostic criteria, it is quite reasonable to refer to HLA-DR2, because all of the researchers accept the value of HLA typing in the diagnosis of narcolepsy. In this case, cataplexy will be accepted as the most important symptom. In narcoleptic patients, sleepiness is often irresistible; however, so-called sleep attacks are not the only type of narcoleptic sleepiness. Sometimes patients can tolerate sleepiness with effort. After many years, so-called sleep attacks may disappear and only mild and tolerable sleepiness remains. Cataplexy is defined as attacks of sudden bilateral loss of muscle tone triggered by strong emotional stimuli

TABLE 7. Clinical Features and DR2 Frequencies

| CAT | HH | SP | REM[a] | Narcolepsy (no.) | Essential Hypersomnia DR2 N+ | Essential Hypersomnia DR2 N− | DR2 Frequency (%) |
|---|---|---|---|---|---|---|---|
| + | + | + | + | 92 | 0 | 0 | 100.00 |
| + | + | + | − | 25 | 0 | 0 | 100.00 |
| + | + | − | + | 8 | 0 | 0 | 100.00 |
| + | + | − | − | 3 | 0 | 0 | 100.00 |
| + | − | + | + | 3 | 0 | 0 | 100.00 |
| + | − | + | − | 1 | 0 | 0 | 100.00 |
| + | − | − | + | 4 | 0 | 0 | 100.00 |
| + | − | − | − | 5 | 0 | 0 | 100.00 |
| − | + | + | + | 0 | 3 | 0 | 100.00 |
| − | + | + | − | 0 | 5 | 7 | 41.67 |
| − | + | − | + | 0 | 0 | 0 | ... |
| − | + | − | − | 0 | 0 | 0 | ... |
| − | − | + | + | 0 | 0 | 0 | ... |
| − | − | + | − | 0 | 1 | 1 | 50.00 |
| − | − | − | + | 0 | 2 | 1 | 66.67 |
| − | − | − | − | 0 | 11 | 7 | 61.11 |
| + | | | | 190 | 0 | 0 | 100.00 |
| | + | | | 169 | 8 | 7 | 96.20 |
| | | + | | 160 | 10 | 8 | 95.51 |
| | | | + | 107 | 5 | 1 | 99.12 |

ABBREVIATIONS: CAT = cataplexy; HH = hypnagogic hallucinations; SP = sleep paralysis; REM = sleep-onset rapid eye movement.

unaccompanied by loss of consciousness. Drug treatment as with clomipramine or imipramine is effective in preventing attacks of cataplexy. These characteristics of narcoleptic cataplexy are useful in the differential diagnosis.

HLA antigens play a critical role in regulating interactions between immunocompetent cells. Without these cellular interactions, the generation of immune responses is impossible. It is possible to speculate on the same regulatory role of HLA antigens in cell-to-cell interactions in the central nervous system. However, this speculation seems unreasonable, because HLA class II antigens are expressed on very limited types of cells. It is also difficult to speculate on the possible immunologic mechanisms of a sleep disorder; however, Krueger et al.[17] reported that interleukin-1, which is a product of macrophages and a potent lymphocyte-activating factor, showed sleep-promoting effects in addition to its original activity. Further investigations are expected. If it is assumed that HLA antigen molecules are a direct cause of narcolepsy, it is interesting to question whether or not the molecular structure of the HLA antigen causing narcolepsy differs from the molecule of the same specificity in healthy subjects. If the difference in the molecular structure could be confirmed, the hypothesis in which HLA antigen directly causes narcolepsy, would be proved.

The other explanation for the association of HLA and narcolepsy is linkage disequilibrium. In this hypothesis, a gene causing narcolepsy is independent but is closely linked to HLA genes in the HLA-D region. The HLA genes serve as markers for the narcoleptic gene, because there is no direct method to identify this pathogenic gene.

For the time being, HLA-Dw2 is the most informative marker of the narcoleptic gene, because the frequency of this antigen among the markers in the HLA-D region, such as Dw2, DR2, DQw1, 2.4-kb band of DQ$\beta$[18] and 6.0-kb band of DQ$\alpha$, is lowest in normal subjects. Progress in this field of science will in the future provide the more polymorphic markers in each of these alleles; the associations of the disease with these markers will be stronger. Simultaneously, it is very important to estimate the frequency of the HLA-linked narcoleptic gene in normal subjects. If a genetic marker, which is found in 100% of narcoleptic patients, is defined in the same frequency as the aforementioned estimated frequency of the narcoleptic gene in normal subjects, all healthy carriers of this gene will be identified by this genetic marker. Recently, the presence of DR2-negative narcolepsy was reported. These cases are not only interesting but also very valuable. It is necessary to organize an international committee to collect the clinical information and materials of these rare cases and to evaluate these cases properly. To better understand the role of HLA in narcolepsy, it is extremely important to investigate these exceptionally rare and valuable cases extensively.

## SUMMARY

Narcolepsy is characterized by excessive daytime sleepiness and cataplexy. It had been reported that 100% of Japanese and Caucasian narcoleptic patients are HLA-DR2 and HLA-DQw1 positive; last year, however, exceptionally rare cases of DR2-negative narcolepsy were reported. Conversely, we tested 190 Japanese narcoleptic patients, and all were still DR2 and DQw1 positive. Among several symptoms in narcoleptic patients, HLA-DR2 showed the strongest association with cataplexy. Exclusive association has been demonstrated between narcolepsy and a specific band of *Eco*RI-digested DQ$\beta$ fragments. In this paper Taq I-digested genomic DNAs were hybridized with a DQ$\alpha$ probe, and five specific bands were observed to associate strongly with particular HLA-DR or D specificities. Interestingly, the 6.0-kb band

TABLE 8. HLA Alleles Associated with Narcolepsy

| HLA Alleles | Narcolepsy (%) | Controls (%) | Chi Square | Relative Risk |
|---|---|---|---|---|
| A2 | 54.8 | 41.0 | 9.30 | 1.75 |
| B35 | 33.5 | 17.7 | 16.47 | 2.34 |
| Bw67 | 8.6 | 1.6 | 14.29 | 5.76 |
| C2*AT | 17.8 | 6.5 | 7.7 | 3.1 |
| BF*F | 56.5 | 35.3 | 8.1 | 2.4 |
| DR2 | 100.0 | 33.5 | 217.8 | 780.6[a] |
| Dw2 | 100.0 | 10.0 | 49.0 | 479.3[a] |
| DQw1 | 100.0 | 68.7 | 74.2 | 180.4[a] |
| DQ:*Eco*RI (2.4 kb) | 100.0 | 39.7 | 37.6 | 150.0[a] |
| DQ:*Pst*I (12 kb) | 100.0 | 82.7 | 6.5 | 20.9[a] |
| DQ:*Taq*I (6.0 kb) | 100.0 | 53.6 | 14.4 | 49.6[a] |

[a]Approximate values calculated by a modified formula because one of the values in the 2 × 2 table was 0.

was found in 100% of 28 narcoleptic patients and in 54% of DR2-positive normal control subjects. For the time being, HLA-Dw2 is the better marker of the HLA-associating narcoleptic gene than is DR2, DQw1, 2.4-kb band of *Eco*RI-digested DQβ, and 6.0-kb band of Taq I digested DQα, because the frequency of DW2 is the lowest in normal control subjects.

## REFERENCES

1. SCHLOSSTEIN, L., P. I. TERASAKI, R. BLUESTONE & G. M. PEARSON. 1973. High association of an HL-A antigen, w27, with ankylosing spondylitis. N. Engl. J. Med. **288:** 704-706.
2. BREWERTON, D. A., M. CAFFREY, F. D. HART, D. C. D. JAMES, A. NICHOLLS & R. D. STURROCK. 1973. Ankylosing spondylitis and HL-A27. Lancet **i:** 904-907.
3. HONDA, Y., Y. DOI, T. JUJI & M. SATAKE. 1984. Positive HLA-DR2 finding as a prerequisite for the development of narcolepsy. *In* Proceedings of the 9th meeting of Japanese Society of Sleep Research, May 11, p. 8.
4. JUJI, T., M. SATAKE, Y. HONDA & Y. DOI. 1984. HLA antigens in Japanese patients with narcolepsy. All the patients were DR2 positive. Tissue Antigens **24:** 316-319.
5. LANGDON, N., K. I. WELSH, M. V. DAM, R. W. VAUGHAN & D. PARKES. 1984. Genetic markers in narcolepsy. Lancet **ii:** 1178-1180.
6. BILLIARD, M. & J. SEIGNALET. 1985. Extraordinary association between HLA-DR2 and narcolepsy. Lancet **i:** 226-227.
7. GUILLEMINAULT, C. & C. GRUMET. 1986. HLA-DR2 and narcolepsy: Not all narcoleptic-cataplectic patients are DR2. Human Immunol. **17:** 1-2.
8. LANGDON, N., C. LOCK,, K. WELSH, D. VERGANI, R. DOROW, H. WACHTEL, D. PALENSCHAT & J. D. PARKES. 1986. Immune factors in narcolepsy. Sleep **9:** 143-148.
9. ANDREAS-ZIETZ, A., E. KELLER, S. SCHOLZ, E. D. ALBERT, B. ROTH, S. NEVSIMALOVA, K. SONKA, P. DOCEKAL, E. IVASKOVA, H. SCHULZ & P. GEISLER. 1986. DR2 negative narcolepsy. Lancet **ii:** 684;-685.
10. MULLER-ECKHARDT, G., K. MEIER-EWERT, D. J. SCHENDEL, F. B. REINECKER & C. MEULLER;.HYECKHARDT. 1986. HLA and narcolepsy in a German population. Tissue Antigens **28:** 163-169.
11. ALPER, C. A., R. BOENISCH & L. WATSON. 1972. Genetic polymorphism in human glycine-rich beta-glycoprotein. J. Exp. Med. **135:** 68-80.
12. TOKUNAGA, K., K. OMOTO, C. ARAKI & T. JUJI. 1980. Genetic polymorphism of the second component of human complement (C2) in Japanese. Jpn. J. Hum. Gent. **25:** 287-283.
13. MAUFF, G., C. A. ALPER, Z. L. AWDEH, J. R. BATCHELOR, J. BERTRAMS, G. BRUNN-PETERSEN, R. L. DAWKINS, *et al.* 1983. Statement on the nomenclature of human C4. Immunobiology **164:** 184-191.
14. FUGII, Y., T. JUJI & S. KAIHARA. 1983. Family study of HLA-A,B,C, and DR in Japanese. Ishoku **18:** 189-203.
15. REINSMOEN, N. L., T. SASAZUKI, N. KANEOKA, H. OHTA, H. J. NOREEN, L. J. GREENBERG & J. H. KERSEY. 1978. Two distinct HLA-D specificities (DHO and Dw2) in linkage with HLA-DRw2 as defined in white and Japanese populations. Transplant. Proc. **10:** 789-791.
16. SASAZUKI, T., H. KANEOKA, K. TSUJI, Y. NOSE, N. KASHIWAGI & T. KANEKO. 1980. HLA-D in Japan. *In* P. I. Terasaki, Ed. Histocompatibility Testing 1980. UCLA Tissue Typing Laboratory, Los Angeles, pp. 274-276.
17. KRUEGER, J. M., J. WALTER, C. A. DINARELLO, S. M. SOLFF & L. CHEDID. 1984. Sleep-promoting effects of endogenous pyrogen (interleukin-1) Am. J. Physiol. **246:** R994-R999.
18. INOKO, H., A. ANDO, K. TSUJI, K. MATSUKI, T. JUJI & Y. HONDA. 1986. HLA-DQ beta chain DNA restriction fragments can differentiate between healthy and narcoleptic individuals with positive HLA-DR2. Immunogenetics **23:** 126-128.

# Neurologic Complications of Collagen Vascular Diseases

ROBERT P. LISAK,[a] PATRICIA M. MOORE,[a]
ARNOLD I. LEVINSON,[b] AND BURTON ZWEIMAN [b]

[a]*Department of Neurology*
*Wayne State University*
*School of Medicine*
*Detroit, Michigan 48201*

[b]*Section of Allergy and Immunology*
*Department of Medicine*
*University of Pennsylvania School of Medicine*
*Philadelphia, Pennsylvania 19104*

The collagen vascular or connective tissue diseases are diverse disorders in which multiple organ systems are usually affected and immunologic mechanisms seem to be of primary pathogenic importance. Neurologic dysfunction involving the central nervous system (CNS), peripheral nervous system (PNS), and muscle is frequent in systemic lupus erythematosus (SLE),[1,2] mixed connective tissue disease (MCTD),[3] and the primary vasculitides[4,5] and unusual in scleroderma and juvenile rheumatoid arthritis (JRA).[6] Neurologic abnormalities may herald the onset of SLE, MCTD, polyarteritis nodosa, and giant cell arteritis or occur much later in long-standing highly expressed disease such as rheumatoid arthritis (RA). Isolated or granulomatosus angiitis of the CNS, an exception to the usual multisystem diseases, is defined as being limited to the CNS.[7]

The neurologic manifestations of some diseases are protean. Patients with neurologic involvement from SLE typically develop encephalopathy, changes in mood, psychosis, seizures, and strokes. One of several types of polyneuropathy, myelopathies, aseptic meningitis, myopathies, and trigeminal sensory neuropathies also occur. The specific neurologic abnormality sometimes suggests a particular collagen vascular disease such as the trigeminal sensory neuropathy seen with SLE, MCTD, and scleroderma. Entrapment and compression of peripheral nerve, nerve roots, and spinal cord occur in disorders in which severe joint or thickening of soft tissue involvement, or both, is frequent, as in RA, ankylosing spondylitis, Reiter's disease, and rarely scleroderma.[8]

Problems confronting the clinician and investigator include: (1) categorizing and defining the heterogeneous neurologic manifestations and correctly diagnosing the particular collagen vascular disorder; (2) distinguishing primary neurologic involvement from involvement due to drugs, opportunistic infections, toxins, and involvement of other organ systems; (3) assessing the effect of therapy in diseases with variable natural history; and (4) determining immunologic mechanisms responsible for different neurologic abnormalities. The occurrence of multiple immunopathogenic mechanisms may be important in some diseases, and the possibility that more than one mechanism could cause the same neurologic syndrome must be considered.

## CATEGORIZING THE NEUROLOGIC DISORDER

Symptoms of nervous system involvement in collagen vasular diseases are manifestations of involvement of particular parts of the nervous system. Even when neurologic and psychiatric manifestations are categorized by suitably experienced specialists, there clearly are difficulties in making clinicopathologic correlations, especially in SLE. Some difficulties may relate to pathogenic mechanisms that do not result in obvious pathologic lesions (see below). Other problems may relate to inadequate analysis of neurologic symptoms, that is, distinguishing diffuse polyneuropathy from a subtle mononeuropathy multiplex and distinguishing a multifocal CNS syndrome from a diffuse encephalopathy. However, it must be admitted that even with the most detailed clinical evaluation and laboratory support (see below), there are clearly limitations to the approach of detailed clinical analysis. Detailed physiologic analysis is often not performed or described in large studies of patients even for standard techniques such as nerve conduction velocities and EMG or evoked responses.

Detailed brain mapping has not been employed to investigate cerebral dysfunction in collagen vascular disease. Standard imaging techniques have been of some help in defining involvement of the nervous system but not in precisely defining the anatomic defects responsible for particular focal, multifocal, or diffuse syndromes.[9] Magnetic resonance imaging (MRI), especially combined with injection of paramagnetic material that can cross an abnormal blood-brain barrier and combined with detailed clinical and neuropsychologic testing, may provide useful data.

The lack of clear-cut pathologic abnormalities in several entities, most particularly cerebral involvement in SLE and Sjögren's syndrome, suggests that techniques that assess physiologic and metabolic changes may prove of value. Evoked potentials and brain mapping have already been mentioned. A few studies have employed measurement of cerebral blood flow using inhalation techniques.[12] Rectilinear or proton emission tomography (PET) scanning with its capacity to detect and localize rapid changes in cerebral metabolism and blood flow needs to be combined with detailed clinical, neurophysiologic, and psychologic tests.[13] Nuclear magnetic resonance spectroscopy also could be employed in correlative studies.

## DISTINGUISHING PRIMARY FROM SECONDARY INVOLVEMENT

Patients with collagen vascular disease frequently develop neurologic symptoms secondary to medication such as corticosteroids, gold, chloroquine, and penicillamine. Metabolic abnormalities such as those accompanying renal failure may cause encephalopathies, seizures, and neuropathies. In addition, treatment with potent antiinflammatory and immunosuppressive agents frequently results in opportunistic infections that commonly affect the nervous system. At times the clinical picture or results of laboratory tests readily allow a distinction between secondary and primary involvement. However, many times this distinction is not possible.[8,14] As discussed earlier, part of the problem is the difficulty in defining the various neurologic syndromes. The other major problem is the lack of laboratory, physiologic, or imaging techniques that readily predict or mirror active nervous system involvement.

## EFFECTS OF THERAPY

The clinical course of many collagen vascular diseases is variable as are the neurologic manifestations. The uncertainty of the prognosis confounds therapeutic studies which are rarely, if ever, randomized, prospective, or controlled. Our incomplete understanding of the pathogenesis of many syndromes has also contributed to the controversy in planning appropriate therapy.

## IMMUNOPATHOLOGIC MECHANISMS

Entrapment and compression of nerves and roots, as noted, clearly are important mechanisms in some disorders. In most other instances of neurologic involvement there is only an incomplete understanding of the relative importance of the major immunopathologic mechanisms.

## ANTIBODIES TO NEURONS

The role of antibodies in the production of symptoms in clinical and experimental myasthenia gravis has been well established. Important to our discussion is that antibodies to acetylcholine receptor clearly can affect the target cell without necessarily producing irreversible cytotoxic effects in that cell. Indeed, it is clear that antibodies to cell surface receptors can stimulate as well as down-regulate. A potential for antibody-mediated changes in neurologic function in collagen vascular diseases exists, particularly in SLE, but a causal relationship is not yet established. There are numerous reports of antineuronal IgG and IgM antibodies in the sera and CSF of patients with SLE.[15-18] Assays demonstrating neuron reactive antibodies include indirect immunofluorescence on frozen brain sections, cross-reactivity with lymphocytes, cytotoxic effects on neuroblastoma cells, and more recently the isolation of a cytoplasmic protein antigen.[19] The latter finding parallels that of antibodies to cytoplasmic and nuclear antigens in some of the remote effects of carcinoma affecting the nervous system. Are these antibodies markers of disease caused by other pathologic antibodies directed against surface components or an epiphenomenon resulting from damage to that cell type caused by other mechanisms perhaps not immune in nature? Can antibodies to a nonsurface component be internalized by a non-Fc receptor-bearing cell and cause cellular dysfunction? What are the relationships of these cytoplasmic antibodies to anti-Ro seen in: (1) infants with congenital heart block born to SLE patients; (2) patients with neurologic syndromes that resemble multiple sclerosis; and (3) cognitive disorders in Sjögren's syndrome? Is there a parallel to two of the myositis-associated antibodies, anti-Jo-1 and anti-PL-7? Some subsets of neurologic disease are reported to have an increased association with antineuronal antibody, notably neuropsychiatric changes and seizures. What are the antigens that serve as the target epitope? Are there shared specificities with other tissues? An unresolved question is whether these antibodies originate in the sera and/or the CSF.[15] Reports of intrathecal synthesis of IgG usually depend on calculations fraught with error when the blood-brain barrier is disrupted. Do antibodies cross the blood-brain barrier by an active or a passive mechanism? Is there a role for antineuronal antibodies in collagen vascular diseases other than SLE? What are other pathogenic mechanisms of neuro-SLE? The vasculopathies in SLE may not have an inflammatory component; there are data suggesting that the development of vascular inflammation in association with antibody deposition in blood vessels depends on the level and duration of circulating immune complexes as well as host factors. Are the same features applicable in CNS as well as non-CNS vasculopathy?

## ROLE OF IMMUNE COMPLEXES

Immune complex disease is well defined in animals and is clearly associated with organ system damage in SLE, serum sickness, and some of the vasculitides. Immune complex deposition or deposition of aggregated immunoglobulin and complement with subsequent inflammation and damage to the vessel wall is likely responsible for some instances of vasculitis involving the nervous system in both primary and secondary vasculitides.[6,8] There is also evidence that immune complex deposition may be associated with the development of a degenerative noninflammatory vasculopathy as occurs in murine models of SLE. In human and murine SLE, immune complex deposition in the choroid plexus is well described as is the presence of immune complexes in the CSF.[21–25] Granular localization of immunoglobulins and complement components in the choroidal epithelium and choroidal blood vessels may be associated with neuropsychiatric abnormalities, seizures, and aseptic meningitis in SLE,[15,21] but similar histopathologic changes occur in neurologically normal patients. What are the clinical correlations of these serologic abnormalities? In addition, both encephalopathies and some polyneuropathies associated with SLE and vasculopathies indicate diffuse rather than multifocal disease. Are the clinical features accurate reflections of anatomic localization in these processes? Do hemodynamic factors principally control the site of immune complex deposition or do altered endothelial and astrocytic immune receptors guide deposition.

The role of immune complex deposition in inflammatory myopathies, temporal arteritis, and other vasculitides is less clear. Because demyelinating neuropathies are seen in SLE, hepatitis, and other postviral syndromes, it is possible that they play a direct or indirect role in the production of these syndromes. However, experimental vascular lesions of the PNS do not produce primary demyelination.[14] Although immune complex deposition is thought more likely to be important in the production of focal neurologic deficits, it is of interest that *in vivo* immune complexes have been reported to alter hypothalamic function, leading to changes in behavior and in fluid and electrolyte balance.[26,27]

Other possible consequences of immune complex deposition also include alterations in blood-brain and blood-nerve barrier that could allow larger proteins, including antibodies, access to the nervous system.[28]

*Vasculopathy Without Vasculitis*

Abnormalities of small vessels in the brain of patients with SLE with resulting microhemorrhagic infarcts are the most common pathologic finding at autopsy.[1,2]

However, frank vasculitis is distinctly uncommon. The development of a degenerative vasculopathy in some murine models of SLE has already been noted. The role, if any, of antibodies to endothelial antigens is uncertain in SLE and other disorders.[28] It has been demonstrated *in vitro* that complement components as well as cytokines can have adverse effects on endothelium. There is recent interest in the pathogenic role of circulating lupus procoagulant (anti-cardiolipin) in the production of cerebral infarction in patients with SLE as well as in those without collagen vascular disease.[31]

*Cell-Mediated Mechanisms*

Cell-mediated immunopathologic reactions have been the subject of investigation in polymyositis, dermatomyositis, and the acquired demyelinating neuropathies that can be seen in patients with collagen vascular disease.[8,14,33] Indeed, polymyositis is a frequent part of the picture of MCTD. There has been interest in the role of cells in the pathogenesis of vasculitis, especially isolated angiitis of the nervous system, a vasculitis not associated with detectable circulating immune complexes.

Some studies of vasculitis suggest a pathologic classification into neutrophilic inflammatory vascular disease (NIVD) and monocytic inflammatory vascular disease (MIVD), although some reports claim that these are merely stages in the development of the infiltrate.[34,35] Neutrophilic inflammatory vascular disease is the prototype immune-complex-mediated vasculitis. Although ischemia is thought to be important in the production of symptoms, the role of cell products, including free radicals, in the production of tissue damage is not known.

Isolated angiitis of the nervous systems appears predominantly to be an example of MIVD. Cellular mechanisms contributing to neurologic disease in the presence of systemic inflammation may be explored in the model of mononuclear cell vasculitides. Class I major histocompatibility complex (MHC) antigens, which are widely distributed in the body and are present on both the usual antigen presenting cells (APC) and endothelial cells, appear to have little specific role in the development of vasculitis. Class II MHC antigens, narrowly expressed as they are, provide a mechanism to maintain tolerance.[36] Gamma interferon or viral infection induces expression of MHC class II antigens on endothelial cell surfaces, thus providing a second signal that in combination with unregulated T help to autologous antigens may result in vascular inflammation. Questions arise regarding factors that incite class II antigens on endothelial cells, vascular smooth muscle, and astrocytes. Are the reactions evidence of antigen-specific hypersensitivity?

Other questions concern the role of cytokines. Little is currently known about interleukin-1, interleukin-2, and gamma interferon in *in vivo* lesions. The potential role of cytokines has not been explored, although it is clear that mediators may profoundly affect the function of cells of the nervous system. Alterations of lymphokines have been implicated in human and murine models of SLE. In SLE interleukin-2 from blood cells is decreased, but gamma interferon is normal.[37] Gamma interferon in CSF was reported to be increased in several patients with CNS involvement with SLE, although vasculitis, as noted, is unusual.

# SUMMARY

Despite the importance of neurologic manifestations of the collagen vascular diseases, it is clear that there are more questions than answers. The use of *in vitro* culture systems, *in vivo* models, and clinical and laboratory study of patients that attempt to correlate these findings with immunologic abnormalities, including parallels with animal models, should increase our understanding of these syndromes.

## REFERENCES

1. JOHNSON, R. T. & E. P. RICHARDSON. 1968. The neurological manifestations of systemic lupus erythematosus: A clinical pathological study of 24 cases and review of the literature. Medicine **47:** 337-369.
2. ELLIS, S. G. & M. A. VERITY. 1979. Central nervous system involvement in systemic lupus erythematosus: A review of neuropathologic findings in 57 cases, 1955-1977. Semin. Arthritis Rheum. **8:** 212-221.
3. BENNETT, R. M., D. M. BONG & B. H. SPARGO. 1979. Neuropsychiatric problems in mixed connective tissue disease. Am. J. Med. **65:** 955-962.
4. ALEXANDER, E. L., M. B. STEVEN, T. T. PROVOST & G. E. ALEXANDER. 1982. Neurologic complications of primary Sjögren's syndrome. Medicine (Baltimore) **61:** 247-257.
5. MOORE, P. M. & A. S. FAUCI. 1981. Neurologic manifestations of systemic necrotizing arteritis: Clinical and pathologic features in 24 cases. Am. J. Med. **71:** 517-524.
6. MOORE, P. M. & T. R. CUPPS. 1983. Neurologic complications of vasculitis. Ann. Neurol. **14:** 155-167.
7. CUPPS, T. R., P. M. MOORE & A. S. FAUCI. 1983. Isolated angiitis of the central nervous system. Am. J. Med. **74:** 97-105.
8. LISAK, R. P. 1986. Neurologic manifestation of systemic disease: Collagen vascular diseases. *In* Diseases of the Nervous System, Vol. 2. A. K. Asbury, G. M. McKhann, & W. I. McDonald, Eds. Ardmore Medical Books (WB Saunders Co.), Philadelphia: 1499-1509.
9. GONZALEZ-SCARANNO, F., R. P. LISAK, L. T. BILANIUK, R. A. ZIMMERMAN, P. C. ATKINS & B. ZWEIMAN. 1979. Cranial computerized tomography in the diagnosis of systemic lupus erythematosus. Ann. Neurol. **5:** 158-165.
10. VERMESS, M., R. M. BERNSTEIN, G. M. BYDDEN, R. E. STEINER, I. R. YOUNG & G. R. V. HUGHES. 1983. Nuclear magnetic resonance (NMR) imaging in systemic lupus erythematosus. J. Comp. Assist. Tomograph **7:** 461-467.
11. AISAN, A. M., T. O. GABRIELSEN & W. S. MCCUNE. 1985. MR imaging of systemic lupus erythematosus involving the brain. Am. J. Radiol. **144:** 1027-1031.
12. KUSHNER, M. J., J. CHAWLUK, F. FAZEKAS, B. MANDELL, A. BURKE, J. JOGGI, M. ROSEN & M. REIVICH. 1987. Cerebral blood flow in systemic lupus erythematosus with or without cerebral complications. Neurology **37:** 1596-1598.
13. PINCHING, A. J., R. L. TRAVERS, G. R. V. HUGHES, T. JONES & S. MOSS. 1978. Oxygen-15 brain scanning for detection of cerebral involvement in systemic lupus erythematosus. Lancet 898-900.
14. LISAK, R. P. & A. I. LEVINSON. 1984. Neuropathy in connective tissue disorders. *In* Neurology, Vol. 4. Peripheral Nerve Disorders: A Practical Approach. A. K. Asbury & R. Gilliat, Eds.: 154-183. Butterworth, London.
15. WINFIELD, J. B., M. SHAW, L. M. SILVERMAN, R. A. EISENBERG, H. A. WILSON & D. KOFFLER. 1983. Intrathecal IgG synthesis and blood-brain impairment in patients with systemic lupus erythematosus and central nervous system dysfunction. Am. J. Med. **74:** 837-844.
16. BLUESTEIN, H. & N. J. ZVAIFLER. 1983. Antibodies reactive with central nervous system antigens. Hum. Pathol. **14:** 424-428.
17. BLUESTEIN, H. G., G. W. WILLIAMS & A. D. STEINBERG. 1981. Cerebrospinal fluid antibodies to neuronal cells: Association with neuropsychiatric manifestations of systemic lupus erythematosus. Am. J. Med. **70:** 240-246.
18. DENT, P. B., S. K. LIAO & J. A. DENBURG. 1985. Antineuronal antibodies in neuropsychiatric systemic lupus erythematosus. Arthritis Rheum. **28:** 789-795.

19. BONFA, E., S. J. GOLOMBEK, L. D. KAUFMAN, S. SKELLY, H. WEISSBACH, N. BROT & K. B. ELKON. 1987. Association between lupus psychosis and ribosomal protein antibodies. N. Engl. J. Med. **317:** 265-271.
20. BERDEN, J., HM, L. HANG, P. J. MC CONAHEY & F. J. DIXON. 1983. Analysis of vascular lesions in murine SLE 1. Association with serologic abnormalities. J. Immunol. **130:** 1699-1705.
21. KEFE, E. B., E. F. BARDONA JR., R. J. HARBECK, B. PIROFSKY & R. I. CARR. 1974. Lupus meningitis antibodies to deoxyribonucleic acid (DNA): Anti-DNA complexes in cerebrospinal fluid. Ann. Int. Med. **80:** 58-60.
22. BOYER, R. S., N. C. J. SUN, A. VERITY, K. M. NIES & J. S. LOUIE. 1980. Immunoperoxidase staining of choroid plexus in systemic lupus erythematosus. J. Rheumat. **7:** 645-650.
23. PERRES, N. S., V. A. ROXBURGH & M. C. GELFAND. 1981. Binding sites for immune components in human choroid plexes. Arth. Rheum. **24:** 300-326.
24. SEIBALD, I. R., R. B. BUCKINGHAM, T. A. MEDSGER & R. H. KELLY. 1982. Cerebrospinal fluid immune complexes in systemic lupus erythematosus involving the CNS. Sem. Arthritis Rheum. **12:** 68-76.
25. SCHWARTZ, M. M. & J. L. ROBERTS. 1983. Membranous and vascular choroidopathy: Two patterns of immune deposits in systemic lupus erythematosus. Clin. Immunol. Immunopathol. **29:** 369-380.
26. HOFFMAN, S. A., D. W. SHUCARD, R. J. HARBECK & A. A. HOFFMAN. 1987. Chronic immune complex disease. Behavioral and neurologic correlates. J. Neuropathol. Exp. Neurol. **37:** 426-430.
27. HOFFMAN, S. A., D. W. SHUCARD, H. A. BRODIE, C. REIFENRETH & R. J. HARBECK. 1982. Suppression of water intake by immune complex formation in the hypothalamus. Implications for systemic lupus erythematosus. J. Neuroimmunol. **2:** 167-170.
28. HOFFMAN, S. A., D. N. ARBOGAST, T. T. DAY, D. W. SHUCARD & R. J. HARBECK. 1983. Permeability of the blood cerebrospinal fluid barrier during acute immune complex disease. J. Immunol. **130:** 1695-1698.
29. BEVILACQUA, M. P., J. S. POBER, M. E. WHEELER, R. S. COTRAN & M. A. GIMBRONE. 1985. Interleukin I acts on cultured human vascular endothelium to increase the adhesion of polymorphonuclear leukocytes, monocytes and related leukocyte cell lines. J. Clin. Invest. **76:** 2003.
30. COTRAN, R. S., M. A. GIMBRONE, M. P. BEVILACQUA, D. L. MENDRICK & J. S. POBER. 1986. Induction and detections of a human endothelial activation antigen in vivo. J. Exp. Med. **164:** 661-666.
31. MUEH, J. R., K. D. HERBERT & S. I. RAPAPORT. 1980. Thrombosis in patients with lupus anticoagulant. Ann. Intern. Med. **92:** 156-159.
32. DERKSEN, R. H., B. N. BOUMA & L. KATER. 1986. The association between lupus anticoagulant and cerebral infarction in SLE. Scand. J. Rheumat. **15:** 179-184.
33. LISAK, R. P. 1987. Immunology of neuromuscular disease. *In* Disorders of Voluntary Muscle, 5th Ed., J. N. Walton, Ed. Chap. 9,: 345-371. Churchill Livingston, Edinburgh.
34. SOTER, N. A., M. C. MIHN, L. GIGI, H. F. DVORAK & K. F. AUSTEN. 1976. Two distinct cellular patterns in cutaneous necrotising angiitis. J. Inv. Derm. **66:** 344-350.
35. ALEXANDER, E. L., C. MAYER, G. S. TRAVLAS, J. B. ROTHS & E. D. MURPHY. 1985. Two histopathologic types of inflammatory vascular disease in MRL/LPR autoimmune mice. Arth. Rheum. **28:** 1146-1155.
36. COWING, C. 1985. Does T cell restriction to Ia limit the need for self-tolerance? Immunol. Today **6:** 72-74.
37. SIBBITT, K. C. & C. W. SPELLMAN. 1984. Lymphokines in autoimmunity: Relationship between interleukin-2 and interferon-gamma production in systemic lupus erythematosus. Clin. Immunol. Immunopathol. **32:** 166-173.

# Immune Mechanisms in Inflammatory Polyneuropathy[a]

## H. P. HARTUNG,[b,c] K. HEININGER,[b] B. SCHÄFER,[b] W. FIERZ,[c] AND K. V. TOYKA[b]

[b]Department of Neurology
University of Düsseldorf
Düsseldorf, 1 FRG

[d]Division of Immunology
Department of Medicine
University of Zürich
Zürich, Switzerland

This paper reviews the recent advances in the understanding of the pathogenesis of inflammatory polyneuropathies and outlines new therapeutic aspects. Reference will be made to clinicopathologic, electrophysiologic, and immunologic findings obtained in the human diseases and to experimental observations made in animal models of these disorders.

## ACUTE DEMYELINATING INFLAMMATORY POLYNEUROPATHY—THE GUILLAIN-BARRÉ SYNDROME

It has been increasingly recognized that a small proportion of patients with the acute Guillain-Barré syndrome (GBS) have a severe form of the disease with a poor prognosis. Clinical, pathologic, and electrophysiologic studies have demonstrated that axonal degeneration characterizes nerve pathology in these cases.[1-5] Clinically, the disease reaches peak severity much earlier in these patients than in most other GBS patients, and they require ventilatory assistance more often.

In some patients, conduction block occurred at distal sites, whereas in others there was electrophysiologic evidence of widespread muscle denervation. Thus, patients that fulfill all of the established diagnostic criteria for GBS may either—in the majority—have a demyelinating polyneuropathy with conduction slowing or block that is milder and yields better recovery, or have axonal damage with conduction failure, signaling severe disease with slower recovery (TABLE 1).

It is unclear at present whether the axonal form is part of the spectrum of GBS

---

[a]This work was supported by grants from Deutsche Forschungsgemeinschaft SFB 200/B5, Gemeinnützige Hertie-Stiftung and Ministerium für Wissenschaft und Forschung NRW.

[c]Address for correspondence: Neurologische Klinik, University of Düsseldorf, Moorenstr. 5, 4000 Düsseldorf, FRG.

or represents a separate entity. The patients reported on by Feasby et al.[3,6] all had extensive axonal degeneration without significant demyelination or inflammation on nerve biopsy or autopsy.

Although occasional axonal degeneration is encountered in most GBS patients, it is usually proportional to the amount of demyelination and is traditionally considered to be due to a "bystander effect."[7] However, morphologic studies in the intraneural transfer model indicate that axonal degeneration and demyelination can occur independently, and axonal damage was attributed to an intense inflammatory response with prominent edema formation.[8,9] It is of interest that the same spectrum of clinical, electrophysiologic, and histologic disease severity can be observed in experimental autoimmune neuritis (EAN), the animal model of GBS. In adoptive transfer-EAN (AT-EAN), injection of myelin protein $P_2$-specific T lymphocytes of the W3/25 helper phenotype into naive Lewis rats can produce either fulminant neuritis characterized electrophysiologically by conduction failure that resembles acute nerve transection and morphologically by axonal degeneration and prominent endoneurial edema (high cell dose), or upon transfer of a smaller number of line cells a milder condition with later onset of signs of conduction slowing and, histologically, of predominant demyelination[10,84] (FIGS. 1 and 2). Thus, disease severity is strictly cell-dose dependent.

Similarly, it is possible to produce a mild and almost entirely demyelinating form

TABLE 1. Guillain-Barré Syndrome—Spectrum of the Disease

| Demyelinating | Axonal Damage |
|---|---|
| Conduction Slowing Block | Conduction Failure |
| Less Severe Better Recovery | Severe Poorer Recovery |

of actively induced EAN by immunization of rats with a small dose of myelin, and a more severe variety with more extensive demyelination and significant axonal damage in animals that received a larger dose of the immunogen[11] (B. Schäfer, H.-P. Hartung, K. Heininger, and K. V. Toyka, in preparation; FIG. 3). The conclusion that can be drawn from these animal experiments is that the existence of profound axonal degeneration, as observed in the hyperacute forms of GBS, is nonetheless in keeping with an autoimmune reaction to a myelin antigen and does not necessarily imply a different antigen and etiology.

## Pathogenesis of GBS

Viruses have long been suspected to be of etiologic importance in GBS based on the time-honored observation that viral infections frequently precede the onset of the disease and on the reportedly increased incidence of GBS after influenza vaccination. In this context, it is noteworthy that inflammatory polyneuropathies, both acute and chronic, have recently been identified as one of the protean manifestations of HIV infection.[12-15a] Both forms are clinically and electrophysiologically indistinguishable from polyneuropathies not associated with HIV infection. A distinctive laboratory feature of the seropositive cases is CSF pleocytosis. Some also have oligoclonal bands and raised MBP levels.[15,16] All cases so far reported have occurred early in the course of HIV infection, that is, during stage I or II of the CDC classification, some even around seroconversion for HIV.[12-15] All patients responded to steroid or plasmapheresis treatment with concomitant reversal of neurographic and CSF abnormalities. At 20 months' follow-up, most had not yet developed signs or symptoms of stage III or IV HIV disease.[15,15b]

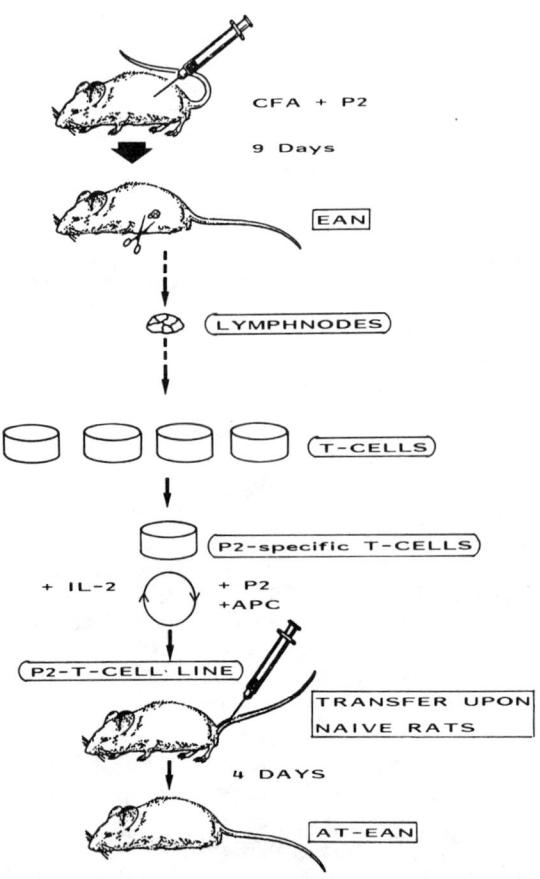

**FIGURE 1.** Adoptive transfer-experimental autoimmune neuritis (EAN). Apart from active immunization with neuritogenic myelin basic proteins, EAN can be induced by passive transfer of autoreactive T-line cells of the CD4 helper phenotype. T lymphocytes obtained from lymph nodes of rats afflicted with EAN can be specifically selected for their exclusive reactivity with the neuritogenic $P_2$ protein of peripheral myelin. After repetitive cycles of stimulation with antigen and interleukin-2, these cell lines can be transferred to naive syngeneic Lewis rats (see ref. 10 and 66).

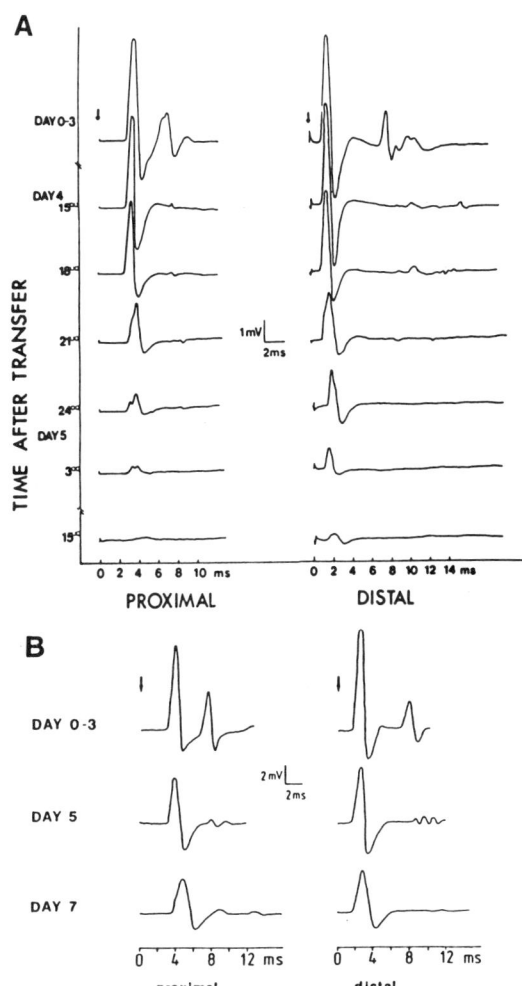

**FIGURE 2.** Cell-dose-dependent functional deficits in adoptive transfer-experimental autoimmune neuritis (AT-EAN). (**A**) Representative time course in a rat developing fulminant and complete paraplegia 5 days after injection with a high dose of $2 \times 10^6$ $P_2$-specific T cells. *Acute phase:* redrawn original recordings of compound muscle action potentials (CMAPs) and of F waves are shown from *top to bottom: left,* after stimulation at the sciatic notch (proximal); *right,* after stimulation at the malleolus (distal). Note that a fall in F-wave amplitude and an increase in F-wave latency preceded changes in the amplitudes of CMAPs. Within 24 hours, CMAPs become barely detectable, but they are completely absent thereafter. *Arrows* denote stimulation artifact. (**B**) Low cell dose: AT-EAN was induced with $5 \times 10^5$ T-line cells. Representative redrawn original recordings of compound muscle action potentials obtained after stimulation at the malleolus (distal) and at the sciatic notch (proximal). Adapted from Heininger et al.[10]

Are there lessons to be learned in determining the etiology of GBS? The histologic lesions found on nerve biopsy in HIV-seropositive patients with the disease were identical to those described in seronegative patients, and immunohistologic characterization of the cellular infiltrate revealed a distribution of CD4/CD8 lymphocytes corresponding to the ratio found in the peripheral blood.[15,17] Direct infection of the nerve by HIV is unlikely, although the virus has been cultivated from a sural nerve in one patient.[18] *In situ* hybridization failed to identify viral genome in Schwann cells, infiltrating lymphocytes, or perineurial cells.[15] Furthermore, the almost uniformly good outcome argues against retrovirus infection as the primary mechanism of nerve damage in these patients. Cytomegalovirus inclusions, however, have been found in the Schwann cells of sural nerves of four HIV-positive patients with GBS.[13,19]

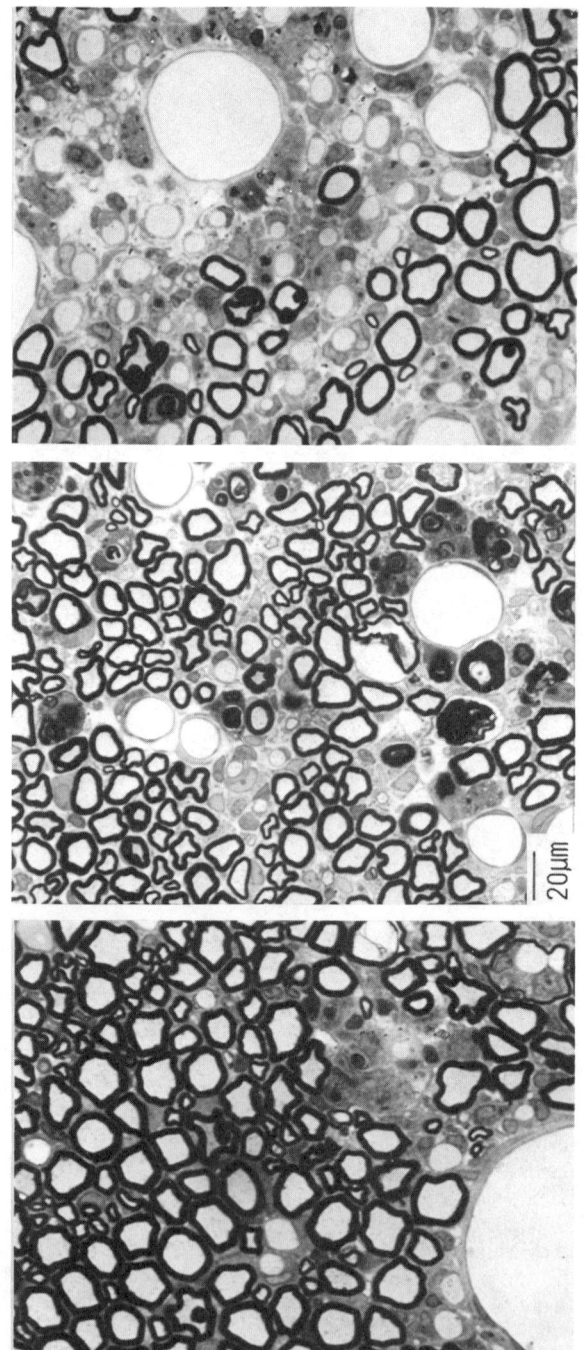

**FIGURE 3.** Immunogen dose determines the severity of myelin-induced EAN. Lewis rats were immunized with complete Freund's adjuvant and indicated amounts of purified bovine dorsal root myelin. Displayed are representative 1 μm Epon sections at the S1 root level from animals sacrificed on day 21 after immunization: *left*, 1.5 mg; *center*, 3 mg; *right*, 5 mg. Note the dose-dependent severity of perivascular demyelination.

The recognition of acute and chronic inflammatory polyneuropathy as a manifestation of HIV infection is therefore of prime importance, because it may be the presenting symptom of early disease and it is excellently amenable to therapy. However, these associations do not provide further clues as to how viral infection may relate to the pathogenesis of inflammatory polyneuropathies.

There are a few naturally occurring equivalents of human acute GBS in animals: Marek's disease in the chicken, Coonhound paralysis in dogs, and inflammatory cauda equina disease in horses.[20] In these disorders as in human GBS a similar dilemma exists, that is, the exact etiologic role of the viral infection is not clear.

*Pathogenic Humoral Factors*

*Antibodies and Complement*

Studies on the pathogenesis of GBS have also focused on the role of humoral factors (TABLE 2). Observations from a number of laboratories on demyelinating

TABLE 2. Guillain-Barré Syndrome—Search for Pathogenic Humoral Factors

- Antibodies to neural glycolipids
- Intraneural passive transfer demyelinates peripheral nerve
- Complement activation in CSF and serum
- Complement neoantigen deposition on myelin sheaths
- Plasma exchange effective
- Other proinflammatory humoral mediators?

properties of sera from GBS patients *in vitro* and *in vivo* prompted an intensive search for the identification of possible pathogenic antibodies directed to peripheral nerve antigens. Most investigators agree that humoral immune responses to myelin antigens MBP, $P_0$, $P_2$, and galactocerebroside, which have all been identified as neuritogens in EAN, do not play a significant role in the pathogenesis of GBS.[21-23] Early evidence implicating circulating factors in the pathogenesis of GBS relied on studies *in vitro* on myelinotoxic properties of patients' sera.[24] The strength of arguments in favor of the pathogenicity of circulating factors in these studies was mitigated by the lack of specificity of the myelin-damaging effects observed in culture. Likewise, both GBS and control sera were found to contain factors capable of exerting cytotoxic actions on cultured Schwann cells.[25] Binding of immunoglobulins to peripheral nerve tissue was studied by a number of groups and yielded divergent results with positive findings ranging from 13-80%.[24,26-28] Our own studies employing newer immunocytochemical techniques (PAP and ABC) have been inconclusive in over 30 patients.[29] However, immunoglobulins may nonspecifically bind to nerves,[30] and intraneural deposits are found in both inflammatory and degenerative polyneuropathies.[31,32]

An extensive study showing demyelinating activity in sera from normal individuals and employing a well-myelinated mouse cerebellum culture system underscores this caveat.[33] Complement components located along myelin sheaths were observed in biopsies from GBS patients.[27,28] More recently, deposits of C3d and the membrane attack complex were identified on peripheral nerve myelin in biopsy specimens of patients with GBS, indicating local activation of the complement cascade at the lesional sites.[34,35]

Koski et al.[36,37] consistently detected elevated levels of complement-fixing anti-PNS-myelin antibodies that correlate closely with disease activity, being highest at the peak of the disease and decreasing in titer along with clinical improvement. Such antibodies were also found in some patients with HIV-associated GBS. There is evidence that the complement system is activated in the CSF[34,38,39] of GBS patients (FIG. 4). Recent studies relating levels of complement-fixing anti-PNS-myelin antibodies with the quantity and kinetics of soluble complexes of terminal complement components in serum suggest that specific IgM antibodies participate in myelin destruction by recruitment of the membrane attack complex, C5b-9. In sections of peripheral nerve and nerve roots of a GBS patient obtained at autopsy, focal and segmental staining for C9 neoantigen, coincident with anti-IgM binding, and some immunostaining for C3 were observed.[34] All these studies suggest that the complement system with its highly potent activation products, namely, C3a, C3b, C5a, and C5b-9, which exert a multitude of proinflammatory actions, contributes to tissue damage in GBS. It was shown earlier *in vitro* that myelin, in particular the $P_0$ protein, can initiate complement activation even in the absence of myelin-specific antibodies.[40] By this mechanism, a vicious circle may be started, adding to the damaging activity of complement split products once myelin is set free from its intracellular compartment. Although these findings taken together strongly implicate humoral factors in the pathogenesis of GBS, their importance so far is confined to the effector phase of the disease.

What is the target antigen to which these antibodies are directed? There is evidence that these complement-fixing antibodies may be directed to neural glycolipids. In a small proportion of GBS patients, antibodies of IgG or IgM class were shown to react with different neutral or acidic glycolipids.[41-43]

After it was demonstrated that intraneural injection of experimental allergic neuritis serum can transfer demyelinative activity to normal recipient animals,[44,45] similar experiments were carried out in which serum from GBS patients was injected into rat sciatic nerves.[46-49] The reported differences in the percentage of sera capable of evoking demyelination on passive transfer and in the specificity of effects as well as the completely opposite results obtained in electrophysiologic studies[50,51] have been attributed to different storage conditions of the sera employed and the technique of injection. Furthermore, Brown et al.[49] recently reported the distinct early and late effects of GBS and control serum passively transferred. They found that only GBS patients' sera could induce vesicular demyelination within 24-48 hours after intraneural injection. Delayed demyelination, mediated by macrophages, was first observed on day 2 after injection, and it became more prominent over the next 3-5 days. This type of demyelination was produced on transfer of both GBS-specific and GBS-unspecific serum. Obviously, the latter result contrasts with those of earlier reports. The macrophage-mediated demyelination found in animals that had received control sera could be due to a chemotactically active constituent of serum such as antibody or complement that is bound to Schwann cells but does not cause lysis. Other mediators including lymphokines, proteases, and eicosanoids could evoke a nonspecific inflammatory response. It was concluded that passive transfer of demyelination by GBS serum, in contrast to EAN serum, apparently was not complement dependent. On the basis of these passive transfer studies, it appears that human serum-induced demyelination results from at least two distinct processes, acute demyelination occurring in the absence of contact with inflammatory cells and delayed demyelination mediated by host macrophages.

The rapid conduction block produced by GBS serum on intraneural transfer, first described by Sumner et al.,[50] resembles that seen with hyperimmune serum of rabbits with galactocerebroside-induced EAN which is thought to alter paranodal cable properties of nerve fibers.[52] In contrast to intraneural transfer experiments, attempts with

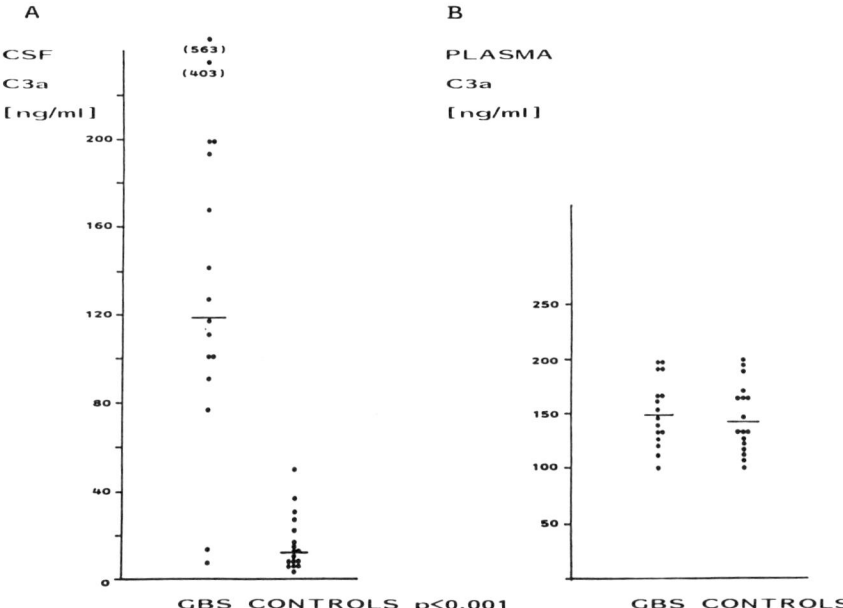

FIGURE 4. Guillain-Barré syndrome: Complement activation in the cerebrospinal fluid. To search for evidence of complement activation in the CSF of GBS patients, CSF and plasma samples were drawn within an average of 4 days of disease onset. Concentrations of the complement activation product, anaphylatoxic peptide C3a, were determined by radioimmunoassay. CSF levels of C3a and C5a (not shown) were markedly elevated in 16 patients with the Guillain-Barré syndrome, whereas plasma concentrations did not differ. Adapted from reference 39.

systemic transfer of GBS serum and purified IgG have generally failed,[29] although transferred human IgG can cross the blood-nerve barrier in monkeys and mice.[53,54]

Apart from circulating antibodies, other humoral factors could conceivably contribute to the pathogenesis of GBS: mediators such as lymphokines, arachidonic acid metabolites, oxygen-free radicals, or lysosomal enzymes. Studies on their role in GBS are not available, but recent work in animal models provides strong evidence of their involvement in lesion development (TABLE 3; see section on *Other Humoral Factors*).

TABLE 3. Proinflammatory Mediators in Experimental Autoimmune Neuritis

Eicosanoids
    Prostaglandin E   (cyclooxygenase pathway)
    Leukotriene $C_4$   (lipoxygenase pathway)

Oxygen Radicals
    Metabolically active oxygen intermediates

Proteases

Vasoactive Amines

## Humoral Factors in EAN

### Antigens and Circulating Antibodies

In EAN, neuritogenic constituents of peripheral nerve myelin that differ in part of their sequence from species to species have been identified.[56-60] The main neuritogen in the experimental animal most commonly studied, the Lewis rat, is the 14-kd basic protein, $P_2$ (FIG. 5). Recently, $P_0$ that had been conformationally changed by lysophosphatidylcholine treatment was also shown to elicit EAN in Lewis rats.[56] The 30-kd $P_0$ protein contains a hydrophobic region of 19 kd buried in the lipid bilayer and a single nine residue-containing carbohydrate chain bound to the other part of the molecule. It was proposed that the addition of lysophosphatidylcholine allows exposure of immunogenic and antigenic carbohydrate structures on the surface of $P_0$. $P_2$ is a minor component of peripheral nerve myelin comprising 131 amino acids. Its highly ordered conformation determines its neuritogenic properties. The soluble purified $P_2$ protein apparently assumes a partially denatured conformation and is only a little effective in causing EAN. Conversely, treatment with mercaptoethanol enhances the immunogenic potency of $P_2$, as do lipids. Nuclear magnetic resonance spectroscopic studies indicate that changes in the conformation of the $P_2$ protein occur in a lipid environment. A more unfolded conformation for the $P_2$ protein in myelin, compared with the isolated protein, would be consistent with the increased neuritogenicity of peptides derived from the $P_2$ protein or of PNS myelin compared to isolated $P_2$ protein.[61] These observations indicate that critical antigenic determinants must be present in a distinct configuration within the $P_2$ protein for it to act as a neuritogen. To define further epitopes within the $P_2$ protein, it was cleaved into several peptide fragments by cyanogen bromide digestion. Three fragments were identified as: CB-1, an internal peptide comprising residues 21-113; CB-2, containing C-terminal acids 114-131; and CB-3, comprised of the N-terminal amino acids 1-20[60] (FIG. 5). The neuritogenic potency of $P_2$ resides within the CB-1 peptide, probably in amino acid sequence 66 (Leu)-78 (Arg).[60,63] A study on the distribution of the target antigen $P_2$ in various species including human, rabbit, guinea pig, and Lewis rat yielded a good correlation between $P_2$ localization and the clinicopathologic findings in GBS and EAN. For example, the highest content of $P_2$ was found in ventral spinal roots, the site of predilection for lesions in inflammatory polyneuropathy. In the Lewis rat, $P_2$

was detected only in spinal roots and peripheral nerves but not in the CNS. These findings contrast with those in guinea pigs whose spinal cord also contains some $P_2$, explaining why immunization with $P_2$ in guinea pigs causes both EAN and EAE.[64]

Intraneural injection into rat sciatic nerve has been performed with polyclonal antisera raised to several myelin antigens. Specific demyelination was produced only by antisera to galactocerebroside and $P_0$. The addition of complement had no effect.[55] These findings are of particular importance because both galactocerebroside and $P_0$ are major antigenic determinants of the Schwann cell surface and in view of the recent observation that immunization with $P_0$, altered by lysophosphatidylcholine, results in EAN.[56]

Antibodies directed to the $P_2$ protein have been detected in the circulation of animals with EAN. However, neither antibody titers nor antibody kinetics correlated with disease activity, casting doubts on a simple cause and effect relationship.[60,65] Further evidence against a primary role for humoral antibodies in the pathogenesis of EAN comes from studies in which the disease was produced by adoptive transfer of $P_2$-specific T-lymphocyte line cells.[66,67] As mentioned earlier, recipient rats come down with the disease on day 4 or 5 after transfer of $P_2$-specific CD4 T cells. This interval is too short for a significant antibody response to be elicited. In fact, circulating antigen-$P_2$ antibodies were not detectable in the sera of these recipient animals. Yet they developed a polyneuropathy clinically, electrophysiologically, and histologically resembling actively induced EAN.[10,84]

A possible role for complement in EAN is suggested by the recent demonstration that systemic complement depletion achieved through administration of cobra venom factor delays the onset of clinical signs and reduces the degree of demyelination observed histologically.[68] These findings are not necessarily indicative of either an exclusively cell-mediated or an exclusively humoral immunopathogenesis.

It is an attractive hypothesis, based on recent findings in EAE, to envision a requirement of both $P_2$-specific T cells and anti-PNS myelin antibodies in concert for the full production of the disease. In EAE, it was shown that small doses of MBP-specific T-line cells synergize with an antibody directed against a surface antigen present on oligodendrocytes (MOG) to cause inflammatory demyelination.[69] One major function of the T cells in EAN may be to open up the blood-nerve barrier and allow circulating antibodies to reach their target antigen on the peripheral nerve more readily.

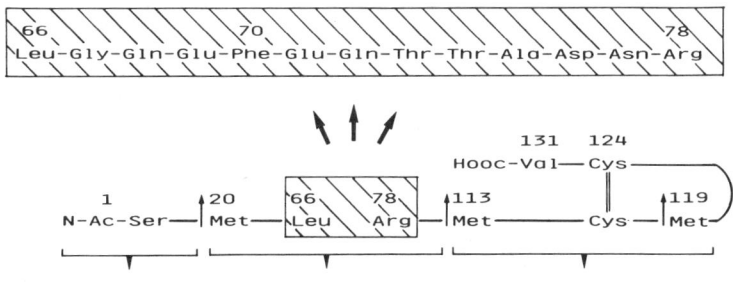

**FIGURE 5.** Schematic structure of bovine basic protein $P_2$ and peptides CB-1, CB-2, and CB-3 derived from the parent molecule by cleavage with cyanogen bromide. In the Lewis rat, the sequence 66 (Leu)-78 (Arg) is neuritogenic. Modified from reference 20.

*Other Humoral Factors*

The role of humoral mediators other than antibodies was recently examined in great detail in EAN and may provide clues to the pathogenesis of GBS. It was well established by morphologic investigation that as the nerve lesion in EAN progresses, macrophages emerge as the predominant cellular constituent.[70-72] Ultrastructural observations revealed that macrophages strip off and phagocytose myelin. Global blockade of macrophages with silica quartz dust by either physical elimination or functional inactivation was documented to suppress EAN and AT-EAN.[73-76] In addition to the well-documented ability of macrophages to effect phagocytic breakdown of myelin in GBS and EAN, these major cellular components of the inflammatory lesion could conceivably damage the myelin sheath by a number of other actions. Macrophages can elaborate a range of highly potent mediators that cause tissue damage in other model systems of inflammation. In our laboratory, we focused on the possible pathogenic role of macrophage-derived oxygen-free radicals and eicosanoids (FIGS. 6 and 7). Following univalent reduction of molecular oxygen, macrophages in a sequence of events termed the oxidative burst can form highly reactive oxygen metabolites, such as superoxide anion, hydrogen peroxide, and hydroxyl radicals. Some were shown to produce lipid peroxidation of myelin membranes with consequent breakdown *in vitro*. To examine a possible role of these metabolically active oxygen intermediates, we applied inactivators, so-called oxygen radical scavengers, to Lewis rats with EAN and demonstrated that application of the enzymatic scavengers superoxide dismutase and catalase effectively reduces disease activity assessed both clinically and electrophysiologically.[77] Morphometric and immunocytochemical analyses in these treated animals revealed that clinical efficacy was mirrored by a reduction or even a lack of perivenular demyelination and macrophage infiltration when the scavengers were administered early in the course of disease. Delayed treatment still led to marked suppression of the disease despite the presence of macrophages in the lesion. Furthermore, we demonstrated that macrophages collected from rats with EAN generated a markedly higher chemiluminescent response and released larger amounts of superoxide anion and hydrogen peroxide *ex vivo* than did macrophages from nonimmunized rats or those inoculated with complete Freund's adjuvant only (FIG. 8). Taken to-

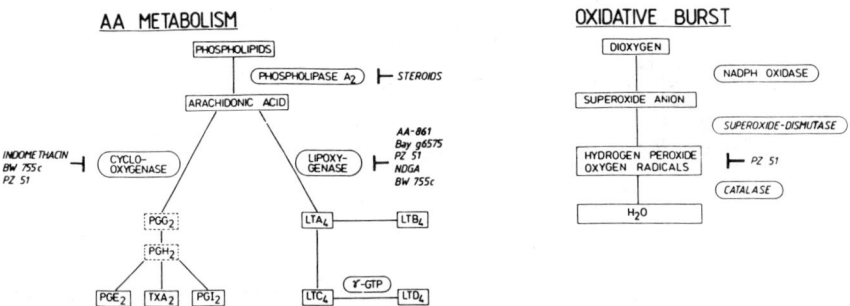

**FIGURE 6.** Biosynthetic pathways yielding macrophage-derived proinflammatory mediators. Biosynthesis of prostaglandins, leukotrienes, and metabolically active oxygen intermediates. The major enzymatic steps and their end products are displayed. Also indicated are the sites at which pharmacologic and physiologic inhibitors act. BW 755c (Wellcome): derivative of pyrazoline jointly blocking cyclooxygenase and lipoxygenase. PZ51: Ebselen (Nattermann). Bay g6575: Nafazatrom (Bayer). NDGA: Nordihydroguaretic acid, both predominant lipoxygenase blockers.

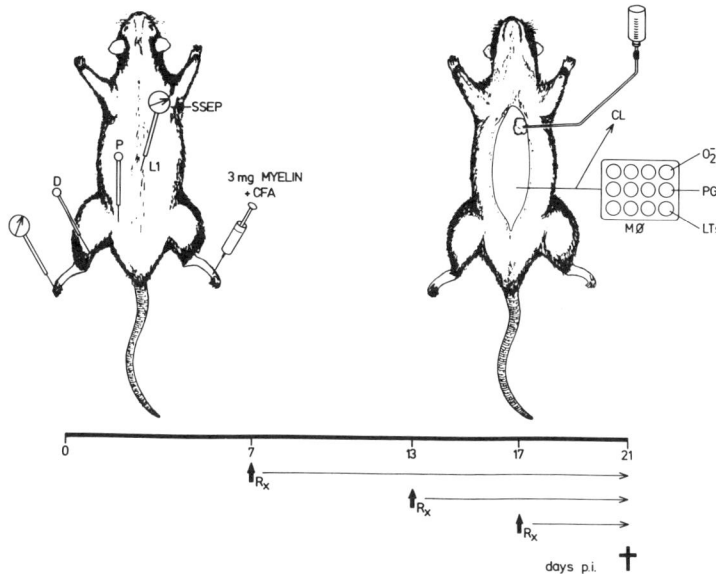

**FIGURE 7.** Serial clinical, electrophysiologic, histologic, and biochemical observations in myelin-induced EAN: Evaluation of immunopharmacologic treatment. EAN was induced in Lewis rats with 3 mg of myelin plus complete Freund's adjuvant. Treatment with any one of the tested pharmacologic compounds was initiated at three different time points: day 7 postinjection (early amplification phase, no clinical signs); day 13 postinjection (first clinical signs: amplification and early effector phase); day 17 postinjection (manifest disease: late effector phase). The course of the disease was followed throughout by electrophysiologic monitoring. Rats were killed on day 21. Peritoneal macrophages were collected and evaluated for the release of eicosanoids and reactive oxygen intermediates (CL = chemiluminescence, $O_2^-$ = superoxide anion, PGs = prostaglandins, LTs = leukotrienes). Animals were perfused, and sections were taken for histologic and immunohistochemical evaluation.

gether, these results prove an involvement of macrophage-derived oxidants in the production of functional deficits and tissue damage in EAN. The mechanisms by which oxygen radical scavengers achieve their protective effects may involve the prevention of direct peroxidative injury to myelin, the restriction of secondary cellular immigration by inhibiting production of the chemotactic signals focusing hematogenous macrophages into the PNS tissue, and the reduction in the amount of blood-nerve barrier damage.

Eicosanoids are lipid mediators derived by oxidative conversion from arachidonic acid, a C20 polyunsaturated fatty acid. The major pathways leading to the synthesis of prostaglandins and leukotrienes are given in FIGURE 6. Among leukocytes, macrophages are the predominant source of these physiologically active compounds. To examine a possible pathogenic role of these mediators, we took the same experimental approach as already outlined (FIG. 7) and examined the effects of pharmacologic inhibitors of eicosanoid formation. Treatment with inhibitors of the cyclooxygenase pathway (indomethacin, BW755C, Ebselen) largely reduced signs of EAN, whereas predominant blockers of lipoxygenase (e.g., Nafazatrom) did not substantially suppress disease activity in EAN[75] (FIGS. 9-12). These findings were corroborated by electro-

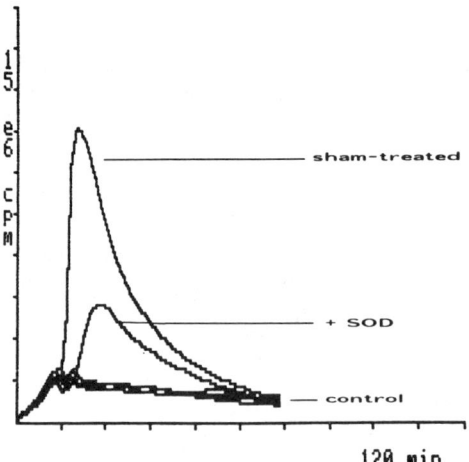

**FIGURE 8.** Release of reactive oxygen intermediates from macrophages. Before perfusion, peritoneal macrophages were collected from nonimmunized (control) and sham-treated rats. The phorbol myristate acetate (PMA)-elicited chemiluminescent response (a general measure of oxidative burst activity) indicates *in vivo* activation of macrophages. It can be suppressed *in vitro* by adding SOD (300 U/ml) simultaneously with PMA (100 ng/ml) to cell suspensions. Ordinate: counts per minute (cpm); abscissa: time after addition in minutes. From reference 77.

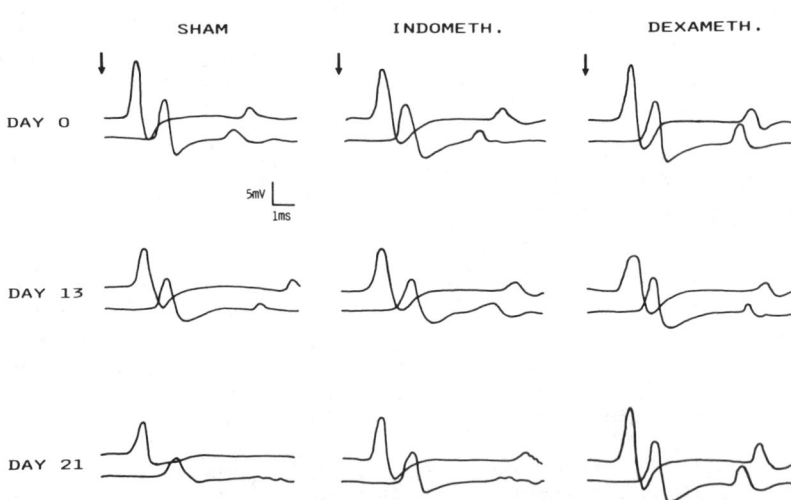

**FIGURE 9.** Pharmacologic intervention in EAN: The role of macrophage-derived eicosanoids. Serial motor nerve conduction studies in animals with myelin-induced EAN. Displayed are representative redrawn original recordings of compound muscle action potentials obtained from the small foot muscles after stimulation of the sciatic nerve distally (*upper traces*) and proximally (*lower traces*). Lewis rats were sham treated or received indomethacin (1 mg/kg) or high-dose dexamethasone (4 mg/kg) from day 13 through day 21 after immunization. Note failures of F waves, conduction block, and conduction slowing in sham-treated rats. These changes are less pronounced after indomethacin treatment and absent after dexamethasone on day 21. Adapted from reference 75.

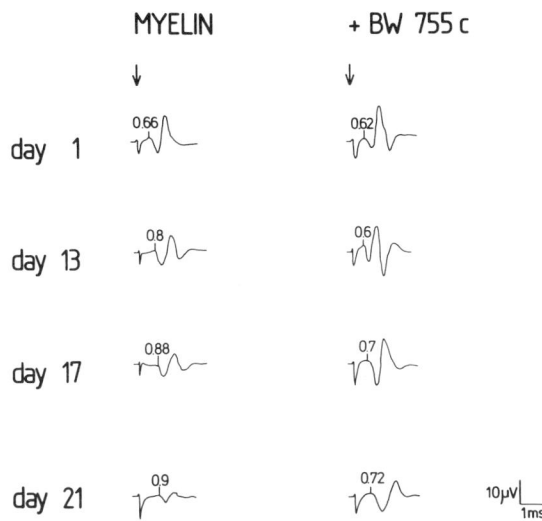

**FIGURE 10.** Role of eicosanoids in EAN: Effects of combined cyclooxygenase and lipoxygenase blockade. Animals immunized with myelin were either sham treated (myelin) or received the joint cyclooxygenase and lipoxygenase blocker BB755c from postinjection day 7. Displayed are mixed afferent nerve potentials of the sciatic nerve obtained after stimulation at the malleolus and recorded with near-nerve needle electrodes at the sciatic notch. Note delayed latencies and reduction in amplitude in the sham-treated group and only slight changes in the treated group. Adapted from reference 75.

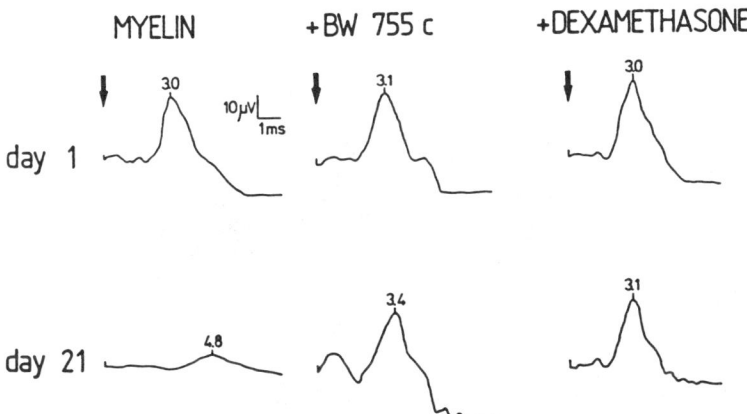

**FIGURE 11.** Pharmacologic intervention in EAN: Lumbar somatosensory evoked potentials (SSEP). Rats with EAN were treated from postinjection day 7 with BW755c (50 mg/kg per day) or dexamethasone (4 mg/kg per day). Changes of lumbar SSEP recorded at the D12/L1 spinal level are illustrated in representative redrawn original recordings. Numbers indicate latencies of the S response. Myelin-sham-treated animals.

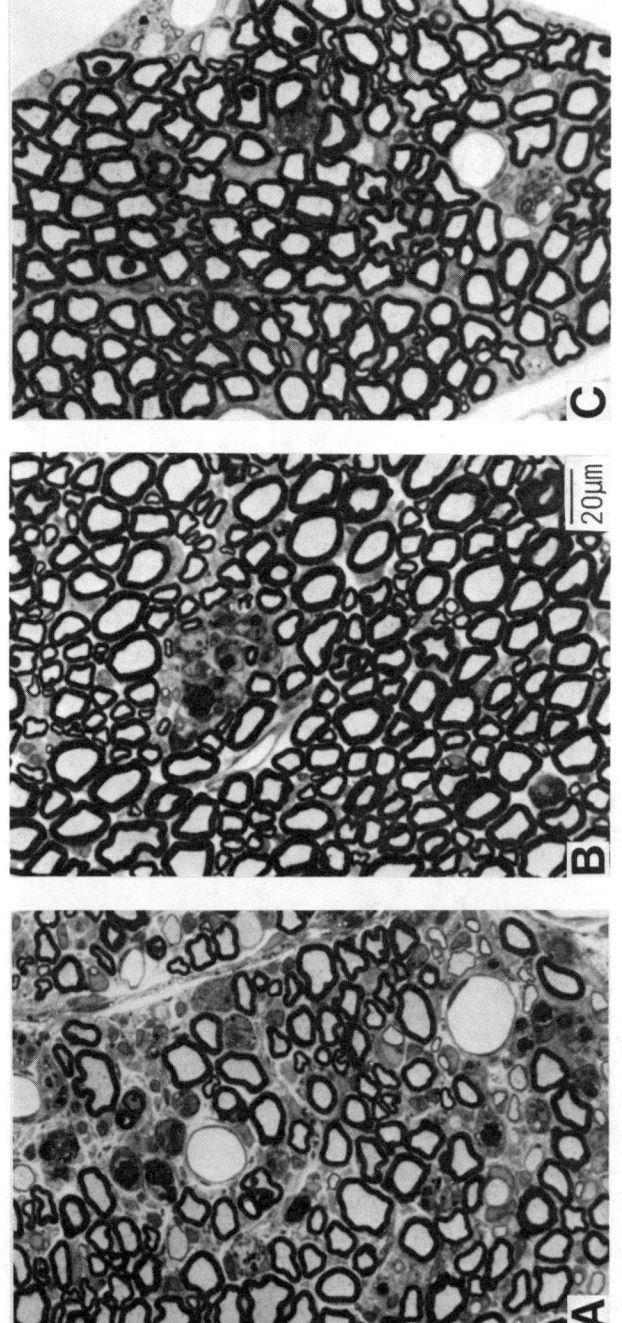

FIGURE 12. Pharmacologic intervention in EAN: morphology. Displayed are micrographs of 1 μm Epon sections at the S1 root level from EAN rats that had received sham treatment (**A**) or were administered dexamethasone (**B**) or BW755c (**C**). Note the extensive cellular infiltration and demyelination both in the immediate vicinity as well as at a distance from intraneural vessels in **A**. There are only occasional cells and few demyelinated fibers in sections from the dexamethasone- or BW755c-treated group.

physiologic, morphologic, and immunohistologic studies. Again, it was found that the production of eicosanoids *in vitro* is increased in EAN. The role of lysosomal enzymes, yet another example of highly active biosynthetic products in macrophages, was examined by looking at their tissue distribution. It was found that activity was elevated in the spinal roots and sciatic nerves of animals with EAN compared with controls. The topographic distribution of the increased enzyme activities closely corresponded to the histologic distribution of EAN lesions.[78]

Macrophage-derived neutral proteases and phospholipid enzymes have also been implicated in myelin damage in an *in vitro* system.[79,80] An observation of particular interest was that cultured peritoneal macrophages, when preincubated with EAN serum, agglutinated and phagocytosed purified peripheral nerve myelin.[78] Similarly, opsonization of macrophages with anti-MBP antibody induced heightened metabolic activity, leading to augmented myelin digestion.[81] The specificity of these phenomena, however, remains to be explained (effects are reportedly mediated by the antigen-unspecific Fc fragment of antibodies).

Finally, a role for vasoactive amines elaborated in the course of mast cell degranulation has emerged. Occasional mast cells have been identified in sural nerve biopsies from GBS patients.[28] Degranulated mast cells were found in both actively induced and adoptive transfer EAN.[82-84] This may be the consequence of a T-cell-initiated delayed-type hypersensitivity reaction. Suggestive evidence for the role of mast cell-derived vasoactive amines is based on studies in which treatment of immunized rats with reserpine, an agent that among other actions depletes vasoactive amine stores, delayed the onset of EAN.[85] Evidence is available that peripheral nerve myelin can degranulate cultured mast cells *in vitro*.[86] Vasoactive amines may be instrumental in opening up the blood-nerve barrier, an event that occurs very early in the course of EAN.[70,71,82,87,89]

*Lymphokines and Monokines*

Lymphokines and monokines are important chemical messengers of cell-cell interaction during inflammatory responses. In particular, interleukin-1, interleukin-2, tumor necrosis factor (TNF), and gamma-interferon (IFN-$\gamma$) may be pathogenic factors in EAN. We have examined the effects of recombinant rat IFN-$\gamma$ in myelin-induced EAN. When given from day 1-10 after active immunization during the induction phase, peak disease on day 21, the time of sacrifice, was more severe than that in sham-treated rats with EAN as evidenced by clinical, electrophysiologic, and morphometric analysis (FIG. 13). However, when administration of IFN-$\gamma$ was initiated on day 11 and given until sacrifice, disease severity was alleviated. This experimental observation supports the notion that immunomodulatory lymphokines may have contrasting net effects depending on the immune mechanisms activated at a given time. Recent evidence suggests that IFN-$\gamma$ induces expression of class II molecules on Schwann cells.[90,191] It is currently not clear which of the various immunomodulatory mechanisms account for the net effects observed *in vivo*.

*Cellular Immunity in GBS*

There has been a long search for evidence of cellular immunity in GBS. Most investigators have found no consistent increase in T-lymphocyte-mediated responses

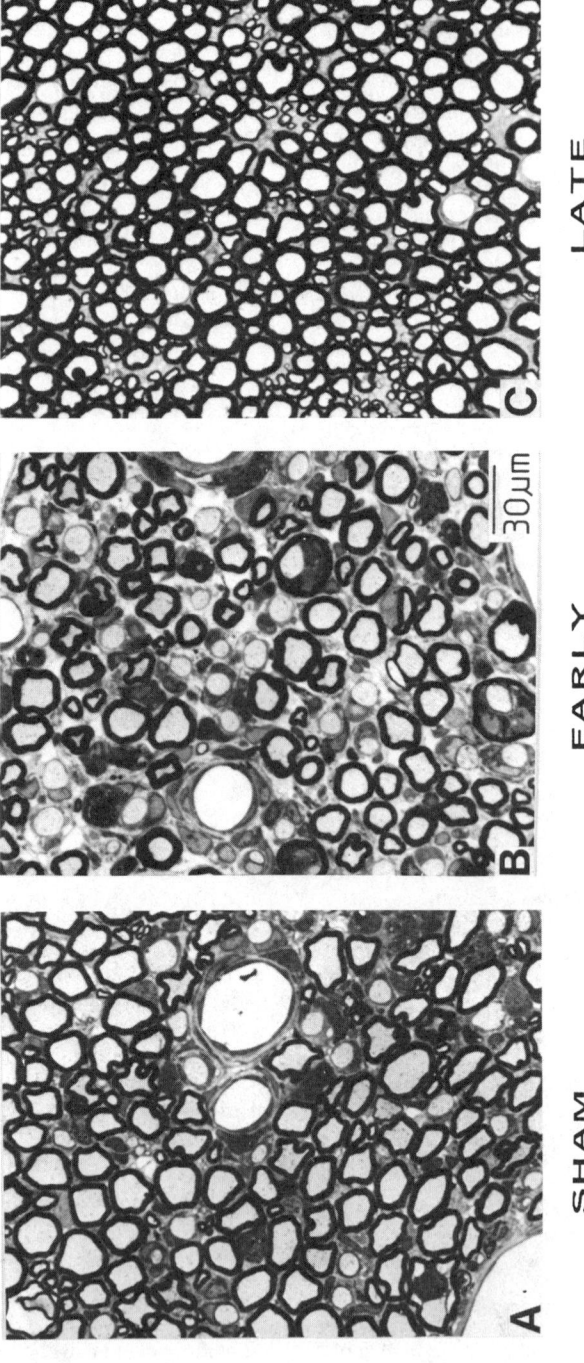

**FIGURE 13.** EAN: The role of gamma-interferon. IFN-γ (100,000 U per animal per day) was administered either early in the course of the disease (through postinjection days 1-10) or late (days 11-19). Rats were killed on day 21. Representative micrographs (1 μm Epon sections) at S1 root level. Early administration of IFN-γ resulted in enhanced severity of the disease assessed clinically, electrophysiologically, and, as shown here, morphologically. However, when IFN-γ was given later in the course of the disease, the severity of EAN was reduced on the day of sacrifice.

to $P_2$ protein or other putative neuritogens.[91-93] In one report employing lymphokine-induced procoagulant synthesis by macrophages as a measure of antigen sensitization, cellular immunity to this neuritogen of EAN was claimed to be demonstrable almost exclusively in GBS patients.[94] In another study, $P_2$ sensitization of peripheral T lymphocytes was found, and $P_2$-reactive T-cell lines were isolated from one GBS patient and from normal controls, a situation reminiscent of what is found with MBP T-cell lines.[95] The implication of the latter study is that in the T-cell repertoire of man, autoantigen-reactive cells may exist that are usually under restraint by precisely operating immunoregulatory mechanisms that normally prevent the emergence of autoimmune disease.

Cellular immunoreactivity may be governed by additional factors such as the specific epitope of autoantigen recognized by the T cells or the actual number of autoantigen-reactive cells in the peripheral blood or lymphatic tissues and the efficacy of immunoregulation. Circulating T-cell subsets have been studied in GBS. Whereas in the first series of 12 patients no significant changes in the distribution of T-helper/inducer (CD4) versus T-cytotoxic/suppressor (CD8) cells were noted,[96] subsequent reports noted a definite decrease in the level of either CD4 or CD8 cells in the peripheral blood of GBS patients.[97,98] No evidence of a deficit in T-cell suppressor function was found in the latter study. Thus, there is no uniform pattern of T-cell subset derangement in GBS. It is unclear if this lack of uniformity is due to different experimental technology or reflects disease heterogeneity in GBS. Because peripheral blood lymphocytes constitute only a small proportion in relation to lymphatic tissues, counts of circulating subsets may not represent the body's overall immune reactivity. A decrease in OX8-positive (suppressor/cytotoxic) T cells was also observed in the blood of animals with EAN during the most severe phase of clinical disease.[99] However, no changes were found by Feasby et al..[100]

Preliminary evidence has been advanced that B cells are reduced in the CSF of patients with GBS.[101]

Further clues on cell-mediated immunologic responses in GBS come from immunohistologic studies. The pathologic hallmarks of GBS, segmental demyelination and mononuclear cell infiltration, were established early by light microscopy and electron microscopy. It was found that peripheral blood lymphocytes initially accumulate around interneurial and epineurial venules. With progression of disease, these cells traverse the endoneurium. Full-blown demyelination is found when activated macrophages are present in the endoneurium later on and strip myelin lamellae off axons.[102]

In one study, immunostaining of cells in frozen sections of sural nerve biopsies from four patients with GBS revealed a predominance of T cells. Interestingly, in one biopsy from an HIV-seropositive GBS patient, three times as many T cells as in the other GBS biopsies were counted. Monocytes and macrophages were present in all biopsies, whereas only occasional B cells were seen. The CD4/CD8 ratio in nerve mirrored the ratio in peripheral blood, suggesting that there is nonspecific trafficking of T lymphocytes from blood to the site of pathology during the inflammatory process.[16] In the second study of sural nerve biopsies in two GBS patients, only small numbers of T cells were present without significant differences between the number of CD4 and CD8 lymphocytes.[103] The predominant component of the cellular infiltrate consisted of cells of the monocyte/macrophage lineage, in accordance with earlier morphologic observations.[102] The most important finding, however, was the demonstration by light and electron microscopy that various proportions of Schwann cells were positive for MHC class II antigen.[103] This finding implicates the Schwann cell as a potential autoantigen presenter in the peripheral nervous system.

## Cell-Mediated Immunity in EAN

Sensitization of lymphocytes to PNS myelin, isolated $P_2$, and its neuritogenically active peptide sequences was demonstrated in rats applying skin testing and lymphocyte transformation assays.[60,63,65,104,105]

The capacity to mount a significant cell-mediated response to $P_2$ was found to differ between high responder Lewis and low responder Sprague-Dawley and Brown Norway (BN) rats.[104,105]

Apparently the cellular response to $P_2$ is under the control of the RT-I locus.[104] However, recent experimental evidence obtained in the AT-EAN model indicates that resistance of so-called low responder BN rats to actively induced EAN is not due to the lack of $P_2$-specific autoreactive T-cell clones in the T-cell repertoire of these animals, because BN T cells specifically reactive with bovine $P_2$ protein could be selected that were capable of evoking EAN upon transfer in naive BN recipients.[106] A common neuritogenic epitope for both the Lewis and BN strains was contained in the CB2 peptide. In contrast, neuritogenic BN T lines failed to mount a response to the sequence 53-78 (SP4) which is part of an epitope neuritogenic for Lewis rats. Only Lewis $P_2$-specific T cells could transfer EAN to (Lewis X BN) $F_1$ hybrids, suggesting that only the neuritogenic epitopes for the parental Lewis strain are active in the $F_1$ hybrid.

The role of predominant cellular immune reactions underlying the pathogenesis of EAN was suggested by the passive transfer to naive Lewis rats of EAN with lymph node cells obtained from animals that had been actively immunized with myelin or $P_2$.[65] The role of T cells was formally established by adoptive transfer of the disease with $P_2$ reactive CD4-T-lymphocyte line cells.[66,67] Recipient animals became ill within 4 days of transfer, discounting a role for humoral antibodies in the initiation of autoimmune disease. The requirement of T cells for the development of EAN was also demonstrated by the reduced susceptibility of rats rendered T-cell deficient by adult thymectomy and lethal irradiation to induction of the disease.[107]

The availability of autoreactive T-cell lines has allowed a more direct approach to the question: by which mechanisms do T cells cause autoimmune disease in the peripheral nervous system?[108] This involves the question of how a systemic autoaggressive T-cell response to $P_2$ protein results in local organ-specific tissue damage. Breakdown of the blood-nerve barrier was observed to be an initial event in EAN, but exactly how this is brought about has not been worked out yet. With regard to autoreactive T-line cells, it is possible that a major derangement of the blood-nerve barrier is not a prerequisite if the analogy with the situation in T-cell-induced EAE is accepted. In AT-EAE it was shown that activated T cells, irrespective of their antigenic specificity, can easily traverse the blood-brain barrier to execute immune surveillance in the CNS.[109] Whether homing of the T cells to a specific site in the vascular tree requires expression of Ia antigen on endothelium, induced by IFN-$\gamma$ during an inflammatory response, or specific receptors for activated T-cell blasts is not clear. Once activated $P_2$-specific T cells have invaded the peripheral nervous system, they would have to interact with cells that could present $P_2$ antigen in context with MHC class II antigen. Although Schwann cells do not constitutively express Ia antigens on their surface,[110] they can be induced to do so upon treatment with IFN-$\gamma$.[90] Cocultivation of IFN-$\gamma$-treated Schwann cells from newborn rats with autoaggressive syngeneic MBP-specific T-cell lines resulted in spontaneous T-cell blastogenesis in the absence of exogenous MBP. T-cell proliferation was inhibited by the addition of anti-Ia monoclonal antibodies. These studies indicate that Schwann cells can function as antigen-presenting cells and interact with autoaggressive T cells in the peripheral nervous system. They may also present endogenous neural autoantigens on their surface as targets for a pathologic autoimmune response.[90] The induction of both MHC class I and II antigens on Schwann cells would mark them as targets not only for T helper cells but also for T effector cells, and the possibility exists that, as with AT-EAE, neuritogenic $P_2$-specific T-cell lines may cause Schwann cell death. Alternative mechanisms of demyelination could be envisaged. Although the role of specific humoral antibodies can be excluded in early AT-EAN, other antigen-unspecific humoral factors may be operative, such as cytotoxic activated complement components (see section on Antibodies and Complement). As referred to earlier, autoreactive $P_2$ T-cell lines not only can initiate demyelination but apparently in a dose-dependent manner also can produce significant axonal damage evidenced both electrophysiologically and histologically.[10,84] Endoneurial edema, prominent in EAN but even more so in severe AT-EAN, could elevate intraneural pressure to levels that would induce nerve ischemia.[82] Under such conditions, both primary demyelination due to Schwann cell injury and secondary demyelination due to axonal damage would ensue. The extremely rapidly occurring conduction failure in the inflammatory phase of high cell dose AT-EAN could be accounted for by edema formation or soluble factors released from autoreactive T cells.[108,111]

As in actively induced EAN, macrophages in AT-EAN may also play an important role as effector cells.[76] Although their role in the early amplification and effector phase of EAN and AT-EAN has been clarified, their importance in the initiation of autoimmune diseases of the peripheral nervous system has yet to be elucidated.

*Immunocytochemical Studies in EAN*

Some aspects of the cellular composition of nerve lesions during the course of EAN were investigated immunocytochemically using monoclonal and polyclonal antibodies.[75, 112-115] As far as can be concluded from thick sections and a few electron microscope studies, cells appearing early seem to be macrophages and they have been noted 8 days after immunization. With the onset of clinical signs (day 13), the influx of T cells started with a predominance of the T-helper/inducer (CD4) phenotype. At the peak of disease, CD4-positive T cells and macrophages were most numerous, whereas during recovery, CD8-positive cells prevailed. Using macrophage-specific monoclonal antibodies (ED1), it was possible to identify unequivocally macrophages within EAN lesions.[75] The proximity of CD4-positive T cells and Ia-expressing cells, mostly macrophages, provides a local environment for T-cell activation. There is a debate as to the expression of class II antigens on endothelial cells in the nerve capillaries.

Recently the presence of class I and the absence of class II antigens were documented in normal rats. Class II expression was seen in the endoneurium 11 days after induction of EAN.[110] Electron microscope identification on thin cryosections is needed to localize definitely the surface markers on a given cell population.

*Electrophysiologic Studies in EAN*

The electrophysiologic changes in rats actively immunized with myelin or $P_2$ and inoculated with autoreactive $P_2$-specific T-cell lines have been worked out by serial monitoring of a number of relevant peripheral nerve functions.[10,75-77,116,117]

### Immunogenetics

So far no convincing linkage between the susceptibility to GBS and HLA-haplotypes has been demonstrated.[118-120]

### Hypothesis

Summarizing the direct experimental and circumferential evidence from studies on GBS patients, the following chain of events may characterize the pathogenesis of GBS. The initial event and the autoantigen are not yet known in GBS. A viral infection preceding the onset of the disease may start an immune reaction and because of some sequence homology between viral proteins and peptide sequences of basic proteins of the myelin sheath, cross-reactive immunization to peripheral nervous system antigens may take place.[121] The viral infection may also induce production of IFN-$\gamma$ which in turn may cause MHC class II antigen expression on vascular endothelium. Activated autoreactive T cells cross the blood-nerve barrier and recognize MHC class II antigen and peripheral nerve autoantigen on Schwann cells or on other antigen-presenting cells (monocytes/macrophages). This leads to further peripheral activation of autoreactive T cells, delayed-type hypersensitivity with mast cell degranulation and additional vasoactive amine-elicited blood-nerve barrier breakdown, and invasion of monocytes/macrophages and other leukocytes with subsequent production of chemotactic signals. These further promote secondary cellular immigration into the lesion. Demyelination may be caused by activated macrophages as a consequence of direct phagocytic attack or through secreted inflammatory mediators (oxygen-free radicals, eicosanoids, lysosomal enzymes, and complement). These reactions may be further enhanced by systemic or local antibody formation, complement, or lymphokines. Functional deficits (conduction failure or block) may result from demyelination (damage of myelin sheath) or increased intraneural pressure due to edema.

FIGURE 14 attempts to summarize schematically some of the experimental findings obtained in EAN and AT-EAN pertinent to the pathogenesis of these autoimmune model disorders.

### Treatment

Presently, there is only one treatment for GBS, the efficacy of which was convincingly proven by large controlled studies. In the North American multicenter study, 245 patients were randomized in a nonblinded design into conventional and plasmapheresis arms. A total of 200-250 ml of plasma per kilogram of body weight were exchanged in 7-14 days. Groups were compared with regard to clinical outcome at 4 weeks, time required to walk unaided, time required to improve one grade on a disability scale, and outcome at 6 months. By all criteria, plasma exchange was superior to conventional treatment. Plasmapheresis was particularly effective in patients who received this treatment within 7 days of onset and in those who required mechanical ventilation.[122] These results were confirmed in the French multicenter study (220 patients) which also revealed that there were no advantages of fresh frozen plasma over albumin as replacement fluid. Because of increased risks and side effects in the group that received plasma, the use of albumin was advocated.[123] Results of two earlier controlled studies were reviewed by Pollard.[124] Multivariate analysis of factors influencing patient outcome in the North American trial revealed that four factors correlated with poor recovery: reduced distal motor amplitude to less than 20% of normal, older age, less than 7 days from the onset of disease to its peak, and the need for ventilatory support. The most powerful electrophysiologic predictor of outcome was the abnormal summed distal motor amplitude.[125,125a] Young age and near normal distal motor amplitudes were also found to correlate with a beneficial response in a smaller

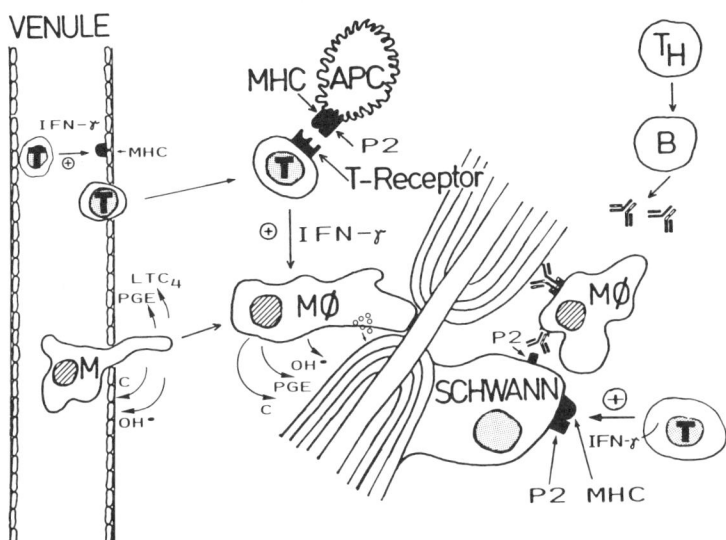

**FIGURE 14.** Simplified scheme depicting major putative immune mechanisms in immunoinflammatory polyneuropathies. APC = antigen-presenting cell; IFN-$\gamma$ = gamma-interferon; $T_H$ = T-helper lymphocyte; B = B-lymphocyte producing antibodies to peripheral nerve antigens. OH• = Hydroxyl radical; PGE = prostaglandin E; C = complement. Granules in the macrophage cytoplasm represent lysosomal enzymes that can attack the myelin sheath (cf. section on Hypothesis.)

study of 24 patients with severe GBS who underwent plasmapheresis.[126] Corticosteroids were used earlier in the treatment of GBS. Two controlled trials yielded divergent results.[124] In the first study[127] on 16 patients with mild or moderate disease, the administration of ACTH begun after the progressive phase of the illness showed a significant reduction in the duration of the disease in the treated versus the placebo group. Hughes et al.[128] studied more severely affected patients who needed respiratory assistance. Twenty-one patients were treated with prednisolone at a starting dose of 60 mg, whereas 19 patients did not receive treatment. These investigators found a detrimental effect of steroid treatment. However, a possible beneficial effect of steroids cannot be excluded on the basis of this study, first, because of its small sample size which does not allow valid statistical statements; second, because only severely affected patients were included; third, because treatment was instituted late after the onset of disease; and finally, because comparatively moderate doses of steroids were employed. Studies in EAN unequivocally demonstrated that steroids are efficacious, as will be discussed herein. In a new British multicenter study, one treatment arm will include high-dose methylprednisolone.

So far, there is no conclusive evidence that immunosuppressive agents such as azathioprine or cyclophosphamide have any benefit in GBS.[124] In the Netherlands, a large-scale clinical trial of high-dose intravenous gammaglobulin treatment based on preliminary results of a pilot study is under way.[129]

*Experimental Approaches to Treatment (TABLE 4)*

As already discussed, the administration of inhibitors of arachidonic acid conversion is highly effective in reducing disease activity in myelin-induced EAN.[75] Oxygen radical scavengers (superoxide dismutase and catalase) also suppress the disease.[77] Even late initiation of treatment was shown to alleviate the manifestations of EAN. Dexamethasone prevents or dramatically ameliorates disease severity in both EAN and AT-EAN.[75,76] Corticosteroids have profound inhibitory effects on all immune cells, but their main antiinflammatory actions are due to inhibition of the enzyme phospholipase. This enzyme liberates arachidonic acid from membrane-bound phospholipids, and by its inhibition the supply of substrate for further conversion to proinflammatory eicosanoids is curtailed. The organoselenic drug, Ebselen, which interferes with the production of arachidonic acid metabolites and possibly exerts immunosuppressive actions on lymphocytes, also prevents EAN.[130]

TABLE 4. Treatment

| Guillain-Barré Syndrome | Experimental Autoimmune Neuritis |
|---|---|
| • Plasma exchange<br>• Corticosteroids? | • *Macrophage depletion:* Silica corticosteroids cyclooxygenase, blockers (e.g. indomethacin, BW755c, Ebselen) |
| | • Oxygen radical scavengers (SOD, catalase, Ebselen) |
| | • *Mast Cells:* Depletion of vasoactive amines (reserpine); membrane stabilization (cromoglycate) |
| | • Complement depletion |
| | • Plasma exchange |
| | • *T-cell directed:*<br>Cyclosporin A<br>Anti-CD4 monoclonals<br>Anti-IL-2 receptor antibodies (ART 18) |

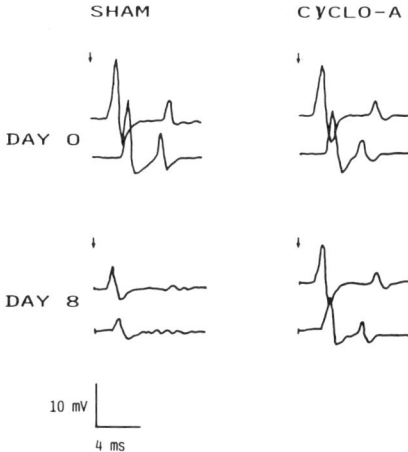

**FIGURE 15.** Immunopharmacologic intervention in AT-EAN: Effects of cyclosporin A. Representative redrawn original recordings of motor nerve conduction studies. Compound muscle action potentials (M) and F waves (F) obtained from small foot muscles on stimulation of the sciatic nerve proximally at the sciatic notch (*lower traces*) or distally at the malleolus (*upper traces*). Note the marked fall in M response and F-wave amplitudes and the delayed and dispersed F waves in sham-treated rats. The treatment group received 1.5 mg/kg per day of cyclosporin A from day 0 until sacrifice on day 9 after transfer of $P_2$-reactive T-helper line cells. Adapted from reference 119.

These agents can be used in the effector phase of the disease. Immunopharmacologic suppression of both EAN and AT-EAN has been achieved with cyclosporin A, which inhibits T-helper/inducer cell-dependent immune reactions by interfering with synthesis of and responsiveness to interleukin 2 (IL-2) and gamma interferon (IFN-$\gamma$)[116,131] (FIGS. 15 and 16). Monoclonal antibodies to T-cell differentiation markers and to MHC class II molecules have been used as immunomodulating agents in various autoimmune animal models and in a prospective trial of multiple sclerosis. Data are not yet available in GBS. In EAN application of monoclonal antibodies directed to the T-helper/inducer subset were shown to reduce disease activity.[132] Rather than functionally blocking or physically eliminating entire T-cell subsets, a more selective way to inhibit only recently activated proliferating T cells is to apply monoclonal antibodies directed to the IL-2 receptor which is expressed on activated T cells only. In $P_2$ T-cell line mediated EAN, prophylactic treatment with the rat monoclonal antibody ART 18 directed at the IL-2 receptor during the latent phase of the disease markedly mitigated its severity.[133] However, it was not effective when applied after the onset of clinical disease. Although strictly prophylactic therapy as demonstrated in this adoptive transfer model does at first seem inappropriate for a human disorder, it could well be of value because in the naturally occurring disease, ongoing immune reactions take place in a much less synchronous pattern.

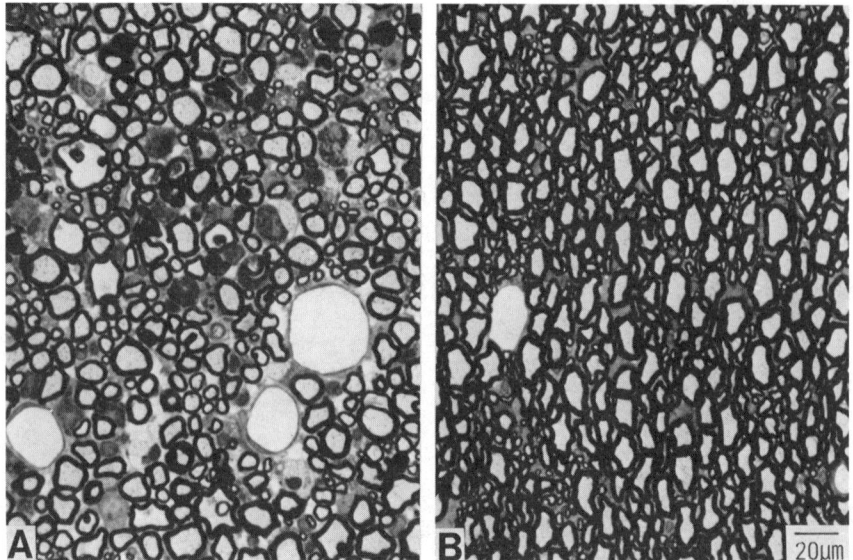

**FIGURE 16.** Immunopharmacologic intervention in AT-EAN: The effects of cyclosporin A. Representative micrographs of 1 μm Epon sections at S1 root levels from sham-treated (**A**) and cyclosporin A-treated animals (**B**). Note extensive cellular infiltration and demyelination in **A** and the almost complete absence of such findings in **B**.

## CHRONIC INFLAMMATORY DEMYELINATING POLYNEUROPATHY

*Pathogenic Humoral Mechanisms (TABLE 5)*

Chronic inflammatory demyelinating polyneuropathy (CIDP) has been separated from acute polyneuritis on clinical grounds, the main difference being the time course of the illness. It may follow a subacute, chronic progressive, or remitting and relapsing course similar to that of multiple sclerosis.[134]

In contrast to GBS, there is a less frequent association with preceding infections in CIDP. Pathologically, frank inflammatory infiltration of peripheral nerve is less common and, if present (45% of biopsies in one series), milder than demyelination. Correspondingly, there is usually profound slowing of nerve conduction. Low level immunoreactive MBP was detected in the CSF of 65% of patients with CIDP, suggesting a breakdown of nerve root myelin.[16] CSF cell typing disclosed a moderately increased percentage of macrophages/monocytes compared with that in control patients.[101] As in GBS, Koski *et al.*[36] demonstrated in three of four patients with CIDP the presence of complement-fixing antiperipheral myelin antibodies, probably recognizing neutral glycolipids.[36] A possible role of circulating humoral factors has been directly investigated by passive transfer experiments. Long-term injection of physiologic amounts of crude or purified IgG from patients with CIDP to marmoset monkeys resulted in significant slowing of nerve conduction in the recipient animals. The most active immunoglobulin fractions were derived from patients who had responded to therapeutic plasma exchange. However, in none of the animals was overt polyneuropathy noted on morphologic examination.[53] Intraneural injection of purified IgG from the serum of 1 of 12 patients with CIDP produced demyelination of rat sciatic nerve, and immunofluorescent studies on the patient's sural nerve demonstrated IgG bound to surviving myelin sheaths.[124] An earlier study reported IgM and IgG deposition on the external surface of the Schwann cell plasma membrane in sural nerve biopsies from nine patients with CIDP.[135] In one case of chronic relapsing demyelinating polyneuritis associated with hepatitis B infection, immunofluorescent deposits of hepatitis B antigen, IgG, and C3 were detected in the endoneurium throughout the vessel wall of the vasa nervorum in a histologically typical demyelinative lesion. Suggestive evidence for immune complexes containing GBS antigen was obtained by electronmicroscopy.[136]

Immunohistology of sural nerve biopsies from six patients showed prominent class II antigen staining within nerve fascicles, in capillary endothelial cells, and within the perineurium. Most Ia antigen staining occurred on mononuclear and Schwann cells. Only a few T lymphocytes were present.[137] CIDP is also an early manifestation of HIV infection and cannot be separated from HIV-negative patients on clinical, electrophysiologic, or morphologic grounds, with the exception of CSF pleocytosis in the former.[15]

It is of interest that recently two small series of cases were reported in which CIDP was associated with multiple lesions in the central nervous system as evidenced by magnetic resonance imaging and electrophysiologic studies, raising the question of cross-reactive immune responses to central and peripheral nervous system autoantigens.[138,139]

## *Autoimmune Animal Models of CIDP*

Early attempts to induce chronic polyneuritis by immunization with peripheral nerve antigens met with only partial success. An easily reproducible chronic monophasic and self-limited chronic EAN was established in rabbits by immunization with galactocerebroside. The clinical, electrophysiologic, and morphologic signs with de- and remyelination resemble CIDP in some, but not all, aspects.[140-142]

TABLE 5. Chronic Inflammatory Demyelinating Polyneuropathy

Humoral factors are operative
- Plasma exchange effective
- Functional defect on passive transfer to monkeys
- Activated complement

Gal C - EAN MODEL

Humoral factors (? antibody to Gal C)
- Block and demyelinate rat nerve on intraneural transfer
- No inhibition of myelination *in vivo*

Intraneural passive transfer of hyperimmune serum from these rabbits may lead to acute conduction block with rapid paranodal demyelination.[143] This process is complement dependent. It is not clear if antibody to galactocerebroside or other peripheral nerve antigens, for that matter, are responsible for this fulminant nerve dysfunction, or if other unspecific humoral factors are the causative agents. An alternative hypothesis favors the view that the antimyelin antibodies target adjacent macrophages that are preactivated by complement split products and in turn produce proinflammatory compounds. In the chronic de- and remyelination observed in this model and in CIDP, it was further speculated that circulating anti-nerve antibodies inhibit remyelination rather than produce demyelination as suggested earlier in multiple sclerosis. This hypothesis varies with recent experimental findings in galactocerebroside-induced EAN: regenerating sprouts of the crushed tibial nerve myelinate normally despite the presence of high titers of circulating antibodies to galactocerebroside.[144] A chronic relapsing animal model has been induced in Lewis rats. More recently, an easily reproducible model was induced by immunizing rabbits at multiple sites with myelin.[145] Little data on the immunology of this chronic relapsing model disease are available, but it is possible that continuous release of or challenge with autoantigen plays a role.

To date the conclusions that can be drawn from these chronic EAN models of CIDP are limited to a better understanding of the nerve pathology rather than the underlying immune mechanisms. Because of the chronic course of the model diseases, experimental approaches to immunomodulation appear more difficult to test than in the acute models of EAN.

*Therapy*

Because CIDP is even less frequent than GBS and has a variable natural history, validation of therapeutic modalities is difficult. Only three controlled trials of therapy have been conducted in CIDP.[124] In the first, 28 patients were treated with prednisone (initially 120 mg on alternate days) or placebo for 3 months.[146] There was on average only moderate improvement in clinical disease with prednisone treatment. The second study tested alternate-day decremental prednisone therapy alone versus prednisone plus azathioprine (2 mg/kg of body weight) for 9 months, and no statistically significant alterations were achieved with these treatment regimens.[147] The disease variability and the small number of patients limit the conclusive evidence of the latter study. In the third prospective double-blind trial 15 patients with CIDP received plasma exchange for 3 weeks; 14 patients were assigned to sham exchange. One third of patients treated with plasma exchange showed greater clinical improvement than did the sham-treated group as corroborated by corresponding changes in nerve conduction studies.[148] The latter study confirmed observations from open but well-controlled smaller trials.[29,135] No conclusive data on the efficacy of immunosuppressive treatment with cyclosporin A or cyclophosphamide are available. The HIV-associated form of CIDP may also respond favorably to plasma exchange.[15]

## PARAPROTEINEMIC POLYNEUROPATHIES (TABLE 6)

Monoclonal gammopathies arise from proliferation of a single clone of B lymphocytes generating a homogeneous immunoglobulin. Both malignant and nonmalignant gammopathies (also termed monoclonal gammopathies of undetermined significance) are associated with clinical polyneuropathy in at least 10-15% of cases. Patients with the osteosclerotic form of multiple myeloma have a much higher incidence of associated neuropathy.[149] Clinical and pathologic features of the neuropathies in patients with monoclonal gammopathies are heterogeneous, and biopsies from affected nerves may show primary demyelination, axonal degeneration, or selective involvement of motor fibers. Polyneuropathies associated with nonmalignant IgM paraproteinemia appear to have a relatively uniform clinical presentation with slow progression over years and decades and involvement of both motor and sensory functions. Motor nerve conduction velocity is severely reduced. Pathologically, primary demyelination with widening of myelin lamellae at the minor dense line and deposition of IgM on the myelin sheath can be demonstrated.[150-154] Immunoglobulin deposits of the appropriate class and light chain type have been detected on sural nerve biopsies.[155,156] Immunoblotting first revealed that monoclonal IgM antibodies in these patients bind to a carbohydrate determinant shared by central and peripheral myelin-associated glycoprotein. Approximately 50% of the monoclonal IgM proteins show this specificity. Thin-layer chromatography allowed the identification of binding of some IgM monoclonals to glycolipids and several low molecular weight glycoproteins of human peripheral nerve.[151,152,157,158] Evidence of shared idiotypy among neuropathy-associated paraproteins has been obtained in some series but not in others, suggesting

TABLE 6. Paraproteinemic Polyneuropathy

Humoral factors are operative
- m-IgM abs to MAG and other glycolipids demyelinate cat nerve on intraneural transfer
- m-IgG abs to unknown myelin antigens damage mouse nerve on systemic transfer (some)
- Plasma exchange effective in some

polymorphism in the human anti-MAG IgM system.[152] A pathogenic function of these anti-MAG monoclonal antibodies can be inferred from several observations. As just stated, deposits of the monoclonal paraprotein are found on the myelin sheath of affected nerves, and their antimyelin activity correlates with the degree of demyelination.[156] Intraneural injection of anti-MAG IgM from three patients with neuropathy produced demyelination of cat sciatic nerve.[159] Myelin damage in that model was dependent on the presence of human complement, and immunofluorescent studies showed that the anti-MAG IgM reacted with epitopes of myelin exposed to the extracellular space. In a proportion of patients, treatment to reduce IgM led to clinical improvement.[151,152] It should be noted that systemic passive transfer of human monoclonal IgM kappa directed to MAG for up to 3 months failed to cause a neuropathy in adult and newborn guinea pigs and in the monkey possibly because the integrity of the blood-nerve barrier prevented access of the transferred IgM to the nerve,[160] whereas direct intraneural passive transfer circumvents this barrier. In most patients with IgM paraproteinemia-associated polyneuropathy, in particular those with Waldenstrom's disease, however, antigen specificity is unknown. In one case of demyelinating neuropathy in which the IgM paraprotein did not react with MAG, the epitope recognized appeared to involve disialosyl groups on gangliosides.[161] In patients with axonal neuropathy, IgM monoclonal antibodies were bound by chondroitin sulfate and proteoglycans.[151,152,158] In yet another group with IgM monoclonal gammopathy-associated polyneuropathy, distinct clinical features are pure motor involvement with selective degeneration of ventral roots and chromatolytic alterations of anterior horn cells.[151] In one patient with this form of lower motor neuron disease, ganglioside $GM_1$ and $GD_{1b}$ are the antigens recognized by the IgM monoclonal antibody (cf., A. Steck, this volume). The C57BL mouse may serve as an animal model of monoclonal gammopathy-associated inflammatory demyelinating polyneuropathy.[162]

## PARANEOPLASTIC POLYNEUROPATHY

Subacute sensory polyneuropathy is a recognized paraneoplastic complication of various cancers.[163] Little is known about the immunology of this group of peripheral nerve disorders. In sural nerve biopsies of four patients with bronchial and breast carcinoma-associated polyneuropathies, myelin vacuolation and fiber loss were present. Immunostaining revealed IgM and C3 deposits in the inner layers of the perineurium.[164] In patients with subacute sensory neuronopathy associated with small cell carcinoma of the lung, an autoantibody reactive with a 35-38 kd basic nucleoprotein of neurons was identified that as evidenced by immunoblotting also stained a 35-36 kd antigen of tumor extract.[165,166] In these cases, cross-reaction of an antibody to a tumor cell antigen with a neuronal nucleoprotein could cause the polyneuropathy, but direct evidence is lacking.

## INFLAMMATORY NEUROPATHIES IN INFECTIOUS DISEASES

### Garin-Bujadoux-Bannwarth Syndrome—Lyme Disease

Infection with the spirochete *Borrelia burgdorferi,* the causative agent of Lyme disease, a multisystem disorder, can affect both the central and peripheral nervous systems.[167] Lymphocytic meningoradiculoneuritis (Garin-Bujadoux-Bannwarth syndrome), often bilateral facial nerve palsy, painful polyradiculoneuritis, a Guillain-Barré-like syndrome, mononeuritis multiplex, or brachial neuritis are manifestations of peripheral nervous system involvement.[167-169] Tick bite by the vector *Ixodes dammini* (in the United States) or *rizinus* (in Central Europe) is followed by a characteristic skin lesion, erythema chronicum migrans, after 1-3 weeks. Neurologic symptoms start after an average interval of 4 weeks. Serum and CSF contain antibodies to *B. burgdorferi.* Apart from lymphocytic pleocytosis, there is evidence of an intense intrathecal humoral immune response as mirrored by elevated CSF IgM and IgG indices with oligoclonal bands not present in serum.[170] In one series, histologic examination of sural nerve biopsies showed perivascular inflammatory infiltrates made up of lymphocytes and plasma cells and a significant loss of myelinated and unmyelinated fibers. Spirochetes were not detected, and immunofluorescent studies failed to demonstrate antibody, immune complex, or complement deposition.[168] In another series of patients, no inflammatory cells were seen in the endoneurial space. Minimal abnormalities were suggestive of a mild axonal process with secondary demyelination.[169] Microinjection of patients' serum into rat sciatic nerve did not produce lesions.[168] It must be concluded that the pathogenesis of peripheral nervous system involvement in borreliosis currently is elusive. The condition generally responds well to antibiotic treatment.

### Chagas' Disease-Associated Polyneuropathy

In chronic Chagas' disease caused by the protozoan *Trypanosoma cruzi,* which follows the acute phase after months or years, autonomic nervous system lesions with attendant gastrointestinal and cardiac complications are prominent. Muscle denervation and atrophy are due to peripheral neuropathy. The demonstration of circulating antibodies to Schwann cell epitopes absorbable by *T. cruzi* epimastigotes suggests an autoimmune etiology of Chagasic neuropathy.[171] It was further studied in an experimental model induced in mice by inoculation with trypomastigotes.[172,173] In the early phase, mononuclear cell infiltration in the endoneurium, the perineurium, and the epineurium of sciatic nerves was encountered and *T. cruzi* mastigotes were seen in macrophages. The lesion in chronically infected mice had a distinct histologic appearance. Prominent inflammatory infiltrates composed of lymphocytes, monocyte/macrophages, and mast cells were observed in the vicinity of endoneurial capillaries resembling granulomas.[172-174] There was also some degree of axonal degeneration, and later in the course of the disease Wallerian degeneration with subsequent regeneration ensued. The random distribution of demyelinative lesions in the spinal roots, plexuses, and nerve trunks argues against the notion that they are due to autoantibodies. Intraneural passive transfer of serum from chronically infected mice did not reproduce the disease in naive recipient animals. However, injection of trypomastigotes into sciatic nerves evoked focal inflammatory demyelination similar to that observed in chronically infected animals.[175] The critical importance of cellular immune reactions in the pathogenesis of chagasic neuritis has been highlighted by transfer experiments.[172,175] Purified T helper cells from chronically infected mice, when injected into naive recipients, produced granulomatous inflammatory infiltrates. These cells and CD4 T-helper cell lines obtained from chronically infected mice specific for either *T. cruzi* or peripheral nerve antigen were able to transfer a delayed-type hypersensitivity reaction in the presence of the relevant antigen. Furthermore, intraneural injection of T-helper line cells reproduced the nerve lesions found in chronically infected mice. Adoptive passive transfer by T-cell lines was H-2 restricted. Although the antigenic specificities of the T-line cells have not been clearly identified, some of the cells appeared to recognize determinants shared between *T. cruzi* and peripheral nerve. In this context, it is noteworthy that common determinants on *T. cruzi* and mouse cerebellum have been demonstrated.[176] Thus, during the acute phase, it is possible that parasites perturb immunoregulatory mechanisms with ensuing emergence of autoreactive helper T cells which induce delayed-type hypersensitivity, eventually leading to the formation of granulomatous infiltrates of the nerves in chronic Chagas' disease.

### Leprous Polyneuropathy

Leprosy, a chronic granulomatous infection of man caused by *Mycobacterium leprae,* has a propensity to affect the peripheral nervous system.[177] Epidemiologically, leprous polyneuropathy is the most common treatable neuropathy in the world. Cellular immunocompetence in combatting the invading microorganism determines the manifestations of the disease which form a broad spectrum.[178] At one end, *M. leprae* produces lepromatous leprosy characterized by the absence of a significant immunoinflammatory response to the infectious agent with subsequent massive invasion of skin and peripheral nerves. Owing to the compromised cellular immune reactivity, nerve destruction does not occur until late in the disease. At the other end of the spectrum, tuberculoid leprosy is characterized by the presence of a few well-localized skin and nerve lesions.[179,180] (For detailed information on nerve pathology, see references 177, 181-184.) Because there is a vigorous immune response against the microorganisms that invaded the PNS, nerves are damaged at the outset.[185]

In the lepromatous form of the disease there is a predominance of CD8 suppressor/cytotoxic T cells in both peripheral blood and the lesions.[179,186] Macrophages are engorged with *M. leprae* and are unable to kill or degrade the microorganism. This inability has been attributed to a deficit in IL-2 production, which in turn leads to defective expansion of specifically sensitized T cells capable of releasing IFN-$\gamma$ or failure to trigger them for IFN-$\gamma$ release.[186] This lymphokine is the major macrophage-activating factor. Cloned suppressor T cells were recently obtained from patients with lepromatous leprosy that exerted suppression of *M. leprae* reactive T-helper cell responses.[187,188] Conversely, in tuberculoid leprosy, CD4-positive helper cells greatly outnumber CD8 cells in cutaneous lesions.[179]

There is no evidence of specific T-cell sensitization to a peripheral nerve myelin antigen, the lesions probably the result of a delayed-type hypersensitivity reaction.[189,190]

The nerve lesion in lepromatous leprosy features endoneurial and perineurial invasion of foamy macrophages filled with numerous bacilli.[177,181] In contrast, in tuberculoid leprosy there is macroscopically a conspicuous enlargement of cutaneous nerves and nerve trunks. Microscopically, nerves are invaded and destroyed by giant cell granulomas, with only scarce occurrence of bacilli.

In all forms of leprosy, Schwann cells are a prime target for *M. leprae*. Their involvement results in segmental demyelination. When infected with *M. leprae*, Schwann cells can express MHC class II antigens upon treatment with IFN-$\gamma$, suggesting that they may be able to present *M. leprae* antigens to T lymphocytes.[191,192] As a result, an immune response against the bacteria could be elicited, which however requires that cellular immunity is not depressed. As already mentioned, it is intact in tuberculoid leprosy.

Specific cellular immune unresponsiveness in lepromatous leprosy, however, could then be accounted for by failure of MHC class II antigen expression on infected Schwann cells due to a deficit of IFN-$\gamma$ production.[192] Humoral immune responses do not appear to play a major pathogenic role in leprosy-associated neuropathy. In general, no circulating antibodies to peripheral nerve myelin antigens can be detected.[193] Recently described antineural antibodies in the sera of patients with leprosy seem to be directed against intermediate filament proteins released as breakdown products upon *M. leprae*-induced nerve damage.[194]

In conclusion, circumstantial evidence is available that links *M. leprae* infection of the PNS to disordered immune responsiveness, but the precise sequence of events culminating in peripheral nerve damage is not yet clear.

## REFERENCES

1. LÖFFEL, N. B., L. N. ROSSI, M. MUMENTHALER, J. LÜTSCHIG & H.-P. LUDIN. 1977. The Laundry-Guillain-Barré syndrome. Complications, prognosis and natural history in 123 cases. J. Neurol. Sci. **33:** 71-79.

2. BROWN, W. F. & T. E. FEASBY. 1984. Conduction block and denervation in Guillain-Barré polyneuropathy. Brain **107**: 219-239.
 3. FEASBY, T. E., J. J. GILBERT, W. F. BROWN, C. F. BOLTON, A. F. HAHN, W. F. KOOPMAN & D. W. ZOCHODNE. 1986. An acute axonal form of Guillain-Barré polyneuropathy. Brain **109**: 1115-1126.
 4. ROPPER, A. H. 1986. Severe acute Guillain-Barré syndrome. Neurology **36**: 429-432.
 5. MILLER, R. G., C. PETERSON & N. L. ROSENBERG. 1987. Electrophysiologic evidence of severe distal nerve segment pathology in the Guillain-Barré syndrome. Muscle & Nerve **10**: 524-429.
 6. FEASBY, T. E., A. F. HAHN, J. J. GILBERT, W. F. BROWN, C. F. BOLTON & W. J. KOOPMAN. 1987. Severe acute axonal degeneration in Guillain-Barré syndrome (abstract). Neurology **37**: 252-253.
 7. MADRID, R. E. & H. M. WISNIOWSKI. 1977. Axonal degeneration in demyelinating disorders. J. Neurocytol. **6**: 103-117.
 8. POWELL, H. C., S. L. BRAHENY, R. A. C. HUGHES & P. W. LAMPERT. 1984. Antigen-specific demyelination and significance of the bystander effect in peripheral nerves. Am. J. Pathol. **114**: 443-453.
 9. SAID, G., K. SAIDA, T. SAIDA & A. K. ASBURY. 1981. Axonal lesions in acute experimental demyelination: A sequential teased nerve fiber study. Neurology **31**: 413-421.
10. HEININGER, K., G. STOLL, C. LININGTON, K. V. TOYKA & H. WEKERLE. 1986. Conduction failure and nerve conduction slowing in experimental allergic neuritis induced by $P_2$-specific T-cell lines. Ann. Neurol. **19**: 44-49.
11. HAHN, A. F., T. E. FEASBY & J. J. GILBERT. 1987. Axonal degeneration in experimental allergic neuritis (EAN) is related to the immunizing dose of myelin (abstract). Neurology **37**: 362.
12. LIPKIN, W. I., G. PARRY, D. KIPROV & D. ABRAMS. 1985. Inflammatory neuropathy in homosexual men with lymphadenopathy. Neurology **35**: 1479-1483.
13. EIDELBERG, D., A. SOTREL, H. VOGEL, P. WALKER, J. KLEEFIELD & C. S. CRUMPACKER III. 1986. Progressive polyradiculopathy in acquired immune deficiency syndrome. Neurology **36**: 912-916.
14. PIETTE, A. M., F. TUSSEAU, D. VIGNON, A. CHAPMAN, G. PARROT, J. LEIBOWITCH & L. MONTAGNIER. 1986. Acute neuropathy coincident with seroconversion for LAV/HTLV-III. Lancet **1**: 852.
15. CORNBLATH, D. R., J. C. MCARTHUR, P. G. E. KENNEDY, A. S. WITTE & J. W. GRIFFIN. 1987. Inflammatory demyelinating peripheral neuropathies associated with human T-cell lymphotropic virus type III infection. Ann. Neurol. **21**: 32-40.
15a. PARRY, G. J. 1988. Peripheral neuropathies associated with human immunodeficiency virus infection. Ann. Neurol. **23**(suppl.): 49-53.
15b. CORNBLATH, D. R. 1988. Treatment of neuromuscular complications of human immunodeficiency virus infection. Ann. Neurol. **23**(suppl.): 88-91.
16. CORNBLATH, D. R., J. W. GRIFFIN & G. I. TENNEKOON. 1986. Immunoreactive myelin basic protein in cerebrospinal fluid of patients with peripheral neuropathies. Ann. Neurol. **20**: 370-372.
17. CORNBLATH, D. R., D. E. GRIFFIN, M. CHUPP, J. W. GRIFFIN & J. C. MCARTHUR. 1987. Mononuclear cell typing in inflammatory demyelinating polyneuropathy nerve biopsies (abstract). Neurology **37**: 253.
18. HO, D. D., T. R. ROTA, R. T. SCHOOLEY et al. 1985. Isolation of HTLV-III from cerebrospinal fluid and neural tissues of patients with neurologic syndromes related to the acquired immunodeficiency syndrome. N. Engl. J. Med. **313**: 1493-1497.
19. BISHOPRIC, G., J. BRUNER & J. BUTH. 1985. Guillain-Barré syndrome with cytomegalovirus infection of peripheral nerves. Arch. Pathol. Lab. Med. **109**: 1106-1108.
20. LEIBOWITZ, S. & R. A. C. HUGHES. 1983. Immunology of the nervous system. Chap. 5, pp. 101-130. E. Arnold, London.
21. HUGHES, R. A. C., I. A. GRAY, N. A. GREGSON, M. KADLUBOWSKI, M. KENNEDY, S. LEIBOWITZ & H. THOMPSON. 1984. Immune responses to myelin antigens in Guillain-Barré syndrome. J. Neuroimmunol. **6**: 303-312.
22. ZWEIMAN, B., A. ROSTAMI, R. P. LISAK, A. R. MOSKOVITZ & D. E. PLEASURE. 1983. Immune reactions to $P_2$ protein in human inflammatory demyelinative neuropathies. Neurology **33**: 234-237.

23. ROSTAMI, A. M., J. B. BURNS, P. A. ECCLESTON, M. C. MANNING, R. P. LISAK & D. H. SILBERBERG. 1987. Search for antibodies to galactocerebroside in the serum and cerebrospinal fluid in human demyelinating disorders. Ann. Neurol. **22:** 381-383.
24. COOK, S. D. & P. C. DOWLING. 1981. The role of autoantibody and immune complexes in the pathogenesis of Guillain-Barré syndrome. Ann. Neurol. **9:** 70-79.
25. LISAK, R. P., D. KUCHMY, P. J. ARMATI-GULSON, M. J. BROWN & A. J. SUMNER. 1984. Serum-mediated Schwann cell cytotoxicity in the Guillain-Barré syndrome. Neurology **34:** 1240-1243.
26. NYLAND, H. & J. A. AARLI. 1978. Guillain-Barré syndrome: Demonstration of antibodies to peripheral nerve tissue. Acta Neurol. Scand. **58:** 35-43.
27. LUIJTEN, J. A. F. M., D. E. L. A. BAART & E. H. FAILLE-KUYPER. 1972. The occurrence of IgM and complement factors along myelin sheaths of peripheral nerves: An immunohistochemical study of the Guillain-Barré syndrome. J. Neurol. Sci. **15:** 219-224.
28. NYLAND, H., R. MATRE & S. MORK. 1981. Immunological characterization of sural nerve biopsies from patients with Guillain-Barré syndrome. Ann. Neurol. **9** (suppl.): 80-86.
29. TOYKA, K. V. & K. HEININGER. 1987. Humoral factors in peripheral nerve disease. Muscle & Nerve **10:** 222-232.
30. VAN LIS, J. M. J. & F. G. I. JENNEKENS. 1977. Plasma proteins in human peripheral nerve. J. Neurol. Sci. **34:** 329-341.
31. LIEBERT, U. G., R. J. SEITZ, T. WEBER & W. WECHSLER. 1985. Immunocytochemical studies of serum proteins and immunoglobulins in human sural nerve biopsies. Acta Neuropathol. (Berl.) **68:** 39-47.
32. NEUEN, E., R. J. SEITZ, M. LANGENBACH & W. WECHSLER. 1987. The leakage of serum proteins across the blood nerve barrier in hereditary and inflammatory neuropathies. Acta Neuropathol. (Berl.) **73:** 53-61.
33. SILBERBERG, D. H., M. C. MANNING & A. D. SCHREIBER. 1984. Tissue culture demyelination by normal human serum. Ann. Neurol. **15:** 575-580.
34. KOSKI, C. L., M. E. SANDERS, P. T. SWOVELAND, T. J. LAWLEY, M. L. SHIN, M. M. FRANK & K. A. JOINER. 1987. Activation of terminal components of complement in patients with Guillain-Barré syndrome and other demyelinating neuropathies. J. Clin. Invest. **80:** 1492-1497.
35. HAYS, A. P., S. S. L. LEE & N. LATOV. 1988. Immune reactive C3d on the surface of myelin sheaths in neuropathy. J. Neuroimmunol. **18:** 231-244.
36. KOSKI, C. L., R. HUMPHREY & M. L. SHIN. 1985. Anti-peripheral myelin antibody in patients with demyelinating neuropathy: Quantitative and kinetic determination of serum antibody by complement component 1 fixation. Proc. Natl. Acad. Sci. USA **82:** 905-909.
37. KOSKI, C. L., E. GRATZ, J. SUTHERLAND & R. F. MAYER. 1986. Clinical correlation with anti-peripheral-nerve myelin antibodies in Guillain-Barré syndrome. Ann. Neurol. **19:** 573-577.
38. SANDERS, M. E., C. L. KOSKI, D. ROBBINS et al. 1986. Activated terminal complement in cerebrospinal fluid in Guillain-Barré syndrome and multiple sclerosis. J. Immunol. **136:** 4456-4459.
39. HARTUNG, H. P., C. SCHWENKE, D. BITTER-SUERMANN & K. V. TOYKA. 1987. Guillain-Barré syndrome: Activated complement components C3a and C5a in CSF. Neurology **37:** 1006-1009.
40. KOSKI, C. L., P. VANGURI & M. L. SHIN. 1985. Activation of the alternative pathway of complement by human peripheral nerve myelin. J. Immunol. **134:** 1810-1814.
41. KOSKI, C. L., D. CHOU & F. B. JUNGALWALA. 1987. Myelin lipids bound by serum antibodies to peripheral myelin (a-PNM Ab) in patients with Guillain-Barré syndrome (abstract). Neurology **37:** 253.
42. QUARLES, R. H., A. A. ILYAS & H. J. WILLISON. 1986. Antibodies to glycolipids in demyelinating diseases of the human peripheral nervous system. Chem. Phys. Lipids **42:** 235-248.
43. ILYAS, A. A., H. J. WILLISON, R. H. QUARLES et al. 1988. Serum antibodies to gangliosides in Guillain-Barré syndrome. Ann. Neurol. **23:** 440-447.
44. SAIDA, T., K. SAIDA, D. H. SILBERBERG & M. J. BROWN. 1978. Transfer of demyelination with experimental allergic neuritis serum by intraneural injection. Nature **272:** 639-641.

45. SUMNER, A. J., K. SAIDA, T. SAIDA, D. H. SILBERBERG & A. K. ASBURY. 1982. Acute conduction block associated with experimental anti-serum mediated demyelination of peripheral nerve. Ann. Neurol. **11:** 469-477.
46. FEASBY, T. E., A. F. HAHN & J. J. GILBERT. 1982. Passive transfer studies in Guillain-Barré polyneuropathy. Neurology **32:** 1159-1167.
47. SAIDA, T., K. SAIDA, R. P. LISAK, M. J. BROWN, D. H. SILBERBERG & A. K. ASBURY. 1982. In vivo demyelinating activity of sera from patients with Guillain-Barré syndrome. Ann. Neurol. **11:** 69-75.
48. HARRISON, B. M., L. A. HANSEN, J. D. POLLARD & J. G. MCLEOD. 1984. Demyelination induced by serum from patients with Guillain-Barré syndrome. Ann. Neurol. **15:** 163-170.
49. BROWN, M. J., J. L. ROSEN & R. P. LISAK. 1987. Demyelination in vivo by Guillain-Barré syndrome and other human serum. Muscle & Nerve **10:** 263-271.
50. SUMNER, A., G. SAID, I. IDY & S. METRAL. 1982. Syndrome de Guillain-Barré: Effets electrophysiologiques et morphologiques du serum humain introduit dans l'espace endoneural du nerf sciatique du rat: resultats preliminaires. Rev. Neurol. (Paris) **138:** 17-24.
51. LOW, P. A., J. SCHMELZER, P. J. DYCK & J. J. KELLY. 1982. Endoneurial effects of sera from patients with acute inflammatory polyradiculoneuropathy: Electrophysiologic studies on normal and demyelinated rat nerves. Neurology **32:** 720-724.
52. LAFONTAINE, S., M. RASMINSKY, T. SAIDA & A. J. SUMNER. 1982. Conduction block in rat myelinated fibres following acute exposure to anti-galactocerebroside serum. J. Physiol. (Lond.) **323:** 282-306.
53. HEININGER, K., U. G. LIEBERT, K. V. TOYKA et al. 1984. Chronic inflammatory polyneuropathy: Reduction of nerve conduction velocities in monkeys by systemic passive transfer of immunoglobulin G. J. Neurol. Sci. **66:** 1-14.
54. SEITZ, R. J., K. HEININGER, G. SCHWENDEMANN, K. V. TOYKA & W. WECHSLER. 1985. The mouse blood-brain-barrier and blood-nerve-barrier for IgG: A tracer study by use of the avidin-biotin system. Acta Neuropathol. (Berl.) **68:** 15-21.
55. HUGHES, R. A. C., H. C. POWELL, S. L. BRAHENY & S. BROSTOFF. 1985. Endoneurial injection of antisera to myelin antigens. Muscle & Nerve **8:** 516-522.
56. MILNER, P., C. A. LOVELIDGE, W. A. TAYLOR & R. A. C. HUGHES. 1987. $P_o$ myelin protein produces experimental allergic neuritis in Lewis rats. J. Neurol. Sci. **79:** 275-285.
57. BROSTOFF, S. W., S. LEVIT & J. M. POWERS. 1977. Induction of experimental allergic neuritis with a peptide from myelin $P_2$ basic protein. Nature **268:** 752-753.
58. KADLUBOWSKI, M. & R. A. C. HUGHES. 1979. Identification of the neuritogen for experimental allergic neuritis. Nature **277:** 140-141.
59. UYEMURA, K., M. SUZUKI, K. KITAMURA et al. 1982. Neuritogenic determinant of bovine $P_2$ protein in peripheral nerve myelin. J. Neurochem. **39:** 895-898.
60. MILEK, D. J., J. M. CUNNINGHAM, J. M. POWERS & S. W. BROSTOFF. 1983. Experimental allergic neuritis: Humoral and cellular immune responses to the cyanogen bromide peptides of the $P_2$ protein. J. Neuroimmunol. **4:** 105-117.
61. LEES, M. B. & S. W. BROSTOFF. 1984. Proteins of myelin. In Myelin, 2nd ed.: 197-224. P. Morell, Ed. Plenum, New York.
62. BROSTOFF, S. W. 1984. Immunological responses to myelin and myelin components. In Myelin, 2nd ed. P. Morell, Ed.: 405-439. Plenum, New York.
63. NOMURA, K., K. HAMAGUCHI, R. OHNO et al. 1987. Cell-mediated immunity to bovine $P_2$ protein and neuritogenic synthetic peptide in experimental allergic neuritis. J. Neuroimmunol. **15:** 25-35.
63a. ROSTAMI, A. M., E. VENTURA, H. KIMURA, M. J. & D. PLEASURE. 1988. Induction of severe experimental allergic neuritis (EAN) with a synthetic peptide corresponding to the 53-78 amino acid sequence of the myelin $P_2$ protein. Neurology **38**(suppl.): 375.
64. KADLUBOWSKI, M., R. A. C. HUGHES & N. A. GREGSON. 1984. Spontaneous and experimental neuritis and the distribution of the myelin protein $P_2$ in the nervous system. J. Neurochem. **42:** 123-129.
65. HUGHES, R. A. C., M. KADLUBOWSKI, I. A. GRAY & S. LEIBOWITZ. 1981. Immune responses in experimental allergic neuritis. J. Neurol. Neurosurg. Psychiatry **44:** 565-569.

66. LININGTON, C., S. IZUMO, M. SUZUKI, K. UYEMURA, R. MEYERMANN & H. WEKERLE. 1984. A permanent rat T cell line that mediates experimental allergic neuritis in the Lewis rat in vivo. J. Immunol. **133:** 1946-1950.
67. ROSTAMI, A., J. B. BURNS, M. J. BROWN, J. ROSEN, B. ZWEIMAN, R. P. LISAK & D. E. PLEASURE. 1985. Transfer of experimental allergic neuritis with $P_2$-reactive T-cell lines. Cell Immunol. **91:** 354-361.
68. FEASBY, T. E., J. J. GILBERT, A. F. HAHN & M. NEILSON. 1987. Complement depletion suppresses Lewis rat experimental allergic neuritis. Brain Res. **419:** 97-103.
69. FIERZ, W., K. HEININGER, B. SCHÄFER, K. V. TOYKA, C. LININGTON & H. LASSMANN. 1988. Synergism in the pathogenesis of EAE induced by an MBP-specific T cell line and monoclonal antibodies to galactocerebroside or to a myelin oligodendroglial glycoprotein. Ann. N. Y. Acad. Sci, this volume.
70. BALLIN, R. H. M. & P. K. THOMAS. 1968. Electron microscope observations on demyelination and remyelination in experimental allergic neuritis. Part I. Demyelination. J. Neurol. Sci. **8:** 1-18.
71. LAMPERT, P. W. 1969. Mechanisms of demyelination in experimental allergic neuritis—electronmicroscopic studies. Lab. Invest. **20:** 127-138.
72. RAINE, C. S. 1985. Experimental allergic encephalomyelitis and experimental allergic neuritis. *In* Handbook of Clinical Neurology, Vol. 47: 429-466. P. J. Vinken *et al.*, Eds. Elsevier, Amsterdam.
73. TANSEY, F. A. & C. F. BROSNAN. 1983. Protection against experimental allergic neuritis with silica quartz dust. J. Neuroimmunol. **3:** 169-179.
74. CRAGGS, R. I., R. H. M. KING & P. K. THOMAS. 1984. The effect of suppression of macrophage activity on the development of experimental allergic neuritis. Acta Neuropathol. (Berl.) **62:** 316-323.
75. HARTUNG, H. P., B. SCHÄFER, K. HEININGER, G. STOLL & K. V. TOYKA. 1988. The role of macrophages and eicosanoids in the pathogenesis of experimental allergic neuritis. Serial clinical, electrophysiological, biochemical, and morphological observations. Brain **111:** in press.
76. HEININGER, K., B. SCHÄFER, H. P. HARTUNG, W. FIERZ, C. LININGTON & K. V. TOYKA. 1988. The role of macrophages in experimental autoimmune neuritis induced by a $P_2$-specific T-cell line. Ann. Neurol. **23:** 326-331.
77. HARTUNG, H. P., B. SCHÄFER, K. HEININGER & K. V. TOYKA. 1988. Suppression of experimental autoimmune neuritis by the oxygen radical scavengers superoxide dismutase and catalase. Ann. Neurol. **23:** 453-460.
78. SOBUE, G., S. YAMATO, M. HIRAYAMA, Y. MATSUOKA, H. UEMATSU & I. SOBUE. 1982. The role of macrophages in demyelination in experimental allergic neuritis. J. Neurol. Sci. **56:** 75-87.
79. CAMMER, W., B. R. BLOOM, W. T. NORTON & S. S. GORDON. 1978. Degradation of basic protein in myelin by neutral proteases secreted by stimulated macrophages: A possible mechanism of inflammatory demyelination. Proc. Natl. Acad. Sci. **75:** 1554-1558.
80. TROTTER, J. & M. E. SMITH. 1986. The role of phospholipases from inflammatory macrophages in demyelination. Neurochem. Res. **11:** 349-361.
81. TROTTER, J., L. J. DEJONG & M. E. SMITH. 1986. Opsonization with antimyelin antibody increases the uptake and intracellular metabolism of myelin in inflammatory macrophages. J. Neurochem. **47:** 779-789.
82. POWELL, H. C., S. L. BRAHENY, R. R. MYERS, M. RODRIGUEZ & P. W. LAMPERT. 1983. Early changes in experimental allergic neuritis. Lab. Invest. **48:** 332-338.
83. BROSNAN, C. F., W. D. LYMAN, F. A. TANSEY & T. H. CARTER. 1985. Quantitation of mast cells in experimental allergic neuritis. J. Neuropathol. Exp. Neurol. **44:** 196-203.
84. IZUMO, S., C. LININGTON, H. WEKERLE & R. MEYERMANN. 1985. Morphologic study on experimental allergic neuritis mediated by T-cell line specific for bovine $P_2$ protein in Lewis rats. Lab. Invest. **53:** 209-218.
85. BROSNAN, C. F. & F. A. TANSEY. 1984. Delayed onset of experimental allergic neuritis in rats treated with reserpine. J. Neuropathol. Exp. Neurol. **43:** 84-93.
86. JOHNSON, D., P. A. SEELDRAYERS & H. L. WEINER. 1988. The role of mast cells in demyelination. 1. Myelin proteins are degraded by mast cell proteases and myelin basic protein and $P_2$ can stimulate mast cell degranulation. Brain Res. **444:** 195-198.

87. ASTRÖM, K. E., H. DE F. WEBSTER & B. G. W. ARNASON. 1968. The initial lesion in experimental allergic neuritis. J. Exp. Med. **128:** 469-495.
88. HAHN, A. F., T. E. FEASBY & J. J. GILBERT. 1985. Blood-nerve-barrier studies in experimental allergic neuritis. Acta Neuropathol. (Berl.) **68:** 101-109.
89. LAMPERT, P., R. GARRETT & H. POWELL. 1977. Demyelination in allergic and Marek's disease virus-induced neuritis. Comparative electron-microscopic studies. Acta Neuropathol. (Berl.) **40:** 103-110.
90. WEKERLE, H., M. SCHWAB, C. LININGTON & R. MEYERMANN. 1986. Antigen presentation in the peripheral nervous system: Schwann cells present endogenous myelin autoantigens to lymphocytes. Eur. J. Immunol. **16:** 1551-1557.
91. IQBAL, A., J. J.-F. OGER & B. G. W. ARNASON. 1981. Cell-mediated immunity in idiopathic polyneuritis. Ann. Neurol. **9**(suppl.): 65-69.
92. ZWEIMAN, B., A. ROSTAMI & R. P. LISAK. 1983. Immune responses to $P_2$ protein in the human inflammatory demyelinative neuropathies. Neurology **33:** 234-237.
93. HUGHES, R. A. C., I. A. GRAY & N. A. GREGSON. 1984. Immune responses to myelin antigens in Guillain-Barré syndrome. J. Neuroimmunol. **6:** 303-312.
94. GECZY, C., R. RAPER, I. M. ROBERTS, P. MEYER & C. C. A. BERNARD. 1985. Macrophage procoagulant activity as a measure of cell-mediated immunity to $P_2$ protein of peripheral nerves in the Guillain-Barré syndrome. J. Neuroimmunol. **9:** 179-191.
95. BURNS, J., L. J. KRASNER, A. ROSTAMI & D. PLEASURE. 1986. Isolation of $P_2$ protein-reactive T-cell lines from human blood. Ann. Neurol. **19:** 391-393.
96. HAUSER, S. L., A. H. ROPPER, V. P. PERLO, E. L. REINHERZ, S. F. SCHLOSSMANN & H. L. WEINER. 1982. T-cell subsets in human autoimmune diseases. Neurology **32:** 1321-1322.
97. LISAK, R. P., B. ZWEIMAN, F. GUERRERO & A. R. MOSKOVITZ. 1985. Circulating T-cell subsets in Guillain-Barré syndrome. J. Neuroimmunol. **8:** 93-101.
98. HUGHES, R. A. C., S. ASLAN & I. A. GRAY. 1983. Lymphocyte subpopulations and suppressor cell activity in acute polyradiculoneuritis (Guillain-Barré syndrome). Clin. Exp. Immunol. **51:** 448-454.
99. BROSNAN, J. V., R. FELLOWES, R. I. CRAGGS, R. H. M. KING, T. J. BOWLEY & P. K. THOMAS. 1985. Changes in lymphocyte subpopulations during the course of experimental allergic neuritis. Brain **108:** 315-334.
100. FEASBY, T. E., R. MAZAHERI, A. F. HAHN, J. J. GILBERT, C. R. STILLER & P. A. KEOWN. 1984. Circulating T lymphocyte subpopulations in experimental allergic neuritis. J. Neuroimmunol. **6:** 209-214.
101. CORNBLATH, D. R., D. E. GRIFFIN, J. C. MCARTHUR, D. WELCH & J. W. GRIFFIN. 1987. Cerebrospinal fluid and peripheral blood mononuclear cell typing in inflammatory demyelinating polyneuropathy (abstract). Ann. Neurol. **22:** 117.
102. PRINEAS, J. W. 1981. Pathology of the Guillain-Barré syndrome. Ann. Neurol. **9**(suppl.): 6-19.
103. POLLARD, J. D., J. BAVERSTOCK & J. G. MCLEOD. 1987. Class II antigen expression and inflammatory cells in the Guillain-Barré syndrome. Ann. Neurol. **21:** 337-341.
104. STEINMAN, L., M. E. SMITH & L. S. FORNO. 1981. Genetic control of susceptibility to experimental allergic neuritis and the immune response to $P_2$ protein. Neurology **31:** 950-954.
105. HOFFMANN, P. M., J. M. POWERS, M. J. WEISE & S. W. BROSTOFF. 1980. EAN: 1. Rat strain differences in the response to bovine myelin antigens. Brain Res. **195:** 355-362.
106. LININGTON, C., A. MANN, S. IZUMO, K. UYEMURA, M. SUZUKI, R. MEYERMANN & H. WEKERLE. 1986. Induction of experimental allergic neuritis in the BN rat: $P_2$ protein-specific T cells overcome resistance to actively induced disease. J. Immunol. **137:** 3826-3831.
107. BROSNAN, J. V., R. I. CRAGGS, R. H. M. KING & P. K. THOMAS. 1987. Reduced susceptibility of T cell-deficient rats to induction of experimental allergic neuritis. J. Neuroimmunol. **14:** 267-282.
108. LININGTON, C., H. WEKERLE & R. MEYERMANN. 1986. T lymphocyte autoimmunity in peripheral nervous system autoimmune disease. Agents Actions **19:** 256-265.
109. WEKERLE, H., C. LININGTON, H. LASSMANN & R. MEYERMANN. 1986. Cellular immune reactivity within the CNS. TINS **9:** 271-277.
110. LISAK, R. P., M. HIRAYAMA, D. KUCHMY, A. ROSENZWEIG, S. U. KIM, D. E. PLEASURE

& D. H. SILVERBERG. 1983. Cultured human and rat oligodendrocytes and rat Schwann cells do not have immune response gene-associated antigen (Ia) on their surface. Brain Res. **289:** 285-292.

111. YAROM, Y., Y. NAPARSTEK, V. LEV-RAM, J. HOLOSHITZ, A. BEN-NUN & I. R. COHEN. 1983. Immunospecific inhibition of nerve conduction by T lymphocytes reactive to basic protein of myelin. Nature **303:** 246-247.

112. OLSSON, T., R. HOLMDAHL, L. KLARESKOG, U. FORSUM & K. KRISTENSSON. 1984. Dynamics of Ia-expressing cells and T lymphocytes of different subsets during experimental allergic neuritis in Lewis rats. J. Neurol. Sci. **66:** 141-149.

113. HUGHES, R. A. C., P. F. ATKINSON, I. A. GRAY & W. A TAYLOR. 1987. Major histocompatibility antigens and lymphocyte subsets during experimental allergic neuritis in the Lewis rat. J. Neurol. **234:** 390-395.

114. KIYOSHI, O., H. IRIE & K. TAKAHASHI. 1987. T cell subsets and Ia-positive cells in the sciatic nerve during the course of experimental allergic neuritis. J. Neuroimmunol. **13:** 283-292.

115. STRIGARD, K., T. BRISMAR, T. OLSSON, K. KRISTENSSON & L. KLARESKOG. 1987. T-lymphocyte subsets, functional deficits, and morphology in sciatic nerves during experimental allergic neuritis. Muscle & Nerve **10:** 329-337.

116. HARTUNG, H. P., B. SCHÄFER, W. FIERZ, K. HEININGER & K. V. TOYKA. 1987. Ciclosporin A prevents $P_2$ T cell line-mediated experimental autoimmune neuritis (AT-EAN) in rat. Neurosci. Lett. **83:** 195-200.

117. ROSTAMI, A., M. J. BROWN, R. P. LISAK, A. J. SUMNER, B. ZWEIMAN & D. E. PLEASURE. 1984. The role of myelin $P_2$ protein in the production of experimental allergic neuritis. Ann. Neurol. **16:** 680-685.

118. ADAMS, D., J. D. GIBSON, P. K. THOMAS et al. 1977. HLA antigens in Guillain-Barré syndrome. Lancet **2:** 504-505.

119. STEWART, G. J., J. D. POLLARD, J. G. MCLEOD & C. M. WOLNIZER. 1978. HLA antigens in the Landry-Guillain-Barré syndrome and chronic relapsing polyneuritis. Ann. Neurol. **4:** 285-289.

120. LATOVITZKI, N., N. SUCIA-FOCA, A. S. PENN, M. R. OLARTE & A. M. CHUTORIAN. 1979. HLA typing and Guillain-Barré syndrome. Neurology **29:** 743-745.

121. JAHNKE, U., E. H. FISCHER & E. C. ALVORD. 1985. Sequence homology between certain viral proteins and proteins related to encephalomyelitis and neuritis. Science **229:** 282-284.

122. The Guillain-Barré Syndrome Study Group (1985). Plasmapheresis and acute Guillain-Barré syndrome. Neurology **35:** 1096-1104.

123. French Cooperative Group on Plasma Exchange in Guillain-Barré syndrome. 1987. Efficiency of plasma exchange in Guillain-Barré syndrome: Role of replacement fluids. Ann. Neurol. **22:** 753-;761.

124. POLLARD, J. D. 1987. A critical review of therapies in acute and chronic inflammatory demyelinating polyneuropathies. Muscle & Nerve **10:** 214-221.

125. MCKHANN, G. M., J. W. GRIFFIN, D. R. CORNBLATH et al. 1988. Plasmapheresis and Guillain-Barré syndrome: Analysis of prognostic factors and the effect of plasmapheresis. Ann. Neurol., **23:** 347-353.

125a. CORNBLATH, D. R. et al. 1988. Motor nerve conduction studies in Guillain-Barré syndrome: Description and prognostic value. Ann. Neurol. **23:** 354-359.

126. GRUENER, G., E. P. BOSCH, R. G. STRAUSS, M. KLUGMAN & J. KIMURA. 1987. Prediction of early beneficial response to plasma exchange in Guillain-Barré syndrome. Arch. Neurol. **44:** 295-298.

127. SURIK, H. M. & M. P. MCQUILLEN. 1976. The use of steroids in the treatment of idiopathic polyneuritis. Neurology **26:** 205-212.

128. HUGHES, R. A. C., J. NEWSOM-DAVIS, G. D. PERKINS & J. M. PIERCE. 1978. Controlled trial of prednisolone in acute polyneuropathy. Lancet **2:** 750-753.

129. VERMEULEN M., F. G. A. VAN DER MECHE, J. D. SPEELMAN, A. WEBER & H. F. M. BUSCH. 1985. Plasma and gamma-globulin infusion in chronic inflammatory polyneuropathy. J. Neurol. Sci. **70:** 317-326.

130. HARTUNG, H. P., B. SCHÄFER, K. HEININGER & K. V. TOYKA. 1986. Interference with arachidonic acid metabolism suppresses experimental allergic neuritis (abstract). Ann. Neurol. **20:** 168.

131. KING, R. H. M., R. I. CRAGGS, L. P. GROSS, C. TOMKINS & P. K. THOMAS. 1983. Suppression of experimental allergic neuritis by cyclosporin A. Acta Neuropathol. (Berl.) **59:** 262-268.
132. HOLMDAHL, R., T. OLSSON, T. MORON & L. KLARESKOG. 1985. In vivo treatment of rats with monoclonal anti T-cell antibodies. Immunohistochemical and functional analysis in normal rats and in experiment allergic nerutis (EAN). Scand. J. Immunol. **22:** 157-169.
133. HARTUNG, H. P., B. SCHÄFER, T. DIAMANTSTEIN, W. FIERZ, K. HEININGER & K. V. TOYKA. 1988. Suppression of $P_2$-T cell line mediated experimental autoimmune neuritis by interleukin-2 receptor blockade. Ann. N. Y. Acad. Sci., this volume.
134. MCCOMBE, P. A., J. D. POLLARD & J. G. MCLEOD. 1987. Chronic inflammatory demyelinating polyradiculoneuropathy. Brain **110:** 1617-1630.
135. DALAKAS, M. C. & W. K. ENGEL. 1981. Chronic relapsing (dysimmune) polyneuropathy: Pathogenesis and treatment. Ann. Neurol. **9**(suppl.): 134-145.
136. INOUE, A., N. TSUKADA, C. S. KOH & N. YANAGISAWA. 1987. Chronic relapsing demyelinating polyneuropathy associated with hepatitis B infection. Neurology **37:** 1663-1666.
137. POLLARD, J. D., P. A. MCCOMBE, J. BAVERSTOCK, P. A. GATENBY & J. G. MCLEOD. 1986. Class II antigen expression and T lymphocyte subsets in chronic inflammatory demyelinating polyneuropathy. J. Neuroimmunol. **13:** 123-134.
138. THOMAS, P. K., R. W. H. WALKER, P. RUDGE et al. 1987. Chronic demyelinating peripheral neuropathy associated with multifocal central nervous system demyelination. Brain **110:** 53-76.
139. MENDELL, J. R., S. KOLKIN, J. T. KISSEL, K. L. WEISS, D. W. CHAKERES & K. W. RAMMOHAN. 1987. Evidence for central nervous system demyelination in chronic inflammatory demyelinating polyradiculoneuropathy. Neurology **37:** 1291-1294.
140. SAIDA, T., K. SAIDA & S. H. DORFMAN. 1979. Experimental allergic neuritis induced by sensitization with galactocerebroside. Science **204:** 1103-1106.
141. SAIDA, T., K. SAIDA, D. H. SILVERBERG & M. M. BROWN. 1981. Experimental allergic neuritis induced by galactocerebroside. Ann. Neurol. **9**(suppl): 87-101.
142. STOLL, G., G. SCHWENDEMANN, K. HEININGER, W. KÖHNE, H.-P. HARTUNG, R. J. SEITZ & K. V. TOYKA. 1986. Relation of clinical, serological, morphological and electrophysiological findings in galactocerebroside-induced experimental allergic neuritis. J. Neurol. Neurosurg. Psychiatry **49:** 258-264.
143. SAIDA, K., A. J. SUMNER & T. SAIDA. 1980. Antiserum-mediated demyelination: Relationship between remyelination and functional recovery. Ann. Neurol. **8:** 12-24.
144. STOLL, G., K. REINERS, G. SCHWENDEMANN, K. HEININGER & K. V. TOYKA. 1986. Normal myelination of regenerating peripheral nerve sprouts despite circulating antibodies to galactocerebroside in rabbits. Ann. Neurol. **19:** 189-192.
145. HARVEY, G. K., J. D. POLLARD, K. SCHINDHELM & J. ANTONY. 1987. Chronic experimental allergic neuritis: An electrophysiological and histological study in the rabbit. J. Neurol. Sci. **81:** 215-225.
146. DYCK, P. J., P. C. O'BRIEN, K. F. OVIATT et al. 1982. Prednisone improves chronic inflammatory demyelinating polyradiculoneuropathy more than no treatment. Ann. Neurol. **11:** 136-141.
147. DYCK, P. J., P. O'BRIEN, C. SWANSON, P. LOW & J. DAUBE. 1985. Combined azathioprine and prednisone in chronic inflammatory-demyelinating polyneuropathy. Neurology **35:** 1173-1176.
148. DYCK, P. J., J. DAUBE, P. O'BRIEN, A. PINEDA, P. A. LOW, A. J. WINDEBANK & C. SWANSON. 1986. Plasma exchange in chronic inflammatory demyelinating polyradiculoneuropathy. N. Engl. J. Med. **314:** 461-465.
149. KELLY, J. J. 1985. Peripheral neuropathies associated with monoclonal proteins. A clinical review. Muscle & Nerve **8:** 138-150.
150. SMITH, I. S., S. N. KAHN, B. W. LACEY, R. H. M. KING, R. A. EAMES, D. J. WHYBREW & P. K. THOMAS. 1983. Chronic demyelinating neuropathy associated with benign IgM paraproteinaemia. Brain **106:** 169-195.
151. LATOV, N. 1987. Peripheral neuropathy and IgM monoclonal gammopathy. *In* Clinical Neuroimmunology. J. A. Aarli, W. M. H. Behan & P. O. Behan, Eds. Oxford, Blackwell, pp. 214-224.

152. STECK, A. J., N. MURRAY, K. DELLAGI, J. C. BROUET & M. SELIGMANN. 1987. Peripheral neuropathy associated with monoclonal IgM autoantibody. Ann. Neurol. **22:** 764-767.
153. NOBILE-ORAZIO, E., P. MARMIROLI, L. BALDINI et al. 1987. Peripheral neuropathy in macroglobulinemia: Incidence and antigen-specificity of M proteins. Neurology **37:** 1506-1514.
154. HAFLER, D. A., D. JOHNSON, J. J. KELLY, H. PANITCH, R. KYLE & H. L. WEINER. 1986. Monoclonal gammopathy and neuropathy: Myelin-associated glycoprotein reactivity and clinical characteristics. Neurology **36:** 75-78.
155. ABRAMS, G. M., N. LATOV, A. P. HAYS, W. SHERMAN & E. A. ZIMMERMAN. 1982. Immunocytochemical studies of human peripheral nerve with serum from patients with polyneuropathy and paraproteinemia. Neurology **32:** 821-826.
156. TAKATSU, M., A. P. HAYS, N. LATOV et al. 1985. Immunofluorescence study of patients with neuropathy and IgM M proteins. Ann. Neurol. **18:** 173-181.
157. O'SHANNESSY, D. J., A. A. ILYAS, M. C. DALAKAS, J. R. MENDELL & R. H. QUARLES. 1986. Specificity of human IgM monoclonal antibodies from patients with peripheral neuropathy. J. Neuroimmunol. **11:** 131-136.
158. FREDDO, L., T. ARIGA, M. SAITO, L. C. MACALA, R. K YU & N. LATOV. 1985. The neuropathy of plasma cell dyscrasia: Binding of IgM M-proteins to peripheral nerve glycolipids. Neurology **35:** 1420-1424.
159. HAYS, A. P., N. LATOV, M. TAKATSU & W. H. SHERMAN. 1987. Experimental demyelination of nerve induced by serum of patients with neuropathy and an anti-MAG IgM M-protein. Neurology **37:** 242-256.
160. STECK, A. J., N. MURRAY, J. C. JUSTAFRE, C. MEIER, K. V. TOYKA, K. HEININGER & G. STOLL. 1985. Passive transfer studies in demyelinating neuropathy with IgM monoclonal antibodies to myelin associated glycoprotein. J. Neurol. Neurosurg. Psych. **48:** 927-929.
161. ILYAS, A. A., R. H. QUARLES, M. C. DALAKAS, P. H. FISHMAN & R. O. BRADY. 1985. Monoclonal IgM in a patient with paraproteinemic polyneuropathy binds to gangliosides containing disialosyl groups. Ann. Neurol. **18:** 655-659.
162. DIB, M., A. VITAL, C. VITAL, D. GEORGESCAULT, A. BAQUEY & J. BEZIAN. 1987. The C57BL mice: An animal model for inflammatory demyelinating polyneuropathy. J. Neurol. Sci. **81:** 101-111.
163. MCLEOD, J. G. 1984. Carcinomatous neuropathy. In Peripheral Neuropathy, vol. 2. P. J. Dyck, P. K. Thomas, E. H. Lambert & R. Bunger, Eds. Saunders, Philadelphia, pp. 2180-2191.
164. ONGERBOER DE VISSER, B. W., T. M. FELTKAMP-VROOM & C. A. FELTKAMP. 1983. Sural nerve immune deposits in polyneuropathy as a remote effect of malignancy. Ann. Neurol. **14:** 261-266.
165. GRAUS, F., C. CORDON-CARDO & J. B. POSNER. 1985. Neuronal antinuclear antibody in sensory neuronopathy from lung cancer. Neurology **35:** 538-543.
166. GRAUS, F., K. B. ELKON, C. CORDON-CARDO & J. B. POSNER. 1986. Sensory neuronopathy and small cell lung cancer: Antineuronal antibody that also reacts with the tumor. Am. J. Med. **80:** 45-52.
167. PACHNER, A. R. & A. C. STEERE. 1985. The triad of neurologic manifestations of Lyme disease: Meningitis, cranial neuritis and radiculoneuritis. Neurology **35:** 47-53.
168. VALLAT, J. M., J. HUGON, M. LUBEAU, M. J. LEBOUTET, M. DUMAS & R. DESPROGES-GOTTERON. 1987. Tick-bite meningoradiculoneuritis: Clinical, electrophysiologic and histologic findings in 10 cases. Neurology **37:** 749-753.
169. HALPERIN, J. J., B. W. LITTLE, P. K. COYLE & R. J. DATTWYLER. 1987. Lyme disease: Cause of a treatable peripheral neuropathy. Neurology **37:** 1700-1706.
170. HENRIKSSON, A., H. LINK, M. CRUZ & G. STIERNSTEDT. 1986. Immunoglobulin abnormalities in cerebrospinal fluid and blood over the course of lymphocytic meningoradiculitis (Bannwarth's syndrome). Ann. Neurol. **20:** 337-345.
171. KHOURY, E. L., V. RITACCO, P. M. COSSIO, R. P. LAGUENS, A. SZARFMAN, C. DIEZ & R. M. ARANA. 1979. Circulating antibodies to peripheral nerve in American trypanosomiasis (Chagas' disease). Clin. Exp. Immunol. **36:** 8-15.
172. SAID, G., M. JOSKOWIEZ, A. A. BARREIRA & H. EISEN. 1985. Neuropathy associated with experimental Chagas' disease. Ann. Neurol. **18:** 676-683.

173. CAPPA, S. M. G., O. P. SANZ, L. A. MULLER, H. A. MOLINA, J. FERNANDEZ, M. T. RIMOLDI & R. E. P. SICA. 1987. Peripheral nervous system damage in experimental chronic Chagas' disease. Am. J. Trop. Med. Hyg. **36:** 41-45.
174. MOLINA, H. A., R. L. CARDONI & M. T. RIMOLDI. 1987. The neuromuscular pathology of experimental Chagas' disease. J. Neurol. Sci. **81:** 287-300.
175. HONTEBEYRIE-JOSKOWIEZ, M. H., G. SAID, G. MILON, G. MARCHAL & H. EISEN. 1987. L3T4$^+$ T cells able to mediate parasite-specific delayed-type hypersensitivity play a role in the pathology of experimental Chagas' disease. Eur. J. Immunol. **17:** 1027-1033.
176. WOOD, J. N., L. HUDSON, T. M. JESSELL & M. YAMAMOTO. 1982. A monoclonal antibody defining antigenic determinants on subpopulations of mammalian neurones and Trypanosoma cruzi parasites. Nature **296:** 34-38.
177. SABIN, T. D. & T. R. SWIFT. 1984. Leprosy. In Peripheral Neuropathy, 2nd ed., vol. 2. P. J. Dyck, P. K. Thomas, E. H. Lambert & R. Bunge, Eds. Saunders, Philadelphia, pp. 1955-1987.
178. SANSONETTI, P. & P. H. LAGRANGE. 1981. The immunology of leprosy: Speculations on the leprosy spectrum. Rev. Infect. Dis. **3:** 422-469.
179. VAN VOORHIS, W. C., G. KAPLAN, E. N. SARNO et al. 1982. The cutaneous infiltrates of leprosy. N. Engl. J. Med. **307:** 1593-1597.
180. BODDINGIUS, J. 1981. Mechanisms of nerve damage in leprosy. In Immunological Aspects of Leprosy, Tuberculosis, and Leishmaniasis. D. Humber, Ed. Excerpta Medica, Amsterdam, pp. 64-73.
181. JOB, C. K. 1971. Pathology of peripheral nerve lesions in lepromatous leprosy—a light and electron microscopic study. Int. J. Lepr. **39:** 251-267.
182. MSHANA, R. N., D. P. HUMBER, M. HARBOE & A. BELEHU. 1983. Demonstration of mycobacterial antigens in nerve biopsies from leprosy patients using peroxidase-antiperoxidase immunoenzyme technique. Clin. Immunol. Immunopathol. **29:** 359-368.
183. BUDDINGIUS, J. 1984. Ultrastructural and histophysiological studies on the blood-nerve barrier and perineurial barrier in leprosy neuropathy. Acta Neuropathol. (Berl.) **64:** 282-296.
184. JACOBS, J. M., V. P. SHETTY & N. H. ANTIA. 1987. Myelin changes in leprous neuropathy. Acta Neuropathol. (Berl.) **74:** 75-80.
185. DASTUR, D. K., G. L. PORWAL, J. S. SHAH & C. R. REVANKAR. 1982. Immunological complications of necrotic, cellular and vascular changes in leprous neuritis: Light and electron microscopy. Lepr. Rev. **53:** 45-65.
186. NOGUIERA, N., G. KAPLAN, E. LEVY et al. 1983. Defective gamma-interferon production in leprosy. Reversal with antigen and interleukin 2. J. Exp. Med. **158:** 2165-2170.
187. OTTENHOFF, T. H. M., D. G. ELFERINK, P. R. KLATSER & R. P. DEVRIES. 1986. Cloned suppressor T cells from a lepromatous leprosy patient suppress Mycobacterium leprae reactive helper T cells. Nature **322:** 462-464.
188. MODLIN, R. L., H. KATO, V. MEHRA et al. 1986. Genetically restricted suppressor T-cell clones derived from lepromatous leprosy lesions. Nature **322:** 459-461.
189. MSHANA, R. N., D. P. HUMBER, M. HARBOE & A. BELEHU. 1983. Immune responses to bovine neural antigens in leprosy patients. II. Absence of in vitro lymphocyte stimulation to peripheral myelin proteins. Lepr. Rev. **54:** 217-227.
190. MSHANA, R. N., D. P. HUMBER, M. HARBOE & A. BELEHU. 1983. Nerve damage following intraneural injection of Mycobacterium leprae damage into rabbits pre-sensitized to mycobacteria. Clin. Exp. Immunol. **52:** 441-448.
191. SAMUEL, N. M., K. R. JESSEN, J. M. GRANGE & R. MIRSKY. 1987. Gamma interferon, but not Mycobacterium leprae, induces major histocompatibility class II antigens on cultured rat Schwann cells. J. Neurocytol. **16:** 282-287.
192. SAMUEL, N. M., R. MIRSKY, J. M. GRANGE & K. R. JESSEN. 1987. Expression of major histocompatibility complex class I and class II antigens in human Schwann cell cultures and effects of infection with Mycobacterium leprae. Clin. Exp. Immunol. **68:** 500-509.
193. MSHANA, R. N., M. HARBOE, G. L. STONER, R. A. C. HUGHES, M. KADLUBOWSKI & A. BELEHU. 1983. Immune responses to bovine neural antigens in leprosy patients. I. Absence of antibodies to an isolated myelin protein. Int. J. Lepr. **51:** 33-40.
194. ESTIS-TURF, E. P., J. A. BENJAMINS & M. J. LEFFORD. 1986. Characterization of the anti-neural antibodies in the sera of leprosy patients. J. Neuroimmunol. **10:** 313-330.

# Infection of the Central Nervous System by Human Immunodeficiency Virus

## Role of the Immune System in Pathogenesis[a]

RICHARD W. PRICE AND BRUCE BREW

*Department of Neurology
Memorial Sloan-Kettering Cancer Center
New York, New York*

Infection by the retrovirus causing the acquired immune deficiency syndrome (AIDS), now designated human immunodeficiency virus type 1 (HIV-1), is complicated by an array of central nervous system (CNS) disorders. (For reviews, see references 1 to 3.) Although some of these are well-characterized opportunistic infections (e.g., cerebral toxoplasmosis, cryptococcal meningitis, and progressive multifocal leukoencephalopathy) or opportunistic neoplasms (e.g., primary CNS lymphoma), others are seemingly unique to HIV-1 infection and are now known or suspected to be caused by direct CNS infection by this retrovirus. The most common and clinically most important of these is a progressive dementing illness that afflicts both adults and children and has been described by a variety of terms, including subacute encephalitis or encephalopathy, AIDS dementia or encephalopathy, and, more recently, the AIDS dementia complex (ADC).[3-9]

Not long after the retroviral etiology of AIDS was established, HIV-1 proviral DNA was identified within the brains of demented AIDS patients by Southern blot hybridization.[10] This result was soon confirmed and extended using a variety of other techniques to detect evidence of HIV-1 in brain.[11-19] More recently, it was shown that HIV-1 infection of the CNS, or at least the leptomeninges, is common and additionally may occur early in the course of systemic infection.[20-26] Thus, in a short time it was recognized that infection of the CNS is a central aspect of the biology of HIV-1 infection and that AIDS is accompanied by an important and unique neurologic disorder caused, at least in part, by direct retrovirus brain infection. However, despite this rapid progress in recognizing, characterizing, and establishing the etiology of this new CNS disease, a number of its fundamental aspects remain poorly understood. In this essay we briefly review some of the essential clinical and pathologic features of the ADC and introduce some of the central pathogenetic questions that remain to be addressed, emphasizing the possible contribution of the immune system. It seems clear

---

[a]Our studies of the AIDS dementia complex are supported by Grants AR-074 from the New York State AIDS Institute, NS-21703 from the U.S. Public Health Service, The Life and Health Insurance Medical Research Fund, and the Rudin Foundation.

to us that clarifying the contributions of the immune system, which include elements of immunosuppression, infection of immunocytes, and perhaps immunopathology, will be important to the clear understanding of CNS HIV infections and the ADC, and that such understanding may help in formulating strategies to prevent and treat the disorder. Additionally, as with other "experiments of nature," analysis of this condition may provide novel insights into the interactions of the immune system and the brain, with or without viral pathogens, that will prove to be pertinent to other important CNS disorders as well.

## CLINICAL ASPECTS OF THE ADC AND CNS HIV INFECTION

### Clinical Presentation

By virtue of its frequency and morbidity, the ADC is the most important CNS complication of HIV-1 infection.[7] Its clinical picture is that of "subcortical dementia" and is characterized by a constellation of cognitive, motor, and behavioral dysfunction.[7,9] Earliest patient complaints most frequently relate to difficulty with concentration, forgetfulness, and diminished mental agility, with slowing or difficulty in manipulating complex tasks. The onset is often insidious, as cognitive difficulty gradually begins to interfere with the more difficult demands of work or daily living. Motor symptoms usually begin with clumsiness of the legs or less commonly the hands, with progression to overt ataxia or weakness. Because of frequent concomitant behavioral apathy, the disorder may be misconstrued by the patient, his associates, or even the physician as due to depression, but dysphoria is surprisingly uncommon. At this early stage patients may perform normally on the relatively insensitive mental status screening tests routinely applied by clinicians, although their responses are often slow. Indeed, combined mental and motor slowing is perhaps the salient feature of the disorder. This slowing becomes more evident when patients are confronted with more demanding timed tasks involved in formal neuropsychologic testing.[27] Additionally, patients often exhibit ancillary findings on neurologic examination, including motor slowing that affects oculomotor function (slowed saccades or interrupted smooth pursuits) and performance of rapid movements of the extremities. Pathologic reflexes are frequent and include snout, glabellar, and, less commonly, grasp responses. Generalized hyperreflexia with a prominent jaw jerk is also common unless there is concomitant peripheral neuropathy.

The disease usually is steadily progressive but with a varying tempo, so that some patients may sustain a period of stabilization or slow progression, whereas others experience subacute onset or worsening. Spontaneous improvement is unusual, and characteristically slowing of both mentation and motor performance worsens and eventually leads, in the most severe cases, to profound global intellectual impairment, to virtual immobility as ataxia gives way to paraparesis, and to urinary and fecal incontinence. In the end stage of the disease the patient is left with only rudimentary cognition and is bedridden, requiring full-time nursing care. Similar, but age-related findings accompany pediatric AIDS with loss of motor milestones as the disease affects the developing brain; as in the adult, these changes then progress to global cognitive loss, mutism, and spastic immobility.[5,6]

Diagnosis of the ADC is based on the characteristic clinical findings, the documentation of systemic or CNS HIV-1 infection, and the exclusion of other CNS disorders. In defining the presence and, more particularly, the severity of the ADC as well as in following its course and possible response to therapy, appropriate neuropsychologic testing may be valuable. For evaluating these patients we have outlined a scheme involving a standardized neurologic history and examination along with a screening and supplementary battery of neuropsychologic tests sensitive to the range of abnormalities noted in these patients.[28,29] Neurodiagnostic studies are also helpful in diagnosing the ADC and, perhaps more importantly, in ruling out alternative CNS disorders to which these patients are susceptible, a number of which require timely specific therapy. In the ADC patient the computed tomographic (CT) scan is characterized by cerebral atrophy with both sulcal and ventricular enlargement, and in perhaps one fifth of patients magnetic resonance imaging (MRI) will additionally show abnormalities in the white matter of either a diffuse or a patchy nature.[7] Nonspecific cerebrospinal fluid (CSF) changes include mildly elevated protein in a majority of patients and mild pleocytosis in a lesser number. Oligoclonal bands are probably also common. Local (intrathecal) antibody production in the CNS as well as the presence of HIV-1 demonstrated by virus isolation also characterizes these patients, although the diagnostic importance of these findings is diminished by similar abnormalities in asymptomatic HIV-1-infected individuals.[11,12,19-26]

*Pathologies*

In general, subcortical structures are more frequently and severely affected in patients with the ADC, although the pathologic findings are variable.[8,30-35] At least three prominent and overlapping pathologies are noted in these patients: (1) diffuse white matter pallor, (2) inflammatory infiltration by macrophages and multinucleated cells, and (3) vacuolar change afflicting particularly the spinal cord. Diffuse white matter pallor is the most common microscopic pathology of the CNS noted in HIV-1 infected individuals with its severity generally paralleling that of the clinical dementia. In our own series all demented patients exhibited this finding, and pallor was also detected in patients with mild or no (?subclinical) ADC.[8] The pallor is most prominent in the deep white matter adjacent to the ventricles, whereas the fibers underlying the cortex are relatively spared. Other than an increase in the prominence of astrocytes and an inconspicuous increase in perivascular or parenchymal lymphocytes and macrophages, there is minimal inflammation. In a subset of ADC patients, and generally those with the most severe progressive dementia, the neuropathologic findings are notable for the presence of prominent perivascular or parenchymal infiltrates of mononuclear inflammatory cells, including foamy macrophages and multinucleated cells. In our own series, these findings were present in about one quarter of autopsied AIDS patients and were generally confined to those with severe symptoms.[8] The cellular infiltrates are surrounded by focal rarefaction of the white matter that is superimposed on the diffuse background pallor; as will be noted, these multinucleated cells are virtually pathognomonic of HIV brain infection.

A vacuolated or spongiform appearance may be noted in the brain, either diffusely or focally, but this finding is generally a minor component of the brain histopathology. More common is the presence of a prominent vacuolar myelopathy in some patients.[8,35] In these cases vacuolation is generally most notable in the thoracic spinal cord and most commonly affects the lateral and posterior funiculi. This process may also extend into the long tracts of the brain stem. Other than phagocytic macrophages noted within vacuoles, inflammation is absent. By electron microscopy, the process appears to involve splitting of the myelin lamellae with formation of intramyelin vacuoles. Clinically, the vacuolar changes in the spinal cord correlate with the development of paraparesis, but these patients are also frequently demented.

### Epidemiology of CNS HIV-1 Infections

Studies using a variety of methodologies have implicated direct brain HIV-1 infection in causing the ADC, at least in part. A direct retroviral cause was initially suspected on the basis of: (1) the clinical frequency of the disorder in HIV-1-infected individuals, (2) its unique clinical and pathologic features, and (3) the precedence of retrovirus brain infection in animals, particularly visna, a slow virus infection of sheep caused by an agent subsequently shown to be related to HIV-1.[36,37] This suspicion has now been clearly confirmed in a subset of patients, those with macrophage and multinucleated cell infiltrates noted pathologically,[13-18] and it is suspected that the virus is also involved in causing the other pathologic forms of the clinical ADC syndrome. Before considering the etiopathogenesis of the ADC, it is worthwhile to review more broadly the natural history and spectrum of HIV-1 infections of the CNS.

Central nervous system HIV-1 infections can be considered to occur in four clinical stages: (1) "acute" monophasic CNS syndromes; (2) asymptomatic (leptomeningeal) infection; (3) aseptic meningitis; and (4) AIDS dementia complex. In what is probably a small minority of patients, the CNS may be clinically affected very early in the course of systemic HIV-1 infection. Although described only in scattered individual case reports and therefore not yet well characterized, it is evident that monophasic neurologic syndromes may develop early in patients infected by HIV-1.[38-40] Acute or subacute CNS disorders have been described in the setting of the acute systemic mononucleosis-like disorder accompanying seroconversion and also somewhat later after virus exposure, but still before even minor systemic disease. In their epidemiology and timing in relation to systemic complications, these syndromes appear to parallel certain peripheral neuropathies, including the demyelinating and vasculitic neuropathies,[41,42] complicating HIV-1 infection. Our own experience includes patients in whom focal brain disease has evolved over a matter of days or a few weeks at most, and then has regressed with a variable amount of recovery and residua. These syndromes need to be further clarified with respect to their frequency, clinical characterization, pathology, relationship to the timing of virus exposure and evolving immune dysfunction, and overall pathogenesis. They appear to occur during the initial immune response to the virus or the early "proliferative" phase of immune dysfunction which includes polyclonal B-cell activation.[43]

In contrast to the rarity of these early CNS syndromes, accumulating evidence indicates that early asymptomatic infection of the CNS, or at least of the leptomeninges, is relatively common and may even be the rule. Such early infection has been demonstrated in asymptomatic seropositive subjects by: (1) abnormal findings in "routine" laboratory studies including cell count, protein, and immunoglobulin, (2) detection of local, "intrablood-brain barrier" synthesis of anti-HIV-1 antibody, and (3) isolation of virus from the CSF.[19-26]

Aseptic meningitis represents an additional distinct clinical manifestation of HIV-1 infection. It was recognized early as a complication of AIDS by Snider et al.[3] and recently was further characterized by Hollander and Stringari.[44] Patients may present with acute or chronic symptoms in the context of minor HIV-1-related disease or after full-blown AIDS. They suffer typical meningitic symptoms, with headache the most prominent; CSF examination reveals mild mononuclear pleocytosis, and virus can be isolated from this fluid.

Finally, the most important sequela of CNS HIV-1 infection is the ADC. This clinical syndrome most commonly develops after the major systemic complications of immunosuppression that define AIDS clinically. However, the ADC can also antecede these complications,[7,45] and the recognition that the ADC can precede "systemic AIDS" has resulted in the inclusion of moderate to severe ADC in HIV-1 seropositive subjects within the newest Centers for Disease Control case definition of AIDS.[46] In some patients the ADC may be the first, and less commonly, the only major clinical complication of HIV-1 infection, although virtually all have laboratory evidence of altered immunity. Even those without major systemic disease have suffered "minor" complications of HIV-1 infection such as oral candidiasis, weight loss, malaise, lymphadenopathy, and herpes zoster.

As alluded to earlier, evidence continues to accumulate implicating direct HIV-1 infection as the cause of this major CNS disorder. The virus has now been well

TABLE 1. Pathologies Associated with the AIDS Dementia Complex

| Histopathology | Etiopathogenesis |
|---|---|
| White matter pallor | ? Low level or nonproductive HIV-1 infection |
|  | ? Indirect toxic effect of virus- or cell-coded products |
|  | ? "Hit and run" with intermittent productive HIV-1 infection |
| Multinucleated cell infiltrates | Productive HIV-1 infection |
| Vacuolar myelopathy | ? Low level or nonproductive HIV-1 infection |
|  | ? Indirect toxic effect of virus- or cell-coded products |
|  | ? Other virus, systemic metabolic toxin |

documented in brains of the subset of patients with the pathologic findings of multinucleated cell infiltration using a variety of methods, including Southern blot and *in situ* hybridization, direct virus isolation, immunohistochemical detection of viral antigens, and electron microscopy.[10-18] In accord with the clinical character of the dementia and the distribution of histopathology, HIV-1 has been noted predominantly in subcortical areas including the deep white matter, basal ganglia, thalamus, and brain stem.[18]

It should be cautioned, however, that the relationship between CNS infection and both the clinical syndrome and the various brain pathologies is not yet fully characterized, and although it is suspected that the brain infection by the virus underlies the entire spectrum of the ADC, a direct etiology has not been confirmed in all patients with the clinical syndrome. In particular, neither the diffuse white matter pallor nor the vacuolar myelopathy has clearly been shown to be caused by direct CNS retrovirus infection (TABLE 1). Only in the subset of patients with macrophage and multinucleated infiltrates has brain HIV-1 infection been consistently demonstrated. For this reason we continue to use the designation ADC to refer to the broad clinical syndrome and restrict the term "HIV encephalitis" to that pathologic subset consisting of multinucleated cells or confirmed parenchymal infection.

Even in "virus-positive" cases some controversy remains regarding the cells infected by HIV-1 within the brain; however, there is an emerging consensus that the major cell type exhibiting productive infection is the macrophage and multinucleated cells, the latter representing the product of virus-induced cell fusion of macrophages.[13-18,48] Our own recent studies have focused on infection of brain microglia (Michaels, Rosenblum, & Price, unpublished). Using combined immunocytochemical localization of a viral protein (p24 core protein) with a monoclonal antibody and both morphologic analysis and identification of microglia using a lectin (*Ricinis comminis* agglutinin I), we have confirmed the observations of Vazeux and colleagues[16] that microglia participate in HIV-1 encephalitis in some patients. Microglia thus comprise one of the infected process-bearing cell types found in these brains and very likely participate in cell fusion and formation of multinucleated cells. Whether other glial elements, including astrocytes and oligodendrocytes, or neurons participate in infection is less certain, and the evidence to date is equivocal.[18,49] Wiley and colleagues[14] have additionally stressed infection of vascular endothelial cells.

## PATHOGENESIS OF THE ADC AND HIV BRAIN INFECTIONS

The nature and mechanisms involved in HIV brain infections and the evolution of clinical syndromes and pathologies are presently not well understood.[50] As just described, HIV-1 infection may occur early in the course of systemic infection. In most this infection remains asymptomatic for some time, seemingly for several years. In a small number there is an early monophasic CNS disease, whereas in others the later course is punctuated by symptomatic aseptic meningitis. In the majority, the ADC subsequently develops. What determines progression through these stages of disease in relation to HIV-1 infections, with early sparing of the brain despite infection and later transition to a devastating parenchymal encephalitis? Among related cardinal questions are: (1) What factors contribute to the variability noted from patient to patient in the evolution of the CNS disease in relation to the systemic complications of HIV-1 infection? (2) What determines the clinical and more particularly the pathologic heterogeneity of the ADC? (3) What is the full spectrum of cells infected, the nature of infection in each cell type, and the pathophysiologic importance of each of these targets? (4) Finally, what are the mechanisms causing brain injury and dysfunction? AIDS is characterized by a panoply of immune disturbances (for a recent review see Ref. 43), and, of course, profound suppression of cell-mediated defenses is the hallmark of end-stage disease. It is therefore likely, as with systemic complications in general, that the evolving disturbance of the immune system contributes importantly to the pattern of interaction between HIV-1 and the CNS and to the genesis and form of neurologic manifestations of infection. TABLE 2 outlines some ways in which the immune system might contribute to the character of HIV-1 brain interaction.

### *Contribution of Immunosuppression*

In classifying the ADC among CNS complications of AIDS, we have segregated the disorder from opportunistic infections and neoplasms.[1,9] However, from a mechanistic point of view this separation may not be entirely justified. The ADC may, in fact, be an opportunistic CNS infection caused by an organism that "creates the opportunity" by first causing systemic immunosuppression. Invasion of the brain parenchyma may proceed only when host defenses, which normally would prevent viral invasion and spread, are depleted. As already discussed, one of the fundamental questions involving HIV-1 brain infection is: what causes an asymptomatic CNS infection to be punctuated in some by symptomatic aseptic meningitis, and even more frequently to eventually evolve into a devastating encephalitis? One possible explanation is that invasion of and spread within the brain parenchyma depend on depletion of host antiviral responses that normally stop infection by what is a relatively nonpathogenic virus, at least with respect to the CNS. This possibility is in keeping with

TABLE 2. Immune System Involvement in HIV-1 CNS Infection and the AIDS Dementia Complex

Immunosuppression
   HIV-1 is an opportunistic brain infection

Infection of Immune Cells
   Cells infected:
      Monocyte/macrophage, microglia — > multinucleated cell
      ? Endothelial cell
      ? Astrocyte, oligodendrocyte (neuron)
   Sequence of brain infection:
      Introduction of virus by monocytes (alternative: direct hematogenous route or the CSF)
      ? Low-grade/latent infection of intrinsic glial and neuronal elements
      Amplification and spread by monocyte/macrophages, microglia
   Sequelae of infection:
      Direct lysis of (productively) infected cells
      Indirect toxicity related to release of virus-coded products (e.g., gp120 interference with neuroleukin effect)
      Indirect toxicity related to release of cell-coded factors (transactivation or other dysregulation of cellular gene expression)

Immunopathology
   Bystander effect:
      Release of cytokines and toxic products from infected and reactive cells (e.g., tumor necrosis factor, interferons)
   Autoimmunity: antibody or cell mediated
      Possible role in early "acute" CNS syndromes

the clinical observation that the ADC is a late sequela of HIV-1 infection, occurring only when host defenses are crippled.

Conversely, immunosuppression may not be the only factor determining the development of parenchymal brain infection in HIV-1-infected individuals. There is considerable variability from patient to patient in the comparative development of the ADC versus systemic complications related to immunosuppression. Thus, on the extremes there are patients who, on the one hand, develop inexorably progressive ADC evolving over months in the absence of concomitant systemic problems and, on the other hand, have complicated systemic disease punctuated by recurrent opportunistic infections including *Pneumocystis carinii* pneumonia who remain neurologically spared. These differences may depend, in part, on undefined host factors, perhaps genetically determined,[51] or on accumulated experience with other infections that alter the specific pattern of immunosuppression. However, another, perhaps even more important factor may relate to the polymorphism of HIV-1. It is now clear that this retrovirus has a very high mutation rate and undergoes rapid genetic change, as it spreads not only in the community, but also over time within an individual infected host.[52,53] Differences in virus isolates are readily demonstrated by Southern blot analysis and have been further analyzed by direct comparison of nucleotide sequences. Such studies show that greatest variability occurs in the regions of the viral genome coding for the envelop glycoprotein, and that there are particular "hot spots" that are intensely variable. Because the external viral glycoprotein (gp120) determines initial interaction with the cell, including attachment to the cell receptor and the early steps of internalization and intracellular processing,[54,55] it is possible that one result of HIV-1 polymorphism might be variability in the "neurotropism" of virus strains. In this way it is likely that both waning host immune defenses and the changing virus together determine the development, course, and perhaps the particular clinical and pathologic form of the ADC.

*Role of Infected Immune Cells in the Development and Evolution of the ADC*

A central aspect of HIV-1 infection and development of AIDS is the direct viral infection of immunocytes. Such infection is determined by the interaction of the major external surface glycoprotein of the virus (gp120) with the CD4 surface molecule that serves as the cell receptor for the virus;[54,55] this cell-surface molecule also phenotypically identifies the helper-inducer subset of T lymphocytes. Monocyte/macrophages also are susceptible to infection, which presumably is related to their surface expression of CD4 as well, although the determinant is present in smaller amounts than that on the lymphocyte subset.[56,57] As already discussed, in brains in which productive infection can be demonstrated by immunocytochemistry or *in situ* hybridization, the most prominent infected cells are the invading monocyte-derived macrophages and multinucleated cells that are formed as a result of virus-induced cell fusion of macrophages. Microglia also appear to participate in infection and cell fusion, accounting for some, and perhaps the majority of productively infected process-bearing cells, including some with multinucleation[16] (Michaels, Rosenblum, & Price, unpublished). These infected macrophages and microglia are clearly important in the pathogenesis of overt brain infection underlying severe ADC. We now need to know how these cells come to be infected, their precise role in introducing and amplifying brain infection, and how this infection leads to brain dysfunction (TABLE 2).

It has been proposed that the infected monocyte/macrophage may play a major role in the entry of HIV-1 into the brain, and that systemically infected cells might migrate into the brain carrying the virus, the so-called *Trojan Horse* hypothesis that was first articulated in relation to visna.[58] Pathologically, this possibility is consistent with the finding of infected macrophages located perivascularly and in the parenchyma. Conversely, it is uncertain how this hypothesis is to be reconciled with the early development of the leptomeningeal HIV-1 infection, and it may be just as likely that virus already present in the brain infects entering macrophages, which in turn further replicate and amplify the virus. Microglia are likely infected *in situ*, having entered the brain in the remote past and resided there for some time before infection. Additionally, because infected monocytes in the blood may not be abundant and are not found in similar concentrations in other organs, it is perhaps likely that many, if not most, become infected only after entering the brain; the alternative, that the brain serves as a "sink" for circulating infected monocytes, seems improbable. One can envision a cascade in which brain infection triggers the entry of monocytes from the blood and the activation of resident microglia, both of which then become infected and amplify replication further. How variable permissiveness for replication of virus in these cells contributes to suppressing or enhancing this process remains to be evaluated. The localization of virus to the deep brain with relative cortical sparing suggests factors other than simple hematogenous dissemination and entry of infectious virus or infected macrophages. Entry of virus from the infected ventricular CSF provides one possible explanation for the predilection for infection of deep brain structures.

Whether or not they carry virus into the brain, infected macrophages clearly seem to play a central role in the pathologic subset of patients with multinucleated cells, because these macrophage-derived syncytia are virtually pathognomonic of brain HIV-1 infection of sufficient severity to be detected by Southern or *in situ* hybridization and immunocytochemistry.[8,18,32,34] Do monocyte/macrophages vary in their permissiveness and is such variability important in the development or progression of brain disease? One can speculate that the level of virus replication within these cells might depend on signals from immune T lymphocytes. If this is the case, T-lymphocyte-macrophage interaction and macrophage/microglial infection become central determinants in the evolution of brain infection, with multinucleated-cell pathology and severe progressive ADC occurring when antiviral defenses are exhausted and macrophage and microglia become predominantly disposed to productive infection. Permissive macrophages and microglia may convert low-level productive or latent infection associated with mild symptoms and disease (white matter pallor) to progressive productive infection when they "rescue" virus, amplify HIV-1 leading to further spread, and induce further damage of the surrounding white matter with rarefaction or frank demyelination. This hypothesis views the "virus-negative" cases in which diffuse white matter pallor predominates as also caused by direct HIV-1 infection, but involving only indolent or predominantly latent infection. T-cell-directed permissiveness of macrophages then serves as a pivotal variable in brain disease evolution.

An additional question is whether infection is indeed confined to macrophages and microglia. It has been suggested that astrocytes also may participate in this infection,[18,49,59] and recent studies suggest that a low-grade productive infection of astrocytes can be induced in cell culture.[60-62] This infection likely depends on the CD4 receptor suspected to be present in low quantities on the surface of astrocytic glial cells; CD4 messenger RNA has been detected by Northern blotting in HIV-1-susceptible astrocyte cultures, although CD4 protein has not been clearly detected.[61] Perhaps a similar type infection of astrocytes occurs *in vivo*. Similarly, infection of oligodendrocytes, endothelial cells, and neurons has not been carefully assessed in cell culture and may have a parallel character.

In neither the "virus-negative" brains nor in those with demonstrable productive infection are the mechanisms of brain injury and dysfunction clearly understood. In neither case is there evidence of prominent virus-induced lysis of neurons, oligodendrocytes, or other intrinsic neural elements; injury is therefore not a simple sequela of productive-lytic infection of these cells as occurs in many acute viral encephalitides. Rather it is likely that neurologic dysfunction is due to less direct mechanisms. Again one can speculate that a latent or low-grade infection of native neural elements may occur, but it may not be detected by present histopathologic methods because of limited expression of the viral genome or its products. Such infection might still pervert the metabolism of cells through transactivation or other mechanisms, leading to cellular dysfunction. Alternatively or additionally, infection of macrophages and microglia might alter the metabolism of neighboring noninfected cells by virtue of the secretion of toxic virus-coded products. Recent studies showing functional interference with the activity of a trophic factor, neuroleukin, by the external glycoprotein gp120 provide preliminary concrete support for this speculation.[63] Neuroleukin and gp120 share partial homology, and thus the release of the viral glycoprotein by infected cells may interfere with the integrity of neurons, although the importance of neuroleukin to adult neurons is uncertain. A similar speculation has been advanced regarding homology of gp120 and a peptide (peptide T) with neurotransmitter activity and perhaps the capacity to interfere with HIV-1 infectivity.[64] Because white matter alteration is a prominent component of the pathology of the ADC, the possible parallel indirect toxicity to the myelin or oligodendrocytes rather than the neurons warrants study. Wiley and colleagues[14] have suggested that endothelial infection might alter brain capillary permeability and as a result allow exposure of the brain to circulating toxins.

*Immunopathology*

Immunopathologic mechanisms may also be involved in the pathogenesis of the ADC, although this possibility currently remains almost wholly a matter of speculation. Analogous to the mechanisms just described concerning the indirect toxicity related to the release of virus-coded products, it can be hypothesized that reactive or infected cells might also secrete cell-coded products that alter the function of uninfected cells. Reactive cells may cause bystander pathology by release of various cytokines (e.g., tumor necrosis factor, interleukins, and interferons) or enzymes (e.g., proteases). In the case of infected macrophages, microglia, or even astrocytes, cell metabolism may be altered by transactivation or other mechanisms affecting gene expression, enhancing or suppressing the release of cytokines or trophic factors that are either toxic to or supportive of neuronal or glial function. These alterations may result in injury or dysfunction of neighboring cells.

Direct autoimmunity is less likely to play a role in the ADC, although it may be involved in the acute monophasic CNS syndromes with focal encephalopathy occurring early in the course of HIV-1 infection when other autoimmune phenomena, including peripheral neuropathies, may occur. The pathogenetic significance of oligoclonal immunoglobulin bands in the CSF that are not reactive with viral antigens is uncertain.

# CONCLUSION

Brain infection is a central biologic aspect of human HIV-1 infection. Its sequelae range from asymptomatic infection to severe devastating parenchymal encephalitis. The latter presents as a subcortical dementia with concentration of major histopathologic changes and evidence of productive infection in the white matter and deep gray structures of the brain. The pathogenesis of brain infection and injury is currently uncertain, but it is likely that the immune system is involved in several ways, including loss of immune surveillance and antiviral defenses, direct infection of immunocytes, and perhaps bystander immunopathology. Further studies using the tools of modern neuroimmunology are needed to complement the virologic and neurobiologic investigative approaches currently being undertaken to understand this important disease. It is hoped that such studies may lead to additional approaches to prevention and therapy, complementing those currently under study. Additionally, such studies may also provide important insight into other "neurodegenerative" disorders.

## REFERENCES

1. NAVIA, B. A. & R. W. PRICE. 1986. Central and peripheral nervous system complications in AIDS. Clin. Immunol. Allergy **6:** 543-558.
2. LEVY, R. M., D. E. BREDESEN & M. L. ROSENBLUM. 1985. Neurological manifestations of the acquired immunodeficiency syndrome (AIDS): Experience at UCSF and review of the literature. J. Neurosurg. **62:** 475-495.
3. SNIDER, W. D., D. M. SIMPSON, S. NIELSON, J. W. M. GOLD, C. E. METROKA & J. B. POSNER. 1983. Neurological complications of acquired immune deficiency syndrome: Analysis of 50 patients. Ann. Neurol. **14:** 403-418.
4. BRITTON, C. B. & J. R. MILLER. 1984. Neurologic complications in acquired immunodeficiency syndrome (AIDS). Neurol. Clin. **2:** 315-339.
5. EPSTEIN, L. G., L. R. SHARER, V. V. JOSHI et al. 1985. Progressive encephalopathy in children with acquired immune deficiency syndrome. Ann. Neurol. **17:** 488-496.
6. BELMAN, A. L., M. H. ULTMANN, D. HOROUPIAN et al. 1985. Neurological complications in infants and children with acquired immune deficiency syndrome. Ann. Neurol. **18:** 560-566.
7. NAVIA, B. A., B. D. JORDAN & R. W. PRICE. 1986. The AIDS dementia complex. I. Clinical features. Ann. Neurol. **19:** 517-524.
8. NAVIA, B. A., E.-S. CHO, C. K. PETITO & R. W. PRICE. 1986. The AIDS dementia complex. II. Neuropathology. Ann. Neurol. **19:** 525-535.
9. PRICE, R. W., J. J. SIDTIS, B. A. NAVIA, T. PUMAROLA-SUNE & D. B. ORNITZ. 1988. AIDS dementia complex. *In* AIDS and the Nervous System. R. M. Levy, M. L. Rosenblum, & D. E. Bredesen, Eds.: 203-219. Raven Press, New York.
10. SHAW, G. M., M. E. HARPER, B. H. HAHN, L. G. EPSTEIN, D. C. GAJDUSEK, R. W. PRICE, B. A. NAVIA, C. K. PETITO, C. J. O'HARA, J. E. GROOPMAN, E.-S. CHO, J. M. OLESKE, F. WONG-STAAL & R. C. GALLO. 1985. HTLV-III infection in brains of children and adults with AIDS encephalopathy. Science **227:** 177-182.
11. LEVY, J. A., J. SHIMABUKURO, H. HOLLANDER, J. MILLS & L. KAMINSKY. 1985. Isolation of AIDS-associated retroviruses from cerebrospinal fluid and brain of patients with neurological symptoms. Lancet **2:** 586-588.
12. HO, D. D., T. R. ROTA, R. T. SCHOOLEY, J. C. KAPLAN, J. D. ALLAN, J. E. GROOPMAN, L. RESNICK, D. FELSENSTEIN, C. A. ANDREWS & M. S. HIRSCH. 1985. Isolation of HTLV-III from cerebro-spinal fluid and neural tissue of patients with neurologic syndromes related to the acquired immunodeficiency syndrome. N. Engl. J. Med. **313:** 1493-1497.
13. KOENIG, S., H. E. GENDELMAN, J. M. ORENSTEIN, M. O. DAL CANTO, G. H. PEZESHKPOUR, M. YUNGBLUTH, F. JANOTTA, A. AKSAMIT, M. A. MARTIN & A. S. FAUCI. 1986. Detection of AIDS virus in macrophages in brain tissue from AIDS patients with encephalopathy. Science **233:** 1089-1093.
14. WILEY, C. A., R. D. SCHRIER, J. A. NELSON, P. W. LAMPERT & M. B. A. OLDSTONE. 1986. Cellular localization of human immunodeficiency virus infection within the brains of acquired immune deficiency syndrome patients. Proc. Nat. Acad. Sci. USA **83:** 7089-7093.

15. STOLER, M. H., T. A. ESKIN, S. BENN, R. C. ANGERER & L. M. ANGERER. 1986. Human T-cell lymphotropic virus type III infection of the central nervous system — a preliminary in situ analysis. JAMA **256** 2360-2364.
16. VAZEUX, R., N. BROUSSE, A. JARRY et al. 1987. AIDS subacute encephalitis; identification of HIV-infected cells. Am. J. Pathol. **126:** 403-410.
17. EPSTEIN, L. G., L. R. SHARER, E.-S. CHO, M. MEYENHOFER, B. A. NAVIA & R. W. PRICE. 1985. HTLV-III/LAV-like retrovirus particles in the brains of patients with AIDS encephalopathy. AIDS Research **1:** 447-454.
18. PUMAROLA-SUNE, T., B. A. NAVIA, C. CORDON-CARDO, E.-S. CHO & R. W. PRICE. 1987. HIV antigen in the brains of patients with the AIDS dementia complex. Ann. Neurol. **21:** 490-496.
19. RESNICK, L., F. DI MARZO-VERONESE, J. SCHUPBACH, W. W. TOURTELLOTTE, D. D. HO, F. MULLER, P. SHAPSHAK, M. VOGT, J. E. GROOPMAN, P. D. MARKHAM & R. C. GALLO. 1985. Intra-blood-brain-barrier synthesis of HTLV-III-specific IgG in patients with neurologic symptoms associated with AIDS or AIDS-related complex. N. Engl. J. Med. **313:** 1498-1504.
20. ELOVAARA, I., M. IIVANAINEN, S. L. VALLE, J. SUNI, T. TERVO & J. LAHDEVIRTA. 1987. CSF protein and cellular profiles in various stages of HIV infection related to neurological manifestations. J. Neurol. Sci. **78:** 331-342.
21. MCARTHUR, J. C., H. FARZADEGAN, D. R. CORNBLATH et al. 1987. Cerebrospinal fluid abnormalities in homosexual/bisexual men with and without neuropsychiatric symptoms. Presented at the III International Conference on AIDS, Washington, D.C., June 1-5.
22. APPELMAN, M. E., R. L. BREY, D. W. MARSHALL et al. 1987. Cerebrospinal fluid (CSF) findings in HIV positive patients (pts) without AIDS. Presented at the III International Conference on AIDS, Washington, D.C., June 1-5.
23. COLLIER, A. C., R. W. COOMBS, B. NIKORA et al. 1987. Cerebrospinal fluid (CSF) findings in HIV-infected persons without clinically evident neurologic disease. Presented at the III International Conference on AIDS, Washington, D.C., June 1-5.
24. KATLAMA, C., M. A. REY MA, R. D. SALMON et al. 1987. Cerebrospinal fluid (CSF) study in forty-four HIV-infected patients: Clinical correlation with virus isolation and intrathecal specific antibodies synthesis. Presented at the III International Conference on AIDS, Washington, D.C., June 1-5.
25. GOUDSMIT, J., E. C. WOLTERS, M. BAKKER et al. 1986. Intrathecal synthesis of antibodies to HTLV-III in patients without AIDS or AIDS-related complex. Br. Med. J. **292:** 1231-1234.
26. RESNICK, L., J. R. BERGER, P. SHAPSHAK & W. W. TOURTELLOTTE. 1988. Early penetration of the blood-brain-barrier by HTLV-III/LAV. Neurology **38:** 9-14.
27. TROSS, S., R. W. PRICE, B. NAVIA, H. T. THALER, J. GOLD, D. A. HIRSCH & J. J. SIDTIS. Neuropsychological characterization of the AIDS dementia complex: A preliminary report. AIDS, in press.
28. SIDTIS, J. J., H. AMITAI, D. ORNITZ & R. W. PRICE. 1987. The brief neuropsychological examination for AIDS dementia complex: Correlations with functional status scales and other neuropsychological tests. Presented at the III International Conference on AIDS, Washington, D.C., June 1-5.
29. ORNITZ, D., H. AMITAI, J. J. SIDTIS & R. W. PRICE. 1987. Scales for the neurological examination and history in the AIDS dementia complex. Presented at the III International Conference on AIDS, Washington, D.C., June 1-5.
30. DE LA MONTE, S. M., D. D. HO, R. T. SCHOOLEY, M. S. HIRSCH & E. P. RICHARDSON. 1987. Subacute encephalitis of AIDS and its relation to HTLV-III infection. Neurology **37:** 562-569.
31. KATO, T., A. HIRANO, J. F. LLENA & H. M. DEMBITZER. 1987. Neuropathology of the acquired immune deficiency syndrome (AIDS) in 53 autopsy cases with particular emphasis on microglial nodules and multinucleated giant cells. Acta Neuropathol. **73:** 287-294.
32. PETITO, C. K., E.-S. CHO, W. LEMANN, B. A. NAVIA & R. W. PRICE. 1986. Neuropathology of acquired immunodeficiency syndrome (AIDS): An autopsy review. J. Neuropathol. Exp. Neurol. **45:** 635-646.

33. KLEIHUES, P., W. LANG, P. C. BURGER, H. BUDKA, M. VOGT, R. MAURER, R. LUTHY & W. SIEGENTHALER. 1985. Progressive diffuse leukoencephalopathy in patients with acquired immune deficiency syndrome (AIDS). Acta. Neuropathol. Berl. **68**: 333-339.
34. BUDKA, H. 1986. Multinucleated giant cells in brain: A hallmark of the acquired immune deficiency syndrome (AIDS). Acta. Neuropathol. **69**: 253-258.
35. PETITO, C. K., B. A. NAVIA, E.-S. CHO, B. D. JORDAN, D. C. GEORGE & R. W. PRICE. 1985. Vacuolar myelopathy pathologically resembling subacute combined degeneration in patients with acquired immunodeficiency syndrome (AIDS). N. Engl. J. Med. **312**: 874-879.
36. NATHANSON, N., G. GEORGSSON, P. A. PALSSON, J. A. NAJJAR, R. LUTLEY & G. PETURSSON. 1985. Experimental visna in icelandic sheep: The prototype leniviral infection. Rev. Infect. Dis. **7**: 75-82.
37. GONDA, M. A., M. J. BROWN, J. C. CLEMENTS, J. M. PYPER, J. W. CASEY, F. WONG-STAAL, R. C. GALLO & R. V. GILDEN. 1986. HTLV-III shares sequence homology with a family of pathogenic lentiviruses. Proc. Natl. Acad. Sci. USA **83**: 4007-4011.
38. CARNE, C. A., A. SMITH, S. G. ELKINGTON, F. E. PRESTON, R. S. TEDDER, S. SUTHERLAND, H. M. DALY & J. CRASKE. 1985. Acute encephalopathy coincident with seroconversion for anti-HTLV-III. Lancet **1**: 1206-1208.
39. DENNING, D. W., J. ANDERSON, P. RUDGE & H. SMITH. 1987. Acute myelopathy associated with primary infection with human immunodeficiency virus. Br. Med. J. **294**: 143-144.
40. BREW, B. J., M. PERDICES & D. A. COOPER. 1987. Neurological complications of HIV infection in the absence of significant immunodeficiency. Presented at the III International Conference on AIDS, Washington, D.C., June 1-5.
41. LIPKIN, W. I., G. PARRY, D. KIPROV & D. ABRAMS. 1985. Inflammatory neuropathy in homosexual men with lymphadenopathy. Neurology **35**: 1479-1483.
42. CORNBLATH, D. R., J. C. MCARTHUR, P. G. E. KENNEDY, A. S. WITTE & J. W. GRIFFIN. 1987. Inflammatory demyelinating peripheral neuropathies associated with human T-cell lymphotropic virus type III infection. Ann. Neurol. **21**: 32-40.
43. SELIGMAN, M., A. J. PINCHING, F. S. ROSEN, J. L. FAHEY, R. M. KHAITOV, D. KLATZMANN, S. KOENIG, N. LUO, J. NGU, G. RIETHMULLER & T. J. SPIRA. 1987. Immunology of human immunodeficiency virus infection and the acquired immunodeficiency syndrome. Ann. Intern. Med. **107**: 234-242.
44. HOLLANDER, H. & S. STRINGARI. 1987. Unexplained cerebrospinal fluid pleocytosis in HIV infected individuals: Clinical course, correlations and outcome. Am. J. Med. **83**: 813-816.
45. NAVIA, B. A. & R. W. PRICE. 1987. The acquired immunodeficiency syndrome dementia complex as the presenting or sole manifestation of human immunodeficiency virus infection. Arch. Neurol. **44**: 65-69.
46. SELIK, R., T. J. DONDERO & J. W. CURRAN. 1987. Proposed revision of the AIDS case definition. Presented at the III International Conference on AIDS, Washington, D.C., June 1-5.
47. GARTNER, S., P. MARKOVITS, D. M. MARKOVITZ, R. F. BETTS & M. POPOVIC. 1986. Virus isolation from and identification of HTLV-III/LAV-producing cells in brain tissue from a patient with AIDS. JAMA **256**: 2365-2371.
48. DICKSON, D. W. 1986. Multinucleated giant cells in acquired immunodeficiency syndrome encephalopathy: Origin from endogenous microglia? Arch. Pathol. Lab. Med. **110**: 967-968.
49. GYORKEY, F., J. L. MELNICK & P. GYORKEY. 1987. Human immunodeficiency virus in brain biopsies of patients with AIDS and progressive encephalopathy. J. Infect. Dis. **155**: 870-876.
50. PRICE, R. W., J. J. SIDTIS & M. ROSENBLUM. 1988. The AIDS dementia complex: Some current questions. Ann. Neurol. **23**(suppl): 27-33.
51. EALES, L. J., J. M. PARKIN, S. M. FORSTER SM *et al.* 1987. Association of different allelic forms of group specific component with susceptibility to and clinical manifestation of human immunodeficiency virus infection. Lancet **1**: 999-1002.
52. HAHN, B. H., M. A. GONDA, G. M. SHAW, M. POPOVIC, J. A. HOXIE, R. C. GALLO & F. WONG-STAAL. 1985. Genomic diversity of the acquired immune deficiency syndrome

virus HTLV-III: Different viruses exhibit greatest divergence in their envelope genes. Proc. Natl. Acad. Sci. USA **82:** 4813-4817.
53. HAHN, B. H., G. M. SHAW, M. E. TAYLOR, R. R. REDFIELD, P. D. MARKHAM, S. Z. SALAHUDDIN, F. WONG-STAAL & R. C. GALLO. 1986. Genetic variation in HTLV-III/LAV over time in patients with AIDS or at risk for AIDS. Science **232:** 1548-1553.
54. MCDOUGAL, J. S., M. S. KENNEDY, J. M. SLIGH et al. 1986. Binding of HTLV-III/LAV to T4+ T cells by a complex of the 110K viral protein and the T4 molecule. Science **231:** 382-385.
55. MADDON, P. J., A. G. DALGLEISH, J. S. MCDOUGAL, P. R. CLAPHAM, R. A. WEISS & R. AXEL. 1986. The T4 gene encodes the AIDS virus receptor and is expressed in the immune system and the brain. Cell **47:** 333-348.
56. GARTNER, S., R. C. GALLO & M. POPOVIC. 1987. Isolation of HTLV-III/LAV using monocyte/macrophages as targets for the virus. Presented at the III International Conference on AIDS, Washington, D.C., June 1-5.
57. HO, D. D., T. ROTA & M. HIRSCH. 1986. Infection of monocyte-macrophages by human T-lymphotrophic virus type III. J. Clin. Invest. **77:** 1712.
58. HAASE, A. T. 1986. Pathogenesis of lentivirus infections. Nature **322:** 130-136.
59. MEYENHOFER, M. F., L. G. EPSTEIN, E.-S. CHO & L. G. SHARER. 1987. Ultrastructural morphology and intracellular production of human immunodeficiency virus (HIV) in brain. J. Neuropathol. Exp. Neurol. **46:** 474-484.
60. CHENG-MAYER, C., J. T. RUTKA, M. L. ROSENBLUM et al. 1987. Human immunodeficiency virus can productively infect cultured human glial cells. Proc. Natl. Acad. Sci. USA **84:** 3526-3530.
61. WEBER, J., E. ROBEY, R. AXEL & R. WEISS. 1987. In vitro infection of glial cells with diverse HIV isolates. Presented at the III International Conference on AIDS, Washington, D.C., June 1-5.
62. CHIODI, F., S. FUERSTENBERG, M. GIDLUND et al. 1987. Infection of brain-derived cells with the human immunodeficiency virus. J. Virol. **61:** 1244-1247.
63. LEE, M. R., D. D. HO & M. E. GURNEY. 1987. Functional interaction and partial homology between human immunodeficiency virus and neuroleukin. Science **237:** 1047-1051.
64. PERT, C. B., J. M. HILL, M. R. RUFF et al. 1986. Octapeptides deduced from the neuropeptide receptor-like pattern of antigen T4 in brain potently inhibit human immunodeficiency virus receptor binding and T-cell infectivity. Proc. Natl. Acad. Sci. USA **83:** 9254-9258.

# Strategies for the Treatment of Myasthenia Gravis

DANIEL B. DRACHMAN, KEVIN R. McINTOSH,
SHARI DE SILVA, RALPH W. KUNCL, AND
CAROLYN KAHN[a]

*Neuromuscular Unit
Department of Neurology
Johns Hopkins University
School of Medicine
Baltimore, Maryland 21205*

More than 50 years ago, Walker[1] introduced anticholinesterase (anti-ChE) drugs for the treatment of myasthenia gravis (MG). Her discovery was important for two reasons: it represented the first effective therapy for MG, and it pointed to the neuromuscular junction as the general site of the defect in this disease. Although treatment with anti-ChE drugs produced some improvement in most patients, the prognosis in MG remained poor. By 1958, when anti-ChE drugs were the mainstay of treatment for MG, the mortality rate for generalized MG was still 30%, and more than 60% of the patients either became worse or failed to improve.[2] During the past 25 years, the outlook for myasthenic patients has improved dramatically. With proper treatment, nearly all patients can be returned to full productive lives.[3,4] Nevertheless, the goal of a "cure" has remained elusive. Given the detailed knowledge now available about the pathophysiology, biochemistry, and immunology of MG, it should be possible to design rational therapy leading to a specific and long-lasting or permanent cure.

To appreciate the therapeutic strategies currently being tried in MG, it is important to understand the background of this disease, which I shall briefly summarize. The basic defect is a reduction of acetylcholine receptors (AChRs) at neuromuscular junctions[5-7] brought about by an autoimmune attack, which was shown to be antibody mediated.[8] The mechanisms by which the antibodies may reduce available AChRs include: (1) accelerated degradation of AChRs;[9,10] (2) blockade of the ligand-binding site of the AChR molecule;[11] and (3) complement-mediated damage to the neuromuscular junction.[8,12] The critical antigen, which is also the target of the autoimmune attack, is the AChR molecule, perhaps the best-defined intrinsic membrane receptor. It is a glycoprotein with a molecular weight of about 250,000 daltons and comprised of four different subunits in the proportion $2\alpha$, $\beta$, $\gamma$, and $\delta$. The base sequences for mRNAs of these subunits are known for AChR from torpedo, man, mouse, and calf.[13-15] The amino acid sequences were deduced from the base sequences, and many peptide sequences have been synthesized or expressed *in vitro*.[15-18]

---

[a]The original work from this laboratory was supported by grants from the National Institutes of Health (Grant #1 RO1 NS 23719-01), Muscular Dystrophy Association, and Myasthenia Gravis Foundation.

The origin of MG has remained a matter for speculation. It is believed that the thymus gland may play a role in the initiation of the autoimmune response. This possibility seems likely, because the thymus contains both muscle-like (myoid) cells that bear AChRs[19] as well as immunocompetent cells. Furthermore, removal of the thymus gland produces clinical benefit in up to 85% of patients, with remission in about 35%.[20] However, it is not yet known what triggers the autoimmune response or what permits it to be sustained. An immunoregulatory defect has been postulated,[21] and there is evidence of a genetic predisposition to the development of this[22,23] as well as other autoimmune diseases.

Current treatment, if properly carried out, is usually highly effective.[3,4] It is aimed at (1) enhancing neuromuscular transmission and (2) suppressing the immune system. Pyridostigmine is the anti-ChE drug that is now most widely used to improve the efficiency of neuromuscular transmission. As already noted, thymectomy is often helpful and is conventionally carried out in virtually all patients with generalized weakness due to MG. The immunosuppressive drugs most commonly used are prednisone and azathioprine. Finally, short courses of plasmapheresis are used to decrease

TABLE 1. Experimental Strategies in Myasthenia Gravis

1. Inhibit endocytosis of AChRs
2. "Hot antigen suicide" of AChR-specific B cells
3. Novel immunosuppressive agents:
   a. Cyclosporine A
   b. Total lymphoid irradiation
4. Induction of tolerance
5. Anti-idiotypic approaches:
   a. Antibodies
   b. T-cell "vaccination"
6. Suppressor cells for AChR
7. Knowledge of AChR molecular structure

the circulating antibody level and to produce temporary improvement in patients who are otherwise not doing well.

If properly used, these treatments produce dramatic improvement in over 95% of patients. However, they have certain drawbacks. They must be used continuously in most cases and pose a risk of adverse side effects. Not the least troublesome is the fact that the immunosuppressive measures lack specificity and therefore suppress the entire immune system, increasing the chance of infection or perhaps even the long-term possibility of neoplasia.

Ideally, treatment should: (1) specifically delete the autoimmune response to AChR; (2) leave the immune system otherwise intact; (3) be long lasting or permanent; and (4) have little or no toxicity. As yet, these ideals have not been reached. However, ingenious new experimental strategies that are designed to fulfill these criteria are currently being tried in several laboratories. For the most part, these strategies are being tested in animals with experimental autoimmune myasthenia gravis (EAMG). First described in 1973,[24] EAMG is produced by immunizing animals with purified AChR derived from the electric organs of electric eels or especially electric rays (torpedo). The strategies that I will discuss are listed in TABLE 1.

## REDUCING THE RATE OF DEGRADATION OF ACHRS

One mechanism by which anti-AChR antibodies reduce the number of junctional AChRs is by accelerating their degradation. Normally stable junctional AChRs are endocytosed randomly and degraded at a rather slow rate (half-life is about 12 days in the mouse).[25] The rate-limiting step is endocytosis;[26] degradation, which takes place by lysosomal mechanisms, can handle as many AChRs as are endocytosed. The antibodies cross-link the receptors at the neuromuscular junctions,[27] resulting in acceleration of the process of endocytosis and therefore rapid loss of AChRs. Because the AChR is embedded in a lipid bilayer, it seemed possible that alterations of the lipids might affect the rate of AChR endocytosis. It was previously shown that methylation of membrane phospholipids can alter translocation of substances within the membrane.[28] The process involves stepwise methylation of phosphatidyl ethanolamine to yield phosphatidyl choline. Methyl groups are provided by the methyl donor, S-adenosyl-methionine. The byproduct of the methylation reactions is S-adenosylhomocysteine (SAH). If this byproduct is allowed to accumulate, it inhibits the methylation reaction. Several pharmacologic agents are available that can increase SAH accumulation and produce inhibition of phospholipid methylation by this mechanism. We have examined the effects of such agents on AChR turnover *in vitro* in cultured rat skeletal muscle and have begun preliminary experiments in a passive transfer model of myasthenia in mice *in vivo*. Our findings show that methylation inhibitors cause a highly significant reduction in AChR endocytosis both in normal muscle cultures and in those that have been treated with immunoglobulin from myasthenic patients.[29] Thus, in this system, inhibitors of phospholipid methylation can slow the loss of AChRs that takes place through endocytosis, thereby resulting in a larger remaining number of surface AChRs per muscle culture. In preliminary *in vivo* studies using mice, we found that treatment with inhibitors of phospholipid methylation slows the normal loss of AChRs, resulting in a significantly greater number of receptors per neuromuscular junction. This slowing also occurs in mice that have been treated for as long as 1 week with serum immunoglobulin from myasthenic patients.[30] This novel method of therapy may help to diminish the loss of AChRs in myasthenia, and it may even prove useful in other disorders characterized by accelerated loss of surface receptors.

## ELIMINATION OF SPECIFIC ANTIBODY-PRODUCING B CELLS: "HOT ANTIGEN SUICIDE"

The goal of this strategy is to eliminate B cells that specifically produce anti-AChR antibody (FIG. 1). Because these B cells bear surface receptors for epitopes of the AChR molecule, they are capable of binding these epitopes. If the AChR molecule or appropriate epitopes have been armed with a lethal "warhead," the relevant B cells will bind the lethal antigen and will be killed. In principle, this should produce specific killing of the population of B cells responsible for production of the anti-AChR antibody of MG. Several different kinds of warheads have been coupled to antigens for the purpose of killing specific cells.[31,32] Some of them have proved effective *in vitro* or in naive animals *in vivo*. However, there are serious potential problems in trying to use them in animals (or eventually patients) with ongoing autoimmune diseases.

First, the general toxicity of the warhead may be unacceptable, which seems to be the case with the A chain of Ricin. Second, in ongoing disease, the immunotoxin must "run the gauntlet" of antibodies that are present in the circulation. The immunotoxic molecules may be complexed by the antibodies, and the complexes precipitated in lungs, liver, or kidneys without ever reaching their goal, but with the risk of producing adverse side effects in these organs. Third, if the elimination of specific B cells is incomplete, the remaining cells may subsequently proliferate, resulting in a recurrence of the autoimmune response. In summary, the "hot antigen suicide" strategy requires the development of a toxin-antigen construct that can evade the circulating antibodies and efficiently destroy antigen-specific B cells or T cells or both.

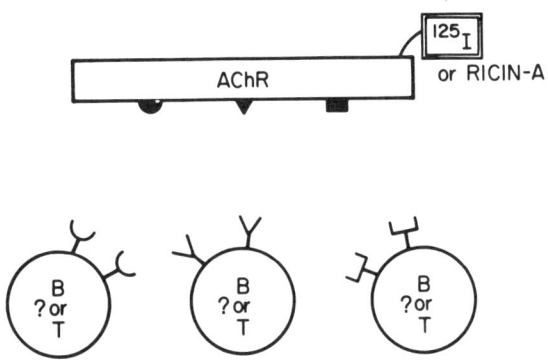

**FIGURE 1.** "Hot Antigen Suicide." The AChR molecule is shown in cartoon form with three epitopes (*black semicircle, triangle, and rectangle*) and a coupled toxic "warhead." When it binds to a relevant B cell (or less likely a T cell), the toxic warhead kills the cell either by radiation (in the case of radioiodine) or after uptake of the A-chain of Ricin.

## NEWER IMMUNOSUPPRESSIVE AGENTS

### Cyclosporin A

Perhaps the most widely used newer immunosuppressive agent is cyclosporin A (CsA). This extraordinary molecule, a novel cyclic peptide, has proven successful in preventing the rejection of transplanted tissue and also has been tried in a number of autoimmune diseases.[33] According to current concepts, it is believed to act chiefly on T lymphocytes through the interleukin-2 (IL-2) pathway. Cyclosporin A was shown to inhibit the release of IL-2 by T cells and in some circumstances to inhibit IL-2 receptors as well. The result is the inhibition of helper T cells and cytotoxic cells, without affecting suppressor cells. In EAMG, cyclosporin was extremely effective in suppressing primary, ongoing, and secondary responses to the antigen AChR.[34] However, large doses of CsA were required. Recently, Tindall and his associates[35] tested

CsA treatment in 10 patients with MG. Though effective, it was relatively toxic, and 6 of the 10 patients discontinued its use. Side effects of CsA chiefly include nephrotoxicity, hepatotoxicity, nausea and vomiting, alopecia, and facial hirsutism. It is most likely that CsA will eventually find its place as an *adjunct* in the treatment of MG, to be used in addition to the other effective immunosuppressive drugs.

### *Total Lymphoid Irradiation*

Total lymphoid irradiation (TLI) has been used for more than three decades in the treatment of Hodgkin's disease and other lymphomas. It was noted to produce profound immunosuppression which began promptly and lasted for a long time, and has therefore recently been used as immunosuppressive treatment in autoimmune diseases.[36] Extensive experience with this therapeutic modality in patients has attested to its overall safety.

The principles underlying TLI include: (1) the use of repeated *fractional doses* of irradiation given daily for up to 6 or 8 weeks in humans; and (2) *shielding* of vital organs and especially the bone marrow. This treatment results in the killing of most mature lymphocytes, while protecting the immunologic precursor cells and other tissues. Following TLI, the immune system is biased towards suppression, and it is considered possible that *tolerance* to antigens present may develop during and after TLI.

We recently tested TLI in a series of rats with EAMG.[37] A total of 3400 Rads were given to rats in 17 fractional doses, while the bone marrow and nonlymphoid organs were shielded with custom-designed blocks. This treatment totally prevented an antibody response to subsequent immunization with AChR. Moreover, it greatly decreased the ongoing response to prior AChR immunization. Finally, TLI greatly inhibited the secondary response to the boost. However, as will be shown, we have not yet succeeded in inducing antigen-specific tolerance to AChR using TLI.

## ANTIGEN-SPECIFIC TOLERANCE

"Tolerance" to antigens occurs naturally during development. It is well known that newborn animals develop the inability to respond to antigens present during the early phases of life. It has also been shown that administration of antigen can, under special circumstances, induce a state of immunologic unresponsiveness to that antigen, or "tolerance."[38] In general, tolerance is most effectively produced by administering the antigen in a manner that bypasses the usual antigen-presenting mechanisms. Thus, for example, the administration of deaggregated antigen (which may not be picked up and presented by antigen-presenting cells) may induce tolerance to that antigen. Another method is to couple the antigen to certain autologous cells, such as peritoneal cells or splenic lymphocytes.[39] Other routes of antigen administration have also been successful. Finally, when antigen is presented to *immature cells*, the chances of developing tolerance are apparently increased.

We wondered whether the administration of AChR to the immature cells present after TLI could induce specific tolerance. We therefore treated rats with TLI and administered AChR in several potentially tolerogenic forms.[40] First, we gave soluble AChR intraperitoneally after TLI. Second, we administered AChR coupled to autologous peritoneal cells after TLI. Third, we gave AChR adsorbed on the adjuvant bentonite. Finally, we reversed the order, treating with TLI *after* the initial immunization with AChR. In no case did we observe specific tolerance produced by any of these methods. In fact, the administration of the "would-be tolerogenic" AChR actually caused some priming, with moderately enhanced responses to a subsequent challenge by AChR. By contrast, human gamma globulin when given in the deaggregated or cell-coupled form induced tolerance which was enhanced by TLI. These results, to be presented in detail elsewhere, suggest that the AChR molecule is a highly immunogenic substance. To induce tolerance it will be necessary to identify some form of the AChR molecule or a fragment of it that is capable of tolerizing rather than stimulating. Based on the work of Oki and Sercarz,[41] this effect may be possible as more becomes known about the critical epitopes on the AChR molecule (see subsequent description).

## ANTI-IDIOTYPIC APPROACH

According to the "network theory,"[42] idiotypes (antibodies directed against specific epitopes) evoke the production of anti-antibodies or anti-idiotypes. The anti-idiotypes may be directed against the *combining sites* of the idiotypes or against a nearby portion of the idiotypic antibody. In some cases, anti-idiotypes are capable of down-regulating the immune response. However, in other instances, the anti-idiotypes may actually enhance the immune response. Several investigators attempted to use an anti-idiotypic strategy in the prevention or treatment of EAMG.[43-48] In some instances, anti-idiotypes prepared in another animal were administered passively,[45-47] whereas in other cases animals were actively immunized with idiotypes in order to induce the production of the anti-idiotypes.[43,48] As expected, the results were variable. In some instances, the anti-idiotypic treatment simply failed to inhibit immune responses to the antigen AChR,[43,44] whereas in others anti-idiotypic strategies inhibited to varying degrees the response to a subsequent challenge with AChR.[45-48] It is of particular interest that the production of anti-idiotypic response to a monoclonal antibody sometimes seemed to *generalize,* that is, it inhibited a broader spectrum of antibody responses than that expected from the single anti-idiotype used.[47,48] These results are intriguing, but they illustrate that anti-idiotypic therapy may be a double-edged sword, sometimes cutting one way and sometimes another. Much more must be known about the specific responses to individual idiotypes before anti-idiotypic therapy can be considered a potential therapeutic modality for MG.

## T-CELL "VACCINATION"

Recently, "vaccination" with T cells immunized against an autoantigen was used to prevent certain experimental autoimmune disorders.[49] It proved effective in preventing experimental autoimmune encephalomyelitis (EAE),[50] adjuvant arthritis,[51] autoimmune nephritis,[52] and thyroiditis.[53] To determine whether a similar strategy could be used in EAMG, we prepared enriched populations of AChR-sensitized T cells from lymph nodes of rats with EAMG. As recently described,[54] these cells were terminally stimulated with concanavalin A, subjected to extremely high pressure in a French press, and used to "vaccinate" rats on three successive occasions. After vaccination, the rats had a low but significant antibody titer against AChR, which we believe was accomplished through an anti-idiotypic route. That is, the AChR-sensitized cells induced an anti-idiotypic response which in turn evoked a minimal immune response against AChR. When challenged with AChR, the vaccinated rats showed a significantly *higher* antibody response to AChR than did control rats, which was the opposite of what we had hoped to produce. However, the spleens of rats that had been vaccinated with AChR-sensitized cells contained lymphocytes that were specifically suppressive for the AChR response. These results, to be reported in detail elsewhere,[55] show that AChR blast-vaccination results in a paradoxic dual response: the *humoral* response is actually enhanced, whereas at the level of the splenic lymphocytes the response to AChR is suppressed. In fact, this response should not be surprising. Previous reports of T-cell vaccination in thyroiditis suggest that the cell-mediated response was inhibited, whereas the antibody response was not.[53] Thus, this anti-idiotypic strategy, like the one just described, may have opposite and conflicting results. Until we learn much more about it, this type of strategy is not suitable for clinical trial.

## SUPPRESSOR CELLS

The immune response to an antigen is a highly self-regulated process. One mechanism by which regulation is known to occur involves suppressor cells that inhibit other cells in the immune system. Complex and sometimes controversial schemes describing the origin and function of these cells have been published and are beyond the scope of this brief review. However, it is believed that suppressive cells may be induced by exposure to antigen, particularly in unusual forms (see tolerance above) as well as under naturally occurring circumstances. Several methods for inducing AChR-specific suppressor T cells or soluble factors have been reported.[56-59] Recently, we used a novel strategy to produce a unique type of suppressor cell that has specificity for the antigen to which it is "trained"—in this case, AChR.[58] To produce these suppressor cells, we first immunized rats with torpedo AChR. Spleen cells were then cultured in a medium containing two major ingredients: (1) CsA to restrain the production of helper and cytotoxic cells, and (2) the *antigen* (usually AChR) to drive the remaining cells. After 1 week in culture under these conditions, the cells were tested for their ability to suppress "responder cultures," consisting of lymphocytes from lymph nodes of AChR-immunized rats. When these responder cultures were stimulated *in vitro* with AChR, they normally produced large amounts of anti-AChR antibody. However, when the cells induced with CsA and AChR were added to the cultures, antibody production was markedly suppressed. This suppression is antigen specific: the cells suppress the AChR response several-fold more powerfully than they suppress other nonrelated responses. Conversely, suppressor cells "trained" to another unrelated antigen, keyhole limpet hemocyanin (KLH), are much more suppressive for the KLH response than they are for AChR.

Recently, we characterized the suppressor cells from these suppressive populations. They are very large (15-30 μm), adherent, and have many of the characteristics of macrophages. We were able to purify them to approximately 95% purity. Under these circumstances, they are extremely suppressive, even at ratios as low as 1 suppressor cell to 320 responder cells. These cells represent an intriguing finding. They are reproducibly antigen specific, yet they are characteristic of macrophages. We speculate that they may be "armed" by some factor derived from a subset of lymphocytes in the same cultures and therefore rendered specific. If suppressor cells can be made in sufficient numbers, they may prove to be a powerful therapeutic measure for the suppression of responses to known antigens.

## HOW CAN WE USE DETAILED KNOWLEDGE OF THE AChR MOLECULE?

As noted herein, the AChR is undoubtedly the most thoroughly studied and best understood membrane receptor molecule. Many critical sites in the AChR have already been defined. "Fusion proteins" constituting large stretches of the α-subunit of the AChR have been made by recombinant DNA techniques,[60] and shorter stretches of peptides have been synthesized in the laboratory. Many laboratories are presently attempting to define "myasthenogenic" sites that will stimulate either the B cells, or, more likely, the T cells (which respond to linear sequences of amino acids, rather than to conformationally defined epitopes). Thus far, only a few stimulatory sequences have been identified. However, prospects for defining portions of the AChR that can then be readily produced and used in any of the aforementioned strategies are very exciting.

Before long, it may be possible to interfere both specifically and safely with the autoimmune reaction in patients with MG.

## ACKNOWLEDGEMENT

We are grateful to Robert N. Adams, Paul Shih, and Donna Maurath for excellent technical assistance, and to Christine F. Salemi for assistance in the preparation of the manuscript.

## REFERENCES

1. WALKER, M. B. 1934. Treatment of myasthenia gravis with physostigmine. Lancet **1**: 1200-1201.
2. GROB, D., N. G. BRUNNER & T. NAMBA. 1981. The natural course of myasthenia gravis and effect of therapeutic measures. Ann. N. Y. Acad. Sci. **377**: 652-669.
3. DRACHMAN, D. B. 1978. Myasthenia gravis. N. Engl. J. Med. **198**: 136-142 and 186-193.
4. DRACHMAN, D. B. 1985. Treatment of myasthenia gravis. In Current Therapy in Neurologic Disease. R. Johnson, Ed.: 366-371. B. C. Decker, Inc., Philadelphia, PA.
5. FAMBROUGH, D. M., D. B. DRACHMAN & S. SATYAMURTI. 1973. Neuromuscular junction in myasthenia gravis: Decreased acetylcholine receptors. Science **182**: 293-295.

6. ITO, Y., R. MILEDI, A. VINCENT & J. NEWSOM-DAVIS. 1978. Acetylcholine receptors and endplate electrophysiology in myasthenia gravis. Brain **101:** 345-368.
7. ENGEL, A. G., J. M. LINDSTROM, E. H. LAMBERT & V. A. LENNON. 1977. Ultrastructural localization of the acetylcholine receptor in myasthenia gravis and in its experimental autoimmune model. Neurology (Minneapolis) **27:** 307-315.
8. TOYKA, K. V., D. B. DRACHMAN, D. E. GRIFFIN, A. PESTRONK, J. A. WINKELSTEIN, K. H. FISCHBECK & I. KAO. 1977. Myasthenia gravis: Study of humoral immune mechanisms by passive transfer to mice. N. Engl. J. Med. **396:** 125-131.
9. KAO, I. & D. B. DRACHMAN. 1977. Myasthenic immunoglobulin accelerates acetylcholine receptor degradation. Science **192:** 527-529.
10. APPEL, S. H., R. ANWYL, M. W. MCADAMS & S. ELIAS. 1977. Accelerated degradation of acetylcholine receptor from cultured rat myotubes with myasthenia gravis sera and globulins. Proc. Natl. Acad. Sci. USA **74:** 2130-2134.
11. DRACHMAN, D. B., R. N. ADAMS, J. F. JOSIFEK & S. G. SELF. 1982. Functional activities of anti-AChR autoantibodies and clinical severity of myasthenia gravis. N. Engl. J. Med. **307:** 769-775.
12. ENGEL, A. G., K. SAHASHI, E. H. LAMBERT & F. M. HOWARD. 1979. The ultrastructural localization of the acetylcholine receptor, immunoglobulin G and the third and ninth complement components at the motor endplate and their implications for the pathogenesis of myasthenia gravis. In Current Topics in Nerve and Muscle Research. A. J. Aguayo and G. Karpati, Eds., pp. 111-122. Excerpta Medica, Amsterdam.
13. NODA, M., Y. FURUTANI, H. TAKAHASI, M. TOYOSATO, T. TANABE, S. SHIMIZU, S. KIKYOTANI, T. KAYANO, T. HIROSE, S. INAYAMA & S. NUMA. 1983. Cloning and sequence analysis of calf cDNA and human genomic DNA encoding α-subunit precursor of muscle acetylcholine receptor. Nature **305:** 818-823.
14. CHANGEUX, J.-P., A. DEVILLERS-THIERY & P. CHEMOUILLI. 1984. Acetylcholine receptor: An allosteric protein. Science **225:** 1335-1345.
15. MISHINA, M., T. KUROSAKI, T. TOBIMATSU, Y. MORIMOTO, M. NODA, T. YAMAMOTO, M. TERAO, J. LINDSTROM, T. TAKAHASHI, M. KUNO & S. NUMA. 1984. Nature **307:** 604-608.
16. LENNON, V., G. A. GRIESMANN, D. J. MCCORMICK, Z.-X. HUANG, H. FENG & E. H. LAMBERT. 1987. Definition of myasthenogenic sites of the human acetylcholine receptor using synthetic peptides. Ann. N. Y. Acad. Sci. **505:** 439-450.
17. J. Neuroimmunol. 1987. **16:** 17, 59, 70, 104.
18. BARKAS, T., A. MAURON, B. ROTH, J.-M. GABRIEL, S. TZARTOS, M. JUILLERAT, C. ALLIOD & M. BALLIVET. 1987. Localization of the main immunogenic region and toxin binding site of the nicotinic acetylcholine receptor. Ann. N. Y. Acad. Sci. **505:** 743-746.
19. KAO, I. & D. B. DRACHMAN. 1977. Thymic muscle cells bear acetylcholine receptors: Possible relation to myasthenia gravis. Science **195:** 74-75.
20. BUCKINGHAM, J. M., F. M. HOWARD, P. E. BERNATZ, W. W. PAYNE, E. G. HARRISON, JR., P. C. O'BRIEN & L. H. WEILAND. 1976. The value of thymectomy in myasthenia gravis: A computer-assisted matched study. Ann. Surg. **184:** 453-457.
21. SHINOMIYA, N., M. SEGAWA & J. YATA. 1981. In vitro study of T-cells regulating anti-acetylcholine receptor antibody formation in myasthenia gravis. Ann. N.Y. Acad. Sci. **377:** 882-883.
22. BEHAN, P. O., & J. SHIELDS. 1982. Genetics. In Myasthenia Gravis. R. Lisak & R. Barchi, Eds. Chap 3: 37-50. W. B. Saunders, Philadelphia, PA.
23. BELL, J. I., L. STEINMAN, K. TOYKA & H. O. MCDEVITT. 1987. HLA-DQ restriction fragment length polymorphisms in myasthenia gravis. Ann. N.Y. Acad. Sci. **505:** 382-387.
24. PATRICK, J. & J. LINDSTROM. 1973. Autoimmune response to acetylcholine receptor. Science **180:** 871-872.
25. STANLEY, E. F. & D. B. DRACHMAN. 1983. Rapid degradation of "new" ACh receptors at neuromuscular junctions. Science **222:** 67-69.
26. DRACHMAN, D. B., R. N. ADAMS, E. F. STANLEY & A. PESTRONK. 1980. Mechanisms of acetylcholine receptor loss in myasthenia gravis. J. Neurol. Neurosurg. Psychiatry **43:** 601-610.
27. DRACHMAN, D. B., C. W. ANGUS, R. N. ADAMS, J. MICHELSON & G. J. HOFFMAN. 1978. Myasthenic antibodies cross-link acetylcholine receptors to accelerate degradation. N. Engl. J. Med. **298:** 1116-1122.

28. HIRATA, F. & J. AXELROD. 1980. Phospholipid methylation and biological signal transmission. Science **209**: 1082-1090.
29. KUNCL, R. W., D. B. DRACHMAN & R. N. ADAMS. 1988. Inhibition of methyltransferase reduces the turnover of acetylcholine receptors. Proc. Nat'l Acad. Sci. USA, in press.
30. KUNCL, R. W. & D. B. DRACHMAN. Unpublished data.
31. KILLEN, J. A. & J. M. LINDSTROM. 1984. Specific killing of lymphocytes that cause experimental autoimmune myasthenia gravis by ricin toxin-acetylcholine receptor conjugates. J. Immunol. **133**: 2549-2553.
32. STERZ, R. K., G. BIRO, K. RAJKI, G. FILIPP & K. PEPER. 1985. Experimental autoimmune myasthenia gravis: Can pretreatment with $^{125}$I-labeled receptor prevent functional damage at the neuromuscular junction? J. Neuroimmunol. **7**: 97-105.
33. SHEVACH, E. M. 1985. The effects of cyclosporin A on the immune system. Ann. Rev. Immunol. **3**: 397-423.
34. DRACHMAN, D. B., R. N. ADAMS, K. MCINTOSH & A. PESTRONK. 1985. Treatment of experimental myasthenia gravis with cyclosporin A. Clin. Immunol. Immunopathol. **34**: 174-188.
35. TINDALL, R. W. A., J. A. ROLLINS, J. T. PHILLIPS, R. G. GREENLEE, L. WELLS & G. BELENDIUK. 1987. Preliminary results of a double-blind, randomized, placebo-controlled trial of cyclosporine in myasthenia gravis. N. Engl. J. Med. **316**: 719-724.
36. SLAVIN, S., S. STROBER, P. FUKS & H. S. KAPLAN. 1980. Immunosuppression and organ transplantation tolerance using total lymphoid irradiation. Diabetes (Suppl. 1) **29**: 121-123.
37. DE SILVA, S., J. E. BLUM, K. R. MCINTOSH, S. ORDER & D. B. DRACHMAN. Treatment of experimental myasthenia gravis with total lymphoid irradiation. Clin. Immunol. Immunopathol. In press.
38. NOSSAL, G. T. V. 1987. Possible strategies for the treatment of myasthenia gravis and other autoimmune diseases. Ann. N.Y. Acad. Sci. **505**: 610-618.
39. PTAK, W., M. BERETA, M. PTAK, G. M. IVERSON & D. R. GREEN. 1985. Suppression and contrasuppression in the induction of contact sensitivity by the administration of cellbound antigen-antibody complexes. J. Immunol. **135**: 2312-2318.
40. DE SILVA, S., K. R. MCINTOSH, J. BLUM, P. J. SHIH, S. ORDER & D. B. DRACHMAN. 1988. Total lymphoid irradiation and antigen-specific tolerance. Neurology **38**(suppl. 1): 376.
41. OKI, A. & E. SERCARZ. 1985. T cell tolerance studied at the level of antigenic determinants. J. Exp. Med. **161**: 897-911.
42. JERNE, N. K. 1984. Idiotypic networks and other preconceived ideas. Immunol. Rev. **79**: 5-24.
43. LENNON, V. A. & E. H. LAMBERT. 1981. Monoclonal autoantibodies to acetylcholine receptors: Evidence for a dominant idiotype and requirement of complement for pathogenicity. Ann. N.Y. Acad. Sci. **377**: 77-95.
44. LINDSTROM, J., S. TZARTOS, W. GULLICK, S. HOCHSCHWENDER, L. SWANSON, P. SARGENT, M. JACOB & M. MONTAL. 1983. Use of monoclonal antibodies to study acetylcholine receptors from electric organs, muscle, and brain, and the autoimmune response to receptor in myasthenia gravis. Cold Spring Harbor Symposium on Quant. Biol. **48**: 89-99.
45. SCHONBECK, S. & D. S. DWYER. 1984. Regulation of the immune response to acetylcholine-receptor after injection of anti-idiotypic antibodies. Immunobiology **168**: 184.
46. DE BAETS, M. H. & P. J. C. VAN BREDA VRIESMAN. 1985. Immunomodulatory effects of anti-idiotypic antibodies in experimental autoimmune myasthenia gravis. Fed. Proc. **44**: 607.
47. AGIUS, M. A. & D. P. RICHMAN. 1986. Suppression of development of experimental autoimmune myasthenia gravis with isogeneic monoclonal antiidiotypic antibody. J. Immunol. **137**: 2195-2198.
48. SOUROUJON, M. C. & FUCHS. 1987. Antiidiotypic antibodies in the regulation of experimental autoimmune myasthenia gravis. Ann. N.Y. Acad. Sci. **505**: 256-270.
49. COHEN, I. R., A. BEN-NUN, J. HOLOSHITZ, R. MARON & R. ZERUBAVEL. 1983. Vaccination against autoimmune disease with lines of autoimmune T lymphocytes. Immunol. Today **4**: 227-230.
50. BEN-NUN, A., A. WEKERLE & I. R. COHEN. 1981. Vaccination against autoimmune

encephalomyelitis with T lymphocyte line cells reactive against myelin basic protein. Nature **292:** 60-61.
51. LIDER, O., N. KARIN, M. SHINITZKY & I. R. COHEN. 1987. Therapeutic vaccination against adjuvant arthritis using autoimmune T cells treated with hydrostatic pressure. Proc. Natl. Acad. Sci. **84:** 4577-4580.
52. NEILSON, E. & M. PHILLIPS. 1982. Suppression of interstitial nephritis by auto-anti-idiotypic immunity. J. Exp. Med. **155:** 179-189.
53. MARON, R., R. ZERUBAVEL, A. FRIEDMAN & I. R. COHEN. 1983. T lymphocyte line specific for thyroglobulin produces or vaccinates against autoimmune thyroiditis in mice. J. Immunol. **131:** 2316-1322.
54. LIDER, O., M. SHINITZKY & I.R. COHEN. 1986. Vaccination against experimental autoimmune diseases using T lymphocytes treated with hydrostatic pressure. Ann. N.Y. Acad. Sci. **275:** 267-273.
55. KAHN, C., K. R. MCINTOSH & D. B. DRACHMAN. In preparation.
56. BOGEN, S., E. MOZES & S. FUCHS. 1984. Induction of AChR-specific suppression: An in vitro model of antigen-specific immunosuppression in myasthenia gravis. J. Exp. Med. **159:** 292-304.
57. SINIGAGLIA, F., C. GOTTI, P. R. CASTAGNOLI & F. CLEMENTI. 1984. Acetylcholine receptor-specific suppressive T-cell factor from a retrovirally transformed T-cell line. Proc. Natl. Acad. Sci. USA **81:** 7569-7573.
58. MCINTOSH, K. R. & D. B. DRACHMAN. 1986. Induction of suppressor cells specific for acetylcholine receptor in experimental autoimmune myasthenia gravis. Science **232:** 401-403.
59. PACHNER, A. R. & F. S. KANTOR. 1987. Suppressor T-cell lines and hybridomas in murine myasthenia. Ann. N.Y. Acad. Sci. **505:** 619-627.
60. BARKAS, T., A. MAURON, B. ROTH & M. BALLIVET. *In* Monographs in Allergy. Karger, in press.

PART IV. VIRUS-INDUCED DISEASE AND AUTOIMMUNITY

# Autoimmune Demyelination in the Central Nervous System[a]

### TAKESHI TABIRA

*Division of Demyelinating Disease and Aging*
*National Institute of Neuroscience*
*National Center of Neurology and Psychiatry*
*Kodaira, Tokyo 187, Japan*

Experimental allergic encephalomyelitis (EAE) is a suitable animal model for studying pathologic and immunologic mechanisms involved in autoimmune demyelination in the central nervous system (CNS). It is induced in genetically susceptible animals by sensitizing them with encephalitogenic antigens in CNS myelin. The clinical form and amount of demyelination differ among species and antigens used. For instance, myelin basic protein (BP) alone induces inflammatory encephalomyelitis with little or no demyelination in rats[1] and guinea pigs,[2] whereas demyelination is the major characteristic of chronic EAE in guinea pigs immunized with whole CNS antigens[3] and in guinea pigs[4] and rabbits[5] immunized with myelin proteolipid apoprotein (PLP). These findings suggest that BP mainly induces inflammatory lesions and that other antigens such as PLP, acting alone or in cooperation with others, are important in eliciting demyelination. However, active challenge with BP or the transfer of BP-sensitized cells induced relapsing EAE with a significant amount of demyelination in mice.[6-8] Therefore, two questions were raised: (1) Is demyelination related more to the species or to antigens? and (2) Is the mechanism of demyelination T-cell mediated or antibody mediated? To answer these questions studies using different antigens and species were performed, and the mechanism of demyelination was studied using T-cell lines and clones.

In addition, in our efforts to understand the mechanism of EAE using T-cell lines and clones, a mechanism of activating effector T cells by allogenic antigens was found and will be described in this report.

## MATERIALS AND METHODS

### Antigens

Basic protein was prepared from several species according to the method of Deibler et al.[9] The method of preparing PLP and its purity were described previously.[4,10]

---

[a] This work was supported in part by grants from the Neuroimmunological Disorder Research Committee and NCNP-86-15 and NCNP-85-17, the Ministry of Health and Welfare, and a Grant-in-Aid for Scientific Research (No. 60480225) from the Ministry of Education, Science and Culture, Japan.

Briefly, total crude proteolipid was extracted from the spinal cord of several species with chloroform (C) and methanol (M) using Folch's method, and it was delipidated and separated by methylated Sephadex G-100 column chromatography. Under these conditions, an electroblot and immunostaining procedure revealed that possible contaminating levels of BP in our PLP were estimated to be less than 0.014%. This insignificant level of contamination was confirmed by the absence of a response of BP-specific T-cell lines to PLP.[11] The PLP was further separated by ion exchange column chromatography with a CM-Trisacryl column into two components: major PLP and DM-20.[10] In this further purified DM-20, possible contaminating levels of BP were less than 0.00%. The PLP and its subcomponents were filtered through an LH-20 column with C/M/0.1 M HCl (10:10:1) to remove salts, and they were converted to water-soluble form and used after filtering them through an 0.45 μm filter. Purified protein derivatives (PPD) from mycobacterium tuberculosis H37Ra (Mitsui Pharmaceutical Co., Tokyo, Japan) and concanavalin A (Con A, Miles-Yeda, Rehovot, Israel) were obtained commercially.

*Animals*

Lewis rats and CBA/J mice were obtained from Charales River Breeding Laboratories (Atsugi, Kanagawa, Japan). SJL/J and A.SW/Sn mice were from Gokita Breeding Service (Tokyo, Japan) and The Jackson Laboratory (Bar Harbor, ME). Hartley guinea pigs and C3H/He, BALB/c, C57BL, B10.BR, B10.D2, AKR/J, and A/J mice were obtained from Sankyo Laboratory Service (Tokyo, Japan). Strain 13 guinea pigs and DBA/2 mice were from Seiwa Experimental Animals (Fukuoka, Japan). A.TL, DDD/1, and DDD/1 nu/nu mice were supplied by the Institute of Medical Science, Tokyo University, and A.TH mice were from Keio University (Tokyo). All mice were used at 6-10 weeks of age except for the source of antigen-presenting cells, and rats were 8-12 weeks old.

*T-Cell Lines and Clones*

Methods to establish T-cell lines and clones were described previously.[11,12] Briefly, single-cell suspensions obtained from BP-sensitized draining lymph nodes were cultured by alternate stimulation with BP and maintenance with interleukin-2 longer than 3 months, and R2 and D1 lines were established from SJL/J and DDD/1 mice, respectively. PLP-specific T-cell lines PL1 and PL3 were similarly established from SJL/J mice. Clones 4b.14a and 6a were established from R2 line and D1 line, respectively, by limiting dilution. Clone 6a.3f is a subclone of clone 6a.

*Assay of Antibodies*

Antibodies to BP and PLP were measured by ELISA.[13,14]

## Assay of Proliferative Response

Proliferative responses were assessed by $^3$H-thymidine incorporation. $10^4$ cells/well were cultured with antigens or mitogens with antigen-presenting cells ($10^6$ cells/well), and 1 µCi of $^3$H-thymidine was added during the last 18 hours of the 4-day culture.

## Induction of EAE

Experimental allergic encephalomyelitis was induced by either active challenge with various antigens in complete Freund's adjuvant (CFA) or adoptive transfer of antigen- or mitogen-activated encephalitogenic T line or clone cells into the tail vein of recipient mice. Some of the recipients were X-irradiated (300-800 R) before transfer and PLP/line-injected mice received X-irradiation and *B. pertussis* vaccine ($2 \times 10^7$).

## Clinical and Pathologic Assessment

The scores of clinical severity were: 0, normal; 1, tail atony; 2, clumsy gait; 3, definite limb weakness; 4, paraplegia or monoplegia; 5, moribund state or death. For pathologic studies glutaraldehyde-fixed tissues were embedded in Epon, and conventional light and electron microscopic observations were made. Toluidine blue staining was used for thick sections. The remaining specimens and formalin-fixed tissues were embedded in paraffin and stained with hematoxylin and eosin. Inflammatory changes were scored as follows; 0, normal; 1, inflammatory cell cuffing limited to the perivascular space or meninges; 2 to 4, mild, moderate, or marked infiltration of inflammatory cells into CNS parenchyma. The amount of axonal damage and demyelination was scored as none ($-$), mild ($+$), moderate ($++$), and severe ($+++$). All slides were read blind.

# RESULTS

## Studies of Antigens and Demyelination in Various Species and Strains

To answer the question of whether autoimmune demyelination depends on species or antigens, experiments were performed and the following results obtained.

1. *Studies in guinea pigs.* Adult and juvenile Hartley and strain 13 guinea pigs were immunized with whole CNS, BP, or PLP in CFA. As shown in TABLE 1 and FIGURE 1, animals immunized with whole CNS antigens or PLP developed chronic EAE with widespread demyelination, but BP never induced significant demyelination. We failed to induce significant demyelination with a mixture of galactocerebroside

and BP (data not shown). Therefore, the responsible antigen for the widespread demyelination seems to be PLP. However, PLP-sensitized guinea pigs developed only chronic progressive EAE, and they did not have a relapse.

2. *Studies in rats.* Lewis rats were sensitized with guinea pig BP (25 µg), whole guinea pig CNS antigens (30 mg), or bovine PLP (100 µg × 1 or × 3) in CFA. In all animals that received BP or whole CNS antigens, acute EAE developed with day 11 being the mean day of onset (TABLE 1). In these animals, only perivascular and subpial inflammatory lesions were observed. Among animals that received a single injection of PLP, 12 of 31 developed clinical signs of EAE with a mean day of onset at day 27, and 18 of 23 showed histopathologic signs of EAE.[15] In these animals the inflammatory change was more widespread and demyelinated axons were frequently observed subpially. The animals that received triple injections developed a similar

TABLE 1. EAE in Guinea Pigs and Rats: Antigens, Clinical Forms, and Demyelination

| Animal Strain | Age | Antigen (Dose) | EAE | Day of Onset | Demyelination | Clinical Course |
|---|---|---|---|---|---|---|
| Hartley | A | Whole (50 mg) | 5/5 | 11 | − | Acute |
| | J | Whole (50 mg) | 9/10 | 20 | −/+++ | Acute/chronic |
| Strain 13 | A | Whole (50 mg) | 4/4 | 11 | − | Acute |
| | J | Whole (50 mg) | 7/7 | 18 | −/+++ | Acute/chronic |
| Hartley | A | BBP (10 µg) | 12/14 | 16 | − | Acute |
| Strain 13 | J | BBP (20 µg) | 8/10 | 19 | − | Acute |
| Hartley | A | BPLP (400 µg) | 1/3 | 45 | +++ | Chronic |
| | J | BPLP (250 µg) | 3/8 | 46 | +++ | Chronic |
| Strain 13 | J | BPLP (250 µg) | 0/4 | ... | − | ... |
| Lewis | A | Whole (30 mg) | 2/2 | 11 | − | Acute |
| Lewis | A | GPBP (25 µg) | 10/10 | 11 | − | Acute |
| Lewis | A | BPLP (100 µg × 1) | 12/31 | 27 | + | Subacute |
| Lewis | A | BPLP (100 µg × 3) | 3/11 | 37 | ++ | Subacute/chronic |
| Lewis | A | BPLP/LNC | 4/5 | 10 | +/− | Acute |

NOTE: Animals were sensitized with the antigens in complete Freund's adjuvant except for the last one which was transferred with primary cultured lymph node cells (LNC). Whole CNS bovine antigens were used for guinea pigs and guinea pig antigens for rats. Onset of EAE is expressed as the mean day of clinical onset. A = adult; BBP = bovine basic protein; BPLP = bovine proteolipid apoprotein; GPBP = guinea pig BP; J = juvenile.

disease with a similar incidence, but demyelination was more profound (FIG. 2). When PLP-sensitized and Con-A-stimulated lymph node cells were transferred to naive X-irradiated (400 R) Lewis rats, four of five developed EAE 9 to 11 days after transfer.[16] The lesion was mainly composed of inflammatory cells with a few demyelinated axons (TABLE 1). Thus, PLP also induces subacute or chronic EAE with significant demyelination in rats, but BP- and whole CNS-induced EAE showed only acute EAE with inflammation.

3. *Studies in mice.* Because BP is known to induce relapsing EAE with significant demyelination,[8] a question was raised whether PLP induces more demyelination as in other species. To answer this question, BALB/cCr, C3H/He, and SJL/J mice were immunized with 100 µg of PLP. All animals received a booster injection with the same amount of PLP on day 7. The incidence of clinical EAE was 3 of 7 (43%),

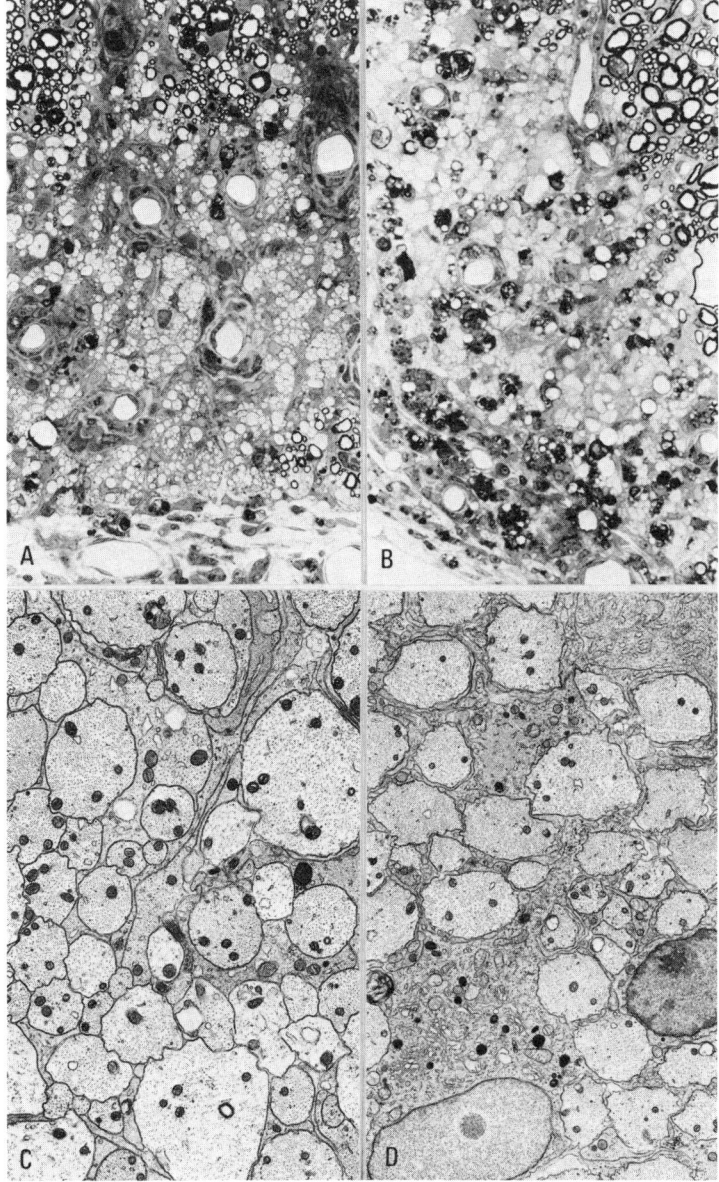

**FIGURE 1.** Whole CNS- and PLP-induced EAE in guinea pigs. **A,** whole CNS-induced EAE in strain 13 guinea pig shows marked demyelination (day 88, toluidine blue stain; original magnification × 280). **B,** bovine PLP induced a similar lesion in Hartley guinea pigs (day 63, toluidine blue stain; original magnification × 280). **C,** electron micrograph of **A** (original magnification × 6150). **D,** electron micrograph of **C** (original magnification × 4300). (Reduced by 10%.)

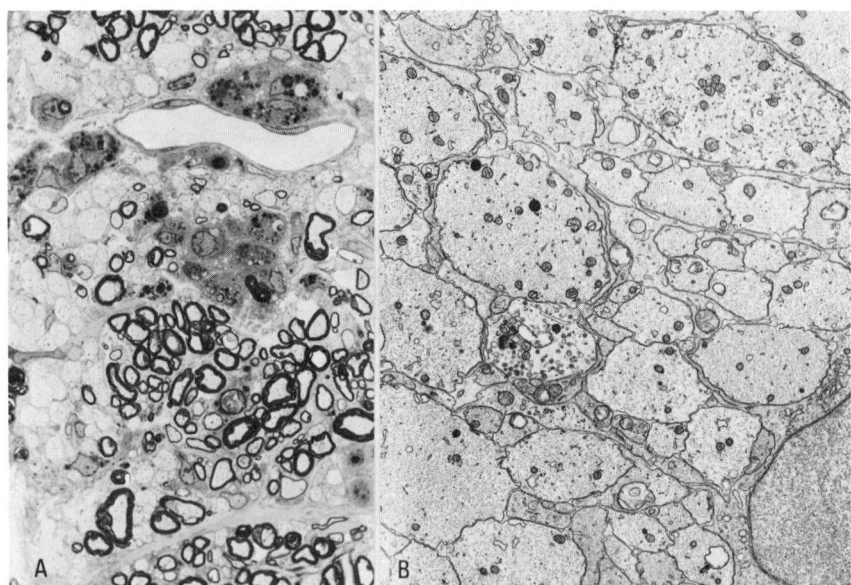

**FIGURE 2.** Proteolipid-apoprotein-induced EAE in Lewis rats. **A**, significant amount of demyelination and lipid-laden macrophages are seen (toluidine blue stain; original magnification × 700). **B**, electron micrograph of A (original magnification × 6200). (Reduced by 15%.)

5 of 5 (100%), and 17 of 19 animals (89%), respectively. The onset of clinical EAE was earliest in SJL/J mice, middle in BALB/c mice, and latest in C3H/He (TABLE 2). In each animal, the pathologic score was taken from six different portions (cerebrum, cerebellum, pons, and cervical, thoracic, and lumbosacral cord). The mean clinical and pathologic scores were not significantly different among these species, but demyelination was more frequent in BALB/c (FIG. 3) and C3H/He mice. The amount of demyelination was significantly greater than that in BP-induced EAE in SJL/J mice.

These results can be summarized as follows;

1. The clinical form and amount of demyelination are different among species and

TABLE 2. PLP-Induced EAE in Mice by Active Challenge: Pathologic Features

| Strain | n | Day of Onset | Day of Sacrifice | Pathologic Score | Demyelination | Axonal Damage |
|---|---|---|---|---|---|---|
| BALB/c | 4 | 38 (20-67) | 28-69 | 1.55 | ++ | ++ |
| C3H/He | 4 | 63 (32-78) | 34-107 | 1.72 | ++ | ++ |
| SJL/J | 4 | 18 (16-19) | 20-21 | 1.56 | +/− | + |
| SJL/J | 4 | 18 (15-22) | 143-166 | 1.21 | + | +++ |

antigens used. Guinea pigs show the greatest amount of demyelination and the least axonal damage.

2. Proteolipid apoprotein induces significantly more demyelination in all species tested.

3. More demyelination is seen in animals with a more chronic disease process.

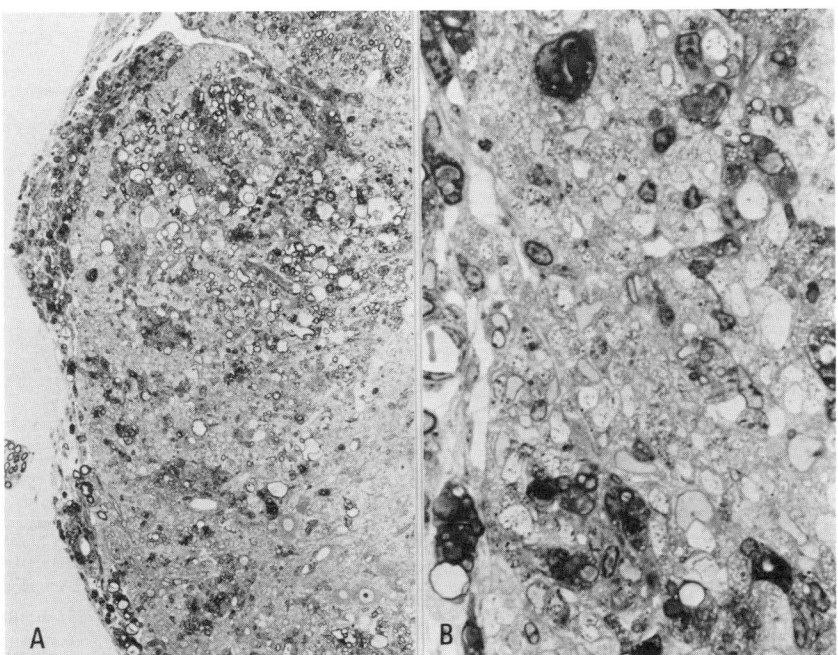

**FIGURE 3.** Proteolipid-apoprotein-induced EAE in BALB/c mice. **A,** widespread demyelinating lesion is seen in the spinal cord where lymphocytes and lipid-laden macrophages were present in the meninges and perivascular parenchyma (toluidine blue stain; original magnification × 140). **B,** higher magnification shows numerous denuded axons (toluidine blue stain; original magnification × 700).

## Mechanism of Demyelination

1. *Role of antibodies.* IgG antibodies to BP and PLP were measured by ELISA in whole CNS-sensitized chronic relapsing EAE in strain 13 guinea pigs. As shown in FIGURE 4, antibody titers to PLP were higher in animals with relapse,[14] although the titer was not related directly in individual cases. Conversely, titers to BP were not significantly different.[16] In rats and mice, antibody titers to PLP were not related at all to clinical or histologic scores.[10,15]

2. *Analysis using T-cell lines and clones.* Basic-protein-specific T-cell lines R2 and D1 were established from SJL/J mice as were PLP-specific T-cell lines PL1 and PL3. Basic-protein-specific T-cell clones 4b.14a and 6a.3f were established from R2 and D1 lines, respectively. Surface phenotypes were examined in R2, 4b.14a, and PL1 cells; all possessed helper and inducer T cells. Lines R2 and D1 and clones 4b.14a and 6a responded to rat, bovine, rabbit, and guinea pig BP. PL1 and PL3 responded well to bovine, rat, and guinea pig PLP, but not to bovine and guinea pig BP (FIG. 5). Major histocompatibility complex restriction was observed in *in vitro* antigen presentation.[11,12]

In SJL/J mice, $3 \times 10^6$ antigen-stimulated R2 line and 4b.14a clone cells constantly induced severe EAE. D1 line and 6a.3f clone behaved similarly. Fewer cells were required to induce EAE in syngeneic recipients with X-irradiation (300-500 R). For comparison, $1 \times 10^7$ antigen-activated R2, D1, 4b.14a, and 6a.3f cells were

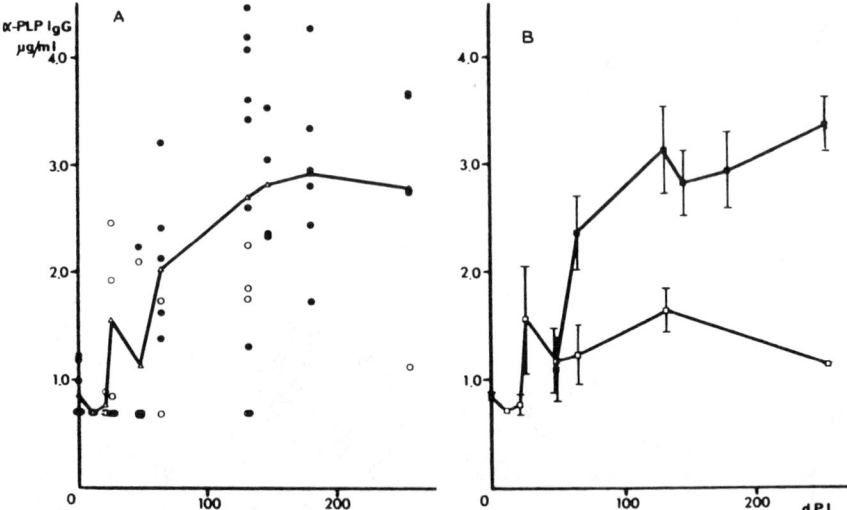

**FIGURE 4.** Antibody titers to PLP in chronic relapsing EAE of the guinea pig. Relapsed animals (*closed circles*) show higher titers to PLP than do nonrelapsed animals (*open circles*). Mean titers in each group are shown in **B**.

transferred to X-irradiated (500 R) SJL/J, DDD/1, and DDD/1 nu/nu mice. They all induced similar disease (TABLE 3).

Severe EAE was induced by $1-3 \times 10^7$ antigen-activated PL1 and PL3 cells in SJL/J mice that were X-irradiated (550 R) and received *B. pertussis* vaccine ($3 \times 10^7$ organisms) immediately after the cell transfer (TABLE 3). A possibility of antigen carry-over was denied by the absence of EAE in animals that received R2 line stimulated with PLP.

The pathology of the T-cell line- and clone-induced EAE was essentially the same as that of EAE induced by active challenge. Lesions were mainly located in the lower part of the spinal cord and were characterized by perivascular and parenchymal cell infiltrates comprised of lymphocytes, macrophages, and polymorphonuclear cells and by edema and fibrin deposits. In severe lesions, axons were markedly affected and decreased in number. However, demyelinated axons were definitely observed especially

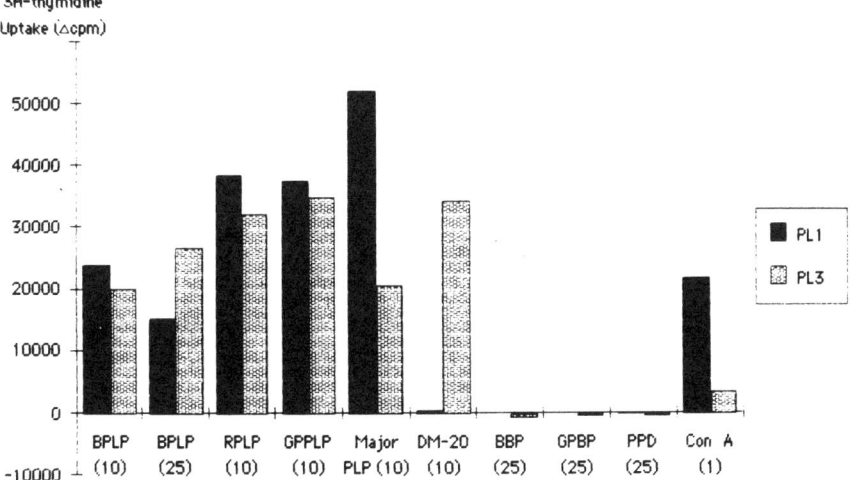

FIGURE 5. Proliferation responses of PLP-specific T-cell lines (PL1, PL3). Both lines responded well to bovine PLP (BPLP), rat PLP (RPLP), guinea pig PLP (GPPLP), and Con A, but not to bovine BP (BBP), guinea pig BP (GPBP), and PPD. PL1 responded to only major PLP, whereas PL3 responded to both major PLP and DM-20.

in X-irradiated allogeneic recipients that were I-A compatible with SJL/J mice[17] (TABLE 4 and FIG. 6). The most common locations of demyelination were root exit and entry zones where cones of CNS myelin extended into the dorsal root. Because a BP-specific T-cell clone induced demyelination in athymic nude mice, there is a method of inducing demyelination by an encephalitogenic single T-cell clone without the aid of recipient-derived T-cell populations. Although active challenge with PLP tended to induce more demyelination than BP, the amount of demyelination in EAE induced by BP- and that by PLP-specific T-cell lines was not significantly different.

TABLE 3. Encephalitogenic T-Cell Line- and Clone-Induced EAE in Euthymic and Athymic Mice

| Line/Clone | Recipient | Incidence | Onset (day) | Severity |
|---|---|---|---|---|
| R2 | SJL/J | 9/9 | 5.1 | 4.2 |
| R2 | DDD/1 nu/nu | 10/10 | 6.6 | 4.3 |
| 4b.14a | SJL/J | 12/12 | 5.1 | 4.5 |
| 4b.14a | DDD/1 nu/nu | 5/5 | 6.2 | 4.4 |
| D1 | DDD/1 | 3/3 | 5.3 | 4.0 |
| D1 | DDD/1 nu/nu | 6/6 | 5.6 | 4.0 |
| 6a.3f | DDD/1 | 3/3 | 5.3 | 4.0 |
| 6a.3f | DDD/1 nu/nu | 9/10 | 6.0 | 4.0 |
| PL1 | SJL/J | 19/21 | 10.2 | 3.4 |
| PL3 | SJL/J | 4/4 | 7.8 | 4.0 |

TABLE 4. Pathologic Features of T-Cell Line- and Clone-Induced EAE in Mice

| Line or Clone | No. of Cells ($\times 10^6$) | Recipient Strain | $n$ | X-R | Day of Sacrifice | Inflammation | Axonal Damage | Demyelination |
|---|---|---|---|---|---|---|---|---|
| R2 | 5 | SJL/J | 5 | − | 7–32 | +++ | +++ | + |
| R2 | 1 | SJL/J | 4 | + | 23 | +++ | +++ | ++ |
| R2 | 3–5 (2×) | SJL/J | 3 | − | 70 | +++ | ++++ | ++ |
| R2 | 10 | A.SW/Sn DDD/1 | 6 | + | 10–13 | +++ | +++ | ++/+++ |
| R2 | 10–15 | DDD/1 nu/nu | 5 | + | 9–25 | +++ | ++ | +++ |
| 4b.14a | 10–15 | SJL/J | 4 | + | 8–10 | +++ | ++ | ++ |
| 6a.3f | 12–15 | DDD/1 nu/nu | 3 | + | 9–15 | ++/+++ | + | +/++ |
| PL1 | 5–20 | SJL/J | 6 | + | 8–79 | ++ | ++ | +/++ |
| PL3 | 5–20 | SJL/J | 2 | + | 7–8 | ++ | + | +/++ |

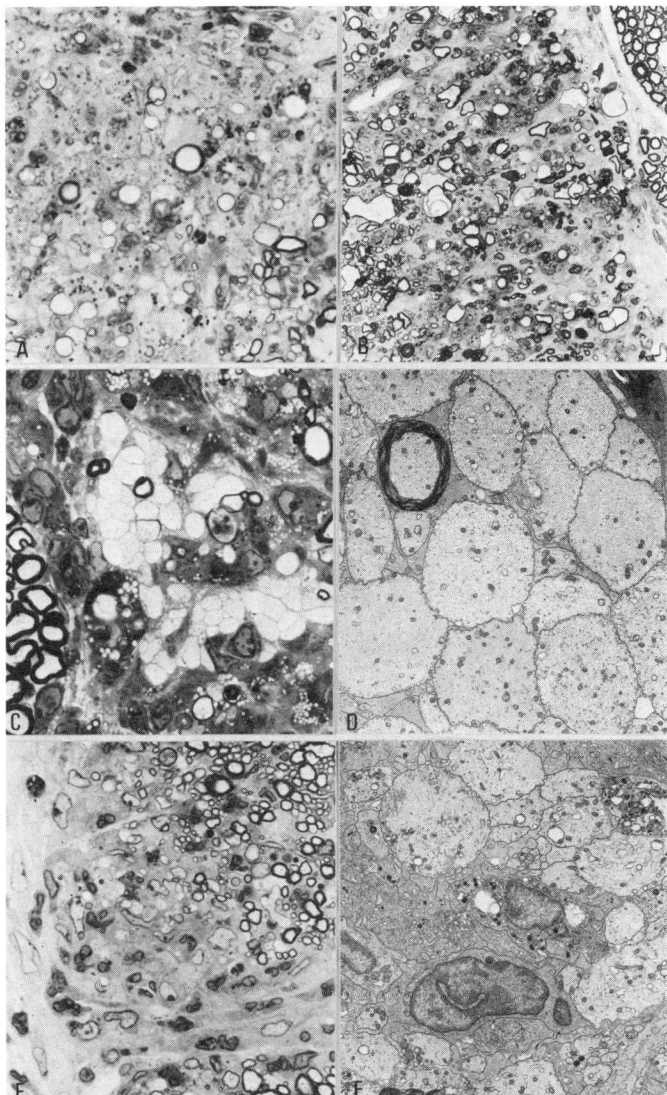

**FIGURE 6.** Encephalitogenic T-cell line- and clone-induced EAE in mice. **A,** R2-line-induced EAE in SJL/J mouse shows marked damage and depletion of axons (toluidine blue stain; original magnification × 880). **B,** PL1 in SJL/J also shows marked axonal damage (toluidine blue stain; original magnification × 280). **C,** R2 line in DDD/1 nu/nu shows a group of demyelinated axons in the cone extending into the dorsal root (toluidine blue stain; original magnification × 700). **D,** electron micrograph of **C** (original magnification × 3000). **E,** PL3 in SJL/J shows mononuclear cell infiltration and a few demyelinated axons (toluidine blue stain; original magnification × 700). **F,** 6a.3f clone in DDD/1 nu/nu shows definite demyelination in ventral column of sacral cord (original magnification × 3000). (Reduced by 20%.)

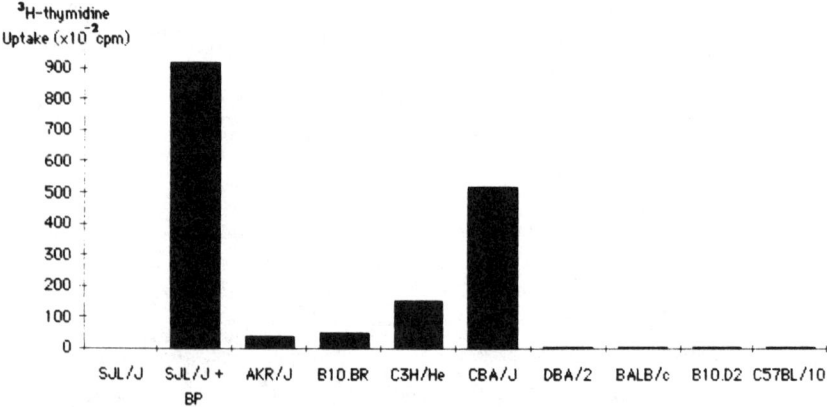

**FIGURE 7.** Alloantigen-activation of clone 4b.14a. Clone 4b.14a (I-A$^s$) responded well to I-A$^{k+}$ antigen-presenting cells from AKR/J, B10.BR, C3H/He, and CBA/J mice, but was not reactive to DBA/2 (I-A$^d$), BALB/c (I-A$^d$), B10.D2 (I-A$^d$), and C57BL (I-A$^b$).

3. *Activation mechanism of effector T cells.* To induce overt EAE with encephalitogenic T-cell lines and clones, the effector T cells must be activated before transfer. For this purpose, the effector T cells are stimulated *in vitro* with the specific antigen and antigen presenting cells (APCs) or lectins such as Con A. However, BP-specific encephalitogenic T-cell clones remain in the local lymph organs such as the spleen where BP is absent. To activate these clones in such places, activation mechanisms by alloantigens[19] or interleukin-2 (IL-2)[20] are postulated. Our BP-specific T-cell clone (I-A$^s$) recognized I-A$^k$ gene product (FIG. 7) and acquired encephalitogenic activity (TABLE 5). When the T-cell clone was cultured with IL-2 without antigenic stimulation, the T cells proliferated well but did not acquire encephalitogenic activity.

## DISCUSSION

We demonstrated that PLP is responsible for widespread demyelination in all species tested. In PLP-sensitized guinea pigs chronic progressive EAE developed without relapse, which suggests that an additional antigen might be required for the relapsing mechanism. However, this is unlikely, because PLP-sensitized mice[10] and rabbits[5] developed chronic relapsing EAE.

TABLE 5. EAE Induced by Alloantigen-Activated T-Cell Clone

| Activation | No. of Cells Transferred | Incidence of EAE | Day of Onset | Severity |
|---|---|---|---|---|
| IL-2 | 1–3 × 10$^7$ | 0/4 | . . . | . . . |
| CBA/J cells | 5–7 × 10$^6$ | 7/7 | 6.0 | 3.4 |

In mice both BP and PLP induce relapsing EAE with demyelination, but the amount of demyelination was significantly greater in PLP-induced EAE especially in BALB/c and C3H mice. SJL/J mice showed early onset of the disease and markedly damaged axons, whereas BALB/c and C3H mice showed later onset of the disease with significant demyelination. Thus, the difference in the disease process is also an important factor in demyelination and axonal damage.

The mechanism of demyelination is still in question. Antibody-mediated demyelination is demonstrated only in traumatic conditions.[21,22] In this study, antibody levels to PLP were higher in relapsed animals than in nonrelapsed animals, but they were not directly correlated in each individual. Therefore, the role of antibodies *in vivo* is still obscure. Because antibodies to myelin components enhance phagocytosis by macrophages as an opsonin,[23] antimyelin antibodies may enhance demyelination.

Conversely, T-cell-mediated demyelination was demonstrated in euthymic mice.[24] As shown in this and in a previous report,[17] a single T-cell clone induced demyelination

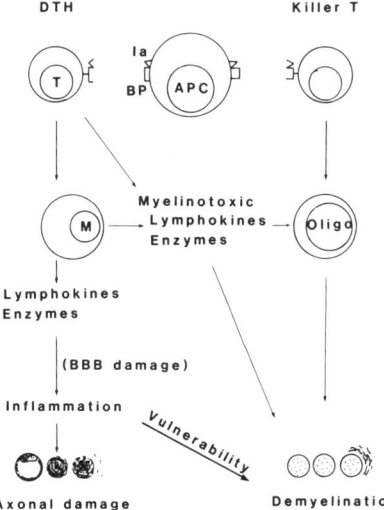

FIGURE 8. Possible mechanisms of BP/T cell line-mediated demyelination. There are possible explanations for T-cell-mediated demyelination, the most probable being differences in vulnerability between axons and myelin.

in congenitally athymic nude mice, which suggests a single T-cell clone-mediated demyelination without the aid of recipient-derived T-cell populations. Because the effector T-cell clone possessed surface phenotypes of T helper and inducer cells, it could be an effector of delayed hypersensitivity or class II-restricted killer T cells. At present, there is no technique to differentiate them. EAE effector T line cells killed Ia-positive astrocytes *in vitro*,[25] but Ia antigens on oligodendrocytes and myelin are negative. Therefore, killer T-cell-mediated demyelination is unlikely. However, because demyelination was more significant in X-irradiated allogeneic mice, the possibility of a graft-versus-host reaction cannot be ruled out because the demyelination was most often seen in root entry and exit zones where axons are closer to neurons and larger in diameter. These axons are no doubt stronger to noxious stimuli. In general, myelin is more susceptible than axon. Therefore, the difference in vulnerability between the axon and myelin may account for the demyelination (FIG. 8) if specific myelinotoxic lymphokines or factors derived from activated macrophages are absent.

Finally, the activation mechanism of the effector T-cell clone by alloantigens is interesting. Previously, we found that effector T cells disappear from the CNS tissue during recovery from acute EAE and remain in the spleen for a long time.[18] Because the spleen has no BP, activation seemed to be mediated by some mechanism other than the specific antigen. Willenborg et al.[19] demonstrated that injection of allogeneic cells in rats after recovery from acute EAE induces relapse. In their experiment, it was not known if the allogeneic cells stimulated the effector clone directly or indirectly. Our study clearly demonstrated this at the monoclonal level.[26] This information will help our understanding of the activation mechanism of effector clones in autoimmune diseases.

## SUMMARY

Autoimmune demyelination was studied in EAE induced by active challenge or by transfer of effector T-cell lines or clones specific for myelin basic protein or proteolipid apoprotein. The following points became clear: (1) Proteolipid apoprotein is responsible for widespread demyelination; (2) demyelination is more significant in EAE with a more chronic disease process; (3) a single T-cell clone can mediate significant demyelination without the aid of recipient-derived T-cell populations; (4) the difference in vulnerability between axons and myelin may account for the T-cell-mediated demyelination; and (5) effector T-cell clones can be activated by allogeneic antigens.

## ACKNOWLEDGMENTS

I thank Drs. T. Namikawa, T. Kunishita, K. Sakai, M. Endoh, J. Satoh, T. Yamamura, and T. Yoshimura who cooperated in this study.

## REFERENCES

1. PANITCH, H. & C. CICCONE. 1981. Induction of recurrent experimental allergic encephalomyelitis with myelin basic protein. Ann. Neurol. **75:** 433-438.
2. KEITH, A. B. & J. R. MCDERMOTT. 1980. Optimum conditions for inducing chronic relapsing experimental allergic encephalomyelitis in guinea pigs. J. Neurol. Sci. **46:** 353-364.
3. RAINE, C. S., D. H. SNYDER, M. P. VALSAMIS & S. H. STONE. 1974. Chronic experimental allergic encephalomyelitis in inbred guinea pigs. An ultrastructural study. Lab. Invest. **31:** 369-380.
4. YOSHIMURA, T., T. KUNISHITA, K. SAKAI, M. ENDOH, T. NAMIKAWA & T. TABIRA. 1985. Chronic experimental allergic encephalomyelitis in guinea pigs induced by proteolipid protein. J. Neurol. Sci. **69:** 47-58.
5. CAMBI, F., M. B. LEES, R. M. WILLIAMS & W. B. MACKLIN. 1983. Chronic experimental allergic encephalomyelitis produced by bovine proteolipid apoprotein. Immunological studies in rabbits. Ann. Neurol. **13:** 303-308.

6. BROWN, A., D. E. MCFARLIN & C. S. RAINE. 1982. Chronologic neuropathology of relapsing experimental allergic encephalomyelitis in the mouse. Lab. Invest. **46:** 171-185.
7. MOKHTARIAN, F., D. E. MCFARLIN & C. S. RAINE. 1984. Adoptive transfer of myelin basic protein-sensitized T cells produces chronic relapsing demyelinating disease in mice. Nature **309:** 356-358.
8. RAINE, C. S., F. MOKHTARIAN & D. E. MCFARLIN. 1984. Adoptively transferred chronic relapsing experimental autoimmune encephalomyelitis in the mouse. Neuropathologic analysis. Lab. Invest. **51:** 534-546.
9. DEIBLER, G. E., R. E. MARTENSON & M. W. KIES. 1972. Large scale preparation of myelin basic protein from central nervous system tissue of several mammalian species. Prep. Biochem. **2:** 139-165.
10. ENDOH, M., T. TABIRA, T. KUNISHITA, K. SAKAI, T. YAMAMURA & T. TAKETOMI. 1986. DM-20, a proteolipid apoprotein, is an encephalitogen of acute and relapsing autoimmune encephalomyelitis in mice. J. Immunol. **137:** 3832-3835.
11. SATOH, J., K. SAKAI, M. ENDOH, F. KOIKE, T. KUNISHITA, T. NAMIKAWA, T. YAMAMURA & T. TABIRA. 1987. Experimental allergic encephalomyelitis by murine encephalitogenic T cell lines specific for myelin proteolipid apoprotein. J. Immunol. **138:** 179-184.
12. SAKAI, K., T. NAMIKAWA, T. KUNISHITA, K. YAMANOUCHI & T. TABIRA. 1986. Studies of experimental allergic encephalomyelitis by using encephalitogenic T cell lines and clones in euthymic and athymic mice. J. Immunol. **137:** 1527-1531.
13. TABIRA, T. & ENDOH, M. 1985. Humoral immune responses to myelin basic protein, cerebroside and ganglioside in chronic relapsing experimental allergic encephalomyelitis of the guinea pig. J. Neurol. Sci. **67:** 201-212.
14. ENDOH, M., T. TABIRA & T. KUNISHITA. 1986. Antibodies to proteolipid apoprotein in chronic relapsing experimental allergic encephalomyelitis. J. Neurol. Sci. **73:** 31-38.
15. YAMAMURA, T., T. NAMIKAWA, M. ENDOH, T. KUNISHITA & T. TABIRA. 1986. Experimental allergic encephalomyelitis induced by proteolipid apoprotein in Lewis rats. J. Neuroimmunol. **12:** 143-153.
16. YAMAMURA, T., T. NAMIKAWA, M. ENDOH, T. KUNISHITA & T. TABIRA. 1986. Passive transfer of experimental allergic encephalomyelitis induced by proteolipid apoprotein. J. Neurol. Sci. **76:** 269-275.
17. TABIRA, T. & K. SAKAI. 1987. Demyelination induced by T cell lines and clones specific for myelin basic protein in mice. Lab. Invest. **56:** 518-525.
18. SAKAI, K., T. TABIRA, M. ENDOH & L. STEINMAN. 1986. Ia expression in chronic relapsing experimental allergic encephalomyelitis induced by long-term cultured T cell lines in mice. Lab. Invest. **54:** 345-352.
19. WILLENBORG, D. O., A. ROLINSON & G. DANTA. 1985. Reactivation of allergic encephalomyelitis by means of allogeneic confrontation. Cell. Immunol. **90:** 614-619.
20. ORTIZ-ORTIZ, L. & W. O. WEIGLE. 1982. Activation of effector cells in experimental allergic encephalomyelitis by interleukin 2 (IL2). J. Immunol. **128:** 1545-1550.
21. SAIDA, T., K. SAIDA, D. H. SILBERBERG & M. S. BROWN. 1978. Transfer of demyelination with experimental allergic neuritis serum by intraneural injection. Nature **272:** 639-641.
22. CARROLL, W. M., A. R. JENNINGS & F. C. MASTAGLIA. 1985. Galactocerebroside antiserum causes demyelination of cat optic nerve. Brain Res. **330:** 378-381.
23. TROTTER, J., L. J. DEJONG & M. E. SMITH. 1986. Opsonization with antimyelin antibody increases the uptake and intracellular metabolism of myelin in inflammatory macrophages. J. Neurochem. **47:** 779-789.
24. ZAMVIL, S., P. NELSON, J. TROTTER, D. MITCHELL, R. KNOBLER, R. FRITZ & L. STEINMAN. 1985. T-cell clones specific for myelin basic protein induce chronic relapsing paralysis and demyelination. Nature **317:** 355-358.
25. SUN, D. & H. WEKERLE. 1986. Ia-restricted encephalitogenic T lymphocytes mediating EAE lyse autoantigen-presenting astrocytes. Nature **320:** 70-72.
26. SAKAI, K. & T. TABIRA. 1987. Recognition of alloantigens of experimental allergic encephalomyelitis by a murine encephalitogenic T cell clone. Eur. J. Immunol. **17:** 955-960.

# Autoimmune Reactions Against Myelin Basic Protein Induced by Corona and Measles Viruses[a]

VOLKER TER MEULEN

*Institut für Virologie und Immunbiologie*
*Universität Würzburg*
*D - 8700 Würzburg, West Germany*

Many major human diseases derive from autoimmune reactions directed against particular organ or tissue antigens, as can be demonstrated by immunohistologic studies. One disease in which a virus-triggered autoimmune phenomenon has been postulated is multiple sclerosis (MS).[1] The strongest evidence in support of a viral etiology of MS comes from epidemiologic studies that suggest that MS derives from environmental factors operating years before the onset of the clinical manifestations of the disease. This evidence consists of age-specific tables, geographic distribution, and patterns of migration and family clustering of the cases of MS. The hypothesis derived from these studies holds that a patient with MS is exposed at puberty, or shortly thereafter, to an infectious agent that triggers the disease. Besides the epidemiologic evidence, many investigators have found an increase in virus-specific antibodies against certain enveloped viruses in patients with MS, suggesting that these viruses could be candidate causative agents. However, thus far, all attempts at isolation or identification of a particular virus as the cause of MS have failed. This failure is the more perplexing, because a number of viruses have been isolated from the brains of patients with MS, none of which could be unequivocally related to the disease.

Despite these failures, the hypothesis of a viral etiology of MS remains viable, because of the available circumstantial evidence. It is reasonable to assume that a virus (or several viruses) can trigger an autoimmune reaction against brain antigens, which can then continue and thus can perpetuate the disease, even when the virus is no longer around.

In an attempt to test the validity of this theory, we developed an animal model, the Lewis rat infected with either the murine coronavirus JHM or a neurotropic measles virus. Both viruses cause central nervous system (CNS) disease and trigger an autoimmune reaction mediated by T cells.

## MURINE CORONAVIRUS JHM INFECTION IN WEANLING LEWIS RATS

When rats are infected with JHM virus at the age of 21 to 35 days, they develop either acute encephalomyelitis (AE) or subacute demyelinating encephalomyelitis

[a] The experiments described in this manuscript were supported by Deutsche Forschungsgemeinschaft.

(SDE).[2,3] The acute disease has an average incubation period of 6-12 days and follows a rapidly progressing clinical course characterized by paralysis and early death. Examination of the neurologic tissues of these animals reveals changes limited to gray matter of both the brain and spinal cord, consisting of necrosis of the neurons and consequent infiltration by granulocytes, lymphocytes, and macrophages. Viral antigen is evident in neurons and glia, and the culprit virus is readily isolated from the brain and spinal cord tissues.

In contrast, SDE has an incubation period of 2 weeks to 8 months, followed by a slow onset of disease characterized by paralysis of the hind legs and ataxic gait, eventually culminating in tetraplegia. The most prominent neuropathologic changes include primary demyelination in the white matter of the optic nerves, midbrain, pons, cerebellum, and spinal cord. Within the demyelinated plaques are well-preserved axons and neurons. There is also perivascular cuffing by lymphocytes and other mononuclear cells, as well as infiltration by macrophages. Here, too, the viral antigen can be recognized in the tissues, but it is primarily found in the glia and in the proximity of the plaques. The virus can also be isolated by conventional techniques, regardless of the length of the incubation period. Many of these animals eventually recover and show evidence of remyelination.

## RELAPSING SUBACUTE DEMYELINATING ENCEPHALOMYELITIS OF LEWIS RATS

Some animals that survive SDE and recover later experience a second attack of the neurologic disease.[4] Between 60 and 120 days following the first episode of disease, the animals get sick again, with identical symptoms that are now more severe. Histopathologic abnormalities consist of new demyelinative lesions infiltrated by mononuclear cells located primarily in the brain stem and the spinal cord. Moreover, there are old lesions where they were previously noted, revealing extensive remyelination indicative of a repair mechanism that had developed after the initial disease. In contrast to the first attack of SDE, following the second attack, isolation of virus is a rarity, even as viral antigen is readily detected in glia and the region surrounding the plaque.

## INFLUENCE OF GENETICS ON CNS INFECTION

Because JHM infection in the Lewis rat resembled some characteristics of experimental allergic encephalomyelitis (EAE), we decided to compare the infection with this virus to that of another inbred rat, BN, which is resistant to EAE. Weanling BN rats can be infected with the JHM virus, but the majority of these animals remain clinically well despite histologic changes of subacute demyelinating encephalomyelitis. Virus can be isolated from their brains, but only up to 10 days after infection, even as fresh CNS lesions continue to develop and viral antigen persists beyond that period. In contrast to SDE in Lewis rats, in BN rats the main neuropathologic lesions consist of small nodular demyelinated plaques predominantly located in the periventricular white matter, an area in which Lewis rats only rarely develop changes. These nodular lesions, which differ from the demyelinated plaque seen in infected Lewis rats, contain microglia, phagocytes, and astrocytes with swollen cytoplasm. In addition, the inflammatory response is expressed mainly by plasma cells.[5] Obviously, therefore, an important pathogenic mechanism in response to the JHM infection depends on the genetic characteristics of the animal.

## MEASLES VIRUS INFECTION OF LEWIS AND BN RATS

Infection of weanling Lewis rats with neurotropic measles virus CAM/RBH results in either acute measles encephalitis or subacute measles encephalitis (SAME).[6] The acute encephalitis is characterized by a short incubation period and focal infiltration by mononuclear cells of gray matter of both cerebral hemispheres and basal ganglia. There are usually few or no degenerative changes. SAME develops in about 20% of the infected animals, after an incubation period of 3 weeks to 3 months. The earliest sign of the disease is an arrest of weight gain or even weight loss. This is followed by generalized hyperexcitability, unsteadiness, abnormal posture, paresis of the limbs, and occasional seizures. This phase of the disease lasts for several days up to 3 weeks and has a case fatality rate of 50%. Histopathologic changes consist of prominent lymphomonocytic perivascular cuffing. There are no demyelinated plaques. The survivors recover completely and remain well for at least 8 months.

Infection of weanling BN rats results in acute encephalitis in a small percentage only; the majority develop clinically silent encephalomyelitis (CSE). The histopathologic lesions in animals with CSE consist of inflammatory lesions, widespread proliferation of the glial cells, and multicystic parenchymal degeneration.

Infectious virus is easily isolated from the cerebral hemisphere of both types of rats with acute encephalitis. However, in contrast, neither in SAME in the Lewis rats nor in CSE in the BN rats could infectious virus be isolated by conventional techniques or by co-cultivation, despite the detection of viral antigen. This failure of isolation could be attributed to restriction of gene expression of the measles virus occurring at the level of virus envelope proteins. As a result, infectious virus particles cannot be assembled, because the matrix protein required for the budding process is not synthesized. At no time during the course of the disease has virus been recovered from their lungs, liver, kidneys, spleen, or thymus.

## IMMUNE REACTION IN INFECTED RATS

Host response, both humoral and cell-mediated immunity (CMI), plays a major role in controlling virus infections. Specific antibodies neutralize extracellular virus and protect against reinfection; in some circumstances they also eliminate infected host cells by antibody-dependent cytotoxicity. CMI reactions, however, are the predominant mechanism that destroys infected cells. Individuals with an inherited defect in the CMI develop severe complications of those infectious diseases that tend to be benign in normal individuals.

In CNS infections, intrathecal synthesis of virus-specific antibodies is an important defense mechanism and is well documented in human patients.[7-12] It is the B lymphocytes that are responsible for the intrathecal synthesis of the antibodies, which are of an oligoclonal nature as determined by agarose electrophoresis or isoelectric focusing. It is possible to determine viral specificity of the IgG clones in the CSF specimens by immunoprint fixation[13] or immunoblot technique.[14] This determination is important in diagnosis.

In rats infected with either JHM or measles virus that develop SDE or SAME, the same diagnostic techniques have been applied by us[15-17] with the following findings. In the Lewis rats there was only an occasional intrathecal virus-specific response despite the presence of oligoclonal IgG. It is therefore probable that these immunoglobulins of restricted heterogeneity are directed against nonviral antigens, which are likely to be antigens of the central nervous tissues. Conversely, in the BN rats the oligoclonal intrathecal antibodies were specific against the virus used in the original infection. It is likely, therefore, that in the BN rat these antibodies tend to play a protective role, whereas in the Lewis rat no such protection is afforded.

An analysis of the CMI response in SDE and SAME revealed a reaction against the JHM, or measles, virus and in the diseased Lewis rats a reaction also against myelin basic protein (MBP).[18,19] Lymphocytes, whether collected from the spleen, thymus, or peripheral blood, all had a proliferative response in the presence of MBP, akin to that in EAE. Moreover, when lymphocytes from rats with SDE or SAME were infused intravenously into normal rats, the recipients developed symptoms of EAE within 5 days, consisting of hypersensitivity to touch and a slightly ataxic gait. Histologic examination of the CNS tissues of these animals revealed perivascular cuffing with mononuclear cells in the white matter of the spinal cord, where the lesions were in the dorsal columns—the pons, the cerebellum, and the thalamus. Infected BN rats did not develop such an autoimmune reaction when tested either by *in vitro* analysis or by the adoptive transfer of lymphocytes.[5,19] We can therefore conclude that the cellular autoimmune reaction is of pathogenic significance in the infected Lewis rat.

## INTERACTIONS OF JHM AND MEASLES VIRUSES WITH ASTROCYTES

Our knowledge of the specific immune responses in the CNS to viral infections is quite incomplete. The CNS is an immunologic island, considered a privileged site. In order for the lymphocytes to find an antigen in the CNS, they must invade its domain and, once there, they must secure a mechanism for identification of the antigens. Recent evidence has been brought forth that astrocytes can act as cells presenting antigens.[20] On the basis of the information, we endeavored to investigate the effects of the two viruses on astrocytes. Both viruses can induce class II molecules on cultured astrocytes,[21,22] a property independent of viral replication in the astrocytes because viruses inactivated by ultraviolet irradiation are also effective. Apparently this capacity to induce the Ia antigen depends on direct interaction of the viruses with the cell membranes of the astrocytes. This interpretation has been derived from the observation that monoclonal antibodies directed against the E2 glycoprotein of the JHM virus or against the hemagglutinin of the measles virus prevent the induction of class II antigens. It appears, therefore, that either the viruses bind to specific receptors on the cell surface or the cells phagocytize the viruses and the expression of the Ia antigen follows. This mechanism is independent of gamma-interferon. It may be similar to the one described for bacterial endotoxin.[23]

The phenomenon of Ia induction by these two neurotropic viruses has important implications on the mechanisms of pathogenesis. Until recently it was assumed that gamma-interferon released by activated T lymphocytes was indispensable to the induction of Ia on certain antigen-presenting cells,[24,25] including astrocytes. Because the brain lacks lymphatic drainage and the so-called blood-brain barrier restricts traffic of lymphocytes and macromolecules, gamma-interferon would not be readily available for the induction of Ia, especially in the early phase of the infection. What apparently happens is that the viruses themselves induce Ia expression on the astrocytes, enabling these cells to present the viral antigens to the lymphocytes and allowing the host to mount an effective immune response to control the infection.

## POSSIBLE MECHANISMS OF VIRUS-INDUCED AUTOIMMUNE REACTIONS

Although the means by which viruses induce T-lymphocyte responses against host antigens are still unclear, there are a number of speculations to account for this phenomenon.

1. The fact that viruses require living cells for replication has major consequences for the host. During replication, the viruses can incorporate into their envelopes host antigens and they insert, modify, or expose internal cellular antigens on the cell surface. These heretofore "hidden" antigens, now exposed, could appear foreign to the host's immune system.

2. The viruses can interact with the immune regulatory systems by destroying subpopulations of lymphocytes or by stimulating generation of lymphocyte clones that are autoreactive. Many viruses are lymphotropic, as exemplified by measles and Epstein-Barr virus. Measles virus replicates in T or B lymphocytes, which leads to lymphocyte destruction and subsequently to an immunosuppressive effect clinically documented by abolition of skin reactions in delayed hypersensitivity. Epstein-Barr virus infects and transforms human B lymphocytes. The transformed, or immortalized, cells could under certain circumstances secrete antibodies reacting with cellular constituents.

3. Molecular mimicry could also be operating. An immune response might be raised against certain viral antigens that cross-react with some native host antigens. A variety of viral sequences, including those of measles virus, were recently compared by computer analysis with myelin basic protein (MBP).[26] The comparison showed amino acid homology between viral proteins and MBP. This observation led to an interesting experiment in which a rabbit was immunized with a synthetic peptide from such a sequence of the hepatitis B virus polymerase.[27] Peripheral blood lymphocytes from the immunized rabbits proliferated in the presence of either MBP or hepatitis B polymerase, and their CNS tissue revealed similar neuropathologic changes similar to those in EAE. In this context it is of interest to note that in postinfectious encephalomyelitis in man associated with rubella, varicella, or measles, an MBP-specific lymphoproliferative response has been observed.[28]

4. An autoimmune response could be triggered by the development of an anti-idiotypic antibody. In a reovirus model these antibodies directed to type III hemagglutinin react with receptors for reovirus on the surfaces of the lymphocytes and nerve cells, and it is possible that this could trigger an autoimmune reaction.[29]

5. The last possible mechanism for the development of an immunopathologic

reaction in the course of a CNS viral infection is the induction by the virus of class II antigens on astrocytes and a consequent delayed type hypersensitivity reaction (DTH) in genetically susceptible animals. In order for the helper T lymphocytes to recognize viral antigens, class II antigens probably have to be present on the astrocytes. However, in extremely high constitutive levels of class II expression on astrocytes, an inappropriate or excessive presentation of self-antigens and viral antigens may develop, similar to that in autoimmune processes directed against the thyroid gland.[30] This mechanism could well play a role in the JHM- and measles-virus-induced CNS disease in Lewis rats, because as recently shown by us,[31] these hyperexpressions of Ia molecules on astrocytes after contact with gamma-interferon or viral particles are genetically regulated.

## CONCLUSIONS

JHM and measles virus infections in rats are models of a persistent viral infection of the CNS with and without demyelination, associated with a cell-mediated immune reaction to MBP. Availability of inbred susceptible and resistant rat strains, which react differentially to viral and host antigens, makes possible a variety of experimental permutations aimed at defining the causal mechanisms of CNS diseases. These mechanisms can be studied from the points of view of molecular biology and immunology, because both viruses used are well characterized and there are appropriate immunologic markers for the lymphocytes and the brain cells of these rats. This approach can be expected to bring us towards an understanding of the pathogenesis of persistent CNS infections that are associated with demyelination and mediated by immunologic reactions. Our hope is that information gained from these animal models will have a bearing on studies of related human diseases, particularly parainfectious encephalitis and multiple sclerosis.

## ACKNOWLEDGMENT

I thank Dr. Michael Katz for helpful discussions and for editing the manuscript. The secretarial assistance of Helga Kriesinger is gratefully acknowledged.

## REFERENCES

1. TER MEULEN, V. & J. R. STEPHENSON. 1983. The possible role of viral infections in MS and other related demyelinating diseases. *In* Multiple Sclerosis. J. F. Hallpike, C. W. M. Adams & W. W. Tourtellotte, Eds.: 241-274. Chapman & Hall, London.
2. NAGASHIMA, K., H. WEGE, R. MEYERMANN & V. TER MEULEN. 1978. Corona virus induced subacute demyelinating encephalomyelitis in rats: A morphological analysis. Acta Neuropathol. (Berl) **44**: 63-70.
3. NAGASHIMA, K., H. WEGE, R. MEYERMANN & V. TER MEULEN. 1979. Demyelinating encephalomyelitis induced by a long-term corona virus infection in rats. Acta Neuropathol. (Berl) **45**: 205-213.

4. WEGE, H., R. WATANABE & V. TER MEULEN. 1984. Relapsing subacute demyelinating encephalomyelitis in rats in the course of coronavirus JHM infection. J. Neuroimmunol. **6:** 325-336.
5. WATANABE, R., H. WEGE & V. TER MEULEN. 1987. Comparative analysis of coronavirus JHM induced demyelinating encephalomyelitis in Lewis and Brown-Norway rats. Lab. Invest. **57:** 375-384.
6. LIEBERT, U. G. & V. TER MEULEN. 1987. Virological aspects of measles virus induced encephalomyelitis in Lewis and BN rats. J. Gen. Virol. **68:** 1715-1722.
7. VANDVIK, B., E. NORRBY, H. J. NORDAL & M. DEGRÉ. 1976. Oligoclonal measles virus-specific IgG antibodies isolated from cerebrospinal fluids, brain extracts, and sera from patients with subacute sclerosing panencephalitis and multiple sclerosis. Scand. J. Immunol. **5:** 979-992.
8. VANDVIK, B., E. NORRBY, J. STEEN-JOHNSON & K. STENSVOLD. 1978a. Mumps meningitis: Prolonged pleocytosis and occurrence of mumps virus-specific oligoclonal IgG in the cerebrospinal fluid. Eur. J. Neurol. **17:** 13-22.
9. VANDVIK, B., M. L. WEIL, M. GRANDIEN & E. NORRBY. 1978b. Progressive rubella virus panencephalitis: Synthesis of oligoclonal virus-specific IgG antibodies and homogeneous free light chains in the central nervous system. Acta Neurol. Scand. **57:** 53-64.
10. VANDVIK, B., F. VARTDAL & E. NORRBY. 1982. Herpes simplex virus encephalitis: Intrathecal synthesis of oligoclonal virus-specific IgG, IgA and IgM antibodies. J. Neurol. **228:** 25-38.
11. VARTDAL, F., B. VANDVIK & E. NORRBY. 1982. Intrathecal synthesis of virus-specific oligoclonal IgG, IgA and IgM antibodies in a case of varicella-zoster meningoencephalitis. J. Neurol. Sci. **57:** 121-132.
12. SKÖLDENBERG, B., K. KALIMO, A. CARLSTRÖM, M. FORSGREN & P. HALONEN. 1981. Herpes simplex encephalitis: A serological follow-up study. Synthesis of herpes simplex virus immunoglobulin M, A and G antibodies and development of oligoclonal immunoglobulin G in the central nervous system. Acta Neurol. Scand. **63:** 273-285.
13. NORDAL, H. J., B. VANDVIK & E. NORRBY. 1978. Demonstration of electrophoretically restricted virus-specific antibodies in serum and cerebrospinal fluid by imprint electraimmunofixation. Scand. J. Immunol. **7:** 381-388.
14. DÖRRIES, R. & V. TER MEULEN. 1984. Detection and identification of virus-specific, oligoclonal IgG in unconcentrated cerebrospinal fluid by immunoblot technique. J. Neuroimmunol. **7:** 77-89.
15. DÖRRIES, R., R. WATANABE, H. WEGE & V. TER MEULEN. 1987. Intrathecal humoral immune response in corona virus induced encephalomyelitis of Lewis and BN rats. *In* Coronaviruses. M. M. C. Lai & S. A. Stohlman, Eds. Adv. Exp. Med. Biol. **218:** 373-381. Plenum Press, New York.
16. DÖRRIES, R., R. WATANABE, H. WEGE & V. TER MEULEN. 1987. Analysis of the intrathecal humoral immune response in Brown Norway (BN) rats, infected with the murine coronavirus JHM. J. Neuroimmunol. **14:** 305-316.
17. DÖRRIES, R., U. G. LIEBERT & V. TER MEULEN. 1988. Comparative analysis of virus-specific antibodies and immunoglobulins in serum and cerebrospinal fluid of subacute measles virus induced encephalomyelitis (SAME) in rats and subacute sclerosing panencephalitis (SSPE). J. Neuroimmunol., in press.
18. WATANABE, R., H. WEGE & V. TER MEULEN. 1983. Adoptive transfer of EAE-like lesions by BMP stimulated lymphocytes from rats with coronavirus-induced demyelinating encephalomyelitis. Nature **305:** 150-153.
19. LIEBERT, U. G., C. LININGTON & V. TER MEULEN. 1988. Induction of autoimmune reactions to myelin basic protein in measles virus encephalitis in Lewis rats. J. Neuroimmunol. **17:** 103-118.
20. FONTANA, A., W. FIERZ & H. WEKERLE. 1984. Astrocytes present myelin basic protein to encephalitogenic T-cell lines. Nature **307:** 273-276.
21. MASSA, P. T., R. DÖRRIES & V. TER MEULEN. 1986. Viral particles induce Ia antigen expression on astrocytes. Nature **320:** 543-546.
22. MASSA, P. T., A. SCHIMPL, E. WECKER & V. TER MEULEN. 1987. Tumor necrosis factor amplifies measles virus-mediated Ia induction on astrocytes. Proc. Natl. Acad. Sci. USA **84:** 7242-7245.

23. MONROE, J. G. & J. C. CAMBIER. 1983. B cell activation. III. B cell plasma membrane depolarization and hyper-Ia antigen expression induced by receptor immunoglobulin cross-linking are coupled. J. Exp. Med. **158:** 1589-1599.
24. STEEG, P. S., R. N. MORE, H. M. JOHNSON & J. J. OPPENHEIM. 1982a. Regulation of murine macrophage Ia antigen expression by a lymphokine with immune interferon activity. J. Exp. Med. **156:** 1780-1793.
25. STEEG, P. S., H. M. JOHNSON & J. J. OPPENHEIM. 1982b. Regulation of murine macrophage Ia expression by an immune interferon-like lymphokine: Inhibitory effect of endotoxin. J. Immunol. **129:** 2402-2406.
26. JAHNKE, U., E. H. FISCHER & E. C. ALVORD. 1985. Sequence homology between certain viral proteins and proteins related to encephalomyelitis and neuritis. Science **229:** 282-284.
27. FUJINAMI, R. S. & M. B. A. OLDSTONE. 1985. Amino acid homology between the encephalitogenic site of myelin basic protein and virus: Mechanism for autoimmunity. Science **230:** 1043-1045.
28. JOHNSON, R. T., D. E. GRIFFIN, R. L. HIRSCH, J. S. WOLINSKY, S. ROEDENBECK, I. LINDO DE SORIANO & A. VAISBERG. 1984. Measles encephalomyelitis: Clinical and immunologic studies. N. Engl. J. Med. **310:** 137-141.
29. NEPOM, J. T., H. L. WEINER, M. A. DICHTER, M. TARDIEU, D. R. SPRIGGS, C. F. GRAMM, M. L. POWERS, B. N. FIELDS & M. I. GREENE. 1982. Identification of a hemagglutinin-specific idiotype associated with reovirus recognition shared by lymphoid and neural cells. J. Exp. Med. **155:** 155-167.
30. LONDEI, M., J. R. LAMB, G. F. BOTTAZZO & M. FELDMANN. 1984. Epithelial cells expressing aberrant MHC class II determinants can present antigen to cloned human T cells. Nature **312:** 639-641.
31. MASSA, P. T., V. TER MEULEN & A. FONTANA. 1987. Hyperinducibility of Ia antigen on astrocytes correlates with strain-specific susceptibility to experimental autoimmune encephalomyelitis. Proc. Natl. Acad. Sci. USA **84:** 4219-4223.

# Virus-Induced Autoimmunity Through Molecular Mimicry[a]

ROBERT S. FUJINAMI

*Department of Pathology*
*University of California, San Diego*
*La Jolla, California 92093*

The fundamental cause of many chronic debilitating diseases is not known. However, host responses to self could play an important role in many of these instances. Microorganisms and/or viruses in coalition with host immune responses are often associated with occurrences of disease. Viruses have been implicated with the initiation of autoimmunity; however, direct cause and effect evidence is often hard to derive.

Immunologic cross-reactions or molecular mimicry, that is, shared determinants between a microorganism and self epitopes, could account for the breaking of tolerance and the initiation of antiself responses, leading to autoimmunity. Advances in current methodology have allowed us to explore the immunologic cross-reactions and determine what epitopes are important in the induction of disease.

The first suggestive evidence that viruses could share common determinants with their hosts came from experiments showing an association between infection and the incidence of autoantibodies in patients with infectious active hepatitis. Ajdukiewicz et al.[1] reported the presence of anti-smooth muscle antibodies. Later Toh et al.[2] extended these observations to include infectious hepatitis, chicken pox, measles, and mumps viruses. They found reactivity to intermediate filament proteins. Over half the sera from infected individuals reacted with intermediate filament proteins. Only 6% of control sera were positive. Similar antibodies were also found in patients with infectious mononucleosis.[3-7] However, in many instances it was not clear if these antibodies reacted with virus and self, or if the antibodies arose through polyclonal B-cell activation, or both.

Reaction to other intracytoplasmic proteins has been described by Sotelo et al.[8] They found autoantibodies against axonal neurofilaments in patients with subacute spongiform encephalopathies such as Kuru and Jakob-Creutzfeldt disease. These sera were tested in *in vitro* central nervous system cultures. Almost two thirds of patients with Jakob-Creutzfeldt disease and approximately one third of patients with Kuru had autoantibodies. These findings were the first evidence of an immune reaction occurring in relation to either of these encephalopathic diseases.

In mouse studies of vaccinia virus infection, Steck et al.[9] demonstrated that inoculation of mice with a neurotropic strain resulted in the production of antibodies that reacted with myelin and oligodendrocytes. No antibodies were found to bind to neurons or thymocytes. Mice injected with a dermotropic strain of vaccinia did not produce autoantibodies to central nervous system elements. The antimyelin and the antioligodendrocyte antibodies could therefore not be removed by absorption using

---

[a] This work was supported by the National Multiple Sclerosis Society and the National Institutes of Health.

whole vaccinia virus. However, not all vaccinia proteins are expressed in the virion. Therefore, the presence of common epitopes between virus and myelin could not be confirmed by this method. In contrast, Dales et al.[10] demonstrated that immunization of mice with vaccinia virus yielded autoantibodies to intermediate filament proteins. One of these intermediate filament proteins, vimentin, was found also to bind to vaccinia hemagglutinin. They found that viral replication was not necessary for the production of autoantibodies.

In another animal model, Webb et al.[11,12] described a system in which infection of mice with Semliki Forest virus led to the production of antibodies to cerebrosides, glucocerebrosides, gangliosides, but not to myelin. Brain-derived or brain-passaged virus was required for the production of autoantibody. The investigators suggest that Semliki Forest virus can incorporate part of the host lipid (myelin glycolipids) into viral envelope, and it is these components that are now immunogenic.

Autoreactive T cells can also play a role during virus infections. Infection of BALB/c mice with a heart-adapted variant of Coxsackie virus led to the production of myocarditis.[13] T cells isolated from infected mice could kill primary cultures of myocytes. Antibodies to cardiac tissue were found in the neurotropic virus-infected mice. However, these antibodies apparently did not play a major role in the disease production.[14] In contrast, in a different mouse system,[15] heart-specific autoantibodies did correspond with the occurrence of disease.

In a human disease of virus-induced immunosuppression, acquired immune deficiency syndrome (AIDS), autoantibodies were found in association with infection by the human immunodeficiency virus (HIV). The reports mostly center on the presence of antilymphocyte antibodies. It has been suggested that these antilymphocytes participate in the suppression of immune responsiveness that is found in AIDS patients.[16] Dorsett et al.[17] found that incubation of normal (uninfected) lymphocytes with sera of patients with AIDS or AIDS-related complex resulted in increased numbers of surface immunoglobulin-positive lymphocytes. Conversely, no such increase occurred when lymphocytes from normal individuals were incubated with sera from patients with diseases unrelated to AIDS or from normal control subjects. These studies[17] demonstrated that cells of the OKT-4 or OKT-11 and not OKT-8 phenotype bound the autoantibodies. Therefore, cells of the helper-suppressor phenotype bound the antilymphocyte antibodies, and alterations in this cell population may be involved in the decreased immune responses observed in AIDS patients.

Evidence that viruses share common antigenic sites with self epitopes was exploited by monoclonal antibody technology. Lane and Hoeffler[18] described a monoclonal antibody that bound to the SV40 T antigen and a 68,000 kd host cell protein. These findings were extended[19,20] to a variety of host cell proteins, ranging in molecular weights from 35,000 to 150,000 daltons. These investigators predicted that the sites shared by the viral T and host proteins reflected similarities of function and shape.[19,20]

Fujinami et al.[21] demonstrated cross-reactions between virus and self, that is, molecular mimicry, in the context of autoimmunity through the use of monoclonal antibodies. The phosphoprotein of measles virus was shown to have a site in common with a cytokeratin protein of normal cells. Monoclonal antibodies have identified similar specificities in other viral systems. Recently, Srinivasappa et al.[22] reported that roughly 3-4% of all antiviral monoclonal antibodies react with host cell components. In addition, Fujinami et al.[21] demonstrated a common determinant between an intermediate filament protein and a herpes virus protein of 146,000 molecular weight. The monoclonal antibody immunoprecipitated this protein during the late phase of herpes virus infection. As mentioned earlier, Dales et al.[10] also found a cross-reacting epitope between vaccinia virus hemagglutinin and vimentin, another intermediate filament protein. Many of the reported monoclonal antibodies cross-react with intracellular determinants in uninfected cells. This finding probably reflects the fact that viruses are intracellular parasites and assemble in association with cytoskeletal proteins within the infected cell.[23] Regions that are common to both virus and intermediate filament proteins would facilitate transport of the virus proteins to compartments occupied by intracellular cytoskeletal proteins and allow viral assembly to occur.

Sheshberadaran and Norrby[24] described monoclonal antibodies against measles virus fusion protein that cross-react with a host cellular stress protein of 79,000 molecular weight. This finding was demonstrated by immunoprecipitation and immunofluorescent staining of infected and uninfected cells. This host stress protein is induced by infection of cells with various paramyxoviruses, heat shock of uninfected HeLa cells, and treatment of various cell lines with 2-deoxyglucose, tunicamycin, or L-canavanine.

Monoclonal antibodies to another paramyxovirus were described. Goswami et al.[25] found that an antibody against the simian virus 5 HN glycoprotein bound to determinants on Purkinje cells and could neutralize virus. Furthermore, this monoclonal antibody could bind to myelin-containing areas after treatment of tissue sections with acetic acid and ethanol. This antibody also reacts with human brain sections or tissue extracts.

Retroviruses have common determinants with host proteins. Haynes et al.[26] reported that a monoclonal antibody bound to a 19,000-dalton HIV protein and a neuroendocrine component found in thymic epithelial cells. This determinant was not found on other normal epithelial or neuroendocrine tissues. Other studies by Sarin et al.[27] demonstrated that antiserum to thymosin alpha-1 could neutralize human T-cell leukemia virus (HTLV)-III/LAV. The reverse transcriptase activity and expression of the p15 and p24 viral proteins were inhibited by purified immunoglobulin preparations from antisera to thymosin alpha-1.

A cross-reacting determinant was also described between murine mammary tumor virus and a subpopulation of B cells.[28] A monoclonal antibody VE7 detects gp52 envelope glycoprotein of murine mammary tumor virus and reacts with a small percentage of lymphocytes and a subpopulation of Thy-1.2-negative surface immunoglobulin positive cells.

Recently, in producing monoclonal antibodies to Theiler's murine encephalomyelitis virus, an antibody was found to react with galactocerebroside. The cross-reacting monoclonal antibody neutralizes the virus and has the ability to cause demyelination in rat sciatic nerve in vivo. The presence of such an antibody could contribute to the demyelinating pattern of this disease observed in chronically infected mice.[29]

Reovirus types 1 and 3 and lymphocytes share common determinants.[30] Tardieu et al.[30] found a monoclonal antibody that binds to the Lyt 2,3 subset of murine lymphocytes. In addition, this monoclonal antibody was shown to mediate complement-dependent lysis of Lyt 2,3 cells.

An alternative scheme to the use of monoclonal antibodies is the direct comparison of amino acid sequences between viruses and host proteins. This approach was used by Fujinami and Oldstone[31] (reviewed in reference 32). A common area was found in myelin basic protein (amino acid 66-75) and the hepatitis B virus polymerase (amino acid 589-598).[31] The amino acid region of myelin basic protein is encephalitogenic for the rabbit, and when injected with adjuvant into a rabbit, it will induce an autoimmune disease known as experimental allergic encephalitis (EAE). Six amino acids in a row were shared with the encephalitogenic site in the rabbit.

The relevant viral polymerase peptide was chemically synthesized and injected with Freund's complete adjuvant into rabbits. The animals were monitored for autoantibody production (antibody to myelin basic protein), cellular reactivity to myelin basic protein, and disease production.[31] Five of seven rabbits immunized with one injection of viral peptide had significant levels of antibody to myelin basic protein. The binding of this antibody to myelin basic protein could be inhibited by the viral peptide. Therefore, sensitization of a rabbit using a viral peptide that cross-reacts with a self protein can lead to autoantibody production. To test for cellular reactivity, peripheral blood lymphocytes from eight rabbits sensitized with the viral peptide were tested for their ability to proliferate when cultured with myelin basic protein or viral peptide. Peripheral blood lymphocytes from four of the eight rabbits responded positively to myelin basic protein. The brains and spinal cords of 11 rabbits sensitized with the viral peptide were examined for histologic lesions characteristic of EAE. In four of these animals cellular infiltrates and lesions in the central nervous system developed that were consistent with the histologic pattern observed in this autoimmune disease.

Kagnoff et al.[33] described an amino acid homology between a 54,000 molecular weight early region E1b protein of human adenovirus type 12 and A-gliadin, a component of wheat. This virus is a common inhabitant of the human intestinal tract. The homologous region includes a 12 amino acid stretch where 8 residues are in common and are in tandem. The common region is hydrophilic. Antibodies induced by the adenovirus 12 region react with A-gliadin. Celiac disease in humans is activated by ingestion of grains containing gliadins or similar proteins. Thus, these investigators suggest that if the common site is important in disease production, then an immune response against a normal intestinal organism, such as adenovirus type 12, could result in manifestations similar to those caused by ingestion of gliadins. Genetic factors also contribute to the expression of celiac disease.

Sequence homologies have been described for retroviruses and self proteins. Clarke et al.[34] describe a homology between the HTLV envelope (env) gene and HLA class I gene. They used molecular clones of HTLV and the human MHC antigen DNA to define a region of homology between the env region of HTLV and a region in the HLA-B locus that encodes the extracellular portion of class I antigens. The authors suggest that T cells expressing the inappropriate HLA antigen would be impaired in mounting a functional immune response. Furthermore, the viral HLA-related antigen would be recognized as self and evade immune responses that would occur if this antigen were recognized as non-self. Similarly, Reither et al.[35] described a region of homology between the env protein of HIV and a portion of the interleukin-2 (IL-2) molecule that purportedly binds to the IL-2 receptor. This homology may explain the characteristic immunosuppression observed in AIDS-infected individuals. The AIDS virus env protein could interfere with IL-2 activity either by competing with IL-2 for the receptor or after binding to the cell. This phenomenon was also apparent for the env proteins of other retroviruses associated with immunosuppression. Weigent et al.[36] found that a peptide from the carboxy terminus of the HIV env protein inhibited the biologic activity of human IL-2 in a murine spleen cell proliferation assay. When the peptide was coupled to a protein carrier, the peptide-carrier combination inhibited the binding of radiolabeled IL-2 to its receptor.

Looking at other retroviruses, Wong and Goldberg[37] produced antibodies to a decapeptide from pp60 src of Rous sarcoma virus (RSV). Peptides to this region inhibited the kinase activities associated with the transforming proteins of pp60 src, p90 of the Y73 avian sarcoma virus, or p140 of Fujinami sarcoma virus. The antipeptide antibody could immunoprecipitate the pp60 src of RSV and p90 of the Y73 avian sarcoma virus. This antiserum could also precipitate a number of high molecular weight phosphoproteins for normal chicken and rat fibroblasts and from several lines of virus-transformed cells that defined a common epitope with the host phosphoproteins. Mathey-Prevot et al.[38] obtained an antiserum specific for the unique sequence of the transforming protein p140 of Fujinami sarcoma virus that bound to a normal cellular protein. This cellular protein was structurally similar to the viral p140 by tryptic peptide mapping and protein kinase activity. Analyzing sequences, Robbins et al.[39] described common regions between the simian sarcoma virus transforming gene product p28 and human platelet-derived growth factor (PDGF). Post-translational processing of the transforming gene produces an 11,000 and 20,000 molecular weight polypeptide. The 20,000-kd polypeptide is similar to an 18,000 molecular weight human PDGF. Antisera to human PDGF recognize the viral transforming polypeptide.

In other transforming viral systems, Ito et al.[40] raised antibodies to an amino acid sequence in the polyoma virus middle T antigen. The sequence is thought to be important in transformation. The antiserum binds to a cellular protein of 130,000 from mouse and rat cells and middle T antigen. By immunofluorescence, this antibody stains uninfected mouse, rat, human, and chicken cell microfilaments. The staining pattern and distribution of antibody binding are similar to those observed with antiactin antibodies.

Viruses are reported to share homologous region to class II molecules. The adenovirus glycoprotein (19,000 molecular weight) is encoded by the E3 region of the virus genome. This protein is expressed on the cell membrane and presumably binds to HLA class I antigen. Chatterjee and Maizel[41] found by structural analysis that the viral glycoprotein resembles the HLA class II antigen in domain structure and amino acid sequence. The alpha chain of the class II antigen domain and intramembrane region is most similar to that of the adenovirus protein. This region has similar regions in common with several HLA proteins and microglobulin. Recently, Fujinami et al.[42] used computer analysis to find a sequence homology and immunologic studies to determine a cross-reactive site between human cytomegalovirus and the HLA-DR beta chain. The sequence homology is encoded by the IE-2 region of human cytomegalovirus.[43] and a conserved domain of HLA-DR. The shared region has similar hydrophilicity and predicted beta turn potential. Antiserum to the viral peptide binds to the HLA beta chain, and this binding is inhibited by the peptide. Reactivity to human cytomegalovirus infection could contribute to graft rejection after transplantation,[44,45] immunosuppression, or both observed in infected individuals.

Recently, Nemerow et al.[46] found sequence homology between the gp350 of the Epstein-Barr virus, and a fragment of C3d complement. Two regions of homology were noted. This finding predicts that a common region on these two unrelated proteins may be involved in Epstein-Barr virus binding to the CR2 receptor on human B cells.

Similarly, many investigators[30,47-49] have looked for homologies between central nervous system proteins and microorganisms. All have suggested that immunologic cross-reactions between virus and myelin could be involved in the pathogenesis of postinfectious encephalopathies or multiple sclerosis. In addition, Lentz et al.[50] found comparable regions in the sequence of rabies glycoprotein and that of snake venom curaremimetic neurotoxins. These neurotoxins are potent ligands of the acetylcholine receptor. The greatest similarity occurred with residues important in neurotoxicity, including those interacting with the acetylcholine binding site of the acetylcholine receptor. This region of the viral glycoprotein may function as a recognition site for the acetylcholine receptor. Direct binding of the rabies virus glycoprotein to the acetylcholine receptor could contribute to the neurotropism of this virus.

Initial infection by a virus leads to an antiviral immune response. A cross-reacting immune response could lead to injury through cytotoxic cells or antibody. This antibody would bind to the common site, activate the complement cascade, and cell damage would ensue. Disease could also occur through the deposition of immune complexes.

## ACKNOWLEDGMENTS

I thank Diana Ferris for her excellent help in manuscript preparation.

### REFERENCES

1. AJDUKIEWICZ, A. B., F. J. DUDLEY, R. A. FOX, D. DONIACH & S. SHERLOCK. 1972. Immunological studies in an epidemic of infective, short incubation hepatitis. Lancet. **1**: 803-806.
2. TOH, H., A. YILDIE, J. SOTELO, O. OSUNG, E. J. HOLBOROW, F. KANAKOUDI & J. V. SMALL. 1979. Viral infectious and IgM autoantibodies to cytoplasmic intermediate filaments. Clin. Exp. Immunol. **37**: 76-82.
3. HOLBOROW, E. J., E. H. HEMSTED & S. V. MEAD. 1973. Smooth muscle autoantibodies in infectious mononucleosis. Br. Med. J. **3**: 323-325.
4. LINDER, E., P. KURKI & L. C. ANDERSSON. 1979. Autoantibodies to "intermediate filaments" in infectious mononucleosis. Clin. Immunol. Immunopathol. **14**: 411-417.
5. WHITEHOUSE, J. M. A., N. FERGUSON & G. A. CURRIE. 1974. Autoantibody to microtubules in infectious mononucleosis. Clin. Exp. Immunol. **17**: 227-235.
6. SUTTON, R. N. P., R. T. D. EDMOND, D. B. THOMAS & D. DONIACH. 1974. The occurrence of autoantibodies in infectious mononucleosis. Clin. Exp. Immunol. **17**: 427-436.
7. ANDERSON, P. & V. FABER. 1978. Antibodies to smooth muscle and other tissue components in infectious mononucleosis. Scand. J. Infect. Dis. **20**: 1-5.
8. SOTELO, J., C. J. GIBBS & D. C. GAJDUSEK. 1979. Autoantibodies against axonal neurofilaments in patients with kuru and Creutzfeldt-Jakob disease. Science **210**: 190-193.
9. STECK, A. J., R. TSCHANNEN & R. SCHAEFER. 1981. Induction of antimyelin and antioligodendrocyte antibodies by vaccinia virus. An experimental study in the mouse. J. Neuroimmunol. **1**: 117-124.
10. DALES, S., R. S. FUJINAMI & M. B. A. OLDSTONE. 1983. Infection with vaccinia favors the selection of hybridomas synthesizing autoantibodies against intermediate filaments, one of them cross-reacting with the virus hemagglutinin. J. Immunol. **131**: 1546-1553.
11. WEBB, H. E., S. MEHTA, N. A. GREGSON & S. LEIBOWITZ. 1984. Immunological reaction of the demyelinating semiliki forest virus with immune serum to glycolipids and its possible importance to central nervous system viral auto-immune disease. Neuropathol. Appl. Neurobiol. **10**: 77-84.
12. WEBB, H. E. & J. K. FAZAKERLEY. 1984. Can viral envelope glycolipids produce autoimmunity, with reference to the CNS and multiple sclerosis. Neuropathol. Appl. Neurobiol. **10**: 1-10.
13. HUBER, S. A. & P. A. LODGE. 1984. Coxsackievirus B-3 myocarditis in BALB/c mice: Evidence for autoimmunity to myocyte antigens. Am. J. Pathol. **116**: 21-29.
14. HUBER, S. A., D. C. LYNDEN & P. A. LODGE. 1985. Immunopathogenesis of experimental coxsackie virus induced myocarditis: Role of autoimmunity. Herz **10**: 1-7.
15. WOLFGRAM, L. J., K. W. BEISEL & N. R. ROSE. 1985. Heart-specific autoantibodies following murine coxsackie-virus B-3 myocarditis J. Exp. Med. **161**: 1112-1121.
16. KLOSTER, B. E., R. H. TOMAR & T. J. SPIRA. 1984. Lymphocytotoxic antibodies in the acquired immune deficiency syndrome (AIDS). Clin. Immunol. Immunopathol. **30**: 330-335.
17. DORSETT, B., W. CRONIN, J. CHUMA & H. L. IOACHIM. 1985. Anti-lymphocyte antibodies in patients with the acquired immune deficiency syndrome. Am. J. Med. **78**: 621-626.
18. LANE, D. P. & W. K. HOEFFLER. 1980. SV40 large T shares an antigenic determinant with a cellular protein of molecular weight 68,000. Nature **288**: 167-170.

19. HARLOW, E., L. V. CRAWFORD, D. C. PIM & N. M. WILLIAMSON. 1981. Monoclonal antibodies specific for the SV40 tumor antigens. J. Virol. **39**: 861-869.
20. CRAWFORD, L., K. LEPPARD, D. LANE & E. HARLOW. 1982. Cellular proteins reactive with monoclonal antibodies directed against simian virus 40 T-antigen. J. Virol. **42**: 612-620.
21. FUJINAMI, R. S., M. B. A. OLDSTONE, Z. WROBLEWSKA, M. E. FRANKEL & H. KOPROWSKI. 1983. Molecular mimicry in virus infection: Cross reaction of measles virus phosphoprotein or of herpes simplex virus protein with human intermediate filaments. Proc. Natl. Acad. Sci. USA **80**: 2346-2350.
22. SRINIVASAPPA, J., J. SAEGUSA, B. S. PRABHAKAR, M. K. GENTRY, M. J. BUCHMEIER, T. J. WIKTOR, H. KOPROWSKI, M. B. A. OLDSTONE & A. L. NOTKINS. 1986. Molecular mimicry: Frequency of reactivity of monoclonal antiviral antibodies with normal tissues. J. Virol. **57**: 397-401.
23. CASJENS, S., ED. 1985. Virus Structure and Assembly. Jones and Bartlett Publish., Inc., Boston.
24. SHESHBERADARAN, H. & E. NORRBY. 1984. Three monoclonal antibodies against measles virus F protein cross-react with cellular stress proteins. J. Virol. **52**: 995-999.
25. GOSWAMI, K. K. A., R. J. MORRIS, S. C. RASTOGI, L. S. LANGE & W. C. RUSSELL. 1985. A neutralizing monoclonal antibody against a paramyxovirus reacts with a brain antigen. J. Neuroimmunol. **9**: 99-108.
26. HAYNES, B. F., M. ROBERT-GUROFF, R. S. METZGAR, G. FRANCHINI, V. S. KALYANARAMAN, T. J. PALKER & R. C. GALLO. 1983. Monoclonal antibody against human T cell leukemia virus p19 defines a human thymic epithelial antigen acquired during ontogeny. J. Exp. Med. **157**: 907-920.
27. SARIN, P. S., D. K. SUN, A. H. THORNTON, P. H. NAYLOR & A. L. GOLDSTEIN. 1986. Neutralization of HTLV-III/LAV replication by antiserum to thymosin a. Science **232**: 1135-1137.
28. TAX, A., D. EWERT & L. A. MANSON. 1983. An antigen cross-reactive with gp52 of mammary tumor virus is expressed on a B cell subpopulation of mice. J. Immunol. **130**: 2368-2371.
29. FUJINAMI, R. S., A. ZURBRIGGEN & H. C. POWELL. 1987. Monoclonal antibody defines determinant between Theiler's virus and galactocerebroside. J. Neuroimmunol., in press.
30. TARDIEU, M., M. L. POWERS, D. A. HAFLER, S. L. HAUSER & H. L. WEINER. 1984. Autoimmunity following viral infection: Demonstration of monoclonal antibodies against normal tissue following infection of mice with reovirus and demonstration of shared antigenicity between virus and lymphocytes. Eur. J. Immunol. **14**: 561-565.
31. FUJINAMI, R. S. & M. B. A. OLDSTONE. 1985. Amino acid homology between the encephalitogenic site of myelin basic protein and virus: Mechanism for autoimmunity. Science **230**: 1043-1045.
32. DYRBERG, T. & M. B. A. OLDSTONE. 1986. Peptides as probes to study molecular mimicry and virus-induced autoimmunity. Current Topics Microbiol. & Immunol. **30**: 25-37.
33. KAGNOFF, M. F., R. K. AUSTIN, J. J. HUBERT, J. E. BERNARDIN & D. D. KASARDA. 1984. Possible role for a human adenovirus in the pathogenesis of celiac disease. J. Exp. Med. **160**: 1544-1557.
34. CLARKE, M. F., E. P. GELMANN & M. S. REITZ, JR. 1983. Homology of human T-cell leukaemia virus envelope gene with class I HLA gene. Nature **305**: 60-62.
35. REITHER, W. E., J. E. BLALOCK & T. K. BRUNCK. 1986. Sequence homology between acquired immunodeficiency syndrome virus envelope protein and interleukin 2. Proc. Natl. Acad. Sci. USA **83**: 9188-9192.
36. WEIGENT, D. A., P. D. HOEPRICH, K. L. BOST, T. K. BRUNCK, W. E. REIHER & J. E. BLALOCK. 1986. The HTLV-III envelope protein contains a hexapeptide homologous to a region of interleukin-2 that binds to the interleukin-2 receptor. Biochem. & Biophys. Res. Comm. **139**: 367-374.
37. WONG, T. W. & A. R. GOLDBERG. 1981. Synthetic peptide fragment of src gene product inhibits the src protein kinase and cross reacts immunologically with avian orc kinases and cellular phosphoproteins. Proc. Natl. Acad. Sci. USA **78**: 7412-7416.
38. MATHEY-PREVOT, B., H. HANAFUSA & S. KAWAI. 1982. A cellular protein is immuno-

logically crossreactive with and functionally homologous to the Fujinami sarcoma virus transforming protein. Cell **28**: 897-906.
39. ROBBINS, K. C., H. N. ANTONIADES, S. G. DEVARE, M. W. HUNKAPILLER & S. A. AARONSON. 1983. Structural and immunological similarities between simian sarcoma virus gene product(s) and human platelet-derived growth factor. Nature **305**: 605-608.
40. ITO, Y., Y. HAMAGISHI, K. SEGAWA, T. DALIANIS, E. APPELLA & M. WILLINGHAM. 1983. Antibodies against a nonapeptide of polyomavirus middle T antigen: Cross-reaction with a cellular protein(s). J. Virol. **48**: 709-720.
41. CHATTERJEE, D. & J. V. MAIZEL. 1984. Homology of adenoviral E3 glycoprotein with HLA-DR heavy chain. Proc. Natl. Acad. Sci. USA **81**: 6039-6043.
42. FUJINAMI, R. S., J. A. NELSON, L. WALKER & M. B. A. OLDSTONE. 1987. Sequence homology and immunologic cross reactivity of human cytomegalovirus with HLA-DR b chain: A means for graft rejection and immunosuppression. J. Virol. **62**: 100-105.
43. STENBERG, R. M., P. R. WITTE & M. F. STINSKI. 1985. Multiple spliced and unspliced transcripts from human cytomegalovirus immediate-early region 2 and evidence for a common initiation site within immediate-early region 1. J. Virol. **56**: 665-675.
44. VAN ES, A., W. M. BALDWIN, P. J. OLJANS, H. J. TANKE, J. S. PLOEM & L. A. VAN ES. 1984. Expression of HLA-DR on T lymphocytes following renal transplantation, and association with graft-rejection episodes and cytomegalovirus infection. Transplantation **37**: 65-69.
45. VON WILLEBRAND, E., E. PETTERSSON, J. AHONEN & P. HAYRY. 1986. CMV infection, class II antigen expression, and human kidney allograft rejection. Transplantation **42**: 364-367.
46. NEMEROW, G. R., C. MOLD, V. K. SCHWEND, V. TOLLEFSON & N. R. COOPER. 1987. Identification of gp350 as the viral glycoprotein mediating attachment of Epstein-Barr virus (EBV) to the EBV/C3d receptor of B cells: Sequence homology of gp350 and C3 complement fragment C3d. J. Virol. **61**: 1416-1420.
47. JAHNKE, U., E. H. FISCHER & E. C. ALVORD, JR. 1985. Sequence homology between certain viral proteins and encephalitogenic and neuritogenic proteins. Science **229**: 282-284.
48. SHAW, S,-Y., R. A. LAURSEN & M. B. LEES. 1986. Analogous amino acid sequences in myelin proteolipid and viral proteins. Febs. Lett. **207**: 266-270.
49. AW, S. E. 1986. Autoimmune disease-pathogenesis through molecular mimicry at the tripeptide level. Ann. Acad. Med. **15**: 546-554.
50. LENTZ, T. L., P. T. WILSON, E. HAWROT & D. W. SPEICHER. 1984. Amino acid sequence similarity between rabies virus glycoprotein and snake venom curaremimetic neurotoxins. Science **226**: 847-848

# Immunobiology of Microglial Cells[a]

KARL FREI, CHRISTINE SIEPL, PETER
GROSCURTH, STEFAN BODMER, AND
ADRIANO FONTANA

*Section of Clinical Immunology and Department of Neurosurgery
University Hospital
Zurich, Switzerland*

Major histocompatibility complex (MHC) class II (Ia) antigens are involved in recognition of antigen by T cells on antigen-presenting cells (APCs). Ia antigens have been found on macrophages, dendritic cells, Kupffer cells, thymic epithelial-reticular cells, and B cells. They have also been detected on certain murine tissue cells with no apparent immune functions, such as normal gut epithelium and mammary gland epithelium during lactation. However, in the brain, Ia expression is confined to some macrophage-like cells in the meninges, especially those around blood vessels, but the brain parenchyma inside of the limiting membrane is free of Ia-positive cells.[1,2] The complete absence of Ia-positive dendritic cells in rat brain tissue is striking as such cells have readily been identified in every other interstitial connective tissue examined (heart, liver, thyroid, pancreas, skin, kidney, ureter, and bladder).[3] In human brain tissue sections, only 1-2% of the cells were shown to express MHC class II antigens.[4]

The absence or only low numbers of Ia-positive cells in brain tissue reflect a severe limit to the expression of immune functions within the central nervous system (CNS). Conversely, damage to the brain tissue occurring in some forms of encephalitis, such as postmeasles encephalitis or multiple sclerosis, is due to an immune-mediated response, which may involve both anti-brain tissue antibodies and activated T cells infiltrating the brain parenchyma through the blood-brain barrier. Once in the brain tissue the future of the intruding T cells may depend on (1) the presence of antigen sensitized towards the T cells, (2) the capacity of the T cells to release gamma interferon (IFN-γ) and (3) the amount of MHC class I and II antigens induced by IFN-γ on APCs within the tissue. (For a review, see reference 5.) As it was shown that viruses can convert Ia-negative APC to Ia-positive cells by IFN-γ independent mechanisms,[6] the capacity of infiltrating T cells to release IFN-γ may not be critical.

Recent observations on astrocytes as APCs provide a new approach towards understanding the pathogenesis of immune-mediated encephalitis. On treatment with IFN-γ, astrocytes were induced to express Ia antigen, to serve as APCs, to release interleukin-3(IL-3)-like factors and interleukin-1, the latter being required for the production of interleukin-2 (IL-2), and to express IL-2 receptors by T cells. (For a review, see reference 5.) Studies of both experimental encephalitis and multiple sclerosis showed Ia-positive astrocytes at the lesion site. Besides astrocytes, the tissue macrophages of the brain, that is, the microglial cells, may also serve as immunoregulatory cells. In general, the highly important role of macrophages as effector cells in cellular

---

[a]This work was supported by grants from the Swiss National Science Foundation (Project No. 3.930-0.87) and the National Multiple Sclerosis Society.

immune reactions has been acknowledged for several years since the observation was made that mononuclear cells with phagocytic properties were essential for resistance to intracellular pathogens. More recently, macrophages were found to be required for antigen-specific activation of T lymphocytes, leading to secretion of various lymphokines and subsequent expansion of T-cell clones. However, macrophages can also reduce the function of lymphocytes, this down-regulatory activity being derived from the release of suppressive molecules, principally prostaglandins of the E series (PGE) and oxygen-reactive species such as superoxide anion and $H_2O_2$.

In the following sections, we will summarize data with respect to functional properties of microglial cells.

## MICROGLIAL CELLS: HISTORICAL PERSPECTIVE AND DEVELOPMENTAL ASPECTS

In 1932, using the silver-carbonate impregnation method Del Rio-Hortega identified microglial cells in the normal brain parenchyma.[7] These cells, now termed resting microglial, were proposed to be mesodermal cells and thought to transform into ameboid microglia, rod cells, or macrophages under degenerative or inflammatory conditions.[7] In such circumstances the cells were termed "activated microglia." However, it was argued that microglia are derived from blood monocytes derived from monocytes infiltrating the brain tissue during the perinatal period.[8-11] Indeed, ameboid microglial cells appear in the CNS during late stages of embryogenesis.[12] The presence of large numbers of such cells in the developing corpus callosum at sites showing a massive loss of axons[13] is consistent with the notion that degenerating cells may act as a stimulus for invasion of the developing CNS by blood-derived mononuclear cells. The ameboid cells disappear by the late postnatal period, but they can be seen in the adult brain in tissue injury.[9,10,11,14,15] Morphologically, the ameboid microglial cells can be distinguished from the resting or "quiescent" microglia, the so-called ramified cell type that has cell processes and lacks hydrolytic enzymes as well as the capacity to engulf particles.[11] Experimental evidence indicates that ameboid cells are transformed into ramified cells during postnatal development.[9,10] Several attempts have been made to demonstrate hematogenously derived cells in the normal and injured brain by immunohistochemical localization using either antisera raised against macrophages or, more recently, antibodies against defined macrophage antigens such as the F4/80 antigen or monoclonal anti-Fc and complement receptor antibodies (description follows). These studies provide further support for the monocytic origin of microglia.

## IMMUNOHISTOCHEMICAL LOCALIZATION OF MICROGLIA IN NORMAL AND PATHOLOGIC CONDITIONS

With the silver-carbonate method, the perikaryon of the resting microglia appears pleomorphic, elongated, or triangular. The cells, which have a round or oval nucleus, possess abundant, thin branches of cytoplasm and contain a few primary lysosomes and varying numbers of secondary lysosomes. The activity of lysosomal and oxireductive enzymes is very low.[16] As judged from light microscopic studies, microglial cells are ubiquitously distributed in the brain, but they represent only a small percentage of the total cell population (<1%). The cells are predominantly localized at perineuronal, perivascular, and interfascicular sites with some variations in their size and shape according to different brain regions. (For a review, see reference 8.) For example, in the cerebral cortex, thalamus, or nuclei of the brain stem, slender processes of the microglial cells radiate in all directions to neurons that are dispersed through the tissue, the pyramidal cell layer of the hippocampus with a more close arrangement of neurons. The interspersed microglial cells have a few polar processes which in some places may reach the surface. Quantitative differences have also been ascertained in a few studies: white matter contains less than gray matter, only low numbers are detectable in the spinal cord of mice, and in the rat optic nerve the figures vary between none and 4-5% of the neuroglial cell population.

Under pathologic conditions, cells with processes and cytoplasmic phagocytosed material accumulate at the lesion site. The cytoplasm is rich in organelles and contains many lysosomes. Histochemically, the cells are positive for nonspecific esterase, acid phosphatase, and peroxidase.[16] Although mitosis or incorporation of $^3$H-thymidine is only rarely seen in resting microglia of undamaged brain, many labeled cells can be identified in inflammatory or degenerative lesions.[8] However, the contribution of dividing resident microglia within the proliferating pool—consisting mainly of macrophages that had invaded the lesion site—is difficult to ascertain. Interestingly, mitotic microglial cells were identified in hypoglossal or facialis nuclei after peripheral hypoglossal or facialis axotomy.[17,18]

With monoclonal antibodies used against Mac-1, the type-3 complement receptor, Mac-1 positive cells were identified in normal adult mouse brain tissue.[19] In the developing CNS, with or without cold lesioning, no Mac-1 staining was detectable.[19] Using Mac-1 antibodies, an antibody recognizing the trypsin-resistant IgG1/IgG2b mouse-Fc receptor as well as a monoclonal antimacrophage antibody (F4/80), two types of F4/80-positive cells became detectable: cells associated with the leptomeninges, the choroid plexus, and the ventricles and the microglia located intraparenchymally.[12] Cells expressing Fc and complement receptors were indistinguishable by their morphology and distribution from those revealed by F4/80 and from classical microglial cells identified by the silver carbonate method.[12] When the effect of injury to the optic nerve within 5 days after having crushed the nerve was investigated, the number of F4/80-positive cells distant to the lesion remained unchanged. By 10 days, the number of F4/80-positive microglial cells had increased slightly.[20]

## MICROGLIAL CELLS IN CULTURE

### Characterization of Isolated Microglial Cells

In 1932, Del Rio-Hortega[7] was the first to recognize microglia as a distinct population of cells within the CNS. His observation was based on light microscopic observations and special silver stains. Aside from morphologic studies, the investigation of microglial biology has been limited because of the lack of appropriate isolation and culture procedures. To investigate the functional properties of microglial cells, we developed methods to obtain highly enriched long-term cultures of such cells.[21] Raff et al.[22] observed phagocytic macrophage-like cells growing on monolayer cultures established from dissociated rat brain. Using a shaking and adhesion procedure, we were able to isolate these macrophage-like cells from brain cell cultures. In investigations of 2-week-old cultures of mouse brain-derived macrophage-like cells, the cells were found to contain nonspecific esterase activity to express the macrophage surface antigen Mac-1 (type three complement receptor) as well as Fc receptors for IgG1/2b. On immunofluorescent staining the cells were negative for glial fibrillary acidic protein and galactocerebroside, established markers for astrocytes and oligodendrocytes, respectively. Furthermore, the cells engulfed 1.1 μm latex beads within 4 hours at 37°C.

Typical microglial cell cultures are shown in FIGURE 1. Both ameboid and ramified microglial cells can be identified. Elongated cells that display at their ends long filipods

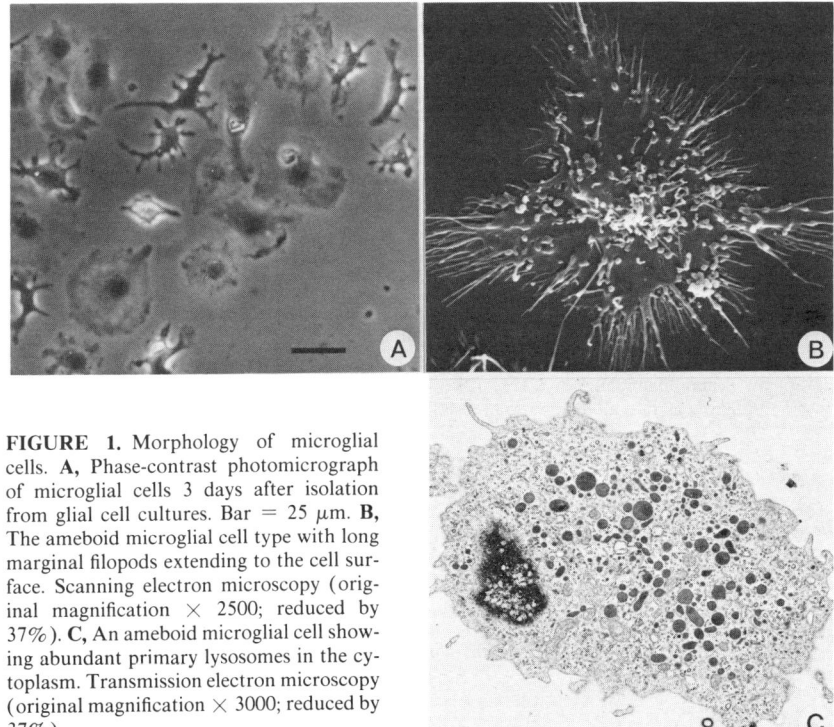

FIGURE 1. Morphology of microglial cells. **A,** Phase-contrast photomicrograph of microglial cells 3 days after isolation from glial cell cultures. Bar = 25 μm. **B,** The ameboid microglial cell type with long marginal filopods extending to the cell surface. Scanning electron microscopy (original magnification × 2500; reduced by 37%). **C,** An ameboid microglial cell showing abundant primary lysosomes in the cytoplasm. Transmission electron microscopy (original magnification × 3000; reduced by 37%).

that extend to the cell surface can be seen in FIGURE 1B. The ramified microglia, characterized by long cytoplasmic processes, were only found occasionally. Transmission electron microscopic studies revealed similar morphology in characteristics of the different microglial cells detected by scanning electron microscopy. They displayed a round-shaped nucleolus rich in euchromatin with a distinct excentrally located nucleus. The cytoplasm contained a few oval-shaped mitochondria of crista type, short profiles of rough endoplasmic reticulum (rER), and a few polyribosomes. The most striking features of the cells were the abundant primary lysosomes scattered throughout the cytoplasm and the large golgi complex (FIG. 1C).

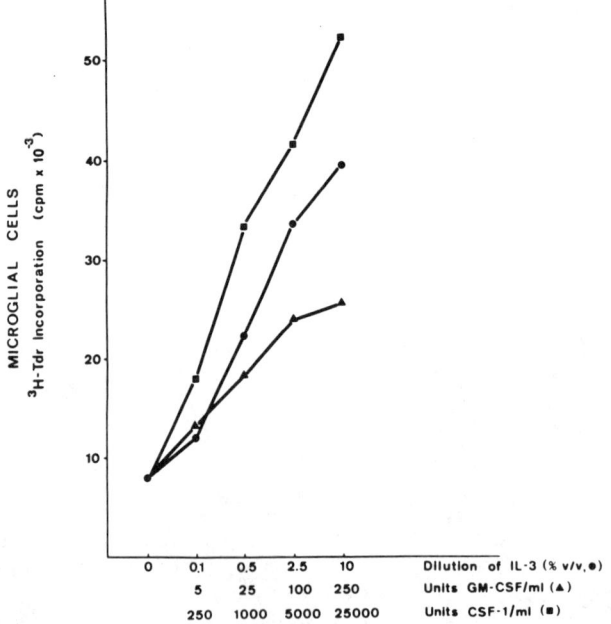

**FIGURE 2.** Stimulation of microglial cells by colony-stimulating factor 1 (CSF-1), granulocyte-macrophage colony-stimulating factor (GM-CSF), and astrocyte-derived interleukin-3 (IL-3). Microglial cells ($1 \times 10^5$ per well) were cultured for 3 days in the presence of astrocyte-derived IL-3 (●), recombinant human CSF-1 (■), and recombinant murine GM-CSF (▲). $^3$H-thymidine uptake was measured for the final 20 hours of incubation.

## Growth Conditions of Microglial Cells

In recent studies using co-cultures of astrocytes and microglial cells, growth conditions of the microglial cells were found to depend on activation of the astrocytes by lipopolysaccharide (LPS), which by their release of an IL-3-like factor,[23] promoted growth of microglial cells.[21] The astrocyte-derived IL-3 induced proliferation of microglial cells in a dose-dependent manner (FIG. 2). Production of this IL-3-like factor by astrocytes *in vivo* may account for the expansion of both resident microglial cells and monocytes having invaded the brain parenchyma in inflammatory lesions. Besides IL-3, colony-stimulating factor 1 (CSF-1) and the granulocyte-macrophage colony-stimulating factor (GM-CSF), two well-known growth factors for macrophages,[24] also caused a pronounced increase in $^3$H-thymidine uptake by microglial cells (FIG. 2). The growth-promoting activity of CSF-1, IL-3, and GM-CSF on microglial cells indicates their relation to the macrophage lineage.

## Functional Properties of Microglial Cells

As described in detail previously,[25] microglial cells were investigated for two macrophage functions thought to be important *in vivo:* antigen presentation and tumor cytotoxicity. Responses of Ia-restricted T lymphocytes to mitogens and antigens depend on accessory cells that have generally been considered to be Ia-positive macrophages and dendritic cells. Whereas untreated microglial cells were found to be Ia negative, treatment with IFN-γ (50 U/ml) for 3 days resulted in the expression of class II (Ia) antigens, as shown by cell radioimmunoassay (FIG. 3). In contrast, class I (H-2) antigens were expressed without IFN-γ treatment. These data agree with the recent report of Suzumura *et al.*,[26] showing both spontaneous expression of MHC class I antigen and induction of class II antigen on cultured microglial cells that were isolated by comparable methods used in our experiments. Furthermore, cultured astrocytes are reported to respond in the same way as shown here with microglial cells.[5] To test if microglial cells can serve as accessory cells in T-cell activation, ovalbumin-specific T cells (H-$2^b$) were added to cultures of either untreated or IFN-

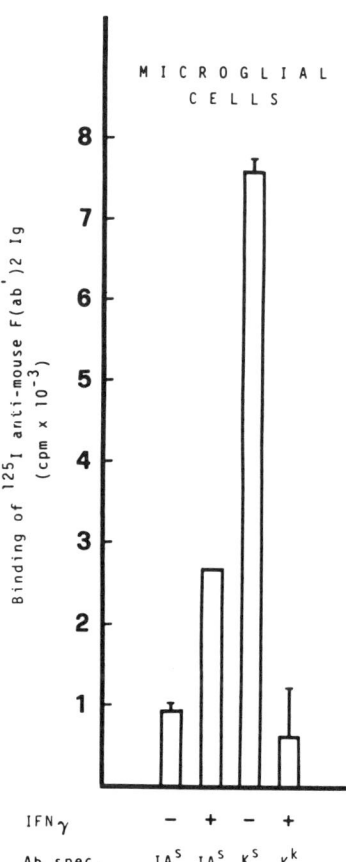

**FIGURE 3.** Induction of major histocompatibility complex (MHC) class II antigens (Ia) and constitutive expression of MHC class I antigens on microglial cells. The cells were seeded in 24-well Petra plates at a density of $5 \times 10^5$ cells per well and stimulated with IFN-γ (12 U/ml) for 72 hours, as described previously. Thereafter, a cell radioimmunoassay was performed in the culture wells using monoclonal anti I-A$^s$ (class II) or anti-H2K (class I) antibodies and 200 μl/well of a $^{125}$I-labeled anti-mouse immunoglobulin F(ab)$_2$ fragment (corresponding to $2 \times 10^5$ cpm). Thereafter, the monolayer was washed, the cells lysed with 5n NaOH, and counted in a gammacounter. Data represent the mean counts per minute (cpm) ± standard deviation of duplicate cultures.

TABLE 1. Antigen Presentation by Microglial Cells to Ovalbumin-Specific T Helper Cells[a]

| Stimulator:Responder Ratio | $^3$H-Thymidine Uptake (cpm ± SD) | |
|---|---|---|
| | − IFN-γ | + IFN-γ (50 U/ml) |
| 0.25:1 | 4,629 ± 296 | 6,383 ± 1,979 |
| 0.5:1 | 5,627 ± 511 | 16,223 ± 4,248 |
| 1:1 | 10,059 ± 3,035 | 61,813 ± 3,238 |
| 2:1 | 12,171 ± 1,798 | 51,275 ± 3,005 |

[a] In this experiment, irradiated microglial cells (H-2$^b$) were cultured at $5 \times 10^3$ to $5 \times 10^4$ cells per well in round-bottom 96-well microtiter plates with or without gamma interferon (IFN-γ). Three days later the medium was removed and both $2 \times 10^4$ Ova-7 T cells (H-2$^b$) and ovalbumin (100 μg/ml) were added. After 48 hours the co-cultures were pulsed with 1 μCi per well of $^3$H-thymidine (5 Ci/mmol) and harvested after an additional 16 hours.

γ pretreated microglial cells of the same H-2 haplotype. Whereas in the absence of microglial cells ovalbumin did not induce proliferation of the OVA-7 T cells, an antigen-dependent T-cell proliferation was noted in co-cultures of T cells and irradiated IFN-γ treated microglial cells (TABLE 1). The response was dependent on the number of microglial cells (stimulator cells), microglia-to-responder ratios of lower than 1 still resulting in T-cell proliferation (TABLE 1). The response was antigen specific and MHC restricted. Besides processing the antigens in the context of MHC class II antigens, the secretion of IL-1 is important in the intercellular communication between the APCs and the T cells. When treated with LPS for 48 hours, microglial cells secrete IL-1 as judged by the property of supernatants of activated microglia to augment the response of mouse thymocytes to phytohemagglutinin (PHA) (TABLE 2). These results confirm the previous findings by Giulian et al.[27] However, we do not agree with their findings that microglial cells are the main source of IL-1 produced intracerebrally. When comparing different species, such as rats and mice or different mice strains, the capacity of IL-1 production by microglial cells is higher or lower than the IL-1 production by astrocytes (TABLE 2).

Another function of activated macrophages is the lysis of tumor cells.[28] Therefore, we also investigated microglial cells for their tumoricidal capacity, using P-815 tumor

TABLE 2. Production of Interleukin-1 (IL-1) by Microglial Cells

| Species/Strain | IL-1 Activity (U/ml)[a] | |
|---|---|---|
| | Astrocytes | Microglial Cells |
| Rat/Holzman | 480 | 5,120 |
| Mice/C57BL/6 | 900 | 320 |
| Mice/SJL | 1,080 | 430 |

[a] Astrocytes and microglial cells were cultured at a cell density of $4 \times 10^5$ cells per well (12-well Linbro plates) in 0.5 ml of culture medium supplemented with lipopolysaccharide (10 μg/ml) and indomethacin (1 μg/ml). After 48 hours the cell supernatants were harvested and tested for IL-1 activity in the classical thymocyte assay.[39] One unit of IL-1 is defined as the amount of supernatant required to give a twofold stimulation of the phytohemagglutinin-induced thymocyte proliferation.

cells. Unstimulated microglial cells expressed no tumor cytotoxicity. However, activation with two signals, IFN-γ and LPS, cytotoxicity became detectable. An effector to target ratio of 0.5:1 resulted in 5.4% specific cytotoxicity and was increased several times to 63.3% at a ratio of 5:1. Interestingly, astrocytes could not be activated to become tumoricidal. In recent years, the killing of tumor cells has been achieved also by soluble factors such as TNF-α and lymphotoxin (TNF-β). Originally discovered in the sera of mice and rabbits injected with mycobacteria followed by endotoxin,[29]

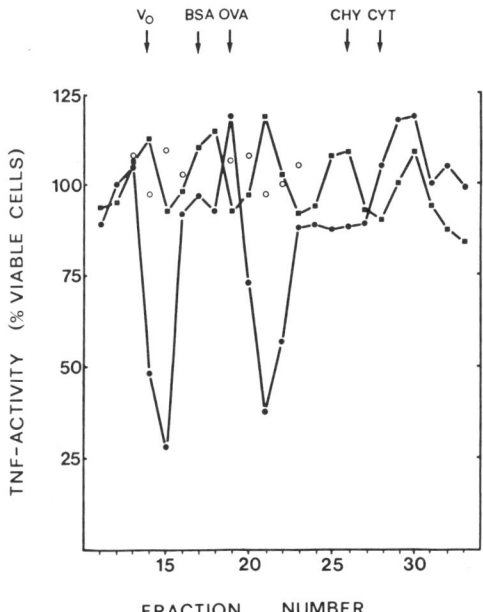

**FIGURE 4.** Secretion of TNF-α by activated microglial cells. Concentrated crude 48-hour supernatants of lipopolysaccharide (10 μg/ml)-treated microglial cells (●) or astrocytes (■) were fractionated on HPLC size exclusion columns. Fractions showing TNF activity were pooled and rechromatographed on an Ultrogel AcA54. Thereafter, fractions (3.8 ml) were assayed again at 1% (v/v) for their cytolytic activity on L-M cells according to described procedures.[25] Fractions of supernatants of microglial cells, obtained by chromatographic procedures, were tested for TNF activity, also in the presence of a polyclonal rabbit anti-murine TNF-α antiserum (○ = final dilution of 1:100). TNF activity was expressed as the percentage of viable cells relative to an untreated control and represents the mean values of triplicate L-M cell cultures ($5 \times 10^4$ cells/well). The AcA54 column was calibrated using the following markers: BSA = bovine serum albumin (67,000); OVA = ovalbumin (45,000). CHYM = chymotrypsinogen (25,000); CYT = cytochrome c (12,300); $V_o$ indicates the void volume.

TNF-α has been identified as a product of activated macrophages.[30] Microglial cells stimulated with LPS release a factor that exhibits cytotoxic activity when tested on murine L-M cells, a well-known target for both TNF-α and TNF-β.[31] To characterize the microglial cell-derived factor we purified concentrated supernatant of LPS-treated microglial cells by gel permeation chromatography. TNF activities were found in both a high molecular weight fraction ($M_r$ 150,000) and a low ($M_r$ 39,000), as in FIGURE 4. Analogous data were reported for murine TNF-α by Haranaka et al.[32] TNF activities of both fractions were completely neutralized by anti-TNF-α antiserum, which does not neutralize TNF-β (FIG. 4). In contrast, LPS-activated astrocytes produced no TNF activity (FIG. 4). Apart from its tumoricidal capacity, TNF produced intracerebrally may also be important in inflammatory processes, as TNF was shown to augment the expression[33] of MHC class I and class II antigens, to induce the release of IL-1[34] and colony-stimulating factors (GM-CSF[35] and G-CSF[36]), as well as to have chemotactic effects on mononuclear cells.[37]

## CONCLUSION

Although microglial cell development and function have been reviewed on several occasions over the years, it seemed pertinent to reevaluate this subject because new methods have been established to isolate and culture microglial cells. In view of the surface characteristics and functional properties of these cells, it is now apparent that microglial cells belong to the macrophage lineage. The cells grow in the presence of macrophage colony-stimulating factors, contain nonspecific esterase activity, express Fc (IgG 1/IgG 2b) and type 3 complement receptors, and mediate tumor cytotoxicity. Furthermore, on stimulation with IFN-γ microglial cells can serve as APCs for Ia-restricted T-cell activation, a property also being described for astrocytes. In regard to antigen presentation in the brain, we believe that the astrocytes play the primary role because: (1) astrocytes outnumber microglial cells by far in the adult brain and are therefore more immediately accessible for antigen presentation functions, and (2) *in vitro* studies demonstrate that the amount of Ia expressed on IFN-γ-treated astrocytes correlates with susceptibility to immune-mediated encephalitis *in vivo*.[38] However, by secreting proteases, TNF-α or IL-1 activated microglial cells may mediate tissue injury, by their release of IL-1 the cells may contribute to astrocytic gliosis, and finally by their phagocytic property the cells may be involved in removal of cell debris.

## REFERENCES

1. WONG, G. H. W., P. F. BARTLETT, I. CLARK-LEWIS, F. BATTYE & J. W. SCHRADER. 1985. Nature (London) **310**: 688-691.
2. FIERZ, W. & A. FONTANA. 1986. Cellular Neurobiology: Astrocytes: Cell Biology and Pathology of Astrocytes, Vol. 3. S. Fedoroff & A. Vernadakis, Eds.: 203-229. Academic Press, Inc., New York, N.Y.
3. HART, D. N. J. & J. W. FABRE. 1981. J. Exp. Med. **153**: 347-361.
4. HAUSER, ST. L., A. K. BHAN, F. H. GILLES, C. J. HOBAN, E. L. REINHERZ, ST. F. SCHLOSSMAN & H. L. WEINER. 1983. J. Neuroimmunol. **5**: 197-203.
5. FONTANA, A., K. FREI, S. BODMER & E. HOFER. 1987. Immunol. Rev. **100**: 185-201.
6. MASSA, P. T., R. DÖRRIES & V. TER MEULEN. 1986. Nature **320**: 543-546.
7. DEL RIO-HORTEGA, P. 1932. *In* Cytology and Cellular Pathology of the Nervous System, Vol. 2. W. Penfield, Ed.: 481-584. Paul P. Hocker, New York, N.Y.
8. CAMMERMEYER, J. 1970. *In* Neurosciences Research, Vol. 3 (S. Ehrenpreis & O. Solnitsky, Eds.: 43-129. Academic Press, New York, N. Y.
9. LING, E. A. 1981. *In* Advances in Cellular Neurobiology, Vol. 2. S. Fedoroff & L. Hertz, Eds.: 33-82. Academic Press, London.
10. MURABE, Y. & Y. SANO. 1982. Cell Tissue Res. **225**: 469-485.

11. OEHMICHEN, M. 1983. Prog. Neuropathol. **5**: 277-325.
12. PERRY, V. H., D. A. HUME & S. GORDON. 1985. Neuroscience **15**: 313-326.
13. VALENTINO, K. L. & E. G. JONES. 1981. Anat. Embryol. **163**: 157-172.
14. BOYA, J., J. CALVO & A. PRADO. 1979. J. Anat. **129**: 177-186.
15. BRIERLEY, J. B. & A. W. BROWN. 1982. J. Comp. Neurol. **211**: 397-406.
16. OEHMICHEN, M. 1982. Immunobiology **161**: 246-254.
17. KREUTZBERG, G. W. 1966. Acta Neuropathol. **7**: 149-161.
18. SUMNER, B. E. H. 1974. J. Neuropathol. Exp. Neurol. **33**: 507-519.
19. MATSUMOTO, Y., K. WATABE & F. IKUTA. 1985. J. Neuroimmunol. **9**: 379-389.
20. PERRY, V. H., M. C. BROWN & S. GORDON. 1987. J. Exp. Med. **165**: 1218-1223.
21. FREI, K., S. BODMER, C. SCHWERDEL & A. FONTANA. 1986. J. Immunol. **137**: 3521-3527.
22. RAFF, M. C., K. L. FIELDS, S. HAKOMORI, R. MIRSKY, R. M. PRUSS & J. WINTER. 1979. Brain Res. **174**: 283-308.
23. FREI, K., S. BODMER, C. SCHWERDEL & A. FONTANA. 1985. J. Immunol. **135**: 4044-4047.
24. METCALF, D. 1986. Blood **67**: 257-267.
25. FREI, K., C. SIEPL, P. GROSCURTH, S. BODMER, C. SCHWERDEL & A. FONTANA. 1987. Eur. J. Immunol. **17**: 1271-1278.
26. SUZUMURA, A., S. G. E. MEZITIS, N. K. GONATAS & D. H. SILBERBERG. 1987. J. Neuroimmunol. **15**: 263-278.
27. GIULIAN, D., T. J. BAKER, N. SHIH & L. B. LACHMANN. 1986. J. Exp. Med. **164**: 594-604.
28. KELLER, R., R. KEIST & P. GROSCURTH. 1986. Int. J. Cancer. **37**: 89-95.
29. CARSWELL, E. A., L. J. OLD, R. L. KASSEL, S. GREEN, N. FIORE & B. WILLIAMSON. 1975. Proc. Natl. Acad. Sci. USA **72**: 3666-3670.
30. RUFF, M. & G. E. GIFFORD. 1981. Lymphokines **2**: 235-272.
31. KRAMER, S. M., M. E. CARVER & S. M. APPERSON. 1986. Lymphokine Res. **5**: 9139-9143.
32. HARANAKA, K., E. A. CARSWELL, B. D. WILLIAMSON, J. S. PRENDERGAST, N. SATOMI & L. J. OLD. 1986. Proc. Natl. Acad. Sci. USA **83**: 3949-3953.
33. PFIZENMAIER, K., P. SCHEURICH, C. SCHLÜTER & M. KRÖNKE. 1987. J. Immunol. **138**: 975-980.
34. NAWROTH, P. P., I. BANK, D. HANDLEY, J. CASSIMERIS, L. CHESS & D. STERN. 1986. J. Exp. Med. **163**: 1363-1371.
35. MUNKER, R., J. GASSON, M. OGAWA & H. P. KOEFFLER. 1986. Nature **323**: 79-82.
36. KOEFFLER, H. P., J. GASSON, J. RANYARD, L. SOUZA, M. SHEPARD & R. MUNKER. 1987. Blood **70**: 55-59.
37. MING, W. J., L. BERSANI & A. MANTOVANI. 1987. J. Immunol **138**: 1469-1474.
38. MASSA, P. T., V. TER MEULEN & A. FONTANA. 1987. Proc. Natl. Acad. Sci. USA **84**: 4219-4223.
39. FONTANA, A., F. KRISTENSEN, R. DUBS, D. GEMSA & E. WEBER. 1982. J. Immunol. **129**: 2413-2419.

# Cell-Mediated Immunity in Virus Infections of the Central Nervous System

PETER C. DOHERTY

*Department of Experimental Pathology*
*The John Curtin School of Medical Research*
*Canberra, Australia*

Virus infections of the central nervous system (CNS) are generally a consequence of systemic exposure, being preceded by replication in other sites throughout the body and thus sensitization of the immune system. The obvious exception is a virus such as the rabies virus, which may progress to the brain by retrograde flow along neuronal processes and consequently avoid immunologic surveillance. The peculiar features of virus-specific cell-mediated immunity (CMI) in the CNS are thus largely a function of the nature of the target organ. The existence of tight endothelial junctions and intimately associated astrocyte processes, the lack (though this is debated) of conventional lymphatic drainage, the low levels of expression of major histocompatibility complex (MHC) glycoproteins,[1] and the complex physiologic and anatomic interactions that are required for normal function all contribute to particular difficulties in the effective operation of host response and lead to unique aspects of pathologic damage.

There can be no doubt, given (for instance) the continuing debate concerning the possible role of viruses in triggering multiple sclerosis (MS)[2-4] and the existence of the somewhat enigmatic dementia associated with human immunodeficiency virus (HIV) infection,[5] that developing a better understanding of the cellular immune response and inflammation in virus infections of the CNS is a priority. The consequences of lymphocyte invasion, the pathologic changes induced by secondarily recruited monocytes and macrophages, and so forth must be addressed using the best available technology. This brief review does not attempt to cover all the relevant literature, but aims simply to highlight some areas of contemporary interest.

## NATURE OF T-CELL RECOGNITION

The basic principle of CMI is that effector T lymphocytes are targeted onto the surface of cells expressing an abnormal phenotype defined by modification of class I or class II MHC glycoproteins,[6,7] the phenomenon known as MHC restriction.[8] Class I MHC-restricted T cells are CD8+, and those that recognize class II molecules are CD4+.[9,10] There is increasing evidence that the CD8 and CD4 molecules play an accessory role in binding together the T cell and target, or stimulator, cell.[11-14] The rules governing the coordinate expression of CD4 or CD8 and the particular T-cell receptor ($TC_r$) genes are not yet understood.

The fact of MHC restriction reflects that the T-cell repertoire is in some way constrained to see variants of self MHC molecules as a consequence of events occurring during thymocyte ontogeny.[15] The role of the thymus in determining self tolerance, on the one hand, and the capacity to mount an immune response, on the other, is currently a subject of intense experimentation by molecular and cellular immunologists.[16-18] This work has been greatly facilitated by the identification of the $TC_r$ genes and by the realization that there are distinct families of these genes. In general, however, it is not yet clear if a particular spectrum of $TC_r$ gene expression is associated with restriction of T-cell effector function to one or another MHC molecule or if the $TC_r$ repertoire is essentially random and depends simply on binding affinities. There are experiments to support both viewpoints.[19-22] It is possible that the MHC-restricted $TC_r$ may have a low affinity for the relevant, unmodified MHC glycoprotein, while being able to bind strongly to one or another allogeneic MHC molecule.[23,24] What is apparent is that the $TC_r$ repertoire is not derived by somatic mutation following a high affinity binding event in the thymus[25,26] along the lines originally suggested by Jerne.[27]

The current paradigm accepted by most investigators is that the two chains of the T-cell receptor combine to form a single, immunoglobulin-like binding site that recognizes a modified MHC molecule.[26-28] Whether an individual T-cell clone is restricted to class I or class II MHC phenotype seems to depend on interactions involving CD8 or CD4 both during ontogeny and in the context of the primary immune response.[10-14] The nature of the entity recognized by the $TC_r$ is now becoming much clearer.[28-30]

Both class I and class II MHC-restricted T cells are apparently recognizing MHC glycoproteins that have been modified by the binding of foreign peptides.[28-30] Whether or not a viral molecule is expressed in an intact form on cell surface may thus be largely irrelevant in CMI; the fact is that the T-cell response to many viruses seems to be directed mainly at essentially "internal" components, such as the matrix and nucleoprotein in influenza.[31,32] The key event is therefore whether a particular viral peptide can bind with sufficient affinity to the relevant MHC glycoprotein. This presumably reflects that viral proteins are being degraded at sites where they encounter MHC molecules. The main characteristic of class II MHC association, which is a function of the less frequent class II MHC-positive cells that tend to have well-recognized antigen-processing functions, may be that such events occur in specialized organelles such as lysosomes. Class I MHC expression is associated with many more cell types, including fibroblasts and tumor cells, and may reflect more generalized degradative processes that are occurring in the cytoplasm. Questions concerning the nature of antigen processing and the recirculation of MHC molecules from the plasma membrane[33,34] are now of great interest. The system must operate in such a way that it does not become saturated with "self" peptides derived from, for instance, "minor" histocompatibility antigens.[35]

The current paradigm concerning the interaction between the peptide and the MHC glycoprotein is, for instance, that the class II molecule has a single peptide binding site of broad specificity[28] which may involve as few as four residues of the peptide. Analysis with a 14-residue peptide of ovalbumin and the class II molecule $Ia^d$ showed that substitution of single amino acids in the peptide changed the binding affinity for $Ia^d$ comparatively rarely, whereas recognition by the $TC_r$ was much less permissive. The model proposed by this group[28] is that T-cell recognition involves the formation of a trimolecular complex in which the peptide is sandwiched in a $\beta$-sheet of extended conformation between Ia and the T-cell receptor.

Sense has thus finally been made of the old proposal that the T-cell receptor recognizes either a virus-induced modification of the H-2 molecule or some complex of virus and H-2,[8,36] with viral peptide being substituted for virus.[28,30] The realization that antigenicity for T cells is a function of peptides associating with MHC glycoprotein also has particular implications when considering CNS pathology. Many candidate neurotransmitters are peptides[37] in the size range that could potentially bind to MHC molecules. This may be part of the reason that at least in the normal physiologic state the CNS is substantially MHC negative.[1]

The low level of MHC expression on normal brain cells can be reversed *in vitro*, at least for a proportion of cells, by culture in the presence of various agents (Table 1). The most potent in this regard is gamma interferon (IFN-$\gamma$), which is produced by activated T cells[44] and causes much higher and more rapid induction of both class I and class II MHC glycoprotein expression than does any other promoter tested.[42] The effect is also seen *in vivo* when IFN-$\gamma$ is injected intracerebrally into normal mouse brain.[37] That we did not observe enhanced class II MHC expression on resident CNS cells in mice with acute lymphocytic choriomeningitis[45] may simply reflect that the disease process proceeded too rapidly.

Work from ter Meulen's laboratory has established that exposure to the inactivated JHM coronavirus is sufficient to induce astrocytes to become class II MHC positive.[42] Astrocytes secrete an interleukin-1-like molecule[46] and can act as both antigen-processing cells and stimulators for T-lymphocyte proliferation.[47] Furthermore, the capacity of JHM virus to cause class II MHC glycoprotein expression on astrocytes is rat-strain dependent and correlates directly with the development of virus-related demyelinating disease in genetically different rats.[48] The general argument that viruses may trigger autoimmune disease by causing aberrant class II expression on potential stimulator cells[49] thus applies clearly to the brain.

## MHC PHENOTYPE AND VIRUS-INDUCED NEUROLOGIC DISEASE

The question of correlation of MHC phenotype with induction of virus-related immunopathology in the CNS has been addressed for two experimental systems:[48] the acute, fatal disease resulting from intracerebral injection of adult mice with LCM virus,[50] and the chronic demyelination associated with persistent infection of the CNS by Theiler's murine encephalomyelitis virus (TMEV).[51-54] The TMEV model is particularly fascinating, as the relationship between MHC gene expression and effector T-cell function would seem, on superficial analysis, to be inappropriate: susceptibility to demyelination is associated with class I MHC phenotype, whereas the T cell responsible for demyelination may be CD4+ and thus class II MHC restricted.[55,56]

The explanation for this may rest in the studies of Rodriguez and colleagues[53] with the H-2$^{dm2}$ mutant. The dm2 mutation results in the expression of a molecule with the extracellular NH$_2$-terminal of H-2D$^d$ associated with the COOH-terminal extracellular portion of H-2L$^d$. This has presumably resulted from the unequal crossing over of the H-2D$^d$ and H-2L$^d$ genes, leaving the N exon and part of the C1 exon of H-2D$^d$ joined to the L$^d$ gene beginning somewhere in the C1 exon.[57] Molecular experiments using "exon-shuffling" protocols[58,59] have shown that such rearrangements often result in the loss of MHC-restricted T-cell recognition directed at, in this case, H-2D$^d$ and H-2L$^d$.

Mice that express both H-2D$^d$ and H-2L$^d$, or have deleted H-2L$^d$ (H-2$^{dm2}$ mutant),

TABLE 1. Induction of MHC Glycoprotein Expression on Brain Cells

| Origin of Cells | Inducing Agent | Cell Type | MHC Class | Reference |
|---|---|---|---|---|
| Cultured cells from baby mice | IFN-γ[a] | Oligodendrocytes<br>Microglia<br>Some neurons<br>Astrocytes | I<br>I<br>I<br>I & II | Wong et al., 1984,[38] 1985[1] |
| Adult human brain, cultured for 10-135 days | Nil | Astrocytes<br>Oligodendrocytes | II(9-24%)<br>II(4-16%) | Kim et al., 1985[39] |
| First passage cells from newborn mice | IFN-γ or Con A Sn[b] | Astrocytes<br>Astrocytes | I & II<br>I & II | Fontana et al., 1986[40] |
| 11-14-day cultures from newborn mice | IFN-γ<br>rec IL-2[b] | Oligodendrocytes<br>Oligodendrocytes | I<br>I | Suzumura et al., 1986[41] |
| Primary cultures from newborn rat | IFN-γ<br>Phorbol ester Ca$^{2+}$ ionophore<br>muramyl dipeptide<br>inactivated JHM virus | Astrocytes<br>Astrocytes | II<br>18% in 4h<br>II<br>10-19% in 5 days | Massa and ter Meulen, 1987[42] |
| Sections of human brain | Abscess or tumor metastasis | Astrocytes and endothelium | II<br>II | Frank et al., 1986[43] |

[a] Type 1 interferon (IFN) may also induce class I expression, but is much less potent than IFN-γ.
[b] Con A Sn = supernates from Con-A-stimulated lymphocyte cultures; rec IL-2 = human recombinant interleukin-2.

clear the virus and do not develop demyelination.[53] The interpretation is therefore that an $H$-$2D^d$-restricted, CD8+ T cell is responsible for clearance of TMEV from the CNS. If this does not occur, persistent viral antigen presentation of class II MHC positive cells (possibly astrocytes or microglia/macrophages) may target the virus-immune CD4+ cells that directly or indirectly cause the demyelination.

The implication is therefore that $H$-$2^{dm1}$ is not an immune response (Ir) gene for CD8+ effectors in TMEV infection. That is to say, $H$-$2^{dm1}$ is unable to associate with any TMEV peptide[28-30] to form a configuration that is recognized by an appropriate $TC_r$. Furthermore, considering the H-2 haplotypes that were used in this study, this would also be true for $H$-$2K^b$ and $H$-$2K^d$. The existence of a very limited spectrum of class I MHC Ir genes has been established for another group of small RNA viruses, the alphaviruses.[60] It may not be a coincidence that the alphaviruses have also been used to develop mouse models for T-cell-mediated demyelination in the presence of viral persistence.[61]

Unfortunately, this simplistic model correlating virus clearance with class I and class II MHC phenotype to explain the TMEV demyelination model is not obviously applicable to the findings of Clatch, Melvold, Lipton, and colleagues.[51,54] This group, using SJL × B10 recombinant mouse strains, exploited the correlation between $H$-$2D^s$ homozygosity and demyelination and found no clear correlation with virus clearance. One parameter that might be worth checking is the anatomic localization of the residual virus in the CNS: the virus titers are low, and it could be worthwhile to use immunohistochemistry to determine exactly where the infection is persisting.

The acute lymphocytic choriomeningitis (LCM) immunopathology model is superficially much more straightforward. The disease is induced by class I MHC-restricted, CD8+-activated T cells.[62,65] Earlier experiments indicated that $H$-$2L^d$ is the sole class I Ir gene for lymphocytic choriomeningitis virus (LCMV) in the $H$-$2^d$ haplotype.[66] This caused us to ask if the $H$-$2^{dm2}$ mutant,[50] which has deleted $H$-$2L^d$,[67] would develop clinical LCM. The answer was in the affirmative, but with a slightly delayed time of onset. Further analysis revealed that in the absence of $H$-$2L^d$, $H$-$2K^k$ emerged as an Ir gene for targeting LCMV-specific cytotoxic T lymphocytes (CTL). This dominance of a strong ($H$-$2L^d$) over a weak ($H$-$2K^d$) class I allele is poorly understood. It could be that they compete for the same viral peptide, with $H$-$2L^d$ having a higher affinity. However, LCMV-infected targets expressing both $H$-$2K^d$ and $H$-$2L^d$ are lysed by $H$-$2K^d$-restricted LCMV-immune CTLs. Similar immunodominant effects have now been observed in several experimental systems[6,68] and must be considered when assessing correlations between class I MHC phenotype and disease susceptibility.

## MHC EXPRESSION AND T-CELL TARGETING TO THE CNS

The LCMV model has been used to examine this question in a systematic way, at least for the induction of viral meningitis. The great advantage of this system is that the severity of inflammation can be determined accurately by counting cells in the CSF. It is thus possible to make a quantitative analysis of cellular extravasation into the site of disease. Early adoptive transfer experiments showed clearly that homology between donor and recipient for class I MHC phenotype was sufficient for the induction of severe meningitis, whereas matching for class II alleles had little effect.[69] More recent studies have confirmed that the key cell is the CD8+ immune lymphocyte, whereas deletion of the CD4+ cells from cytotoxic effector populations, if anything, simply enriches the capacity to cause meningitis.[64]

We then asked if this effect reflected that the transferred lymphocytes were first multiplying in MHC-compatible lymphoid tissue and then localizing nonspecifically to the site of virus growth[70,71]; there is evidence from the experimental allergic encephalomyelitis (EAE) model that any activated lymphocyte can cross the brain endothelium.[72] The alternative was that the capacity of effector T cells to cause meningitis required that there be MHC-restricted T-cell target interactions at the site of pathology,[68] the brain, and the cells of the blood-brain barrier. The experiment was performed by making [(A×B)F1 → (B×C)F1] bone marrow radiation chimeras (A, B, and C are different MHC haplotypes), leaving them for 8-12 weeks, and then using these mice as immunosuppressed, virus-infected recipients for T-cell transfer.[70,71] The situation in such chimeras is that the bone-marrow-derived compartment, including monocyte/macrophages and lymphocytes, is almost entirely of donor origin.[73,74] With time, the same is also true for the microglia.[75] We found that adoptively transferred B virus-immune T cells induced severe pathology, whereas those of the C phenotype were slightly less effective. However, the A LCMV-immune lymphocytes caused little inflammation, though they developed strong, virus-specific CTL activity in recipient spleen and could be shown to be present in blood.

These findings indicate that there is a need for an appropriate, radiation-resistant, MHC-compatible cell in brain if T cells are to be recruited into, and cause severe inflammation at, the site of growth of LCMV. The likely target is the endothelium which can be shown to be infected with this virus.[76] Blood-borne monocytes (either adhering to endothelium or localized in the inflammatory site) are apparently unable to assume this antigen-presenting role, though the inflammatory process in acute LCM consists of approximately 50% monocyte/macrophages. Models proposing that monocytes attach nonspecifically to virally modified endothelium and then target the T cells, or that promotion of the inflammatory process is a consequence of interactions between blood-borne cells that have extravasated nonspecifically into the site of virus growth are not supported by these experiments.

## CHARACTERISTICS OF VIRUS-INDUCED INFLAMMATORY EXUDATE

It is obvious that all categories of immune cells, and a variety of nonspecific effectors, can potentially localize to the site of a virus-induced pathologic process. The brain is no exception, with natural killer (NK) cells often making an early appearance,[77-79] CD8+ cytotoxic T cells and CD4+ lymphocytes being present for a time,[77,80,81] and B cells and plasma cells tending to remain *in situ* for considerable periods especially under conditions of viral persistence. I reviewed the then current situation in this area for the First International Congress of Neuroimmunology,[82] and there is little point in repeating the exercise here. However, more recently there have been two sets of systematic experimental studies with the Sindbis alphavirus, by Moench and Griffin,[80] and with LCMV,[81] in our laboratory.

Sindbis virus-induced meningitis is dominated by T cells,[80] particularly those of the CD8− phenotype (TABLE 2). The opposite situation applies in LCM,[81] where there are numerous monocyte/macrophages and the great majority of T cells are CD8+ CD4−. This finding is intriguing, as most people would consider that the

CD8− CD4+ population is the more potent at mediating monocyte recruitment to a site of pathology. However, it is also true that the CD8+ effectors are the cells that trigger delayed type hypersensitivity (DTH), as measured by footpad swelling, in the LCM model, and that this DTH correlates well with MHC-related patterns of disease susceptibility and CTL activity in CSF.[85,86] The CD8+ cells are also responsible for eliminating the virus from non-neural tissue,[87,88] though clearance from the brain may be incomplete.[89]

The reason for the very low levels of CD4+ T cells in CSF, but not blood, of mice with LCM may be that virus is growing in this T-cell subset[90] and they are thus being eliminated by CD8+ effectors. The dominance of T cells with the CD8+ phenotype applies in all models of LCM,[81] whether induced by direct inoculation of virus or by adoptive transfer of immune spleen cells into immunosuppressed, or unsuppressed, virus-infected recipients. It does not reflect that the majority of these CD8+ cells are LCMV specific. In fact, the preponderant CD8+ population seems to be nonspecifically recruited bystander cells that are not obviously involved directly in the disease process. Fatal LCM may, in fact, be triggered by relatively few specifically

TABLE 2. Characteristics of Meningitis at 6 or 7 Days after Inoculation of Virus

| Cell Phenotype | Percentage of Positive Cells | |
|---|---|---|
| | LCM[81] | Sindbis[80] |
| Thy 1+ | 30 | 85 |
| CD8+ CD4− | 25 | 25 |
| CD8− CD4+ (or Lyt1+) | 25[a] | 40 |
| Pgp,[b,c] or F/480+ | 60 | 0 |

[a] The level of CD4 staining was minimal, and both from this experiment and after nonspecific T-cell expansion *in vitro*, it was concluded that the CD4+ cells were not T lymphocytes.

[b] CD4+ T cells also predominate in the brain of people infected with Japanese encephalitis virus.[85]

[c] Monocyte/macrophages stain brightly for Pgp, whereas activated (but not resting) T cells are more weakly positive.[84]

sensitized, class I MHC-restricted CD8+ effectors that have localized to the site of virus growth in the CNS.

## CONCLUSIONS

This brief review emphasizes the role of specifically sensitized T cells, and the sites of MHC glycoprotein expression, in the cell-mediated immune response to viruses growing in the CNS. Other aspects of this topic are addressed in greater detail elsewhere.[82,91] It should be recognized that virus-immune T cells, both CD4+ and CD8+, are likely to be specific for viral peptide in association with MHC molecules. Whether a particular viral protein is present in an intact form on cell surface may be largely irrelevant to T-cell surveillance, though the level of MHC glycoprotein expression may be crucial.[92] At least in the LCM model the induction of severe T-cell-mediated inflammatory process is totally MHC restricted, though many of the inflammatory cells are secondarily recruited as a consequence of the interaction of a few immune T cells with (perhaps) virus-infected endothelium. It therefore may not be too surprising that it is difficult to find evidence of clonality[93] in, for instance, CSF T cells from patients with multiple sclerosis.[94] Much of the inflammatory process in any acute viral disease of the CNS is likely to be "nonsense," though it would be intriguing to look at a much more chronic virus-induced inflammatory process (e.g., the TMEV model) from this aspect.

## REFERENCES

1. WONG, G. H. W., P. F. BARTLETT, I. CLARK-LEWIS, J. L. MCKIMM-BRESCHKIN & J. W. SCHRADER. 1985. Interferon-$\gamma$ induces the expression of H-2 and Ia antigens on brain cells. J. Neuroimmunol. **7**: 255-278.
2. WAKSMAN, B. H. 1985. Mechanisms in multiple sclerosis. Nature **318**: 104-105.
3. MELNIK, J. L., E. SEIDEL, S.-S. WANG, G. MUCHINK, E. J. RASHTI, L. D. JACOBS, A. I. FREEMAN & J. O.'MALLEY. 1985. Persistence of Inoue-Melnick virus and antibody in cerebrospinal fluid. J. Clin. Microbiol. **22**: 651-653.
4. KOPROWSKI, H., E. C. DE FREITAS, M. E. HARPER, M. SANDBERG-WOLLHEIM, W. A. SHEREMATA, M. ROBERT-GUROFF, C. W. SAXINGER, M. B. FEINBERG, F. WONG-STAAL & R. C. GALLO. Multiple sclerosis and human T cell lymphotropic retroviruses. Nature **318**: 154-160.
5. HO, D. D., R. J. POMERANTZ & J. C. KAPLAN. 1987. Pathogenesis of infection with human immunodeficiency virus. N. Engl. J. Med. **317**: 278-286.
6. ZINKERNAGEL, R. M. & P. C. DOHERTY. 1979. MHC-restricted T cells: Studies on the biological role of polymorphic major transplantation antigens determining T cell restriction specificity and responsiveness. Adv. Immunol. **27**: 51-177.
7. SCHWARTZ, R. H. 1986. Immune response (Ir) genes of the murine major histocompatibility complex. Adv. Immunol. **38**: 31-201.
8. ZINKERNAGEL, R. M. & P. C. DOHERTY. 1974. Immunological surveillance against altered self components by sensitized T lymphocytes in lymphocytic choriomeningitis. Nature **251**: 547-548.
9. REINHERZ, E. L., S. C. MEUER & S. F. SCHLOSSMAN. 1983. The human T cell receptor: Analysis with cytotoxic T cell clones. Immunol. Rev. **74**: 83-112.
10. SWAIN, S. L. 1983. T cell subsets and recognition of MHC cells. Immunol. Rev. **74**: 129-142.
11. DEMBIC, Z., W. HAAS, R. ZAMOYSKA, J. PARNES, M. STEINMETZ & H. VON BOEHMER. 1987. Transfection of the CD8 gene enhances T cell recognition. Nature **326**: 510-511.
12. SLECKMAN, B. P., A. PETERSON, W. K. JONES, J. A. FORAN, J. L. GREENSTEIN, B. SEED & S. J. BURAKOFF. 1987. Expression and function of CD4 in a murine T cell hybridoma. Nature **328**: 351-353.
13. GAY, D., P. MADDON, R. SEKALY, M. A. TALLE, M. GODFREY, E. LONG, G. GOLDSTEIN, L. CHESS, R. AXEL, J. KAPPLER & P. MARRACK. 1987. Functional interaction between human T cell protein CD4 and the major histocompatibility complex HLA-DR antigen. Nature **328**: 626-629.
14. KUPFER, A., S. J. SINGER, C. A. JANEWAY, JR. & S. L. SWAIN. 1987. Coclustering of CD4 (L3T4) molecule with the T cell receptor is induced by specific direct interaction of helper T cells and antigen-presenting cells. Proc. Natl. Acad. Sci. USA **84**: 5888-5892.
15. ZINKERNAGEL, R. M. 1978. Thymus and lymphohemopoietic stem cells: Their role in T cell maturation, in selection of T cells H-2 restriction specificity and in H-2 linked Ir gene control. Immunol. Rev. **42**: 224-270.

16. SNODGRASS, H. R., Z. DEMBIC, M. STEINMETZ & H. VON BOEHMER. 1985. Expression of T cell antigen receptor during fetal development in the thymus. Nature **315:** 232-233.
17. JENKINSON, E. J., P. JHITTAY, R. KINGSTON & J. J. T. OWEN. 1985. Studies of the role of the thymic environment in the induction of tolerance to MHC antigens. Transplantation **39:** 331-333.
18. LO, D. & J. SPRENT. 1986. Identity of cells that imprint H-2-restricted T-cell specificity in the thymus. Nature **319:** 672-675.
19. BLACKMAN, M., J. YAGUE, R. KUBO, D. GAY, C. COLECLOUGH, E. PALMER, J. KAPPLER & P. MARRACK. 1986. The T cell receptor may be biased in favor of MHC recognition. Cell **47:** 349-357.
20. SORGER, S. B., S. M. HEDRICK, P. J. FINK, M. A. BOOKMAN & L. A. MATIS. 1987. Generation of diversity in T cell receptor repertoire specific for pigeon cytochrome C. J. Exp. Med. **165:** 279-301.
21. IWAMOTO, A., P. S. OHASHI, H. PRICHER, C. L. WALKER, E. E. MICHALOPOULUS, F. RUPP, H. HENGARTNER & T. W. MAK. 1987. T cell receptor variable gene usage in a specific cytotoxic T cell response. Primary structure of the antigen-MHC receptor of four hapten-specific cytotoxic T cell clones. J. Exp. Med. **165:** 591-600.
22. MOREL, P. A., A. M. LIVINGSTONE & C. G. FATHMAN. 1987. Correlation of T cell receptor V$\beta$ gene family with MHC restriction. J. Exp. Med. **166:** 583-588.
23. ROCK, K. L. & B. BENACERRAF. 1984. Thymic T cells are driven to expand upon interaction with self class II major histocompatibility gene products on accessory cells. Proc. Natl. Acad. Sci. USA **81:** 1221-1224.
24. KAPPLER, J. W., T. WADE, J. WHITE, E. KUSHNIR, M. BLACKMAN, J. BILL, N. ROEHM, & P. MARRACK. 1987. A T cell receptor V$\beta$ segment that imparts reactivity to a class II major histocompatibility complex product. Cell **49:** 263-271.
25. DAVIS, M. M. 1985. Molecular genetics of the T cell receptor $\beta$ chain. Ann. Rev. Immunol. **3:** 537-560.
26. GOVERMAN, J., T. HUNKAPILLER & L. HOOD. 1986. A speculative view of the multicomponent nature of T cell antigen recognition. Cell **45:** 475-484.
27. JERNE, N. K. 1971. The somatic generation of immune recognition. Eur. J. Immunol. **1:** 1-9.
28. SETTE, A., S. BUUS, S. COLON, J. A. SMITH, C. MILES & H. M. GREY. 1987. Structural characteristics of an antigen required for its interaction with Ia and recognition by T cells. Nature **328:** 395-399.
29. TOWNSEND, A. R. M., J. ROTHBARD, F. M. GOTCH, G. BAHADUR, D. WRAITH & A. J. MCMICHAEL. 1986. The epitopes of influenza nucleoprotein recognized by cytotoxic T lymphocytes can be defined with short synthetic peptides. Cell **44:** 959-968.
30. GOTCH, F., J. ROTHBARD, K. HOLLAND, A. TOWNSEND, & A. MCMICHAEL. 1987. Cytotoxic T lymphocytes recognize a fragment of influenza virus matrix protein in association with HLA-A2. Nature **326:** 881-882.
31. TOWNSEND, A. R. M., A. J. MCMICHAEL, N. P. CARTER, J. A. HUDDLESTON & G. C. BROWNLEE. 1984. Cytotoxic T cell recognition of the influenza nucleoprotein expressed in transfected mouse L cells. Cell **39:** 13-25.
32. YEWDELL, J. W., J. R. BENNINK, G. L. SMITH & B. MOSS. 1985. Influenza A virus nucleoprotein is a major target antigen for cross-reactive anti-influenza A virus cytotoxic T lymphocytes. Proc. Natl. Acad. Sci. USA **82:** 1785-1789.
33. PERNIS, B. 1985. Internalization of lymphocyte membrane components. Immunol. Today **6:** 45-49.
34. MACHY, P., A. TRUNEH, D. GENNARO & S. HOFFSTEIN. 1987. Major histocompatibility complex class I molecules internalized via coated pits in T lymphocytes. Nature **328:** 724-726.
35. DOHERTY, P. C., B. B. KNOWLES & P. J. WETTSTEIN. 1984. Immunological surveillance of tumors in the context of major histocompatibility complex restriction of T cell function. Adv. Cancer Res. **42:** 1-65.
36. DOHERTY, P. C. & R. M. ZINKERNAGEL. 1975. A biological role for the major histocompatibility antigens. Lancet **i:** 1406-1409.
37. HOKFELT, T., O. JOHANSSON, A. LJUNGDAHL, J. M. LUNDBERG & M. SCHULTZBERG. 1980. Peptidergic neurons. Nature **284:** 515-521.

38. WONG, G. H. W., P. F. BARTLETT, I. CLARK-LEWIS, F. BATTYE & J. W. SCHRADER. 1984. Inducible expression of H-2 and Ia-antigens on brain cells. Nature 310: 688-691.
39. KIM, S. U., G. MORETTO & D. H. SHIN. 1985. Expression of Ia antigens on the surface of human oligodendrocytes and astrocytes in culture. J. Neuroimmunol. 10: 141-149.
40. FONTANA, A., P. ERB, H. PIRCHER, R. ZINKERNAGEL, E. WEBER & W. FIERZ. 1986. Astrocytes as antigen-presenting cells. Part II. Unlike H-2K-dependent cytotoxic T cells, H-2 Ia-restricted T cells are only stimulated in the presence of interferon γ. J. Neuroimmunol. 12: 15-28.
41. SUZUMURA, A., D. H. SILDERBERG & R. P. LISAK. 1986. The expression of MHC antigens on oligodendrocytes. Induction of polymorphic H-2 expressions by lymphokines. J. Neuroimmunol. 11: 179-190.
42. MASSA, P. T. & V. TER MEULEN. 1987. Analysis of Ia induction on Lewis rat astrocytes *in vitro* by virus particles and bacterial adjuvants. J. Neuroimmunol. 13: 259-271.
43. FRANK, E. & N. DE TRIBOLET. 1986. Expression of class II major histocompatibility antigens on reactive astrocytes and endothelial cells within the gliosis surrounding metastases and abscesses. J. Neuroimmunol. 12: 26-29.
44. MORRIS, A. G., Y. L. LIN & B. A. ASKONAS. 1982. Immune interferon release when a clones cytotoxic T cell line meets its correct influenza-infected target cell. Nature 295: 150-152.
45. DOHERTY, P. C., J. E. ALLAN, J. E. DIXON, Z. TABI & R. CEREDIG. 1987. Characteristics of the CSF inflammatory exudate in murine lymphocytic choriomeningitis. *In* Proceedings of Workshop on Cellular and Humoral Components of CSF in Multiple Sclerosis. A. Lowenthal & J. Raus, Eds. Plenum Press. In press.
46. FONTANA, A., F. KRISTENSEN, R. DUBS, D. GEMSA & E. WEBER. 1982. Production of prostaglandin E and an interleukin-1 like factor by cultured astrocytes and C-6 glioma cells. J. Immunol. 129: 2413-2419.
47. FONTANA, A., W. FIERZ & H. WEKERLE. 1984. Astrocytes present myelin basic protein to encephalitogenic T cell lines. Nature 307: 273-276.
48. MASSA, P. T., R. BRINKMANN & V. TER MEULEN. 1987. Inducibility of Ia antigens on astrocytes by murine coronavirus JHM is rat strain dependent. J. Exp. Med. 166: 259-264.
49. BOTAZZO, G. F., R. PUJOL-BORRELL, T. HANAFUSA & M. FELDMAN. 1983. Role of aberrant HLA-DR expression and antigen presentation in the induction of endocrine autoimmunity. Lancet 2: 1115-1119.
50. ALLAN, J. E. & P. C. DOHERTY. 1985. Consequences of a single Ir gene defect for the pathogenesis of lymphocytic choriomeningitis. Immunogenetics 21: 581-590.
51. CLATCH, R. J., R. W. MELVOLD, S. D. MILLER & H. L. LIPTON. 1985. Theiler's murine encephalomyelitis virus (TMVE)-induced demyelinating disease in mice is influenced by the H-2D region: Correlation and TMEV-specific delayed type hypersensitivity. J. Immunol. 135: 1408-1414.
52. RODRIGUEZ, M. & C. S. DAVID. 1985. Demyelination by Theiler's virus: Influence of the H-2 haplotype. J. Immunol. 135: 2145-2148.
53. RODRIGUEZ, M., J. LEIBOWITZ & C. S. DAVID. 1986. Susceptibility to Theiler's virus-induced demyelination. Mapping of the gene within the H-2D region. J. Exp. Med. 163: 620-631.
54. CLATCH, R. J., R. W. MELVOLD, M. C. DAL CANTO, S. D. MILLER & H. L. LIPTON. 1987. The Theiler's murine encephalomyocarditis virus (TMEV) model for multiple sclerosis shows a strong influence of the murine equivalants of HLA-A, B and C. J. Neuroimmunol. 15: 121-135.
55. CLATCH, R. D., H. L. LIPTON & S. D. MILLER. 1986. Characterization of Theiler's murine encephalomyelitis virus (TMEV)-specific delayed type hypersensitivity in TMEV-induced demyelinating disease: Correlation with clinical signs. J. Immunol. 136: 920-927.
56. WELSH, C. J. R., P. TONKS, A. A. NASH & W. F. BLAKEMORE. 1987. The effect of L3T4+ T cell depletion on the pathogenesis of Theiler's murine encephalomyelitis virus infection in CBA mice. J. Gen. Virol. 68: 1659-1667.
57. BURNSIDE, S., P. HUNT, K. OZATO & D. W. SEARS. 1984. A molecular hybrid of the H-$2D^d$ and H-$2L^d$ genes expressed in the dm1 mutant. Proc. Natl. Acad. Sci. USA 81: 5204-5208.
58. MURRE, C., E. CHOI, J. WEIS, J. G. SEIDMAN, K. OZATO, L. LIU, S. BURAKOFF & C. S.

REISS. 1984. Dissection of serological and cytolytic T lymphocyte epitopes on murine major histocompatibility antigens by a recombinant H-2 gene separating the first two external domains. J. Exp. Med. **160:** 167-178.
59. ALLEN, H., D. WRAITH, P. PALA, B. ASKONAS & R. A. FLAVELL. 1984. Domain interactions of H-2 class I antigens alter cytotoxic T cell recognition sites. Nature **309:** 279-281.
60. MULLBACHER, A., I. D. MARSHALL & R. V. BLANDEN. 1979. Cross-reactive cytotoxic T cells to alphavirus infection. Scand. J. Immunol. **10:** 291-296.
61. FAZAKERLEY, J. K. & H. E. WEBB. 1987. Semliki Forest virus-induced, immune-mediated demyelination: adoptive transfer studies and viral persistence in nude mice. J. Gen. Virol. **68:** 377-385.
62. BAENZIGER, J., H. HENGARTNER, R. M. ZINKERNAGEL & G. A. COLE. 1986. Induction or prevention of immunopathological disease by cloned cytotoxic T cell lines specific for lymphocytic choriomeningitis virus. Eur. J. Immunol. **16:** 387-393.
63. ALLAN, J. E., J. E. DIXON & P. C. DOHERTY. 1987. Nature of the inflammatory process in the central nervous system of mice infected with lymphocytic choriomeningitis virus. Curr. Top. Microbiol. Immunol. **134:** 131-143.
64. DIXON, J. E., J. E. ALLAN & P. C. DOHERTY. 1987. The acute inflammatory process in murine lymphocytic choriomeningitis is dependent on Lyt2+ immune T cells. Cell. Immunol. **197:** 8-14.
65. LEIST, T. P., S. P. COBBOLD, H. WALDMANN, M. AGUET & R. M. ZINKERNAGEL. 1987. Functional analysis of T lymphocytes in antiviral host defense. J. Immunol. **138:** 2278-2281.
66. ORN, A., R. S. GOODENOW, L. HOOD, P. R. BRAYTON, J. G. WOODWARD, R. C. HARMAN & J. A. FRELINGER. 1982. Product of a transferred H-2L$^d$ gene acts as a restriction element for LCMV-specific killer T cells. Nature **297:** 415-417.
67. HANSEN, T. H., S. E. CULLEN, R. W. MELVOLD & A. I. KOHN. 1977. Mutation in a new H-2-associated histocompatibility gene closely linked to H-2D. J. Exp. Med. **145:** 1550-1558.
68. DOHERTY, P. C. 1986. Virus-immune T cells and the major histocompatibility complex: Evolution of some basic concepts over the past two years. Experientia **42:** 972-977.
69. DOHERTY, P. C., R. V. BLANDEN & R. M. ZINKERNAGEL. 1976. Specificity of virus-immune effector T cells for H-2K or H-2D compatible interactions; Implications for H-antigen diversity. Transplant. Rev. **29:** 89-124.
70. DOHERTY, P. C. & J. E. ALLAN. 1986. Role of the major histocompatibility complex in targeting effector T cells into a site of virus infection. Eur. J. Immunol. **16:** 1237-1242.
71. DOHERTY, P. C. & J. E. ALLAN. 1986. Differential effect of hybrid resistance on the targeting of virus-immune effector T cells to spleen and brain. Immunogenetics **24:** 409-415.
72. WEKERLE, H., C. LININGTON, H. LASSMAN & R. MEYERMANN. 1986. Cell immune reactivity within the CNS. Trends in Neurosci. **9:** 271-277.
73. ZINKERNAGEL, R. M., G. KREEB & A. ALTHAGE. 1980. Lymphohemopoietic origin of the immunogenic, virus-antigen-present cells triggering anti-viral T-cell responses. Clin. Immunol. Immunopathol. **15:** 565-576.
74. DOHERTY, P. C., R. KORNGOLD, D. H. SCHWARTZ & J. R. BENNINK. 1981. The development and loss of thymic-competence in bone marrow radiation chimeras and normal mice. Immunol. Rev. **58:** 38-71.
75. TING, J. P.-Y., D. F. NIXON, L. P. WEINER & J. A. FRELINGER. 1983. Brain Ia-antigens have a bone marrow origin. Immunogenetics **17:** 295-301.
76. MARKER, O., A. R. THOMSEN, M. VOLKERT, B. L. HANSEN & I. H. CLEMMENSEN. 1985. High dose survival in the lymphocytic choriomeningitis virus infection is accompanied by suppressed DTH but unaffected T cell cytotoxicity. Scand. J. Immunol. **21:** 81-91.
77. DOHERTY, P. C. & R. KORNGOLD. 1983. Characteristics of poxvirus induced meningitis: Virus-specific and nonspecific cytotoxic effectors in the inflammatory exudate. Scand. J. Immunol. **18:** 1-7.
78. GRIFFIN, D. E. & J. L. HESS. 1986. Cells with natural killer activity in the cerebrospinal fluid of normal mice and athymic nude mice with acute Sindbis virus encephalitis. J. Immunol. **136:** 1841-1845.

79. ALLAN, J. E. & P. C. DOHERTY. 1986. Natural killer cells contribute to inflammation but do not appear to be essential for the induction of clinical lymphocytic choriomeningitis. Scand. J. Immunol. **24:** 153-162.
80. MOENCH, T. R. & D. E. GRIFFIN. 1984. Immunocytochemical identification and quantitation of the cerebrospinal fluid, meninges and brain during acute viral meningoencephalitis. J. Exp. Med. **159:** 77-88.
81. CEREDIG. R., J. E. ALLAN, Z. TABI, F. LYNCH & P. C. DOHERTY. 1987. Phenotypic analysis of the inflammatory exudate in murine lymphocytic choriomeningitis. J. Exp. Med. **169:** 1539-1551.
82. DOHERTY, P. C. 1984. "Clearance of experimental viral infections of the central nervous system" *In* Proceedings of the First International Congress of Neuroimmunology. P. O. Behan and F. Spreafico, Eds.: 301-310. Plenum Press, New York.
83. JOHNSON, R. T., P. INTRALAWAN & S. PUAPANWATTON. 1986. Japanese encephalitis: Identification of inflammatory cells in cerebrospinal fluid. Ann. Neurol. **20:** 691-695.
84. LYNCH, F., G. CHAUDHRI, J. E. ALLAN, P. C. DOHERTY & R. CEREDIG. 1987. Expression of Pgp-1 (or Ly24) on sub-populations of mouse thymocytes and activated peripheral T lymphocytes. Eur. J. Immunol. **17:** 137-140.
85. ZINKERNAGEL, R. M., C. J. PFAU, H. HENGARTNER, & A. ALTHAGE. 1985. Susceptibility to murine lymphocytic choriomeningitis maps to class I MHC genes—a model for MHC disease associations. Nature **316:** 814-817.
86. ZINKERNAGEL, R. M., T. LEIST, H. HENGARTNER & A. ALTHAGE. 1985. Susceptibility to lymphocytic choriomeningitis isolates correlates directly with early and high cytotoxic T cell activity, as well as with footpad swelling reaction, and all three are regulated by H-2D. J. Exp. Med. **162:** 2125-2141.
87. BRYNE, J. A. & M. B. A. OLDSTONE. 1984. Biology of cloned cytotoxic T lymphocytes specific for lymphocytic choriomeningitis virus: Clearance of virus *in vivo*. J. Virol. **51:** 682-686.
88. MOSKOPHIDIS, D., S. P. COBOLD, H. WALDMANN & F. LEHMANN-GRUBE. 1987. Mechanism of recovery from acute virus infection. Treatment of lymphocytic choriomeningitis virus infected mice with monoclonal antibodies reveals that Lyt2+ T lymphocytes mediate clearance of virus and regulate the antiviral antibody response. J. Virol. **61:** 1867-1874.
89. ALLAN, J. E. & P. C. DOHERTY. 1985. Immune T cells can protect or induce fatal neurological disease in murine lymphocytic choriomeningitis. Cell. Immunol. **90:** 401-407.
90. AHMED, R., C.-C. KING & M. B. A. OLDSTONE. 1987. Virus-lymphocyte interaction: T cells of the helper subset are infected with lymphocytic choriomeningitis during persistent infection *in vivo*. J. Virol. **61:** 1571-1576.
91. DOHERTY, P. C. 1985. T cells and viral infections. Br. Med. Bull. **41:** 7-14.
92. MORRIS, A., P. T. TOMKINS, D. J. MAUDSLEY & M. BLACKMAN. 1987. Infection of cultured murine brain cells by Semliki Forest virus: Effects of interferon $\alpha\beta$ on viral replication, viral antigen display, major histocompatibility complex antigen display and lysis by cytotoxic T lymphocytes. J. Gen. Virol. **68:** 99-106.
93. FLEISCHER, B. & H. KRETH. 1983. Clonal expansion and functional analysis of virus-specific T lymphocytes from cerebrospinal fluid in measles encephalitis. Human Immunol. **7:** 239-248.
94. ROTTEVEEL, F. T. M., I. KOKKELINK, H. H. VAN WALBEEK, C. H. POLMAN, J. J. M. VAN DONGEN & C. J. LUCAS. 1987. Analysis of T cell receptor gene rearrangement in T cells from the cerebrospinal fluid of patients with multiple sclerosis. J. Neuroimmunol. **15:** 243-249.

# Mechanisms of Virus-Induced Demyelination and Remyelination[a]

## MOSES RODRIGUEZ

*Department of Neurology and Immunology
Mayo Clinic and Research Foundation
Rochester, Minnesota*

Animal models of virus-induced demyelination and remyelination have provided one important piece of evidence to suggest that multiple sclerosis is the result of immunopathology induced by a virus.[1] These models provide the framework to study the potential interaction between the immune system, persistent viruses, and glial cells. This review will address major mechanisms considered to be important in the pathogenesis of virus-induced demyelination including:

1. Direct viral cytopathologic effects on oligodendrocytes
2. Virus-induced autoimmune demyelination
3. "Bystander" demyelination
4. Immune-mediated alteration of viral tropism for oligodendrocytes
5. Immune-mediated destruction of persistently infected oligodendrocytes.

Each mechanism will be illustrated by various examples of virus infection. Special emphasis will be given to Theiler's murine encephalomyelitis virus(TMEV)-induced demyelination, a model that exemplifies many potential mechanisms of myelin destruction. In addition, the factors that control new myelin formation after virus-induced demyelination will be discussed.

## DEMYELINATION

### Direct Cytopathology of Oligodendrocytes by Virus

One of the best examples of a virus causing demyelination by direct lytic infection of the myelin-producing cell is the JHM virus, a neurotropic strain of mouse hepatitis virus.[2–6] This coronavirus produces demyelination in susceptible BALB/c mice within the first week of infection. Demyelination in this model is not temporally related to the presence of perivascular inflammatory cells,[2,3] and immunosuppression with cyclophosphamide fails to diminish demyelination in the mouse, strongly suggesting that

---

[a] This work was supported in part by grants from the National Multiple Sclerosis Society (RG 1878-A1) and Searle Foundation. Moses Rodriguez is the recipient of a Teacher Investigator Award (NS-00849) from the National Institutes of Health.

immune mechanisms are not involved. The virus can infect neurons and astrocytes,[6] but oligodendrocytes appear to be the principal target.[2] Experiments by Powell and Lampert[4] demonstrated oligodendrocytes containing intracisternal virions. Virus buds from cytoplasmic vacuoles, leading to pathologic alterations of oligodendrocytes, which then result in abnormal glial connections with myelin sheaths and syncytia formation.

A characteristic feature of JHM-induced demyelination is the rapid recovery of infected animals,[2,5] resulting from proliferation of surviving oligodendrocytes and remyelination of previously demyelinated axons.[5] Myelin sheaths are almost completely restored within 2 to 3 months of infection. Prominent remyelination, observed with this model, indicates that oligodendrocytes within the central nervous system (CNS) have an intrinsic capacity for myelin repair, even when primary injury is directed at the myelin-producing cell. As will be discussed, the extent of remyelination in this model may indicate that immune mechanisms are not important in JHM-induced demyelination.

Papovaviruses also appear to cause demyelination by direct injury of oligodendrocytes.[7-10] The JC virus, a member of the papovavirus family, causes progressive multifocal leukoencephalopathy in immunosuppressed patients.[8] This rare demyelinating disease was seen in patients with lymphoma and leukemia,[7] but it has emerged as an important complication of human immunodeficiency virus (HIV) infection.[9] Pathologically, it is characterized by multiple patches of noninflammatory demyelination without relation to blood vessels.[7] Infected oligodendrocytes are easily recognized by their enlarged nuclei containing papovaviruses. Astrocytes are transformed and develop bizarre, hyperchromatic nuclei. Recent experiments using *in situ* hybridization clearly demonstrated the remarkable propensity of this virus for oligodendrocytes.[10]

## *Virus-Induced Autoimmune Demyelination*

An attractive hypothesis in virus-induced demyelination is that virus infection can trigger a destructive host immune response to self antigens.[11] A basis for this idea comes from observations in patients with postinfectious encephalomyelitis in which perivenular demyelination develops 2 to 3 weeks after virus infection including measles or vaccinia infection and, to a lesser extent, varicella or rubella infection. The pathologic features closely resemble those of acute experimental autoimmune encephalomyelitis.[11] This finding raises the possibility that viruses can cause primary damage to oligodendrocytes or myelin sheaths, or both. This then results in the release of "self" myelin antigens that would be recognized as foreign by immunocytes. This hypothesis would be supported by the demonstration of cellular or humoral immune responses, or both, to myelin antigens after virus infection and by passive transfer of pathologic abnormalities into naive recipients by immune serum or lymphocytes.

Probably the best example of virus-induced autoimmune demyelination is coronavirus infection in rats.[12-13] Watanabe *et al.*[13] inoculated rats with a murine coronavirus and observed late demyelinating disease characterized by perivascular lymphoid infiltration. Early in the disease, viral antigen was found primarily in glial cells in association with small demyelinating plaques. As the animals recovered from the initial infection, late demyelinating disease developed and was associated with intense inflammatory infiltrates. Lymphocytes from infected rats were sensitized against myelin basic protein (MBP) and virus antigen.[13] Lymphocytes from Lewis rats recovering from infection were cultured *in vitro* in the presence of myelin basic protein and injected intravenously in naive syngeneic rats. In a few days, mild clinical disease and perivascular inflammatory infiltrates resembling EAE developed. Interestingly, demyelination was not detectable.

Thus far, autoimmune demyelination has not been confirmed in any other viral model. This hypothesis was tested in the demyelinating disease induced by Theiler's virus (TMEV), a picornavirus that results in chronic immune-mediated demyelination.[14,15] Barbano and Dal Canto[16] failed to produce demyelination *in vitro* when isogenic organotypic brain cultures were exposed to serum or splenocytes from mice persistently infected with TMEV. In addition, disease could not be transferred into naive recipients when splenocytes from infected mice were incubated with myelin basic protein. The studies agree with those of Lampert *et al.*[17] who concluded that MBP-sensitized cells are not elicited in TMEV infection. Also, Miller *et al.*[18] showed that class II-restricted autoimmune responses against syngeneic spinal cord homogenate or MBP are not demonstrable in susceptible SJL/J mice. Finally, experiments using sensitive immunoblotting techniques failed to demonstrate within cerebrospinal fluid an immune response to myelin antigens.[18a] Thus, data do not support a critical role for autoimmune demyelination in TMEV disease.

One other model in which autoimmune demyelination remains a possibility, however, is the late phase of canine distemper virus (paramyxovirus) encephalitis.[19,20] This natural disease in dogs is characterized by central nervous system symptoms and signs in the acute viral phase. Similar to measles virus, the acute syndrome can cause lymphopenia to develop in dogs. Intracellular virus in the absence of inflammatory cells has been demonstrated in acute demyelinating lesions. In contrast, the late demyelinating disease is associated with perivascular cuffs of inflammatory cells, and antimyelin antibodies develop before the onset of symptoms.[20] Thus far, demyelination has not been obtained in rodents infected with the canine distemper virus, making it very difficult to formally test the autoimmune hypothesis in this model.

### *Bystander Demyelination*

Considerable thought has been given to the concept that myelin may be injured "nonspecifically" as a result of an immune response within the nervous system,[21,22] and it would help explain why different viruses may result in myelin destruction.[1] This hypothesis suggests that T cells, macrophages, or both, in reacting to a viral antigen, secrete factors that cause demyelination. For example, myelin is vulnerable to neutral proteases, including plasminogen activator, which can be secreted by activated macrophages.[22] Some experiments suggest that demyelination can occur after local injection of purified protein derivative in the spinal cord of animals previously sensitized to this antigen.[21] However, other similar experiments failed to show a "bystander effect" in the peripheral nervous system.[23] It is possible that "bystander" demyelination may be important in augmenting myelin destruction, especially in a host with latent hypersensitivity to myelin.

The bystander hypothesis was considered by Clatch *et al.*[24] to explain demyelination induced by Theiler's virus. They propose that as a consequence of persistent virus infection, TMEV-specific precursor delayed hypersensitivity (DTH) cells are triggered to expand within the brain. These cells release lymphokines which would lead to recruitment of activated macrophages. Factors released by DTH cells or macrophages would then nonspecifically destroy myelin. In support of this hypothesis is the close relation between skin DTH response and susceptibility to TMEV infection. Also, virus persists within macrophages in the CNS which may predispose to bystander demyelination.[25] Whether this factor contributes significantly to TMEV-induced disease is not yet clear, but there are data to suggest that this may not be the primary mechanism. (1) TMEV-induced demyelinating disease is controlled in part by genes within the major histocompatibility complex.[26–29] However, the disease maps within the H-2D region[27,29] which controls class I-restricted immune responses. If DTH-mediated bystander demyelination were important, restriction to class II genes could be hypothesized. (2) Treatment of TMEV-infected mice with aminomethylcyclohexane carboxylic acid (AMCHA), ϵ-amino caproic acid (EACA), and p-nitrophenyl guanidlinobenzoate (NPGB), which are inhibitors of plasminogen activators and other neutral proteases, fail to suppress TMEV demyelination, even though they diminish demyelination in EAE.[30] Also, pepstatin, an acid protease inhibitor that interferes with cathepsin D, fails to diminish TMEV demyelination.[30] (3) Cyclosporin A fails to diminish demyelination once the disease process is established,[30] indicating that effectors dependent on the production of interleukin-2 are not involved in myelin destruction during late disease. (4) Susceptibility to demyelination does not correlate with proliferative responses of class II-restricted viral antigens.[24] (5) Demyelination occurs in nude mice that are deficient in DTH type responses.[31,32] (6) Demyelinating disease can be suppressed by treatment with mAb to Lyt2 (directed at class I-restricted T cells), whereas mAb to L3T4 (directed at class II-restricted T cells) increases demyelination.[33] (7) Finally, bystander demyelination runs counter to most human neuropathologic observations, because demyelination is not present in most inflammatory responses to CNS viruses.[34] This finding suggests that the presence of primary demyelination in the context of inflammation implies a more specific cellular or humoral reaction directed against virus, myelin, or oligodendrocytes.

*Immune-Mediated Alteration of Viral Tropism for Glial Cells*

Nitayaphan et al.[35,36] proposed a unique hypothesis in which immune cells could change the surface structure of a virus so that it has more propensity to infect myelin-producing cells. Using Theiler's virus to test this concept, they found that proteases secreted by macrophages can cleave one of the major structural proteins of TMEV (VP1) and thereby disrupt an epitope important in neutralization.[35,36] This could promote viral persistence and subsequent infection of oligodendrocytes. Serum from mice with early disease is less effective in neutralizing VP1-cleaved virus than VP1-uncleaved virus. Therefore, immune cells could be critical in demyelination by producing factors that change the structural properties of viruses rather than in mediating disease.

This hypothesis may apply to visna infection in which virus is able to escape host defense mechanisms. This retrovirus causes a slow natural disease of sheep involving the lungs and the CNS.[37] Pathologically, there is subacute encephalitis in which virus antigen is found primarily in macrophages and demyelination is associated with inflammatory infiltrates.[38] A unique aspect of the disease is the failure to neutralize virus by serum as a result of viral "antigenic drift."[39] Virus isolates from sheep years after infection are antigenically different from input virus. It is possible that factors secreted by macrophages may alter virus and contribute to subsequent "antigenic drift."

*Immune-Mediated Destruction of Persistently Infected Oligodendrocytes*

Humoral or cellular immune mechanisms may play a role in injuring oligodendrocytes that have been infected by virus.[40] This hypothesis implies the expression of viral antigens or viral-induced "novel" antigens on the surface of myelin-producing cells. Humoral mechanisms may interact with virus antigens on oligodendrocytes, resulting in immunoglobulin-directed killing, injury by complement, antibody-dependent cell-mediated cytotoxicity, or activation of macrophages through binding of Fc receptors. Cellular immune mechanisms would depend on the recognition of processed viral polypeptides or intact structural viral protein by class II- or class I-restricted T cells in the context of major histocompatibility complex (MHC) glycoproteins.

An example of humoral-mediated destruction of infected oligodendrocytes is subacute sclerosing panencephalitis.[41] This persistent measles virus infection is characterized by infection of neurons and oligodendrocytes. A constant feature of the disorder is high titers of anti-measles antibody in the spinal fluid and brain of infected patients. Lysis of infected oligodendrocytes is associated with antibodies that bind to the nucleocapsid of the virus.[41] Studies in tissue culture have suggested a mechanism by which virus persists in the presence of a competent immune response. If virus antigens are expressed on the cell surface, then lysis of infected cells occurs in the presence of antibody and complement. However, if measles-infected cells are cultured in the presence of antibody without complement, antigens are "modulated" off the cell surface, rendering the cell resistant to subsequent immunopathology. Once the antibody is removed, the persistently infected cell will begin to express viral antigens on the surface so that it is once again susceptible to injury by complement and antibody. Thus, the relative concentration of antibody to measles virus or complement, or both, determines if virus will persist in the nervous system or if oligodendrocytes will be killed.[41]

Theiler's murine encephalomyelitis virus infection may prove to be the result of immune-mediated injury of persistently infected oligodendrocytes.[40] Pathologically, the CNS is characterized by perivascular demyelination in association with mononuclear cellular infiltrates.[42] During the first 2 weeks of infection the infiltrates consist primarily of macrophages and class II-restricted T cells (helper and delayed hypersensitivity cells), but as the demyelinating disease progresses (after 21 days of infection), class I-restricted T cells (cytotoxic and suppressor cells) gradually become more numerous.[43] In every example, demyelination is preceded by perivascular inflammation. In addition, immunosuppression by cyclophosphamide,[44,45] antilymphocyte serum,[45] and monoclonal antibodies to Ia[46,47] diminishes the extent of demyelination. Also, Ia antigens are expressed on astrocytes, oligodendrocytes, and endothelial cells after persistent virus infection,[48] suggesting that the demyelinating process is the result of immune mechanisms.

There is, however, strong evidence that oligodendrocytes are infected persistently by virus. Ultrastructural immunoperoxidase experiments have demonstrated virus antigens within oligodendrocytes.[49,50] Paracrystalline arrays of virus were demonstrated within oligodendrocytes of neonates infected by the WW strain of TMEV.[51] The virus readily infects oligodendrocytes in tissue culture,[52,53] and virus antigens can be detected on the surface of these cells.[54] Finally, *in situ* hybridization studies showed a direct correlation between the presence of viral RNA in the white matter and demyelinating lesions.[55-57] Simultaneous immunoperoxidase and *in situ* hybridization assays have shown that 25-40% of cells expressing viral RNA are also expressing antigenic markers specific for oligodendrocytes.[57] Approximately 10% of infected cells are microglia and macrophages and 5-10% are astrocytes. The identity of the remainder of the cells has not been determined.

There are also strong immunogenetic data that one of the genes that determines susceptibility and resistance to TMEV demyelinating disease maps within the MHC.[26-29] TMEV infection of nonrecombinant H-2 congeneic strains on a common background showed that mice with *s, f, p, r, v,* or *q* haplotypes on C57BL/10 background develop demyelination, whereas mice with *b, k,* or *d* haplotypes are resistant.[28] Infection of mouse strains with congeneic recombinant haplotypes demonstrated that the D region of the H-2 complex determines susceptibility.[29] In addition, the susceptible and resistant gene was mapped to the 3' end of $D^d$ by using mice with mutations within the D region genes.[29] Because the D region controls class I-restricted immune responses, it suggests an important role of T cells in clearing virus (resistance) or in contributing to demyelination (susceptibility).

Rodriguez *et al.*[40] proposed a hypothesis of immune-mediated demyelination that incorporates the beneficial response to immunosuppression, virus persistence in oligodendrocytes, and the immunogenetic data. This hypothesis suggests that resistance to disease is an active immunologic process. In genetically resistant mice, viral replication may be limited by class I-restricted T cells in the context of H-2D gene products, by natural killer cells (preliminary observations by P. Leibson), or by neutralizing antibody to virus. In genetically susceptible mice, virus antigens may fail to be recognized by T cells in association with class I MHC antigens so that virus is not cleared from the CNS and persists in oligodendrocytes. Antibody to virus may fail to neutralize infection, either because it occurs too late or because antigens are sequestered in the cytoplasm.

Once oligodendrocytes become infected, viral infection may directly induce demyelination, which would explain the presence of demyelination in nude mice without a T-cell response.[31,32] However, in immunocompetent mice, antigens not normally expressed by oligodendrocytes may appear on the cell surface and provide the target for an immune response. The nature of the antigen on the cell surface remains to be determined. It may represent a polypeptide on the surface that resides primarily in an unprocessed form within the cytoplasm. Alternatively, the surface antigen may be a "novel" host-derived protein induced by viral infection. Injury to the oligodendrocytes may occur by humoral mechanisms directed at this antigen or by class I- or class II-restricted T cells recognizing the antigen in the context of MHC glycoproteins. Recent experiments showing suppression of demyelination with monoclonal antibodies to Lyt-2[33] suggest that class I-restricted cells may be one important effector in the demyelinating phase of disease.

## REMYELINATION

The factors that control the extent of remyelination after viral-induced demyelination are being evaluated.[58] Some viral infections are characterized by extensive and almost complete myelin repair[5] (i.e., JHM virus infection), whereas in others the extent of remyelination is variable and incomplete[42,59] (i.e., TMEV). Several factors have been considered to explain the extent of new myelin formation after demyelinating conditions, as follows:

1. Degree of oligodendroglial injury or infection
2. Propensity for oligodendroglial proliferation

3. Extent of astroglial "scarring"
4. Intensity of inflammatory response
5. Alteration of demyelinated axon surface
6. Host genetic factors

Of greatest importance is to determine if the original demyelinating process is the result of immune mechanisms. Those disorders in which immune mechanisms play a primary role (chronic experimental autoimmune encephalitis or Theiler's virus) are characterized by abortive attempts at remyelination. In contrast, disorders with minimal immunopathology (JHM infection[2-6] and cuprizone toxicity[60]) show almost completely remyelinated lesions, suggesting that immune factors may be critical in determining the degree of remyelination.

Experiments by Dal Canto and Lipton[42] using the DA strain of TMEV in SJL mice demonstrated abortive attempts at CNS remyelination as early as 21 days after infection. Remyelination was somewhat more prominent in the late phase of chronic infection and was associated with a marked astroglial response. In contrast, experiments with a more attenuated WW strain of TMEV with outbred Swiss male mice resulted in greater remyelination by Schwann cells or oligodendrocytes.[61] This result correlated best with diminution of the inflammatory response in animals infected with WW virus compared to DA virus.

Lang et al.[59] undertook a series of experiments in an attempt to promote remyelination after Theiler's virus-induced demyelination. With the observations of Raine and Traugott[62] in mind, a series of experiments were performed to test the hypothesis that immune factors contribute to the extent of remyelination following infection with the DA strain of TMEV. Lang et al.[59] found that DAV-infected mice treated by injections of MBP plus galactocerebroside in incomplete Freund's adjuvant (IFA) had areas of extensive remyelination. Similar results were obtained with infected mice injected with spinal cord homogenate (SCH) plus IFA. These results were similar to those of Raine and Traugott[62] in promoting remyelination in guinea pigs with chronic EAE.

Rodriguez et al.[64] tested the hypothesis that new myelin formation observed in infected mice treated with myelin components is the result of a humoral factor. Normal syngeneic SJL/J mice were divided into three groups and injected subcutaneously in the flank with a 1-mg dose of SCH in IFA, phosphate-buffered saline (PBS) in IFA (1:1), or PBS alone. Serum was collected and passively transferred into mice chronically infected with DA virus. Of interest is that TMEV-infected animals treated with serum from mice given SCH had extensive areas of remyelination that were 6 to 11 times greater than those in the control groups (FIG. 1). Oligodendrocytes were clustered in groups, suggesting proliferation. The addition of SCH sera to oligodendrocytes grown in tissue culture resulted in three- to fivefold proliferation as measured by the incorporation of tritiated thymidine. This finding suggests that a factor is present in the sera of mice immunized to SCH that promotes new myelin formation and proliferation of oligodendrocytes. The identity of the factor remains to be determined. Preliminary studies suggest that the active factor is in the immunoglobulin fraction of sera. In addition, lymphokines may be important in triggering oligodendrocytes to divide and myelinate.

## SUMMARY

Viral models of demyelination and remyelination provide important clues to the pathogenesis of multiple sclerosis. Determining the precise viral polypeptides recognized by T cells during the demyelinating process will be important in understanding

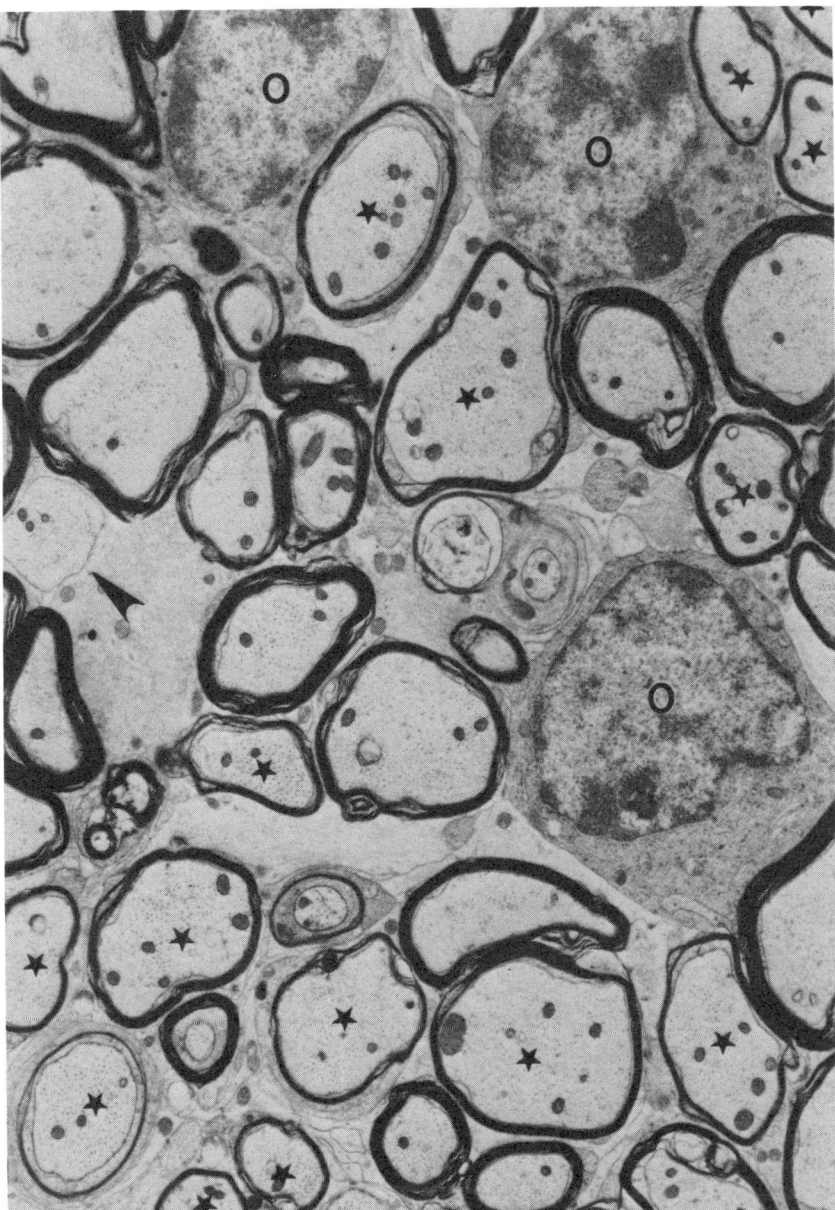

**FIGURE 1.** Extensive remyelination by oligodendrocytes in the spinal cord of an SJL/J mouse infected with the DA strain of TMEV (6 months) and treated for 1 month with sera from a mouse hyperimmunized to spinal cord homogenate (SCH sera). Note three oligodendrocytes (O) making contact with newly synthesized myelin in the area of remyelination. New myelin formation in the CNS is characterized by abnormally thin myelin sheaths compared to axon diameter (**star**). One demyelinated axon that has not undergone remyelination is shown by the **arrow**. The area of remyelination in mice treated with SCH sera was significantly greater ($p <$ 0.01) than that in mice treated with control sera.[64] Similar areas of remyelination were seen in TMEV-infected mice treated with a purified IgG preparation of SCH sera. (Reduced by 35%)

the mechanisms of viral-induced myelin destruction. Isolation, purification, and characterization of factors that promote remyelination and proliferation of oligodendrocytes may provide hope in the treatment of patients with chronic demyelinating disorders.

## ACKNOWLEDGMENT

I wish to thank Kathryn A. Jensen for helping to prepare this manuscript.

## REFERENCES

1. DAL CANTO, M. C. & S. G. RABINOWITZ. 1982. Experimental models of virus-induced demyelination of the central nervous system. Ann. Neurol. **11:** 109-127.
2. LAMPERT, P. W., K. J. SIMS & A. J. KNIAZEFF. 1973. Mechanism of demyelination in JHM virus encephalomyelitis. Electron microscopic studies. Acta Neuropathol. (Berl.) **24:** 76-85.
3. WEINER, L. P. 1973. Pathogenesis of demyelination induced by a mouse hepatitis virus. Arch. Neurol. **28:** 298-303.
4. POWELL, H. C. & P. W. LAMPERT. 1975. Oligodendrocytes and their myelin-plasma membrane connections in JHM mouse hepatitis virus encephalomyelitis. Lab. Invest. **33:** 440-445.
5. HERNDON, R. M., D. L. PRICE & L. P. WEINER. 1977. Regeneration of oligodendroglia during recovery from demyelinating disease. Science **195:** 693-694.
6. KNOBLER, R. L., M. V. HASPEL & M. B. A. OLDSTONE. 1981. Mouse hepatitis virus type 4 (JHM strain)-induced fatal central nervous system disease. I. Genetic control and the murine neuron as the susceptible site of disease. J. Exp. Med. **153:** 832-843.
7. RICHARDSON, E. P. 1961. Progressive multifocal leukoencephalopathy. N. Engl. J. Med. **265:** 815-823.
8. ZU RHEIN, G. M. & S. M. CHOU. 1965. Particles resembling papova viruses in human cerebral demyelinating disease. Science **148:** 1477-1479.
9. KRUPP, L. B., R. B. LIPTON, M. L. SWERDLOW, N. E. LEEDS & J. LLENA. 1985. Progressive multifocal leukoencephalopathy. Clinical and radiographic features. Ann. Neurol. **17:** 344-349.
10. AKSAMIT, A. J., P. MOURRAIN, J. L. SEVER & E. O. MAJOR. 1985. Progressive multifocal leokoencephalopathy. Investigation of three cases using in situ hybridization with JC virus biotinylated DNA probe. Ann. Neurol. **18:** 490-496.
11. LAMPERT, P. W. 1978. Autoimmune and virus-induced demyelinating diseases: A review. Am. J. Pathol. **91:** 176-208.
12. NAGASHIMA, K., H. WEGE, R. MEYERMANN & V. TER MEULEN. 1979. Demyelinating encephalomyelitis induced by a long-term corona virus infection in rats: A preliminary report. Acta. Neuropathol (Berl.) **45:** 205-213.
13. WATANABE, R., H. WEGE & V. TER MEULEN. 1983. Adoptive transfer of EAE-like lesions from rats with coronavirus-induced demyelinating encephalomyelitis. Nature **305:** 150-155.
14. THEILER, M. 1934. Spontaneous encephalomyelitis of mice: A new virus disease. Science **80:** 122.
15. LIPTON, H. L. 1975. Theiler's virus infection in mice: An unusual biphasic disease process leading to demyelination. Infect. Immunol. **11:** 1147-1155.
16. BARBANO, R. L. & M. C. DAL CANTO. 1984. Serum and cells from Theiler's virus-infected mice fail to injure myelinating cultures or to produce in vivo transfer of disease: The pathogenesis of Theiler's virus-induced demyelination appears to differ from that of EAE. J. Neurol. Sci. **66:** 283-293.

17. LAMPERT, P. W., R. S. FUJINAMI, M. RODRIGUEZ, J. L. LEIBOWITZ & W. LANG. 1983. Further studies on the pathogenesis of Theiler's murine encephalomyelitis (abstract). J. Neuropathol. Exp. Neurol. **42:** 326.
18. MILLER, S. D., R. J. CLATCH, D. C. PEVEAR, J. L. TROTTER & H. L. LIPTON. 1987. Class II-restricted T cell responses in Theiler's murine encephalomyelitis virus (TMEV)-induced demyelinating disease. I. Cross-specificity among TMEV substrains and related picornaviruses but not myelin proteins. J. Immunol. **138:** 3776-3784.
18a. RODRIGUEZ, M., C. F. LUCCHINETTI, R. J. CLARK, T. L. YAKSH, H. MARKOWITZ & V. A. LENNON. 1988. Immunoglobulins and complement in demyelination induced in mice by Theiler's virus. J. Immunol. **140:** 800-805.
19. MCCULLOUGH, B., S. KRAKOWKA & A. KOESTNER. 1974. Experimental canine distemper virus-induced demyelination. Lab. Invest. **31:** 216-222.
20. KRAKOWKA, S., B. MCCULLOUGH, A. KOESTNER & R. OLSEN. 1973. Myelin specific autoantibodies associated with central nervous system demyelination in canine distemper virus infection. Infect. Immunol. **8:** 819-827.
21. WISNIEWSKI, H. M. & B. R. BLOOM. 1975. Primary demyelination as a non-specific consequence of a cell-mediated reaction. J. Exp. Med. **141:** 346-359.
22. CAMMER, W., B. R. BLOOM, W. T. NORTON & S. GORDON. 1978. Degradation of basic protein in myelin by neutral proteases secreted by stimulated macrophages: A possible mechanism of inflammatory demyelination. Proc. Natl. Acad. Sci. USA **75:** 1554-1558.
23. POWELL, H. C., S. L. BRAHENY, R. A. C. HUGHES & P. W. LAMPERT. 1984. Antigen-specific demyelination and significance of the bystander effect in peripheral nerves. Am. J. Pathol. **114:** 443-453.
24. CLATCH, R. J., H. L. LIPTON & S. D. MILLER. 1986. Characterization of Theiler's murine encephalomyelitis virus (TMEV)-specific delayed type hypersensitivity responses in TMEV-induced demyelinating disease: Correlation with clinical signs. J. Immunol. **136:** 920-927.
25. DAL CANTO, M. C. & H. L. LIPTON. 1982. Ultrastructural immunohistochemical localization of virus in acute and chronic demyelinating Theiler's virus infection. Am. J. Pathol. **106:** 20-29.
26. LIPTON, H. L. & R. MELVOLD. 1984. Genetic analysis of susceptibility to Theiler's virus-induced demyelinating disease in mice. J. Immunol. **132:** 1821-1825.
27. CLATCH, R. J., R. W. MELVOLD, S. D. MILLER & H. L. LIPTON. 1985. Theiler's murine encephalomyelitis virus (TMEV) induced demyelinating disease in mice is influenced by the H-2D region: Correlation with TMEV-specific delayed-type hypersensitivity. J. Immunol. **135:** 1408-1414.
28. RODRIGUEZ, M. & C. S. DAVID. 1985. Demyelination induced by Theiler's virus: Influence of the H-2 haplotype. J. Immunol. **135:** 2145-2148.
29. RODRIGUEZ, M., J. LEIBOWITZ & C. S. DAVID. 1986. Susceptibility to Theiler's virus-induced demyelination: Mapping of the gene within the H-2D region. J. Exp. Med. **163:** 620-631.
30. RODRIGUEZ, M. & J. QUDDUS. 1986. Effect of cyclosporin A, silica quartz dust and protease inhibitors on virus-induced demyelination. J. Neuroimmunol. **13:** 159-174.
31. ROOS, R. P. & R. WOLLMANN. 1984. DA strain of Theiler's murine encephalomyelitis virus induces demyelination in nude mice. Ann. Neurol. **15:** 494-499.
32. ROSENTHAL, A., R. S. FUJINAMI & P. W. LAMPERT. 1986. Mechanism of Theiler's virus-induced demyelination in nude mice. Lab. Invest. **54:** 515-522.
33. RODRIGUEZ, M. & S. SRIRAM. 1987. Treatment of TMEV-induced demyelination with monoclonal antibodies to T cell subsets (abstract). Neurology 37(Suppl. 1): 344.
34. LAMPERT, P. W. & M. RODRIGUEZ. 1984. Virus-induced demyelination. *In* Viral Pathogenesis, Vol. 1: 260-268. A. L. Notkins & M. B. A. Oldstone, Eds. Springer-Verlag. New York.
35. NITAYAPHAN, S., M. M. TOTH & R. P. ROOS. 1985. Localization of a neutralization site of Theiler's murine encephalomyelitis viruses. J. Virol. **56:** 887-895.
36. NITAYAPHAN, S., M. M. TOTH & R. P. ROOS. 1985. Neutralizing monoclonal antibodies to Theiler's murine encephalomyelitis viruses. J. Virol. **53:** 651-657.
37. SIGURDSSON, B. 1954. Rida, a chronic encephalitis of sheep. Br. Vet. J. **110:** 341-354.

38. PETURSSON, G., N. NATHANSON, G. GEORGSSON, H. PANITCH & P. A. PALSSON. 1976. Pathogenesis of visna. I. Sequential virologic, serologic, and pathologic studies. Lab. Invest. **35**: 402-412.
39. NARAYAN, O., D. E. GRIFFIN & J. CHASE. 1977. Antigenic drift of visna virus in persistently infected sheep. Science **197**: 376-378.
40. RODRIGUEZ, M., L. R. PEASE & C. S. DAVID. 1986. Immune-mediated injury of virus-infected oligodendrocyte: A model of multiple sclerosis. Immunol. Today **7**: 359-363.
41. LAMPERT, P. W., B. S. JOSEPH & M. B. A. OLDSTONE. 1976. Morphological changes of cells infected with measles or related to viruses. In Progress in Neuropathology, Vol. 3: 51-68. H. M. Zimmerman, Ed. Grune and Stratton. New York.
42. DAL CANTO, M. C. & H. L. LIPTON. 1975. Primary demyelination in Theiler's virus infection. An ultrastructural study. Lab. Invest. **33**: 626-637.
43. LINDSLEY, M. D. & M. RODRIGUEZ. 1987. Isolation of inflammatory cells from the CNS of mice persistently infected with Theiler's virus (abstract). J. Neuropathol. Exp. Neurol. **46**: 369.
44. LIPTON, H. L. & M. C. DAL CANTO. 1976. Theiler's virus-induced demyelination: Prevention by immunosuppression. Science **192**: 62-64.
45. ROOS, R. P., S. FIRESTONE, R. WOLLMAN, P. VARIAKOJIS & B. G. W. ARNASON. 1982. The effect of short-term and chronic immunosuppression on Theiler's virus demyelination. J. Neuroimmunol. **2**: 223-234.
46. RODRIGUEZ, M., W. P. LAFUSE, J. LEIBOWITZ & C. S. DAVID. 1986. Partial suppression of Theiler's virus-induced demyelination in vivo by administration of monoclonal antibodies to immune response gene products (Ia antigens). Neurology **36**: 964-970.
47. FRIEDMAN, A., G. FRANKEL, Y. LORCH & L. STEINMAN. 1987. Monoclonal anti-I-A antibody reverses chronic paralysis and demyelination in Theiler's virus-infected mice: Critical importance of timing of treatment. J. Virol. **61**: 898-903.
48. RODRIGUEZ, M., M. L. PIERCE & E. A. HOWIE. 1987. Immune response gene products (Ia antigens) on glial and endothelial cells in virus-induced demyelination. J. Immunol. **138**: 3438-3442.
49. RODRIGUEZ, M., J. L. LEIBOWITZ & P. W. LAMPERT. 1983. Persistent infection of oligodendrocytes in Theiler's virus-induced encephalomyelitis. Ann. Neurol. **13**: 426-433.
50. RODRIGUEZ, M. 1985. Virus-induced demyelination in mice: "Dying back" of oligodendrocytes. Mayo Clin. Proc. **60**: 433-438.
51. PENNEY, J. B., JR. & J. S. WOLINSKY. 1979. Neuronal and oligodendroglial infection by the WW strain of Theiler's virus. Lab. Invest. **40**: 324-330.
52. WROBLEWSKA, Z., S. U. KIM, W. D. SHEFFIELD & D. H. GILDEN. 1979. Growth of the WW strain of Theiler's virus in mouse central nervous system organotypic culture. Acta. Neuropathol. (Berl.) **47**: 13-19.
53. GRAVES, M. C., L. BOLOGA, L. SIEGEL & H. LONDE. 1986. Theiler's virus in brain cell cultures: Lysis of neurons and oligodendrocytes and persistence in astrocytes and macrophages. J. Neurosci. Res. **15**: 491-501.
54. RODRIGUEZ, M., D. HOVANEC-BURNS, L. SIEGEL & M. GRAVES. 1986. Cultured glial cells express Theiler's virus-associated antigen on their surfaces (abstract). Ann. Neurol. **20**: 143.
55. BRAHIC, M., W. G. STROOP & J. R. BARINGER. 1981. Theiler's virus persists in glial cells during demyelinating disease. Cell **26**: 123-128.
56. CHAMORRO, M., C. AUBERT & M. BRAHIC. 1986. Demyelinating lesions due to Theiler's virus are associated with ongoing central nervous system infection. J. Virol. **57**: 992-997.
57. AUBERT, C., M. CHAMORRO & M. BRAHIC. 1987. Identification of Theiler's virus infected cells in the central nervous system of mice during demyelinating disease. Microbiol. Pathogen. **31**: 319-326.
58. LUDWIN, S. K. 1981. Pathology of demyelination and remyelination. In Waxman, S. G. & Ritchie, J. M., Eds. Demyelinating Diseases: Basic and Clinical Electrophysiology. Advances in Neurology, Vol. 31: 123-168. Raven Press, New York.
59. LANG, W., M. RODRIGUEZ, V. A. LENNON & P. W. LAMPERT. 1984. Demyelination and remyelination in murine viral encephalomyelitis. Ann. N. Y. Acad. Sci. **436**: 98-102.
60. LUDWIN, S. K. 1978. Central nervous system demyelination and remyelination in the mouse. An ultrastructural study of cuprizone toxicity. Lab. Invest. **39**: 597-612.

61. DAL CANTO, M. C. & R. L. BARBANO. 1984. Remyelination during remission in Theiler's virus infection. Am. J. Pathol. **116:** 30-45.
62. RAINE, C. S. & U. TRAUGOTT. 1983. Chronic relapsing experimental autoimmune encephalomyelitis: Ultrastructure of the central nervous system of animals treated with combinations of myelin components. Lab. Invest. **48:** 275-284.
63. LANG, W., C. WILEY & P. LAMPERT. 1985. Theiler's virus encephalomyelitis is unaffected by treatment with myelin components. J. Neuroimmunol. **9:** 109-113.
64. RODRIGUEZ, M., V. A. LENNON, E. N. BENVENISTE & J. E. MERRILL. 1987. Remyelination by oligodendrocytes stimulated by antiserum to spinal cord. J. Neuropathol. Exp. Neurol. **46:** 84-95.

WORKSHOP 1. IMMUNOGENETICS AND GENE REGULATION

# Brain Transplantation in Genetic Analysis of Experimental Allergic Encephalomyelitis[a]

FRED D. LUBLIN, ROBERT L. KNOBLER,
JOSEPH MARINI, AND DAN GOLDOWITZ

*Division of Neuroimmunology
Department of Neurology and Department of Anatomy
Jefferson Medical College
Thomas Jefferson University
Philadelphia, Pennsylvania 19107*

Experimental allergic encephalomyelitis (EAE) is an organ-specific autoimmune disorder of the central nervous system (CNS), induced in susceptible strains of mammalian species by immunization with CNS antigens in appropriate adjuvants.[1] This cell-mediated immune response is under genetic control. In the mouse, disease susceptibility is multigenic, with at least one gene for susceptibility residing in the H-2 region (the mouse major histocompatibility complex).[2] The SJL mouse is highly susceptible to induction of EAE, whereas the B10.S mouse is resistant, despite sharing the same H-2 region as the SJL. In previous experiments, using bone marrow transplantation, we showed that the B10.S immune system in an SJL host is capable of mediating EAE, whereas an SJL immune system in a B10.S host had limited capacity to induce EAE.[3,4] This finding suggested that the genetic restriction to development of EAE was being expressed at sites other than the immune system. To investigate if genetic restrictions to development of EAE are expressed in the components of the CNS, we performed fetal brain transplants to the anterior eye chamber between EAE-susceptible SJL and EAE-resistant B10.S mice. Prior studies have demonstrated that these transplants are viable and can, when from a suitable strain, develop pathologic signs of EAE when immunized[5] (FIG. 1).

Host mice bearing either a syngeneic or allogeneic transplant responded to induction of EAE as did mice without brain transplants. SJL mice with either an SJL or B10.S brain transplant *in oculo* had a high incidence of both clinical signs of EAE and pathologic signs of CNS inflammatory demyelination in their native brain and spinal cord. B10.S mice had a low incidence of clinical and pathologic signs of EAE and were unaffected by the presence of a brain transplant *in oculo*.

In experiments with syngeneic brain transplants, the response of the transplants to immunization for EAE was similar to that of native CNS tissue. Thus, SJL brain tissue transplanted into SJL mice had a high incidence of pathologic signs of EAE,

---

[a] This work was supported by Research Grants 1RO1 NS23081-01A1 from NIH/NINCDS and RG 1801-A-3 from the National Multiple Sclerosis Society, and NINCDS Teacher-Investigator Development Award NS 00961.

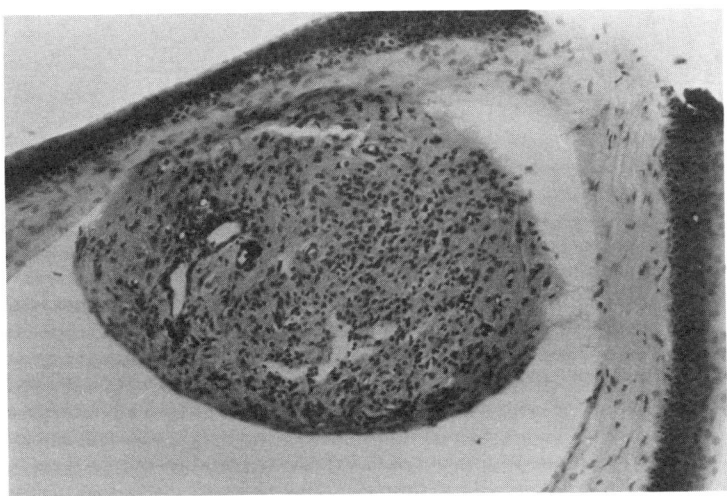

**FIGURE 1.** A photomicrograph of a paraffin section through a mature brain transplant into the anterior eye chamber 2 weeks following immunization for EAE. Perivascular cuffs of inflammatory cells that invade the surrounding tissue are visualized. (Hematoxylin and eosin stain; original magnification × 180. Reduced by 38%.)

whereas B10.S brain tissue transplanted into B10.S mice had a low incidence of EAE. When SJL brain tissue was transplanted into B10.S mice, the incidence of pathologic signs of EAE following immunization with CNS antigens was low, as seen in the B10.S host. When B10.S brain tissue was transplanted into SJL mice, the incidence of EAE was high, as seen in the SJL host's own brain and spinal cord (TABLE 1).

Therefore, the susceptibility of a brain transplant to EAE seems to depend on the susceptibility of the host strain rather than that of the donor. The cells of the CNS do not appear to confer susceptibility or resistance. Others have shown that the vascular endothelial cells of heterotopically transplanted brain tissue are capable of forming a blood-brain barrier. These endothelial cells arise from the host rather than the transplant.[6,7] If this is the case in the transplants described herein, then the B10.S transplant into an SJL host would have SJL endothelial cells forming its blood-brain barrier.

**TABLE 1.** Incidence of Clinical and Pathologic Signs of EAE in the CNS and Transplant of Mice with Brain Transplants

| Donor->Host | N | Clinical Signs | Pathology CNS[a] | Transplant |
|---|---|---|---|---|
| SJL->SJL | 6 | 5/6 | 6/6 (1.4) | 5/6 |
| B10.S->B10.S | 9 | 2/9 | 3/9 (0.8) | 1/9 |
| SJL->B10.S | 6 | 1/6 | 3/6 (0.4) | 1/6 |
| B10.S->SJL | 7 | 5/7 | 6/7 (1.5) | 6/7 |

[a] The pathologic score for each group is provided within parentheses.

Genetic regulation at the level of the cerebral endothelial cell might explain the high incidence of EAE in the B10.S transplant in an SJL host. Studies are underway to determine the genetic origin of the transplant endothelial cells.

## REFERENCES

1. PATERSON, P. Y. 1966. Experimental allergic encephalomyelitis and autoimmune disease. Adv. Immunol. **5:** 131-208.
2. KNOBLER, R. L., D. S. LINTHICUM & M. COHN. 1985. Host genetic regulation of acute MHV-4 viral encephalomyelitis and acute experimental allergic encephalomyelitis in (BALB/cKe × SJL/J) recombinant inbred mice. J. Neuroimmunol. **8:** 15-28.
3. KORNGOLD, R., A. FELDMAN, L. ROURKE, F. LUBLIN & P. DOHERTY. 1986. Acute experimental allergic encephalomyelitis in radiation bone marrow chimeras between high and low susceptible strains of mice. Immunogenetics **24:** 309-315.
4. LUBLIN, F. D., R. L. KNOBLER, P. C. DOHERTY & R. KORNGOLD. 1986. Relapsing experimental allergic encephalomyelitis in radiation bone marrow chimeras between high and low susceptible strains of mice. Clin. Exp. Immunol. **66:** 491-496.
5. GOLDOWITZ, D., R. L. KNOBLER & F. D. LUBLIN. 1987. Heterotopic brain transplants in the study of experimental allergic encephalomyelitis. Exp. Neurol. **97:** 653-661.
6. JANZER, R. C. & M. C. RAFF. 1987. Astrocytes induce blood-brain barrier properties in endothelial cells. Nature **325:** 253-257.
7. STEWART, P. A. & M. J. WILEY. 1981. Developing nervous tissue induces formation of blood-brain barrier characteristics in invading endothelial cells: A study using quail-chick transplantation chimeras. J. Devel. Biol. **84:** 183-192.

# Molecular Identification of Regulatory DNA Sequences for Basal and Gamma-Interferon-Induced Expression of HLA DRα in Human Multiforme Glioblastoma Cell Lines

P. BASTA, P. SHERMAN, AND J. TING

*Department of Microbiology*
*University of North Carolina at Chapel Hill*
*Chapel Hill, North Carolina*

Class II major histocompatibility antigens are essential for antigen presentation and lymphocyte interactions.[1] Therefore, the timing and extent of class II antigen expression are important determining factors in the type and quality of an immune response.

Our laboratory has been interested in the expression of the human class II gene, DRα, in the brain. We and others showed that a small population of cells in the brain endogenously express or can be induced to express class II antigens by gamma-interferon (IFN-γ).[2-4] Recently our laboratory and others have begun analyzing human class II genes for regions involved in IFN-γ induction.[5,6] In this paper, we have mapped the IFN-γ induction region of the human class II gene DRα in brain cell lines to 118 base pairs (bp).

As our model system, we use human multiforme glioblastoma cell lines. We cloned putative IFN-γ regulatory sequences of DRα gene upstream to the indicator gene, chloramphenicol acetyltransferase (CAT), so that expression is driven by the DRα promoter. These recombinant plasmids were transfected into a glioblastoma cell line, U-373-MG, the cells were treated with or without IFN-γ, and the cell extracts were assayed for CAT activity. Using this technique, we previously showed that 266 (bp) of 5′ Drα sequence is sufficient to allow both basal and IFN-γ-induced expression in the glioblastoma line.

To more finely map the region(s) responsible for IFN-γ induction, we prepared a series of deletions in this 266 bp of DRα sequence (FIG. 1). Using these deletions in gene transfer experiments (TABLE 1), we concluded the following: (1) 109 bp of 5′ sequence contain the basic DRα promoter and represent the minimum amount of sequence necessary for basal expression. (2) An additional 9 bp of 5′ sequence (Δ-118) can mediate IFN-γ induction. (3) To obtain maximal induction, at most an additional 23 bp of 5′ sequence is necessary (Δ-141). (4) Sequences between −141 and −266 do not appear to contain any additional positive or negative regulatory elements. (5)

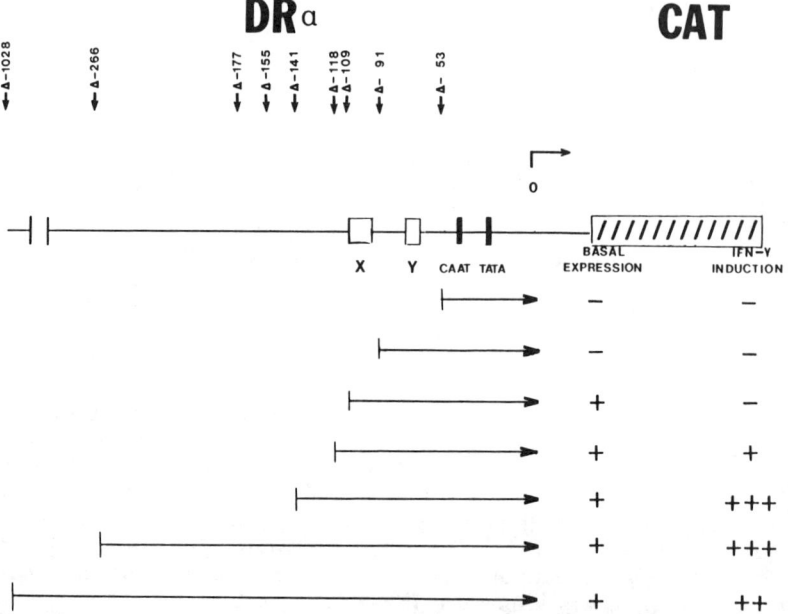

**FIGURE 1.** Map and functional analysis of DRα-chloramphenicol acetyltransferase (CAT) constructs. The 5' deletion mutants used in gene transfer analyses contained DRα sequences extending from positions indicated by *arrows* to +31 bp. Deletions are designated by *arrow* along with their nucleotide position relative to the cap site. Transcriptional regulatory elements including the conserved class II boxes (designated X and Y), a CAAT box-type sequence, a TATA box, and the start of transcription (→) are also labeled. The function of each construct in DNA-mediated gene transfer experiments is shown below the map.

TABLE 1. Basal Expression and Gamma-Interferon Induction Potential of 5' DRα Sequences

| DR-CAT Constructs | IFN-γ Treatment | Percentage of Acetylation | Fold Induction | No. of Experiments |
|---|---|---|---|---|
| 5'Δ-266[a] | − | 0.7 | 13 | 11 |
| | + | 9.2 | | |
| 5'Δ-177 | − | 0.6 | 9 | 6 |
| | + | 5.6 | | |
| 5'Δ-155 | − | 0.4 | 7 | 2 |
| | + | 2.9 | | |
| 5'Δ-141 | − | 0.9 | 8 | 5 |
| | + | 7.6 | | |
| 5'Δ-118 | − | 0.9 | 2 | 3 |
| | + | 2.1 | | |
| 5'Δ-109 | − | 0.7 | 0 | 8 |
| | + | 0.7 | | |
| 5'Δ- 91 | − | 0.1 | 0 | 2 |
| | + | 0.1 | | |
| 5'Δ- 53 | − | 0.2 | 0 | 4 |
| | + | 0.2 | | |
| pD164-2[b] | − | 0.3 | 0 | 10 |
| | + | 0.3 | | |

NOTE: Chloramphenicol acetyltransferase (CAT) analysis of eight DRα-CAT constructs from transfected and IFN-γ treated and untreated cell lines. This table represents a compilation of results from CAT assays from more than 10 transfection experiments. Percentage of acetylation was measured by cutting out appropriate sections of the thin layer chromograph and counting in scintillation fluid.

[a] Formerly designated pDR300 (Basta et al.[5]).

[b] Chloramphenicol acetyltransferase (CAT) structural gene without any known promoter (see Basta et al.[5]).

The sequence between −1028 and −266 contains negative regulatory element(s) that we are in the process of mapping.

In conclusion, we have mapped the regions of the DRα chain gene responsible for basal expression and IFN-γ induction in human multiforme glioblastomas.

## REFERENCES

1. BENACERAF, B. 1981. Science **212:** 1229.
2. TING, J. et al. 1981. Proc. Natl. Acad. Sci. USA **78:** 3170.
3. HAUSER, S. et al. 1983. J. Neuroimmunol. **5:** 197.
4. FONTANA, A. 1984. Nature **307:** 273.
5. BASTA, P. et al. 1987. J. Immunol. **138:** 1275.
6. BOSS, J. & J. STROMINGER. 1986. Proc. Natl. Acad. Sci. USA **83:** 1939.

# Generation of Antibodies to Gangliosides GM1 and GD1b

## Genetic Control of Fine Antigenic Specificity

HIROAKI ITO, ROBERT K. YU, AND
NORMAN LATOV

*Departments of Neurology
Columbia University
New York, New York*

*Yale University
New Haven, Connecticut*

Two patients with lower motor neuron disease and monoclonal gammopathy had IgM lambda M-proteins that bound to gangliosides GM1, GD1b, and asialo-GM1 and cross-reacted with human ovarian cyst blood group polysaccharides and with lacto-N-tetraose-BSA[1,2] (FIG. 1). The monoclonal antibodies are thought to bind to the Gal($\beta$1-3) GalNAc epitope shared by the three gangliosides, and with another, as yet undetermined epitope in lacto-N-tetraose. By immunofluorescence microscopy the M-proteins immunostained both gray and white matter in the spinal cord and motor endplates at the neuromuscular junction. The role of the M-proteins in the neurologic disease and their mechanism of action *in vivo* are currently under investigation.

GM1       Gal( $\beta$1-3) GalNAc( $\beta$1-4) Gal( $\beta$1-4) Glc-Cer
          |( $\alpha$2-3)
          NeuAc

ASIALO-GM1  Gal ( $\beta$1-3) Gal NAc ( $\beta$1-4) Gal( $\beta$1-4) Glc-Cer

GD1b      Gal( $\beta$1-3) GalNAc( $\beta$1-4) Gal( $\beta$1-4) Glc-Cer
          |( $\alpha$2-3)
          NeuAc
          |( $\alpha$2-3)
          NeuAc

LNT-BSA   Gal( $\beta$1-3) GlcNAc( $\beta$1-3) Gal( $\beta$1-4) Glc-BSA

**FIGURE 1.** Structures of antigens that bind to M-proteins from two patients with motor neuron disease and monoclonal gammopathy.

TABLE 1. Serum Antibodies to Gangliosides in Mice Immunized with GM1 or GD1b

| Mouse Strain | Immunizing Antigen | | Antibody Titer (Absorbance at 490 nm) | | |
|---|---|---|---|---|---|
| | | | Anti-GM1 | Anti-GD1b | Anti-Asialo-GM1 |
| BALB/cJ | GM1 | 1 | .032 | .014 | .071 |
| | | 2 | .286 | .031 | .027 |
| | | 3 | .059 | .018 | .033 |
| | | 4 | .308 | .027 | .057 |
| | | 5 | .044 | .023 | .069 |
| | GD1b | 1 | .012 | .188 | .046 |
| | | 2 | .011 | .194 | .061 |
| | | 3 | .022 | .176 | .052 |
| | | 4 | .011 | .054 | .034 |
| | | 5 | .013 | .138 | .028 |
| C57BL/6J | GM1 | 1 | .129 | .039 | .050 |
| | | 2 | .856 | .047 | .063 |
| | | 3 | .135 | .068 | .119 |
| | | 4 (died) | | | |
| | | 5 (died) | | | |
| | GD1b | 1 | .018 | .285 | .044 |
| | | 2 | .034 | .423 | .060 |
| | | 3 | .021 | .361 | .038 |
| | | 4 | .019 | .190 | .031 |
| | | 5 (died) | | | |
| DBA/2J | GM1 | 1 | .638 | .222 | .023 |
| | | 2 | .214 | .096 | .040 |
| | | 3 | .030 | .020 | .037 |
| | | 4 | .405 | .026 | .039 |
| | | 5 | .256 | .017 | .038 |
| | GD1b | 1 | .014 | .541 | .030 |
| | | 2 | .016 | .053 | .039 |
| | | 3 | .017 | .140 | .027 |
| | | 4 | .060 | .324 | .087 |
| | | 5 (died) | | | |
| Normal mouse | | | .011 | .013 | .014 |
| Patient serum | | | .941 | .622 | .927 |

NOTE: BALB/cJ, C57BL/6J, and DBA/2J strains of mice were immunized with 100 μg of gangliosides GM1 or GD1b coated onto *S. Minnesota,* twice, at 3-week intervals. Eight weeks after the first immunization, serum antibodies to GM1, GD1b, or asialo-GM1 were measured by ELISA at serum dilutions of 1:100, using antigen-coated microwells. Results are expressed as absorbance at 490 nm. As controls, serum samples from nonimmunized mice and from a patient with motor neuron disease and monoclonal gammopathy were also tested.

The two M-proteins appear to have identical specificities as defined by their cross-reactivities with the gangliosides and with lacto-N-tetraose. To investigate the occurrence of antibodies with similar specificities, we immunized BALB/cJ, C57BL/6J, and DBA/2J strains of mice with either GM1 or GD1b coated onto S. Minnesota[3] and tested their sera for reactivity by ELISA. All three mouse strains made antibodies that reacted with the immunizing ganglioside. Two of five DBA/2J mice immunized with GM1 also had significant antibody titers to GD1b (TABLE 1). Their sera, however, did not bind to asialo-GM1 or to lacto-N-tetraose-BSA.

These experiments suggest that in mice, antibodies that bind to the Gal($\beta$1-3) GalNAc epitope of gangliosides, or that cross-react with lacto-N-tetraose, are unusual. They also suggest that genetic factors may be important in determining the fine specificities and cross-reactivities of autoantibodies to ganglioside epitopes. Such factors might include the inherited repertoire of genes encoding for major histocompatibility antigens, T-cell receptors. or immunoglobulin variable regions.

## REFERENCES

1. FREDDO, L., R. K. YU, N. LATOV, P. D. DONOFRIO, A. P. HAYS, H. S. GREENBERG, J. W. ALBERS, A. G. ALLESSI, A. LEAVITT, G. DAVAR & D. KEREN. 1986. Gangliosides GM1 and GD1b are antigens for IgM M-proteins in a patient with motor neuron disease. Neurology 36: 454-458, 1986.
2. LATOV, N., A. P. HAYS, P. D. DONOFRIO, J. LIAO, H. ITO, S. MCGINNIS, K. MASNOUSSOS, L. FREDDO, M. E. SHY, W. H. SHERMAN, H. W. CHANG, H. S. GREENBERG, J. W. ALBERS, A. G. ALLESSI, D. KEREN, R. K. YU, L. P. ROWLAND & E. A. KABAT. Monoclonal IgM with unique specificity to gangliosides GM1 and GD1b and to lacto-N-tetraose associated with human neuron disease. Neurology, in press.
3. GALANOS, C., O. LUDERITZ & O. WESTPHAL. 1971. Preparation and properties of antisera against the lipid-A component of bacterial lipopolysaccharides. Eur. J. Biochem. 24: 116-122.

# Quantitation of IgG Subclasses in Cerebrospinal Fluid of Patients with Multiple Sclerosis

P. D. MEHTA

*New York State Institute for Basic Research in Developmental Disabilities*
*Staten Island, New York 10314*

Investigators[1] have used various parameters of reporting cerebrospinal fluid (CSF) IgG levels in multiple sclerosis (MS), but none included the quantitation of IgG subclasses. Human IgG is comprised of four subclasses, $IgG_1$, $IgG_2$, $IgG_3$, and $IgG_4$, which differ in their heavy chain amino acid sequences and in their biologic function. The approximate percentages of the IgG subclasses in normal adult serum are $IgG_1$, 66%; $IgG_2$, 23%; $IgG_3$, 7%; and $IgG_4$, 4%. Attempts to establish a reliable quantitative assay using polyclonal antisera have been frustrated because of the difficulty in producing specific potent antisera. In contrast, many monoclonal antibodies to IgG subclasses have been prepared and evaluated against immunoglobulins. However, their

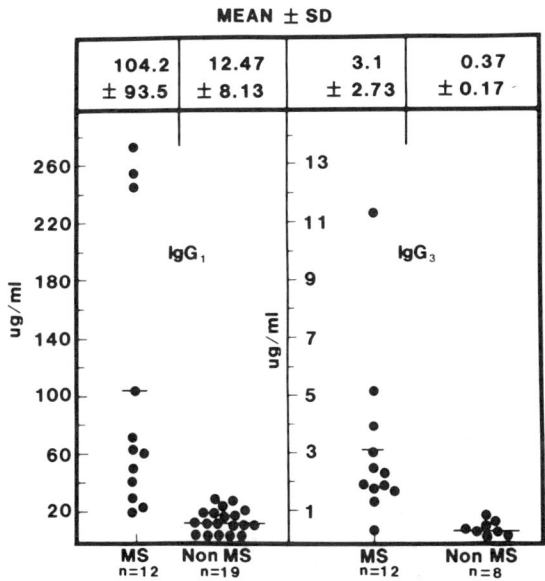

**FIGURE 1.** $IgG_1$ and $IgG_3$ subclass levels in CSF of patients with MS and non-MS controls.

TABLE 1. Cerebrospinal Fluid IgG Subclass Indexes of Patients with MS and non-MS Controls

| Group | n | $IgG_1$ | $IgG_2$ | $IgG_3$ | $IgG_4$ |
|---|---|---|---|---|---|
| MS (acute exacerbation) | 4 | $0.875 \pm 0.712^a$ | $0.613 \pm 0.287$ | $0.511 \pm 0.363^b$ | $0.207 \pm 0.092$ |
| MS (chronic progressive) | 4 | $1.002 \pm 0.485^b$ | $0.507 \pm 0.254$ | $0.440 \pm 0.257^b$ | $0.379 \pm 0.208$ |
| Non-MS controls | 6 | $0.189 \pm 0.215$ | $0.373 \pm 0.205$ | $0.128 \pm 0.059$ | $0.277 \pm 0.259$ |

NOTE: The numbers given represent the mean ± SD.
[a] $p < 0.05$ when compared with non-MS controls.
[b] $p < 0.025$ when compared with non-MS controls.

usefulness in quantitative assays for subclass levels has not been systematically applied to CSF and serum from patients with MS.

Investigators[2,3] using heterospecific antibodies reported the presence of predominant $IgG_1$ subclass in the CSF of patients with MS. The aim of our study is to determine if the findings made with the monoclonal antibodies agree with those made earlier using polyclonal antibodies. IgG subclasses in unconcentrated CSF from 12 patients with clinically definite MS and 19 non-MS control subjects were quantitated using monoclonal antibody and ELISA.[4] Briefly, monoclonal antibodies specific for $IgG_1$ (clone NL16), $IgG_2$ (clone 6014), $IgG_3$ (clone 6050), and $IgG_4$ (clone 6025) in dilutions of 1:500, 1:1000, 1:300, and 1:600, respectively, were immobilized on microtiter plates. The relevant IgG standards or diluted CSF standards were then added. A detection system based on the avidin-biotin reaction was used to enhance the sensitivity of ELISA.

The detection limits to $IgG_1$, $IgG_2$, $IgG_3$, and $IgG_4$ subclasses were 0.25, 0.04, 0.01, and 0.01 $\mu g/ml$, respectively. The mean values and SDs for $IgG_1$ and $IgG_3$ subclasses in the CSF from MS and non-MS controls are shown in FIGURE 1. The CSF values of patients with MS were significantly greater than those of non-MS controls for $IgG_1$ ($p < 0.001$) and $IgG_3$ ($p < 0.02$). The levels of $IgG_2$ and $IgG_4$, respectively, in MS (14.08 ± 9.79; 0.418 ± 0.493) and non-MS (8.1 ± 8.99; 0.044 ± 0.041) groups were not significantly different.

To show if the specific subclasses were synthesized within the CNS, their levels and albumin values were determined in matched pairs of CSF and serum from groups of patients with MS and non-MS controls. The CSF IgG index (CSF IgG ÷ Serum IgG)/(CSF albumin ÷ Serum albumin) for subclasses are given in TABLE 1. The $IgG_1$ and $IgG_3$ indexes were significantly higher in patients with MS than in non-MS controls, whereas those of $IgG_2$ and $IgG_4$ in patients with MS and non-MS controls were not significantly different. The higher $IgG_1$ and $IgG_3$ indexes found in MS are consistent with the humoral immune response of patients to viral infections.

## REFERENCES

1. CAROSCIO, J. T., S. KOCHWA, H. SACKS *et al.* 1983. Arch. Neurol. **40:** 409.
2. VANDVIK, B., J. B. NATVIG & D. WINGER. 1976. Scand. J. Immunol. **5:** 427.
3. KASCHKA, W. P., L. THEILKAES, K. EICKHOFF *et al.* 1979. Infect. Immunity **26:** 933.
4. PAPADEA, C., I. J. CHECK & C. B. REIMER. 1985. Clin. Chem. **31:** 1940.
5. SKVARIL, F. 1986. Monogr. Allergy **19:** 134.

# Gene Activation During Experimental Allergic Encephalomyelitis

## Cloning of New cDNAs

### HERMANN J. SCHLUESENER, KAI W. WUCHERPFENNIG, AND HOWARD L. WEINER

*Center for Neurologic Diseases*
*Brigham and Women's Hospital*
*Harvard Medical School*
*Boston, Massachusetts 02115*

Recently, a new version of rat experimental allergic encephalomyelitis (EAE) was established to study demyelination during autoimmune disease of the CNS. Encephalitis is induced by immunization with MBP/CFA or transfer of encephalitogenic T cells and demyelination by systemic injection of a monoclonal antibody, 8-18C5, specific for a myelin-oligodendrocyte-glycoprotein.[1-3] Antibody injection into EAE rats induces hyperacute disease progression and extensive demyelination throughout the CNS. Because lethal demyelination takes place within 24-48 hours and is spread throughout the white matter, this animal model presents a new way to study the molecular events associated with the development of autoimmune demyelinating inflammatory foci.

A significant increase in total brain RNA of up to 80% was observed in EAE rats as well as in rats treated with antibody 8-18C5 as early as day 9, even before the development of neurologic symptoms. This increase was not due to a differential increase in poly(A)$^+$ RNA, because the relative abundance of poly(A)$^+$ RNA remained unchanged. We examined if it is possible to define brain RNA species that accumulate during the development of autoimmune CNS lesions. *In vitro* translation of poly(A)$^+$ RNA indicated synthesis of distinct RNA species during antibody-mediated demyelination. Therefore, methods were established to clone cDNAs corresponding to such RNAs. A λgt11 rat brain cDNA library was differentially screened with radiolabeled ssDNA probes synthesized from poly(A)$^+$ RNA isolated from normal and demyelinating rat brains. In addition, probes were obtained by subtractive hybridization of ssDNA synthesized from poly(A)$^+$ RNA from demyelinating brains with poly(A)$^+$ RNA from normal rat brain. Sixty-two recombinant phage clones were chosen randomly for further studies. They contained cDNA inserts up to 4 kb in length. Eight of these inserts have been analyzed so far and can be grouped into two categories of homolog sequences. cDNAs of these groups were partially sequenced and do not share significant homologies with any cDNA sequence described so far. The mRNAs corresponding to these cDNAs have a similar pattern of expression during EAE: all are highly abundant during the early phase of disease, even before the appearance of neurologic signs, but decline during later stages of the disease process. This finding suggests that we have isolated two distinct cDNA clones that may encode new brain proteins associated with early phases of the EAE process.

## REFERENCES

1. LINNINGTON, C., M. WEBB & P. L. WOODHAMS. 1984. A novel myelin-associated glycoprotein defined by a mouse monoclonal antibody. J. Neuroimmunol. **6:** 387.
2. SCHLUESENER, H. J., R. A. SOBEL, C. LININGTON & H. L. WEINER. 1987. A monoclonal antibody against a myelin-oligodendrocyte glycoprotein induces relapses and demyelination in central nervous system autoimmune disease. J. Immunol. **139:** 4016.
3. SCHLUESENER, H. J., K. W. WUCHERPFENNIG & H. L. WEINER. 1987. Screening for rat brain cDNA clones as markers for gene-expression during acute demyelinating experimental allergic encephalomyelitis (EAE). J. Immunol., submitted.

# Associations of the Autoimmune Myasthenias with Genetic Markers in the Immunoglobulin Heavy Chain Region[a]

ANDY DEMAINE,[b] NICK WILLCOX,[c] KEN WELSH,[b] AND JOHN NEWSOM-DAVIS[c]

[b]Department of Human Immunogenetics
Guy's Hospital
London, England

[c]Department of Neurological Science
Royal Free Hospital School of Medicine
London, England

In inbred mice, there are many examples of heritable homogeneous antibody responses that depend on variable (V) region genes at the immunoglobulin heavy chain locus ($Ig_H$). In man, disease associations with Gm allotypes (in the heavy chain constant regions) were found in myasthenia gravis (MG) in Japanese[1] and, in Caucasians, in the Lambert-Eaton myasthenic syndrome[2] (LEMS), an autoimmune disorder of acetylcholine (ACh) release from motor nerve terminals. To test whether these associations might indicate $V_H$ susceptibility genes, perhaps encoding particular autoantibody specificities, we are typing patients for three restriction fragment length polymorphisms (RFLPs) in the $Ig_H$ region. One, in the $\mu$ chain switch region (S$\mu$), is relatively close to $V_H$, a second (S$\alpha$1) is nearer the Gm loci, and a third (D14S1) is downstream of the entire $Ig_H$ locus[3] (FIG. 1).

## RESULTS AND DISCUSSION

In the LEMS, there are significantly increased frequencies of 2.6-, 7.6-, and 10.0-kb homozygotes at S$\mu$, S$\alpha_1$, and D14S1, respectively, and of the corresponding alleles (TABLE 1). The associations are seen in patients with and without small cell lung carcinoma (though the numbers are small) and strongly support the suggestion of $Ig_H$ susceptibility genes.[2]

In old onset MG, both 2.6-kb homozygotes and the 2.6-kb allele at S$\mu$ are significantly more common than in the controls. There are no differences at the other two sites. Perhaps these patients have a predisposing gene in the variable—or D or

---

[a]This work was supported by the Medical Research Council, London, England.

TABLE 1. Restriction Fragment Length Polymorphism (RFLP) Phenotype Frequencies (%) in the Lambert-Eaton Myasthenic Syndrome (LEMS) and Myasthenia Gravis (MG) Subgroups

| Patient Group | (n) | Sμ (Sst-I) Phenotype[a] | | | Sα1 Phenotype[a] | | (Sst-I) | (n) | D14S1 (Hind III) Phenotype[a] | | |
|---|---|---|---|---|---|---|---|---|---|---|---|
| | | 2.6 | 2.6 / 2.1 | 2.1 | 7.4 | 7.4 / 6.9 | 6.9 | | 10.0 | 10.0 / 12.0 | 12.0 |
| Controls | (141) | 19.9 | 54.6 | 24.1 | 37.7 | 46.4 | 15.9 | (107) | 23.4 | 56.1 | 20.6 |
| LEMS[b] | (31) | 41.9[c] | 35.5 | 22.6 | 58.1[d] | 35.5 | 6.4 | (30) | 40.0[d] | 50.0 | 10.0 |
| MG Generalized:[b] Onset | | | | | | | | | | | |
| >40 years | (25) | 52.0[e] | 20.0 | 28.0 | 44.0 | 48.0 | 8.0 | (18) | 27.8 | 55.5 | 16.7 |
| <40 years | (39) | 33.3 | 48.7 | 17.9 | 37.5 | 45.0 | 17.5 | (26) | 50.0[d] | 38.5 | 11.5 |
| Thymoma | (17) | 29.4 | 58.8 | 11.8 | 61.5 | 38.5 | 0.0 | (6) | 33.3 | 50.0 | 16.7 |
| MG Ocular | (12) | 25.0 | 66.7 | 8.3 | 50.0 | 50.0 | 0.0 | (7) | 28.6 | 28.6 | 42.9 |

[a] Genomic DNA digested with the indicated restriction endonucleases was electrophoresed in 0.6% agarose, blotted onto nylon membranes, and hybridized to $^{32}$P-labeled probes. The Sμ probe (from clone C57RIB of Dr. T. H. Rabbitts) detects both Sμ and Sα1 RFLPs; the indicated phenotypes refer to the sizes of the bands (e.g., 2.6, 2.6 or 2.1 kb for Sμ, etc.). The D14S1 probe was kindly provided by Dr. R. White.[3]
[b] The LEMS was diagnosed on standard clinical and electrophysiologic grounds; all the generalized MG cases had detectable serum antibodies to the ACh receptor.
[c] $p < 0.01$.
[d] $p < 0.05$.
[e] $p < 0.001$ compared with controls.

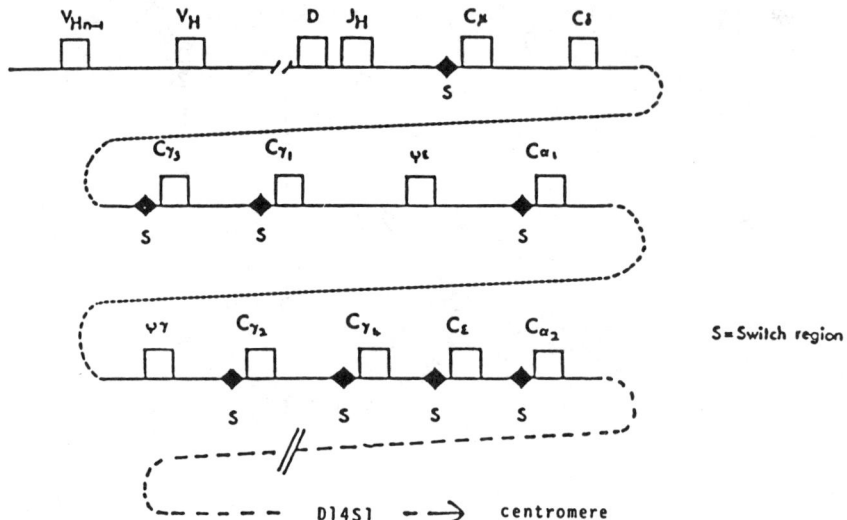

**FIGURE 1.** The human $Ig_H$ locus (chromosome 14). The most informative Gm allotype (2) is located in $C\gamma_1$. Just upstream of each functional constant (c) region gene is the relevant switch region (e.g., $S\mu$, and $S\alpha 1$).

J—regions. In young onset MG, there is also some increase in 2.6-kb homozygotes, but only the D14S1 association is significant. This immunogenetic resemblance between patients with LEMS and MG subgroups is somewhat unexpected in view of the differences in autoantibody specificity. In smaller series of MG plus thymoma, and of ocular MG, there are no significant deviations.

## REFERENCES

1. NAKAO, Y., H. MATSUMOTO, T. MIYAZAKI et al. 1980. Clin. Exp. Immunol. **42**: 20-26.
2. WILLCOX, N., A. G. DEMAINE, J. NEWSOM-DAVIS et al. 1985. Human Immunol. **14**: 29-36.
3. WYMAN, A. R. & R. WHITE. 1980. Proc. Natl. Acad. Sci. USA **77**: 6754-6758.

# Determination of RFLPs Linked to Multiple Sclerosis Susceptibility

VIVIAN H. COHN,[a] DOTY SEARS,[b] MARK HESS,[b]
RICHARD S. SPIELMAN,[c] NORMAN ARNHEIM,[b]
AND LESLIE P. WEINER[a]

[a]*Department of Neurology*
*MCH 142, U.S.C. School of Medicine*
*Los Angeles, California 90033*

[b]*Department of Biology*
*U.S.C.*
*Los Angeles, California 90008*

[c]*Department of Human Genetics*
*University of Pennsylvania, School of Medicine,*
*Philadelphia, Pennsylvania 19104*

Multiple sclerosis (MS) is a human demyelinating disease. The etiology is unknown, but evidence suggests that a genetic component influences MS susceptibility. In studies of monozygotic twins, Ebers *et al.*[1] observed a concordance rate for the development of MS of approximately 26%. Various studies suggest that the rate may be even higher. Dizygotic twins and nontwin siblings, however, displayed a much lower concordance rate of approximately 2%.

Spielman and Nathanson[2] noted an association between MS and certain human leukocyte antigen (HLA) types, especially HLA-DR2. It is of interest to examine the HLA class II region more closely to identify polymorphisms associated with susceptibility to MS. One method of studying genetic variation is to examine restriction fragment length polymorphisms (RFLPs). Analyses at the molecular level offer several advantages over serologic comparisons. Because the number of serologically defined haplotypes is currently limited, RFLPs can provide superior, highly sensitive indicators of the complexity of HLA genes. Furthermore, they may be used to study genes encoding proteins that are not expressed on the cell surface or to identify underlying differences that are silent at the protein level. In MS, RFLPs may be used to identify a polymorphism more closely associated with MS than is the serologically defined HLA-DR2 phenotype.

In this study, DNA from MS-affected or control individuals was examined for the presence of RFLPs, in linkage disequilibrium with MS, detected by HLA class II cDNA probes. The approach taken here was to pool DNA samples from approximately 50 affected or control individuals matched for HLA-DR type and ethnic origin. Pooled DNA was digested with restriction endonucleases; the fragments were separated by agarose gel electrophoresis and transferred to GeneScreen*Plus* or Genentran membranes. These blots were probed with DR beta or DQ beta cDNAs and then examined for evidence of RFLPs in linkage disequilibrium with MS. Pooling of DNA is a powerful technique, allowing rapid, simultaneous screening of many individuals. The

RFLPs in linkage disequilibrium with the disease are readily identified as bands that differ in intensity between the control and the diseased populations. Rare polymorphisms, which are not in linkage disequilibrium and are thus uninformative, are "diluted out," simplifying analysis. Controlling the composition of the two pools normalizes the expected differences between the two populations, so that observed variation reflects novel information. The approach of pooling DNA samples was successfully used previously to study the association between HLA class II loci and susceptibility to insulin-dependent diabetes mellitus (Arnheim et al.[3]). Comparison of MS and control pooled DNAs using either DR beta or DQ beta cDNA probes revealed several RFLPs in linkage disequilibrium. Because HLA-DR serologic types were distributed similarly between control and affected DNA pools, it is unlikely that the detected RFLPs reflect serologically identifiable HLA-DR differences. Thus, there appear to be HLA subtypes associated with MS susceptibility that may be distinguished by major histocompatibility complex class II cDNA probes.

## REFERENCES

1. EBERS, G. C. et al. 1986. N. Engl. J. Med. **315:** 1638.
2. SPIELMAN, R. S. & N. NATHANSON. 1982. Epidemiol. Rev. **4:** 45.
3. ARNHEIM, N. et al. 1985. Proc. Natl. Acad. Sci. **82:** 6970.

# Molecular Genotypes of the T-Cell Receptor Beta Chain in Families with Multiple Sclerosis[a]

T. A. CIULLA,[b] M. A. ROBINSON,[c] E. SEBOUN,[b]
T. H. DOOLITTLE,[b] T. HAYASHI,[b] T. J. KINDT,[c] AND
S. L. HAUSER[b]

[b]*Neuroimmunology Unit*
*Massachusetts General Hospital*
*Boston, Massachusetts*

[c]*Laboratory of Immunogenetics*
*National Institute of Allergy and Infectious Diseases*
*National Institutes of Health*
*Bethesda, Maryland*

The T-cell receptor (TCR) for antigen is a cell-surface heterodimer comprised of alpha and beta chains.[1,2] The human beta-chain gene complex, located on chromosome 7q, consists of a 600-kilobase complex that includes two constant (C) region gene segments, each with linked diversity (D) and joining (J) gene segments and approximately 60 variable (V) gene segments.[3,4] The alpha-chain gene complex consists of one C-gene segment, a cluster of J segments, and many V-gene segments, perhaps numbering greater than 100.[5]

There are several possible mechanisms whereby changes in the germline repertoire of TCR genes might confer a predisposition to autoimmunity in general or to multiple sclerosis in particular. For example, some mouse strains that are prone to autoimmune disease, including experimental allergic encephalomyelitis (EAE), have been shown to contain beta-chain deletions of either C [6] or V [7] gene segments. A deletion resulting in a reduced TCR repertoire might increase the likelihood that, during the course of a normal immune response, clones of cells that are cross-reactive to self-constituents might be activated. The presence of genotypic variations within the TCR complex might also encode molecules that react preferentially with autoantigens.

---

[a]This work was supported by grants from the National Institutes of Health (5R01-NSSS23816-02), The National Multiple Sclerosis Society, and the Upjohn Corporation. S.L.H. is a Harry Weaver Meuroscience Scholar of the National Multiple Sclerosis Society.

# TCR BETA-CHAIN HAPLOTYPES IN PATIENTS WITH MS

## Simplex (Single Affected Member) MS Families

Genotyping was performed in 27 patients with MS and their families and in 10 ethnically diverse control families using probes to both constant and variable gene segments and Southern blot/RFLP analysis of genomic DNA. Both C-region and V-region TCR beta-chain gene probes are derived from murine cDNA lines provided by Mark Davis and Phil Patten. The C-region probe is prepared from cDNA clone 86T1, a 615 bp BamHI-EcoRI fragment that corresponds to 40 bp of the V region and the entire D, J, and C regions.[8] This probe cross-hybridizes with human C-beta but not V-beta genes. (We have obtained identical results using a human C-beta probe provided by Jeff Leiden.) The V-region gene probe is prepared from cDNA clone C5 by PstI and PvuII digestion. This probe, designated V8.1, contains 250 bp of V-beta sequence.[9]

C-region restriction fragment length polymorphism (RFLP) is present following digestion of genomic DNA with BglII and permits detection of two allelic C-region fragments.[10] With a murine V8.1 probe, two allelic fragments are observed in humans following digestion with HindIII or BamHI. Thus, three polymorphisms of two allelic forms each generate a total of eight possible haplotype combinations.[10]

In FIGURE 1, a BglII digest of genomic DNA hybridized with a human C-beta probe reveals restriction fragments of 10.0 and 9.2 kb, named fragments one and two, respectively. With a murine probe V-beta 8.1, HindIII-digested DNA contains a polymorphic doublet at 19 and 20 kb, and BamHI-digested DNA polymorphic fragments at 23 and 23.5 kb. Taking advantage of these polymorphisms, it was possible to assign extended TCR-beta-chain haplotypes in families with MS. Certain assignments were possible using C-region markers, and additional haplotype assignment was possible by making the assumption of C- and V-region linkage.[10]

As shown in FIGURE 2, cumulative data are expressed as the percentage of chromosomes containing a given extended haplotype in each of three groups: (1) MS chromosomes are derived from individuals with MS; (2) Family-normal chromosomes consist of those parental chromosomes in MS families not inherited by MS offspring; and (3) Normal-normal chromosomes are parental chromosomes derived from an ethnically diverse control population.

All eight possible extended haplotypes were present in a group of 54 chromosomes derived from 27 individuals with clinically definite MS. Twenty-two percent of MS chromosomes expressed the 1-1-1 haplotype compared with 12% of control-normal chromosomes and 0 of 28 chromosomes derived from an ethnically diverse control population. There was also a tendency for the 2-1-2 haplotype to be overrepresented in the MS group compared with the control population. Neither of these results reaches statistical significance.

Extended HLA haplotypes were also derived from this population; these results are presented elsewhere (Hauser, S. L. & C. A. Alper, in preparation). It is noteworthy that, in this relatively small series, there was no evident correlation between HLA haplotype and TCR beta-chain haplotype. Thus, no clustering of TCR beta-chain haplotypes was found in the DR2-positive MS population, and the 1-1-1 beta-chain haplotype was present in patients with a variety of HLA-extended haplotypes.

## Southern Blot Analysis of BglII-Digested DNA Using a C-beta TCR Probe

C.Bg1
C.Bg2

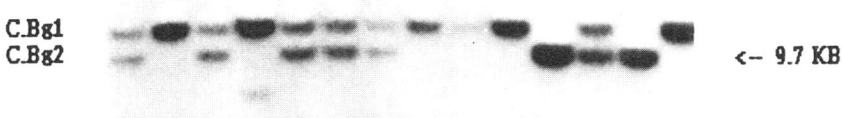

<-- 9.7 KB

## Southern Blot Analysis of HindIII-Digested DNA Using a V8.1 Probe

V8.1Hd1
V8.1Hd2

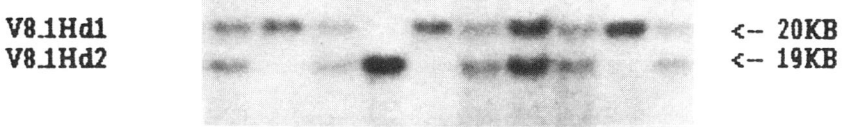

<-- 20KB
<-- 19KB

## Southern Blot Analysis of BamHI-Digested DNA Using a V8.1 Probe

V8.1Ba1
V8.1 Ba2

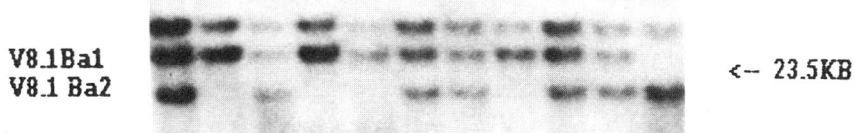

<-- 23.5KB

**FIGURE 1.** Restriction fragment length polymorphism of genomic DNA hybridized with probes to the TCR. DNA from different individuals is digested with *BglII* and hybridized with a C-beta probe (*top*). A V-beta probe reveals polymorphism following DNA digestion with *Hind*III (*middle*) and *Bam*HI (*bottom*). See text for details. The designation of each polymorphic band is given on the left side of the figure.

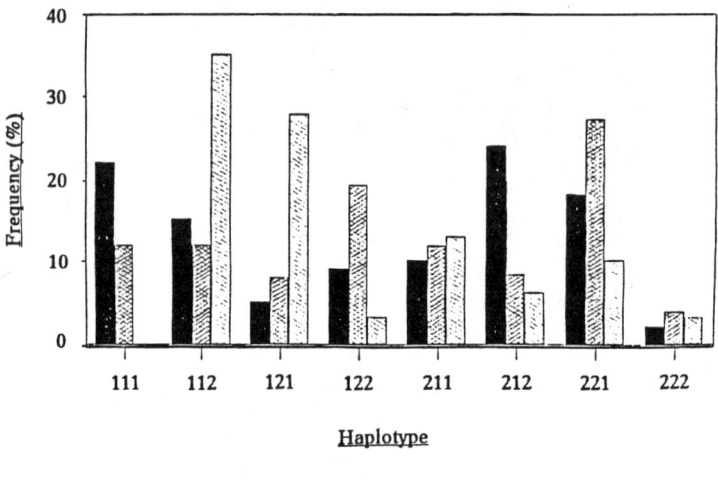

**FIGURE 2.** Distribution of the TCR beta-chain haplotypes in MS chromosomes, family-normal chromosomes, and normal-normal chromosomes. The haplotypes assignment is designated by the allelic fragment present after digestion with *Bgl*II, *Hind*III, and *Bam*HI, respectively. See text and Figure 1. Thus, CBgI, V8.1HdI is designated as the 1-1-1 haplotype, and so on.

## CONCLUSIONS

It is evident that considerable diversity of TCR beta-chain haplotypes is present in individuals with MS. Because of this diversity, larger numbers of MS and control families will need to be studied to determine if specific haplotypes of the TCR beta chain are associated with an increased risk of MS. Other polymorphic markers, in particular other V-gene segment-linked markers, as they are described, might segregate the MS population more definitely than do markers currently available. For the present, the ability to haplotype the TCR beta chain in patients with MS will make possible the analysis of co-inheritance of this gene complex in affected members of multiplex MS kindreds.

## METHODS

### Digestion of Genomic DNA with Restriction Endonuclease

High molecular weight DNA (24-48 µg) extracted from peripheral blood cells is digested with 2 U of enzyme per microgram of DNA for 4 hours at 37°C. Digestion is monitored by adding an aliquot of DNA mixture containing 2 µg of genomic DNA to 1 µg of bacteriophage lambda DNA after the second addition of enzyme.
The lambda test samples are incubated at 37°C for 4 hours, and complete digestion of lambda DNA in each sample is monitored by agarose gel electrophoresis. Digest DNA s samples are serially extracted with phenol and chloroform and then precipitated with ethanol. Precipitated DNA is resuspended in 10 mM Tris pH 7.6, 1 mM EDTA. (*Bg*lII and *Bam*HI are purchased from Bethesda Research Laboratories, Gaithersburg, Maryland, and *Hind*III from New England Biolabs, Beverly, Massachusetts.)

### Labeling of Probes

Probes are prepared by electroblotting onto DEAE paper. Probes (100-200 ng of DNA) are labeled using the random primer method and 80 µCi deoxycytidine 5'-[alpha$^{32}$p] triphosphate (3,000 Ci/mM from Amersham Corporation (Arlington Heights, Illinois) to a specific activity of approximately $10^9$ cpm/µg of DNA.

### Southern Blot Analysis

Restriction endonuclease digested DNA (10 µg/lane) is electrophoresed in 0.6% agarose gels for 36-48 hours in 40 mM tris/10 mM of sodium acetate/1 mM of EDTA brought to pH 7.2 with acetic acid. Lambda DNA digested with *Hind*III is used for size markers. Blots are prepared according to the method of Southern, using nitrocellulose filters (Millipore Corporation, Bedford, Massachusetts).
Following transfer, filters are prehybridized overnight at 42°C using probe at 3.5-5.0 $\times 10^6$ cpm/ml. After three low stringency washes at room temperature, the blots are washed twice in 15 mM of sodium citrate, pH 7.2/0.5% NaDodSo$_4$ at 50°C for 30 minutes. Blots are exposed for 24-72 hours to Kodak Xomat AR film at −70°C using Dupont Lightning Plus Screens.

## REFERENCES

1. HEDRICK, S. M., D. I. COHEN, E. A. NIELSEN & M. M. DAVIS. 1982. J. Neuroimmunol. **2:** 223-234.
2. YANAGI, Y., A. CHAN, B. CHIN et al. 1985. Proc. Natl. Acad. Sci. USA **82:** 5068-5072.

3. CONCANNON, P., L. PICKERING, P. KUNG & L. HOOD. 1986. Proc. Natl. Acad. Sci. USA **83:** 6598.
4. KIMURA, N., B. TOYONAGA, Y. YOSHIKAI et al. 1986. J. Exp. Med. **164:** 739.
5. YOSHIKAI, Y., N. KIMURA, B. TOYONAGA et al. 1986. J. Exp. Med. **164:** 90.
6. NOONAN, D. J., R. KOFLER, P. A. SINGER et al. 1986. J. Exp. Med. **163:** 644-653.
7. BEHLKE, M. A., H. S. CHOU, K. HUPPI & D. Y. LOH. 1986. Proc. Natl. Acad. Sci. USA **83:** 767-771.
8. HEDRICK, S. M., E. A. NIELSEN, J. KAVALER et al. 1984. Nature **308:** 153-158.
9. PATTEN, P., T. YOKUTA, J. ROTHBARD et al. 1984. Nature **312:** 40-46.
10. ROBINSON, M. A. & T. J. KINDT. 1986. Immunogenetics **24:** 259.

# Antibody-Producing Cells in CSF and Peripheral Blood

## A New Principle for Evaluation of B-Cell Response in Inflammatory Nervous System Diseases

H. LINK, S. BAIG, T. OLSSON, AND A. ZACHAU

*Department of Neurology*
*Karolinska Institutet*
*Huddinge University Hospital*
*S-141 86 Huddinge, Stockholm, Sweden*

Determinations of the concentrations of immunoglobulins (Ig) and specific antibodies (Ab) of different isotypes have several limitations that reduce their validity: (1) Concentrations in cerebrospinal fluid (CSF) depend on the functional status of the blood-brain barrier, the level of Ig or Ab in serum, and local production within the CSF-CNS compartment. (2) Results are influenced by the half-life and catabolism of Ab molecules that vary among different classes and subclasses of Ig. (3) *In vivo* absorption of self-reactive Ab by circulating or tissue-bond autoantigens may interfere with their detection, as previously shown in the model of experimental allergic encephalomyelitis.[1] (4) No information is obtained on the precise anatomic location of Ab formation. These limitations may be circumvented by enumeration of cells secreting Ig and specific Ab of different isotypes in CSF and peripheral blood (PB).

We previously employed the hemolytic plaque-forming cell (PFC) assay originally described in 1963 by Jerne and Nordin[2] and modified by Gronowicz *et al.*,[3] who described a PFC assay in which red blood cells were coated with staphylococcal protein A—so-called protein A PFC—for enumeration of IgG-, IgA-, and IgM-secreting cells in CSF and PB from patients with multiple sclerosis (MS) and controls. When employing this assay, we demonstrated that about 90% of patients with MS had in their CSF cells producing IgG, 70% IgA, and 57% IgM; cells producing IgG predominated in CSF in most patients, but IgM- or IgA-producing cells could also predominate; Ig-producing cells were often present in CSF when the corresponding CSF Ig index was normal, indicating that Ig-producing cell enumeration is a more sensitive variable for analysis of immune status within the CNS-CSF compared to determination of free Ig levels; patients with clinically active contra stable MS did not differ in the numbers of IgG-, IgA-, or IgM-producing cells in CSF, which favors continuous immune activity in CNS independent of clinical symptoms.[4,5]

Because of difficulties in coupling various antigens (Ag) to erythrocytes used in the hemolytic PFC assay, this has been less useful for enumeration of cells in body fluids producing specific Ab. We have adopted and modified a nitrocellulose immunospot assay, which is summarized in FIGURE 1. Nitrocellulose-bottomed microtiter plate wells were coated with relevant Ag, such as myelin or myelin basic protein (MBP) considered possible targets for immune attack in the pathogenesis of MS, and *Borrelia burgdorferi* which has been defined as the cause of Lyme disease. Mononuclear cells isolated from CSF (CSF-L) or peripheral blood (PBL) were then cultured directly in the wells for 6 hours or overnight. Secreted Ab bound to Ag were detected with secondary enzyme-labeled antisera, followed by counting of "spots" corresponding to Ab-secreting cells (FIG. 1, right). Total numbers of IgG-, IgA-, and IgM-producing cells were counted in parallel, but in nitrocellulose-bottomed microtiter plate wells initially coated with specific antiserum (FIG. 1, left). Results are presented as numbers of Ab- or Ig-secreting cells per $10 \times 10^3$ CSF-L or PBL.

We applied the nitrocellulose immunospot assay in 17 consecutive patients with clinically definite relapsing-remitting MS not treated with immunomodulatory drugs, 14 patients with other inflammatory nervous system diseases, and 19 with other neurologic disease (OND). Cells producing Ab against bovine myelin prepared according to Kadlubowski *et al.*[6] and in some instances against MBP and virions of Lec measles strain were enumerated. TABLE 1 presents the findings regarding cells producing IgG Ab in patients with MS, and TABLE 2 for the three patient groups. Cells producing IgG Ab against myelin, MBP, and measles are a regular constituent in MS CSF but are not demonstrable in PB with the occasional exception of measles

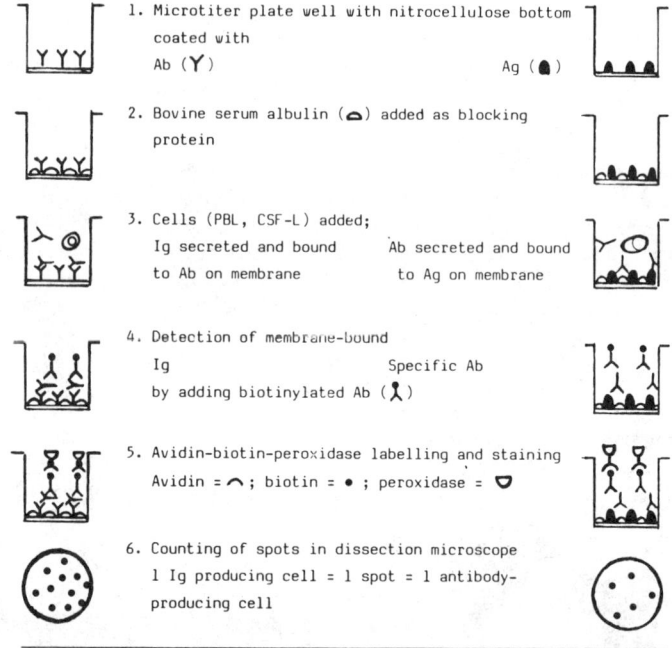

**FIGURE 1.** Schematic presentation of nitrocellulose immunospot assay for enumeration of cells producing Ig (*left*) and specific antibodies (*right*) of different isotypes. Ab = antibodies; Ag = antigen.

TABLE 1. Numbers of Cells Secreting IgG Antibodies Against Myelin, Myelin Basic Protein (MBP) and Measles Virus and Number of IgG-Producing Cells, per 10 × $10^3$ Mononuclear Cells Isolated from CSF and Peripheral Blood (PB) from 17 Patients with MS

| Patient No. | No. of Cells Producing Antibodies Against: | | | | | | No. of IgG-Producing Cells | |
|---|---|---|---|---|---|---|---|---|
| | Myelin | | MBP | | Measles | | | |
| | CSF | PB | CSF | PB | CSF | PB | CSF | PB |
| 1 | 160 | 0 | — | — | — | — | 200 | 4 |
| 2 | 20 | 0 | 6 | 0 | 6 | 2 | 10 | 1 |
| 3 | 13 | 0 | — | — | — | — | 126 | 3 |
| 4 | 10 | 0 | — | — | 2 | 0 | 10 | 2 |
| 5 | 96 | 0 | — | — | — | — | 100 | 6 |
| 6 | 47 | 0 | 36 | 0 | — | — | 14 | 1 |
| 7 | 14 | 0 | 8 | 0 | 20 | 0 | 20 | 2 |
| 8 | 40 | 0 | 5 | 0 | 22 | 0 | 34 | 1 |
| 9 | 3 | 0 | — | — | — | — | 143 | 7 |
| 10 | 33 | 0 | — | — | — | — | 140 | 11 |
| 11 | 25 | 0 | — | — | 0 | 2 | 27 | 4 |
| 12 | 56 | 0 | — | — | — | — | 90 | 3 |
| 13 | 20 | 0 | — | — | 26 | 0 | 48 | 1 |
| 14 | 16 | 0 | — | — | 5 | 0 | 30 | 1 |
| 15 | 14 | 0 | — | — | — | — | 34 | 2 |
| 16 | 22 | 0 | — | — | — | — | 43 | 2 |
| 17 | 35 | 0 | — | — | 20 | 0 | 50 | 5 |

IgG Ab-producing cells. Cells producing myelin IgG Ab predominated and constituted a substantial proportion of the total number of IgG-producing cells in MS CSF. Cells producing myelin Ab of IgA and IgM isotypes were rarely encountered in MS CSF. Interestingly, no cells producing antimyelin or anti-MBP antibodies were demonstrable in peripheral blood.

The occurrence of myelin Ab secreting cells in CSF was not a finding specific for MS, but was also observed in some patients with other inflammatory nervous system diseases (two with neurosyphilis who had cells secreting myelin Ab of all three isotypes; two patients with aseptic meningoencephalitis; and one with the Guillain-Barré syndrome) and also in three among the OND patients (one with hysterical monoparesis, one with oculomotor palsy, and one with epilepsy). These three patients had all oligoclonal IgG bands in CSF and also in serum, probably reflecting a systemic humoral immune response. Among the controls, measles Ab-producing cells were detected in the CSF of only one patient who had aseptic meningitis. Another reference material consisting of patients with aseptic meningoencephalitis had in the CSF cells producing IgG Ab against myelin and MBP at a frequency of only about 30% and comprising only about 10% of IgG producing cells. Our data thus indicate that intrathecal production of Ab against myelin and MBP occurs in MS at a higher frequency than that anticipated previously on the basis of the results from determinations of free Ab levels in CSF,[7] and necessitates a reevaluation of the possible importance of these Ab in the pathogenesis of MS.

Of seven consecutive patients with neuroborreliosis, all had in their CSF cells secreting specific Ab of IgG, IgA, and IgM class. Surprisingly, no such cells were demonstrable in peripheral blood. Thus, the specific B-cell response in these patients seems also to be highly sequestrated to the CNS-CSF compartment. The specificity of *B. burgdorferi* Ab secreting cells enumerated in CSF and peripheral blood was evaluated in 14 controls. Five displayed cells producing *B. burgdorferi* Ab in CSF but never in peripheral blood. Two of them had neurosyphilis, two the Guillain-Barré syndrome, and one Sjögren's syndrome. ELISA revealed marginal elevation of IgM Ab against *B. burgdorferi* in one patient with the Guillain-Barré syndrome, with otherwise normal values. These data, although preliminary, indicate that the three latter patients may in fact have neurologic diseases due to *B. burgdorferi* infection despite normal serology, whereas the positive results in neurosyphilis most probably

TABLE 2. Numbers of Patients with Multiple Sclerosis (MS), Other Inflammatory Nervous System Diseases, and Other Neurologic Disorders (OND) with Cells Secreting Antibodies of Different Classes Against Myelin, Myelin Basic Protein (MBP), and Measles Virus in CSF and Peripheral Blood (PB) per $10 \times 10^3$ Mononuclear Cells[a]

| Diagnosis | | Myelin | | MBP | | Measles | |
|---|---|---|---|---|---|---|---|
| | | CSF | PB | CSF | PB | CSF | PB |
| Multiple sclerosis | IgG | 16 | 0 | 4 (4) | 0 (4) | 7 (8) | 2 (8) |
| ($n = 17$) | IgA | 1 (15) | 0 | 0 (1) | 0 (4) | 0 (7) | 1 (8) |
| | IgM | 1 (14) | 1 | — | 0 (3) | 0 (5) | 0 (7) |
| Other inflammatory | IgG | 5 | 0 | — | — | 1 (6) | 0 (6) |
| nervous system | IgA | 2 | 0 | — | — | 0 (5) | 0 (5) |
| diseases ($n = 14$) | IgM | 2 (13) | 0 | — | — | 0 (5) | 0 (5) |
| Other neurologic | IgG | 3 | 0 | — | — | 0 (17) | 1 (17) |
| disease ($n = 19$) | IgA | 0 | 0 | — | — | 0 (18) | 0 (18) |
| | IgM | 0 | 0 | — | — | 0 (4) | 0 (4) |

[a] Numbers within brackets denote numbers of patients examined.

reflect the well-known cross-reactivity between antibodies against *B. burgdorferi* and those against *Treponema pallidum*. The proportion of cells producing specific Ab usually amounted to 20-30% of the total number of cells producing Ig of corresponding isotype.

In conclusion, the evaluation of B-cell immune response as reflected by numbers of Ab-producing cells enumerated by a nitrocellulose immunospot assay is a sensitive tool that might be used supplementary to conventional determinations of levels of free antibodies in body fluids. In MS, a B-cell response against myelin is demonstrable in CSF more frequently when analyzed at the cellular level than by determinations of free myelin antibody concentrations. In infectious nervous system diseases, evaluation of antibody production at the cellular level might have diagnostic potential in conjunction with conventional serology.

## REFERENCES

1. OLSSON T., A. HENRIKSSON & H. LINK 1985. J. Neuroimmunol. **9:** 293.
2. JERNE, K. & A. A. NORDIN 1963. Science **140:** 405
3. GRONOWICCZ, E., A. COUTINHO & F. MELCHERS 1976. Eur. J. Immunol. **6:** 588.
4. HENRIKSSON, A., S. KAM-HANSEN & R. ANDERSSON 1981. J. Neuroimmunol. **1:** 299.
5. HENRIKSSON, A., S. KAM-HANSEN & H. LINK 1985. Clin. Exp. Immunol. **62:** 176.
6. KADLUBOWSKI, M., R. A. HUGHES & N. A. GREGSON 1980. Brain Res. **148:** 439.
7. CRUZ, M., T. OLSSON, J. ERNERUDH, B. HÖJEBERG & H. LINK 1987. Neurology **37:** 1515.

# Bone Marrow Cells in Multiple Sclerosis

## A Functional and Phenotypic Study

### S. KAM-HANSEN, S. FREDRIKSON, AND C.-Z-LU

*Department of Neurology*
*Karolinska Institutet*
*Huddinge University Hospital*
*Stockholm, Sweden*

Immune mechanisms are thought to be involved in the pathogenesis of multiple sclerosis (MS).[1] Multiple sclerosis is usually classified as an autoimmune disorder, mostly because of certain similarities with the animal model, experimental allergic encephalitis (EAE). Bone marrow may be the site of immune reactions in autoimmune diseases with remote organ pathology.[2]

To investigate if there were signs of bone marrow activation in patients with MS, we studied the morphology, phenotypes, and proliferative response of cells from bone marrow.

## MATERIAL AND METHODS

Thirteen patients (seven female) with clinically definite MS were studied. Six patients undergoing orthopedic surgery because of scoliosis but who were otherwise healthy served as the controls. None showed any signs of infection.

In bone marrow smears differential counting (200 cells) was performed and the ratio of myeloic maturation estimated. Mononuclear cells from bone marrow and peripheral blood were isolated by density gradient centrifugation. Immunochemical staining was performed with monoclonal antibodies[3] as described in TABLE 1.

Proliferative response of mononuclear cells was measured by incorporation of $^3$H-thymidine in cells cultured in microtiter plates with optimal concentrations of phytohemagglutinin (PHA), interleukin-2 (IL-2), PHA + IL-2, or without mitogens. Cultures were harvested from day 1 to day 5.[4]

TABLE 1. Monoclonal Antibodies Used for Phenotypic Characterization of Mononuclear Cells

| Monoclonal Antibody | Predominant Reactivity |
|---|---|
| Leu 2 | Cytotoxic/suppressor T cell |
| Leu 3 | Helper/inducer T cell |
| OKT10 | Lymphoid and myeloic precursor cell, pre-T cell, activated mature lymphocyte |
| HLA-DR | B cell, monocyte, activated T cell |
| OKM1 | Monocyte, macrophage, granulocyte |
| OKB7 | B cell |

## RESULTS

Morphologic observations in each patient are summarized in TABLE 2. In 5 of 11 MS patients, bone marrow showed mild to moderate morphologic signs of activation.

Results from phenotypic characterization are presented in FIGURE 1. OKT10-positive cells were significantly higher in the peripheral blood of MS patients than in the controls ($p < 0.001$).

Bone marrow mononuclear cells (BM-MNC) of MS patients exhibited higher spontaneous proliferation than did BM-MNC from the controls ($p < 0.01$, days 1-5),

TABLE 2. Results from Studies of Bone Marrow Morphology in Patients with Multiple Sclerosis (MS) Given As Percentage of 200 Cells Counted

| Patient No. | Sex | Age (yr) | Disease Activity | Myeloic Maturation Ratio (0.2-0.4) | Lymphocytes (3-17) | Monocytes (<5) | Plasma Cells (<2) |
|---|---|---|---|---|---|---|---|
| 1[a] | Male | 25 | Exacerbation | 0.4 | 14 | 3 | 1 |
| 1a[a] | Male | 25 | Remission | 0.6 | 19 | 3 | 3 |
| 2 | Female | 24 | Exacerbation | 0.4 | 12 | 3 | 1 |
| 3 | Female | 34 | Remission | 0.2 | 16 | 4 | 0 |
| 4 | Female | 23 | Exacerbation | 0.5 | 19 | 6 | 0 |
| 5 | Male | 32 | Remission | 0.4 | 17 | 2 | 1 |
| 6 | Male | 39 | Chronic progressive | 0.5 | 16 | 6 | 1 |
| 7 | Female | 24 | Exacerbation | 0.3 | 12 | 4 | 0 |
| 8 | Female | 21 | Exacerbation | 0.6 | 10 | 4 | 3 |
| 9 | Female | 40 | Remission | 0.5 | 17 | 4 | 0 |
| 10 | Female | 31 | Remission | 0.4 | 21 | 3 | 2 |
| 11 | Male | 36 | Exacerbation | 0.6 | 18[b] | 5 | 1 |

NOTE: Myeloic maturation ratio refers to the ratio between the number of myeloblasts, promyelocytes, and myelocytes and more mature forms including metamyelocytes and granulocytes with staff or segmented nucleus. Numbers within brackets show reference values. nd = not done.

[a] The same patient examined twice within a 7-month interval.
[b] Lymphoid infiltrate.

higher PHA-induced proliferation ($p < 0.01$, days 3-5), and higher PHA + IL-2 induced proliferation ($p < 0.05$, days 4 and 5) (FIG. 2).

Spontaneous proliferation of BM-MNC compared with peripheral blood lymphocytes (PBL) in patients with MS was much higher ($p < 0.001$, days 1-5). When only IL-2 was added, BM-MNC also responded stronger than did PBL ($p < 0.01$, day 1). No such difference was seen in the controls. In contrast, the addition of PHA + IL-2 resulted in much higher proliferation of PBL than of BM-MNC in MS patients ($p < 0.001$, days 2-4). In the controls, the addition of PHA, PHA + IL-2, or IL-2 resulted in higher proliferation of PBL than of BM-MNC.

## CONCLUSIONS

We conclude that in patients with MS—a disease with pathology and symptoms strictly confined to the central nervous system—*in vivo* activated mononuclear cells are present in the bone marrow. The positive response of bone marrow mononuclear cells to IL-2 indicates that at least a part of these *in vivo* activated cells in MS are T cells. This finding so far is unexplained. However, if MS is caused by a lymphotropic agent, such as a retrovirus (RV), RV can be stored in the bone marrow throughout the patient's life. Activation of the immune system by different agents could result in

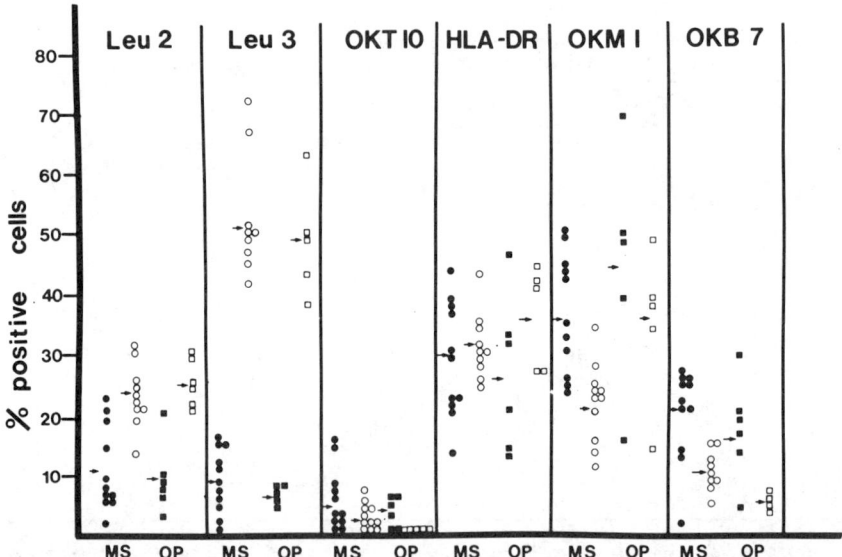

**FIGURE 1.** Percentage of cells stained with different monoclonal antibodies in patients with multiple sclerosis (MS, ●-bone marrow, ○-peripheral blood) and control patients operated on for scoliosis but otherwise healthy (OP, ■-bone marrow, □-peripheral blood). *Arrows* indicate mean values.

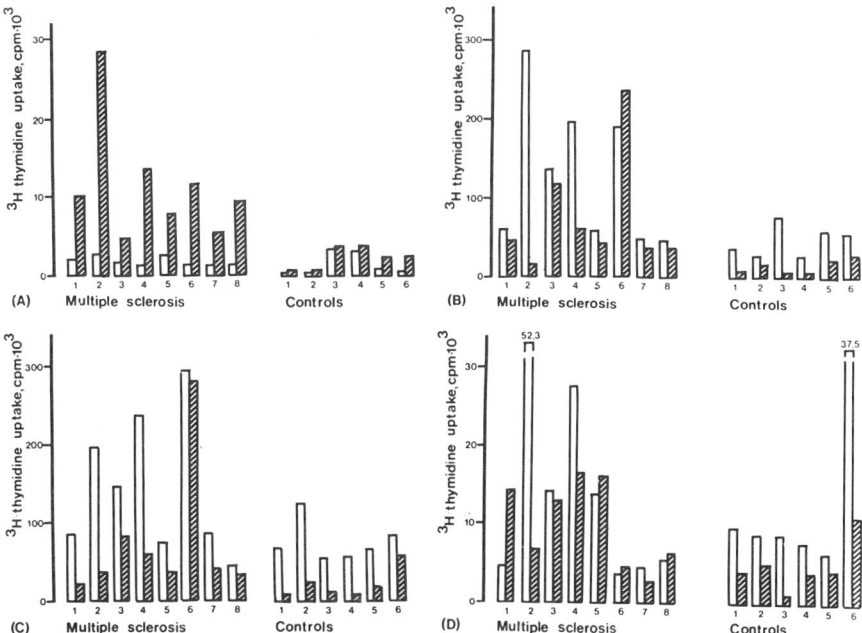

**FIGURE 2.** Proliferative response of peripheral blood lymphocytes (*unfilled bars*) and mononuclear cells from bone marrow (*filled bars*) from eight patients with multiple sclerosis and six subjects control operated on for scoliosis. (**A**) Spontaneous proliferation; proliferations after stimulation with (**B**) PHA, (**C**) PHA and IL-2, and (**D**) IL-2 are shown on day 4, when the responses were highest.

an increase in RV-infected cells which in an activated state can enter the CNS.[5] A presumed neurotropism of this virus could have deleterious effects on the CNS by provoking an immune response that could even destroy the trace of the etiologic agent.

## REFERENCES

1. REDER, A. T. & B. G. W. ARNASON. 1985. *In* Handbook of Clinical Neurology, Vol 3. J. C. Koetsier, Ed. (47) Demyelinating Diseases. Elsevier, Amsterdam: 337-395.
2. FAUCI, A. S. & H. M. MOUTSOPOULOS. 1981. Arth. & Rheumat. **24:** 577.
3. KARLSSON-PARRA, A., U. FORSUM, L. KLARESKOG & O. SJOBERG. 1983. J. Immunol. Meth. **64:** 85-90.
4. FREDRIKSSON, S., S. KAM-HANSEN, C.-Z. LU & L. ERIKSSON. 1988. Submitted.
5. WEKERLE, H., C. LININGTON, H. LASSMAN & R. MEYERMANN. 1986. Trends Neurol. Sci. June: 271.

# Intrathecal Antimeasles Immunity in 140 Patients with Multiple Sclerosis[a]

E. SCHULLER,[b] E. RUZICKA,[c] B. ALLINQUANT,[b]
P. LEBON,[d] A. GOVAERTS,[e] AND J. D. DEGOS[f]

[b]*INSERM U 134*
*Hôpital de la Salpêtriére*
*Paris, France*

[c]*Service de Neurologie*
*Université Charles*
*Prague, Czechoslovakia*

[d]*INSERM U 43*
*Hôpital Saint-Vincent-de-Paul*
*Paris, France*

[e]*Collége de France*
*Paris, France*

[f]*Hôpital Henri Mondor*
*Créteil, France*

Antimeasles intrathecal immunity was analyzed from paired serum and CSF samples of 140 patients with definite multiple sclerosis (MS) (all HLA typed) and compared with paired samples of 18 patients with subacute sclerosing panencephalitis (SSPE) and 27 other neurologic diseases. Intrathecal syntheses of immunoglobulins A, G, and M were calculated using formulas previously described.[1] Complement component (C3, C4, and C3 proA) decreases were also calculated, comparing expected and observed values. Measles and rubella antibodies were determined by HIA and herpes by a neutralization test. The ratio reciprocal of serologic titer/IgG concentration (antibody specific activity, ASA) was calculated in serum and in intrathecally produced IgG as:

$$\text{intrathecal ASA} = \frac{\text{CSF ASA} - (\text{Serum ASA} \times \text{percentage of plasmatic Ig})}{(\text{percentage of intrathecal Ig})}$$

[a]This research was supported by the Institut National de la Santé et de la Recherche Médicale (INSERM) and the Association pour la Recherche sur la Sclérose en Plaques (ARSEP).

TABLE 1. Antiviral Antibodies in the CSF of 140 MS Patients

|  | Antimeasles Antibodies | |
|---|---|---|
|  | Absent (70) | Present (70) |
| Measles only |  | 38 |
| Rubella | 9 | 19 |
| Herpes[a] | 3 | 3 |
| Rubella + herpes | 0 | 10 |

[a] Herpes in 98 patients only.
Statistics:
Measles/rubella: $p < 0.001$
Rubella/herpes: $p < 0.001$
Measles/herpes: $p < 0.05$

## RESULTS

The results are summarized in TABLES 1 to 4.

## DISCUSSION

1. *Intrathecal antimeasles ASA* found in 70 MS patients only and in all SSPE patients (TABLE 3) was:

TABLE 2. CSF Immunity Proteins in 140 Patients with Multiple Sclerosis (MS) and 18 with Subacute Sclerosing Panencephalitis (SSPE)

| Antibody-Specific Activity: | Intrathecal Antimeasles MS | | SSPE Present (18) |
|---|---|---|---|
|  | Absent (70) | Present (70) |  |
| *Intrathecal synthesis* |  |  |  |
| IgG | 51[a] | 69[a] | 18 |
| IgA | 4 | 4 | 1 |
| IgM | 9 | 11 | 2 |
| C3 | 5 | 6 | 2 |
| C4 | 7 | 11 | 4 |
| C3 proA | 15 | 15 | 0 |
| *Decrease* |  |  |  |
| C3 | 18[b] | 33[b] | 2 |
| C4 | 4 | 3 | 1 |
| C3 proA | 6 | 6 | 0 |

[a] $p < 0.001$.
[b] $p < 0.01$.

TABLE 3. Serum, CSF, and Intrathecal Antimeasles Antibody-Specific Activity in 70 Patients with Multiple Sclerosis (MS) and 18 Patients with Subacute Sclerosing Panencephalitis (SSPE)

|  | MS (70) | SSPE (18) |
|---|---|---|
| Serum ASA | $10.5 \pm 0.8^a$ | $22 \pm 9$ |
| CSF ASA | $32.5 \pm 3.5^a$ | $127 \pm 5.6^a$ |
| Intrathecal ASA | $90.2 \pm 15^a$ | $155 \pm 71$ |
| Ratio of intrathecal ASA/serum | 8.6 | 6.4 |
| IgG IS$^b$ (mg/l) | $55 \pm 6^b$ | $207 \pm 58^b$ |
| Correlations $(r)^c$ |  |  |
| Serum ASA/intrathecal ASA | 0.14 | $0.98^a$ |
| Intrathecal ASA/IgG IS | $-0.42^a$ | $-0.13$ |

$^a p < 0.001.$
$^b p < 0.01.$
$^c$ IS = intrathecal synthesis.

- 6 to 9 times higher than serum ASA
- not significantly different in both
- not correlated to serum ASA in MS, but significantly correlated in SSPE
- negatively correlated to the amount of intrathecal IgG in both, a fact suggesting a specific immune answer.

In other neurologic diseases intrathecal antimeasles ASA was observed in seven patients only, all affected by an infectious disease. No correlation with HLA type was found in MS patients.

2. An *intrathecal C3 decrease* was selectively (not observed with rubella or herpes intrathecal ASA) and significantly (0.01) linked to this intrathecal antimeasles ASA in MS and not to a more or less important intrathecal IgG synthesis (TABLE 4).

TABLE 4. Intrathecal Antimeasles ASA and C3 Decrease in 140 Patients with Multiple Sclerosis

|  | Intrathecal Antimeasles ASA | |
|---|---|---|
|  | Absent (70) | Present (70) |
| C3 decrease (51) | $18^a$ | $33^a$ |
| IgG IS$^b$ (mg/l) | $46 \pm 10$ | $50 \pm 6$ |

$^a p < 0.01.$
$^b$ IS = intrathecal synthesis.

CONCLUSION: In MS patients C3 decrease is not linked to the amount of IgG intrathecally produced, but to the presence of intrathecal measles ASA.

## CONCLUSION

These arguments favor a strong intrathecal stimulation by measles or cross-reactive antigens inside the CNS in half of our MS patients, which is not significantly different from that observed in SSPE. The only difference is the correlation between serum and intrathecal ASA observed in SSPE but not in MS, a fact suggesting that measles infection is a general process only in SSPE.

### REFERENCE

1. SCHULLER, E., S. BENABDALLAH, H. J. SAGAR, J. REBOUT L. Tömpe. 1987. IgG synthesis within the central nervous system. Arch. Neurol. **44:** 600-604.

# Autoantibodies in Serum and CSF of Patients with Multiple Sclerosis

A. BLANCHER,[a] P. MATSIOTA,[b] B. GUILBERT,[c]
B. DOYON,[d] M. CLANET,[a] E. KOUVELAS,[e]
A. RASCOL,[a] AND S. AVRAMEAS[c]

[a]*Department of Neurology*
*CHU Purpan*
*31059 Toulouse Cédex, France*

[b]*Department of Medicine*
*University of Patras*
*Patras, Greece*

[c]*Unité d'Immunocytochimie*
*Institut Pasteur*
*Paris, France*

[d]*Unité 230 INSERM*
*Toulouse, France*

[e]*Physiological Laboratory*
*Faculty of Medicine*
*Patras, Greece*

The intrablood-brain barrier (BBB) synthesis of immunoglobulins (Igs) is a well-known feature of multiple sclerosis (MS). However, the specificity of these Igs is still unclear. In previous studies we demonstrated the presence of natural autoantibodies (Nab) in the sera of healthy individuals directed against common antigens.[1]

In this study we attempted to determine the intra-BBB production of antibodies against a panel of 12 antigens. Statistical comparisons were made from the results obtained in three groups: group 1, 38 patients with MS; group II, 42 patients with other neurologic diseases (OND); and group III, 9 control individuals (CONT).

Antibodies against a panel of 12 antigens were investigated by enzyme immunoassay (EIA) in the sera and CSF of patients in three groups. The following antigens were used: actin (calf striated muscle), tubulin (pig brain), myosin (calf), myoglobin (whale skeletal muscle), DNA (from Sigma), myelin basic protein (guinea pig), thyroglobulin (pig), prolactin (man), transferrin (man), albumin (man), peroxidase (horseradish), and $TNP_{25}$/BSA (prepared as described by Little and Eisen).

These antigens were selected because they are highly conserved during evolution (actin, tubulin, myosin, myoglobin, DNA, MBP, and thyroglobulin) or because they are related to self (prolactin, transferrin, and albumin) or non-self antigens (TNP and peroxidase). The EIA was performed as previously described.[2,3] A pool of 10 normal sera was considered the reference standard and was tested under the same conditions as those used for patients' sera or CSF. The values obtained by EIA with a given sample at a given dilution and with a given antigen were compared with the

TABLE 1. Comparison of Index (I) of Intra-BBB Antibody Production

| Antibodies against: | MS | | | OND | | | CONT | | | Analysis of Variance ($p$) | Kruskall and Wallis ($p$) |
|---|---|---|---|---|---|---|---|---|---|---|---|
| | N | M | SD | N | M | SD | N | M | SD | | |
| Thyroglobulin | 18 | 4.8 | 2.9 | 12 | 2.6 | 2.0 | 6 | 4 | 4.5 | NS | <0.05 |
| TNP | 36 | 3.1 | 1.8 | 39 | 1.8 | 1.5 | 9 | 2.0 | 0.9 | <0.01 | <0.01 |
| Tubulin | 37 | 3.2 | 2.5 | 42 | 1.8 | 1.0 | 9 | 2.4 | 1.8 | <0.01 | <0.05 |
| Myoglobin | 18 | 5.2 | 4.0 | 15 | 2.7 | 2.4 | 6 | 2.4 | 3.0 | NS | NS |
| Albumin | 18 | 6.5 | 5.4 | 12 | 4.2 | 4.1 | 6 | 2.5 | 1.4 | NS | NS |
| Myosin | 35 | 3.7 | 3.2 | 41 | 2.2 | 1.9 | 9 | 2.3 | 1.6 | <0.05 | <0.05 |
| Actin | 23 | 3.5 | 2.5 | 27 | 2.0 | 1.6 | 6 | 1.9 | 0.9 | <0.05 | NS |
| DNA | 33 | 2.8 | 2.3 | 36 | 2.0 | 2.6 | 9 | 2.1 | 1.6 | NS | <0.05 |
| Transferrin | 25 | 3.3 | 2.4 | 25 | 1.7 | 1.0 | 7 | 1.7 | 0.9 | <0.01 | <0.05 |
| Peroxidase | 27 | 3.3 | 1.8 | 23 | 2.2 | 1.6 | 7 | 2.3 | 1.4 | NS | <0.05 |
| MBP | 34 | 5.7 | 5.0 | 37 | 3.3 | 2.6 | 7 | 2.8 | 2.5 | <0.05 | <0.05 |
| Prolactin | 18 | 3.2 | 1.6 | 15 | 1.7 | 0.9 | 5 | 2.3 | 0.8 | <0.01 | <0.05 |

ABBREVIATIONS: CONT = control individuals; I = index of intra-BBB antibody (Ab) production = (Ab CSF/Ab serum)/(Albumin CSF/Albumin serum); M = mean value of I; MS = multiple sclerosis; N = sample size; OND = other neurologic diseases; SD = standard deviation.

values obtained with the reference standard. The percentage of absorbance in relation to that found with the reference pool was considered the relative titer of antibody in arbitrary units.

The local synthesis of autoantibodies in the BBB was evaluated by ratios established from the antibodies' titers of serum and CSF and the concentration of albumin. No significant differences were observed among the three groups for antibodies of the sera. However, a significant increase in local synthesis of antibodies was found in group I. The highest index was noted for antialbumin, antimyoglobin, and anti-MBP autoantibodies.

The intra-BBB production was significant in the MS group than in the OND group for the following antibodies: anti-TNP, antitubulin, antitransferrin, antiprolactin, antimyosin, antiactin, and anti-MBP (TABLE 1).

In conclusion, no restricted immunologic reactivity against one antigen of the panel was observed in the patients with MS. On the contrary, a significant intra-BBB production of antibodies against seven antigens of the panel was demonstrated. This study suggests that in MS a general disregulation leads to an expansion of B lymphocytes producing autoantibodies that share reactivities with natural autoantibodies.

## REFERENCES

1. AVRAMEAS, S. 1986. Natural autoreactive B cells and autoantibodies: the "Know thyself" of the immune system. Ann. Inst. Pasteur/Immunol. **137:** 150.
2. MATSIOTA, P., P. DRUET, P. DOSQUET, B. GUILBERT & S. AVRAMEAS. 1987. Natural autoantibodies in systematic lupus erythematosus. Clin. Exp. Immunol. **69:** 79.
3. MATSIOTA, P., S. CHAMARET, L. MONTAGNIER & S. AVRAMEAS. 1987. Detection of natural autoantibodies in the serum of anti-HIV-positive individuals. Ann. Inst. Pasteur/Immunol. **138:** 223.

WORKSHOP 2. T-CELL AND IMMUNE SYSTEM PRODUCT LOCALIZATION IN TARGET TISSUE

# B-Cell Compartment in the Thymus of Patients with Myasthenia Gravis and Control Subjects[a]

B. CHRISTENSSON,[b] P. BIBERFELD,[b] AND
G. MATELL[c]

[b]Immunopathology Laboratory
Department of Pathology
Karolinska Hospital
Stockholm, Sweden

[c]Myasthenia Gravis Center
South Hospital
Stockholm, Sweden

Thymic changes are frequent in myasthenia gravis (MG). Follicular hyperplasia is most frequent. To study the role of the thymus in the pathogenesis of MG and to locate in the thymus a possible precursor cell to the recently described "mediastinal clear cell lymphoma of B-cell type," we studied the distribution of B- and T-cell antigens in thymic follicular hyperplasia associated with MG and in control thymuses and the relation between B cells and medullary epithelial/reticular cells of the thymus.

## MATERIAL AND METHODS

Thymic tissue from 20 patients with MG and 7 patients undergoing cardiac surgery was surgically removed. The material was frozen in liquid nitrogen and subsequently cryosectioned (5-μ sections). Sections fixed in acetone were stained by a three-step immunoalkaline phosphatase method, sometimes in combination with avidin biotin peroxidase. Conjugated antisera to mouse IgG and IgM were obtained from Vector (Burlingame, California, USA) and to rabbit Ig from Dako. The primary antibodies are shown in TABLE 1.

---

[a]This work was supported by grants from the King Gustaf the Vth Jubilee Fund, the Swedish Cancer Society, and the Karolinska Institute.

TABLE 1. Distribution of Immunohistochemically Defined Cells in the Thymic Medulla

| Thymic Tissue: | | | Hyperplastic MG | | | | Controls |
|---|---|---|---|---|---|---|---|
| Antibody | CD n | $MZ^a$ | $GC^b$ | Perivascular/ Interlobular Spaces | Extrafollicular Medulla | Medulla | Perivascular/ Interlobular Spaces |
| | | | Antibodies to Lymphoid and Monocytic Cells | | | | |
| $my^c$ | | +++ | +++ | $(+)^d$ | $(+)$ | − | $(+)$ |
| $delta^c$ | | +++ | − | $((+))^e$ | $(+)$ | − | $(+)$ |
| $gamma^c$ | | − | $(+)$ | − | − | − | − |
| $B4^f$ | 19 | +++ | +++ | ++ | ++ | $(+)$ | ++ |
| $B1^f$ | 20 | +++ | +++ | ++ | ++ | + | + |
| $B2^f$ | 21 | +++ | +++ | − | − | − | − |
| pan-$B^c$ | 22 | $(+)$ | +++ | ++ | ++ | $(+)$ | $(+)$ |
| Leu14$^c$ | 22 | +++ | +++ | ++ | ++ | $(+)$ | $(+)$ |
| PCA-1$^f$ | | − | $((+))$ | + | − | − | − |
| HLA-DR$^f$ | | ++ | ++ | + | + | − | + |
| DRC$^c$ | | − | +$^g$ | − | − | ? | − |
| KiM4$^h$ | | − | +$^g$ | − | − | − | − |
| Leu1$^i$ | 5 | $(+)$ | $(+)$ | $(+)$ | + | + | + |
| Leu2$^i$ | 8 | $((+))$ | $((+))$ | +++ | ++ | ++ | ++ |
| Leu3$^i$ | 4 | $(+)$ | $(+)$ | +++ | +++ | +++ | +++ |
| Leu4$^i$ | 3 | $((+))$ | $(+)$ | +++ | ++ | ++ | ++ |
| Leu9$^i$ | 7 | $(+)$ | − | − | + | + | + |
| T6$^c$ | 1 | − | − | $((+))$ | − | − | − |
| T9$^f$ | | − | + | − | − | − | − |
| Ki-67$^c$ | | − | $(+)$ | − | $(+)$ | − | − |
| IL-2 rec.$^f$ | 25 | − | $((+?))$ | − | $(+)$ | $(+)$ | − |

Antibodies to Stromal and Epithelial Cells

| | | | | | |
|---|---|---|---|---|---|
| cytokeratin[j] | − | − | − | − | + | − |
| Epiderm. ker.[c] | − | − | − | + | + | − |
| MR19[j] | − | − | − | ++ | +++ | − |
| FN[m] | + | ++ | ++ | − | − | + |
| PAL-E[n] | (+) | ++ | ++ | − | − | + |

[a] MZ = mantle zone.
[b] GC = germinal center.
[c] Dako, Copenhagen, Denmark.
[d] Few scattered cells positive.
[e] Very few scattered cells positive.
[f] Coulter, Hialeah, USA.
[g] Follicular dendritic reticulum cells positive.
[h] Dr. A. Feller, Kiel, Germany.
[i] Becton-Dickinson Mountain View, USA.
[j] Ortho, Raritan, USA.
[k] Labsystems, Helsinki, Finland.
[l] Dr. M. Ritter, London, UK.
[m] Sera-Lab, London, UK.
[n] Biozac, Stockholm, Sweden.

## RESULTS

In control thymus, keratin-positive epithelial cells were found in the subcapsular, cortical, and medullar regions. In normal thymus, antifibronectin (FN) stained thin interlobular septa and slender perivascular spaces. The few Ig-positive cells found in control thymus (predominantly IgM and IgD) were mostly located in the septa and perivascularly and only a few in the medulla. However, many cells were positive for B-cell antigens CD19, 20, and 22, both Ig-positive cells in the septa and around the vessels, and cells in the medulla. The immunophenotype of the B cells in control thymus is summarized in TABLE 1. Consistently, more medullary cells were positive for CD20 than for CD22. Because the CD20 staining pattern suggested an epithelial origin for some of the positive cells, double stainings were performed. CD22 staining was not found in cells positive for keratin or MR19. In contrast, anti-CD20 gave double labeling in a small/MR19-positive fraction of the medullary epithelial cells.

Compared to that of the controls, MG thymus with follicular hyperplasia showed deformation of the medullary thymic regions with destruction of medullary epithelium and an increase in fibronectin-rich stroma. In MG thymus, most of the Ig-positive cells (IgM- and/or IgD-positive) were in the follicles. In contrast, using monoclonal antibodies against CD19, 20, and 22 there were also many positive cells outside the follicles, in both the perivascular/interlobular spaces and the medulla, most of which were Ig negative. The B-cell follicles, containing follicular dendritic cells, were most frequent in medullary areas negative for epithelial markers. They were often closely surrounded by keratin and MR19-positive medullary epithelium. There were also follicles in the perivascular spaces. The structure of the follicles as well as the immunophenotype and distribution of B and T cells within these areas was similar to the pattern seen in reactive follicles in lymph nodes (TABLE 1).

## SUMMARY AND CONCLUSIONS

An increased number of CD19, 20, and 22 positive B cells, compared to the number of Ig-positive cells, is regularly found in the thymic medulla of normal thymus, suggesting that a B-cell population normally resides in thymic medulla that lacks Ig expression. However, some of the CD20-positive cells seem to co-express keratin and MR19, suggesting an epithelial origin. The medullary B cells found in normal thymus could be precursors of the tumor cells in "mediastinal clear cell lymphomas of B-cell type." In follicular hyperplasia in MG, the medullary epithelial network is deformed and partly destroyed, and the interlobular/perivascular spaces are expanded. Follicles with follicular dendritic cells are found in both interlobular/perivascular spaces and "punched out" lesions in the medullary epithelium. The B cells are greatly increased in MG thymuses compared with control thymuses. These cells are found mainly in the follicles, but they are also dispersed in the medulla and the interlobular/perivascular spaces. The immunophenotype and distribution of B and T cells as well as the follicular dendritic cells in the hyperplastic follicles are similar to those of reactive follicles in lymph nodes. Our findings are consistent with the contention that in MG there is an autoimmune activation of B cells that normally reside in the thymic medulla. This activation leads initially to follicular hyperplasia in the medullary epithelium with destruction of medullary epithelial cells. The prolonged immune reaction in the autoimmune process induces a fibronectin-rich stroma formation and increased vascularization. The result is a remodeling of the thymic architecture with expansion of the perivascular/interlobular spaces replacing the destroyed medulla.

# Thymopoietin: A Marker of the Human Nicotinic Acetylcholine Receptor

E. MOREL,[a] B. VERNET-DER-GARABEDIAN,[a]
F. RAIMOND,[a] T. K. AUDHYA,[b] G. GOLDSTEIN,[b]
AND J. F. BACH[a]

[a]*INSERM U 25—CNRS UA 122*
*Hôpital Necker 161, rue de Sèvres*
*75730 Paris Cedex 15, France*

[b]*Ortho Pharmaceutical Corporation*
*Raritan, New Jersey*

In myasthenia gravis (MG) the thymus could intervene as an autoantigen or as a site of production of autoantibodies or it could be the site of an immune thymitis associated with the release of a thymic peptide that depresses neuromuscular transmission.[1] The substance that causes impairment of neurotransmission has been fully characterized as thymopoietin (Tpo).[2] It was recently shown that Tpo binds with the characteristics of a specific binding to nicotinic acetylcholine receptor (AChR) obtained from the electric organ of *Torpedo californica*.[3]

In this study we bring the demonstration of Tpo binding to the human AChR and of the recognition of myasthenic sera of the Tpo-AChR complexes, this giving additional arguments implicating the thymus in MG.

*Sera* were collected from patients with MG and from normal donors (NHS). *Thymic hormones* were isolated from human (HTpo) and from bovine (BTpo) origins, and synthesized human (sHTpo), thymopentin (TP5), and thymulin. *Radiolabeled hormones* were $^{125}$I-HTpo (35 µCi/µg) and $^{125}$I-BTpo (38 µCi/µg).

*Preparation of solubilized human acetylcholine receptor (H-AChR):* H-AChR was solubilized from amputated limbs by 0.05 M phosphate buffer containing 1.5% (v/v) of Triton X-100, and its concentration was determined either by using high titered anti-AChR sera (1,000-2,000 nM) from MG patients or by measuring the radioactivity present in $^{125}$I-αbungarotoxin-AChR complexes ($^{125}$I-αBgt-AChR) precipitated by ammonium sulfate.[4]

*Binding of thymic hormones to H-AChR:* The binding of thymic hormones to H-AChR was tested in two sets of experiments.

1. Inhibition of $^{125}$I-αBgt binding to AChR (a) after the addition of the hormones before incubation of the H-AChR preparation with $^{125}$I-αBgt; and (b) by incubating the H-AChR with the hormones in the presence of anti-AChR antibodies, then with $^{125}$I-αBgt.

2. Direct binding of labeled hormones to H-AChR revealed either by ammonium sulfate precipitation or by immunoprecipitation with MG sera.

## RESULTS

The specificity of the binding of Tpo to AChR is demonstrated in the two sets of experiments (TABLE 1). Anti-AChR antibody-positive MG sera were able to bind complexes formed between $^{125}$I-Tpo and human AChR. The specificity of $^{125}$I-Tpo binding to AChR was first demonstrated using an excess of Tpo or αBgt and then with NHS or negative sera. Maximum inhibition was obtained with αBgt, HTpo, and BTpo. The pentapeptide TP5 and other hormones, thymulin and insulin, were unable to inhibit the binding of MG sera to the HTpo-AChR complex. Dose-dependent curves between the amounts of $^{125}$I-Tpo-AChR complexes precipitated and the MG sera dilution were established. Studies on several MG sera revealed that only positive

TABLE 1. Binding of Thymopoietin (Tpo) to Human Acetylcholine Receptor (H-AChR)

| Assays | CPM (mean ± SD) | Inhibition (%) |
| --- | --- | --- |
| Standard assay[a] | 13,424 ± 773 | 0 |
| + αBgt | 2,633 ± 320 | 100 |
| + sHTpo | 2,866 ± 83 | 98 |
| + TP5 | 14,701 ± 357 | 0 |
| + Thymulin | 13,435 ± 690 | 0 |
| Standard assay[b] | 33,222 ± 921 | 0 |
| + αBgt | 18,123 ± 552 | 100 |
| + ACh | 18,080 ± 744 | 100 |
| + DC | 18,171 ± 226 | 100 |
| + sHTpo | 18,650 ± 222 | 97 |
| + TP5 | 35,096 ± 1,008 | 0 |

[a] $^{125}$I-αBgt (1 pmol) is incubated with 56 fmol of human AChR. Precipitation of $^{125}$I-αBgt-AChR complexes is performed with ammonium sulfate. Thymic hormones were used at $10^{-5}$ M.
[b] $^{125}$I-Tpo (38 μCi/μg is incubated with 56 fmol of human AChR. Precipitation of $^{125}$I-Tpo-AChR complexes is performed with ammonium sulfate; αBgt, sHTpo, and TP5 were used at $10^{-5}$ M, and ACh and decamethonium were used at $10^{-3}$ M.

Inhibition is expressed as: $\frac{\text{cpm standard} - \text{cpm assay}}{\text{cpm standard} - \text{cpm } \alpha\text{Bgt}}$ %.

anti-AChR sera gave a significant amount of radioactivity recovered in the radiolabeled Tpo-AChR-antibody complexes (TABLE 2).

When Tpo and MG antibodies were used competitively, the Tpo effect was comparable to that observed with the ACh agonist, decamethonium.[4]

## CONCLUSION

All these data converge to show that Tpo isolated from human or bovine thymuses and synthetic human Tpo interfere with the αBgt binding site of the AChR near the

TABLE 2. Precipitation of $^{125}$I-Tpo-AChR Complexes by MG Sera

| Sera | Anti-AChR Titers (nM) | $^{125}$I-Tpo-AChR Complexes (cpm) |
|---|---|---|
| Normal donors (NHS) | 0-0.53 | 1,478 ± 234[a] |
| Patients with MG | 1-4,000 | 4,680 ± 777 (2,850 − 5,850) |

[a] NHS + 3 SD = 2,180 cpm.

acetylcholine (ACh) binding site on the human receptor. The mechanism of this action remains to be elucidated. Tpo would depress neuromuscular transmission, maybe with autoantibodies to the AChR, a local intrathymic anti-AChR autosensitization stimulated by the AChR-like molecules present on thymus cells would produce a hormone binding to the receptor, or Tpo could contribute to the maturation of T cells involved in the regulation of anti-AChR antibody production.

## REFERENCES

1. GOLDSTEIN, G. & S. WHITTINGHAM. 1966. Lancet ii: 315.
2. AUDHYA, T., D. H. SCHLESINGER & G. GOLDSTEIN. 1981. Biochemistry 20: 6195.
3. VENKATASUBRAMANIAN, K., T. AUDHYA & G. GOLDSTEIN. 1986. Proc. Natl. Acad. Sci. USA 83: 3171.
4. VERNET-DER GARABEDIAN, B., E. MOREL & J. F. BACH. 1986. J. Neuroimmunol. 12: 65.

# Expression and Cellular Localization of Major Histocompatibility Complex Antigens in Active Multiple Sclerosis Lesions[a]

TATSUHIKO HAYASHI,[b] JACK S. BURKS,[c] AND
STEPHEN L. HAUSER [b]

[b]*Neuroimmunology Unit
Massachusetts General Hospital
Boston, Massachusetts*
[c]*Rocky Mountain Multiple Sclerosis Center
Denver, Colorado*

A dual label immunohistochemical method was employed to confirm the identity of the predominant infiltrating cell populations from active multiple sclerosis (MS) lesions obtained at autopsy and to assess the expression of major histocompatibility complex (MHC) antigens *in situ*. Nine fresh-frozen autopsy tissue samples were selected from a collection numbering greater than 60 samples. Each sample was derived from an individual who had a definite premortem diagnosis of MS, and in each case the diagnosis was histologically confirmed postmortem. The nine specimens were selected as representative of active MS lesion edges, defined as regions containing a margin between normal and demyelinating white matter and accompanying inflammation.

The monoclonal antibodies and the immunocytochemical method used is modified from that previously reported for the identification of single antigens in MS brain tissue[1] and is described elsewhere.[2]

## RESULTS

### T-Cell Subpopulations at the MS Lesion Edge

As previously reported,[1] the predominant T-cell population present at the active lesion edge consisted of CD8-positive, CD4-negative cells. Dual label experiments confirmed that this cell co-expresses the CD2,3,8 surface markers, and thus belongs

---

[a] This work was supported by grants from the National Institutes of Health (5R01-23816-02), The National Multiple Sclerosis Society, and the Upjohn Corporation. S.L.H. is a Harry Weaver Neuroscience Scholar of The National Multiple Sclerosis Society.

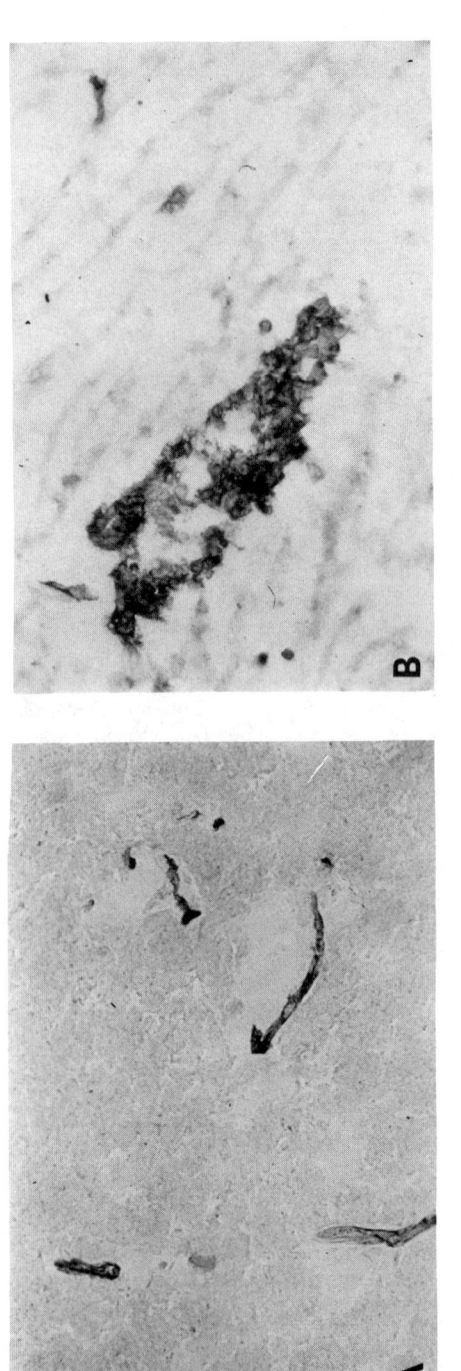

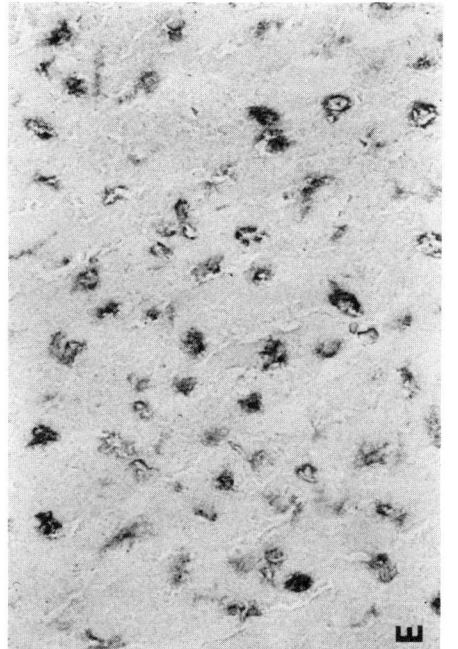
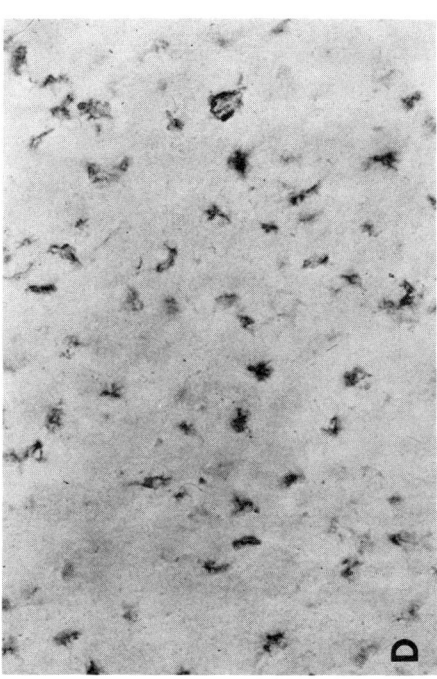

**FIGURE 1.** The distribtuion of immunoreactive cell markers at the active lesion edge in MS. (**A**) Normal human white matter labeled for Class I MHC antigen. Only blood vessel walls are labeled. (**B**) Active MS lesion labeled for Class 2 MHC antigen. In additon to blood vessel walls, perivascular inflammatory cells are identified. Dual-label experiments revealed that most of these cells are T cells. (**C**) Class 2 expression on normal human white matter, demonstrating labeling of some perivascular structures. (**D**) In an active MS lesion, large numbers of parenchymal Class 2-bearing cells are present. (**E**) Large numbers of M5-bearing macrophages are present in an active MS lesion. A subset of these cells coexpresses Class 2 antigen. (Original magnifications × 300 for all.)

to the class I restricted suppressor-cytotoxic subset. These cells do not co-express the HNK-1 natural killer cell marker that is present on aa subset of CD8 cells in peripheral blood.

### MHC Expression

As shown in FIGURE 1A, class 1 MHC expression was detectable only around blood vessel walls in normal central nervous system (CNS) white matter. In active MS lesions, Class 1 was detected, in addition to vessel walls, on perivascular inflammatory cells, but not on parenchymal CNS cells (FIG. 1B). These findings were confirmed using dual label methodology; perivascular T cells were Class 1 positive, whereas astrocytes were uniformly Class 1 negative.

In normal brain, low levels of Class 2 were expressed on some perivascular cells (endothelial and adventitial cells), as previously reported.[3] As shown in FIGURE 1C, this expression was not detectable in all regions of white matter. In active MS (FIG. 1D), large numbers of parenchymal cells expressing Class 2 were present in all cases examined. It was of interest that Class 2 expression on vascular endothelium was not detectably increased in these sections, even in regions where extensive infiltration with inflammatory cells was present.

The cell type responsible for the increased Class 2 expression in active MS white matter was examined by dual labeling of tissue sections for Class 2 antigen combined with label for surface markers specific for T cells, monocyte/macrophage cells, and astrocytes. The great majority of Class 2 bearing cells were monocyte/macrophage in origin (FIG. 1E), and no consistent induction of Class 2 expression on T cells or on astrocytes was present.

## DISCUSSION

The cellular events responsible for the initiation and maintenance of inflammatory responses within the CNS remain largely unknown. There has been considerable interest in the role of the MHC in these events, although most investigators have not found detectable MHC expression in the normal CNS.[3,4] For Class 1 MHC antigens in particular, this lack of MHC expression is in contrast to that found in most other organ systems, where Class 1 expression is easily detected. In the CNS, low or undetectable levels of Class 1 specific mRNA have been found, demonstrating that the absence of MHC gene products in this organ is not due to a translational block.

It might be anticipated that local MHC expression in the CNS is required both for antigen presentation and for the generation of antigen-specific cytotoxic T-cell responses. With regard to the former, Class 2 expression in association with antigen is required to activate T helper or inducer cells, although recent work suggests that cytotoxic function mediated by CD8 effector cells may be triggered in some situations in the absence of a helper signal.[5] In the CNS, candidates for antigen-presenting cell (APC) function include endothelial cells, macrophage/microglial cells, and astrocytes. The first two candidates express Class 2 under normal conditions, and under experimental conditions Class 2 expression can be induced on astrocytes by stimulation with gamma-interferon.[6] Class 2 bearing astrocytes can then be shown to have APC function. Endothelial cells can also *in vitro* be shown to have APC function,[7] although the physiologic importance of Class 2 expression on endothelium is unknown. In this regard, it is of note that the process by which circulating T cells cross the blood-brain barrier and initiate CNS inflammatory responses may not involve recognition of endothelial Class 2.[8]

Because effector T-cell responses also require MHC expression by target cells, expression by intrinsic CNS cells might also appear to be a prerequisite for any cytotoxic T-cell response in the CNS. Most cytotoxic responses are Class 1 restricted and mediated by the CD8 T-cell subset. Class 2 restricted cytotoxicity is mediated by the CD4 subset. Although most antiviral responses are thought to be Class 1 dependent, recent work in humans indicates that it is not universally the case. The virtual absence of Class 1 MHC expression by resident CNS cells might suggest that Class 1 restricted cytotoxic responses do not occur in the CNS, although other experimental data have shown that CNS cells may express levels of Class 1 below those detectable by immunohistochemical methods, yet sufficient for such cells to serve as cytotoxic targets.[9]

In active MS lesions, the striking increase in MHC expression resulted from an influx of cells from the peripheral circulation and not from induction of MHC expression by resident CNS cells. Thus, the Class 1 signal in acute lesions was due to infiltration of Class 1 bearing lymphocytes and, in particular, T cells. The marked increase in Class 2 expression in MS CNS was due to the presence of large numbers of cells of monocyte/macrophage origin as demonstrated by the co-expression of the M5 antigen. Astrocytes, defined immunochemically as GFAP-positive cells, were not induced to express MHC molecules in these lesions.

These results suggest that if antigen presentation does occur in the MS CNS, the macrophage/microglial cell or endothelial cell is the most likely APC candidate. If the mechanism of CNS injury is a cytotoxic response against an intrinsic CNS target, then killing would be effected in the presence of a low density of MHC product on the target cell. As CD8 cells appear to represent the predominant T-cell subpopulation in active lesions, one would speculate that Class 1 gene products might constitute the essential restricting element in this response.

## ACKNOWLEDGMENT

The authors wish to thank Dr. Chikao Morimoto and Douglas Ringler for their helpful advice and criticism.

## REFERENCES

1. HAUSER, S., A. K. BHAN, F. GILLES et al. 1986. Ann. Neurol. **19**: 578.
2. HAYASHI, T., C. MORIMOTO, J. BURKS et al. Ann. Neurol. (in press).
3. HAUSER, S. L., A. K. BHAN, F. H. GILLES et al. 1983. J. Neuroimmunol. **5**: 197.
4. WHELAN, J. P., U. ERIKSSON & L. A. LAMPSON. 1986. J. Immunol. **137**: 2561.
5. INABA, K., J. W. YOUNG & R. M. STEINMAN. 1987. J. Exp. Med. **166**: 182.
6. FONTANA, A. H., W. FIERZ & H. WEKERLE. 1984. Nature (Lond.) **307**: 273.
7. MALE, D. K., G. PRYCE & C. C. W. HUGHES. 1987. Immunology **60**: 453.
8. HINRICKS, D. J., K. W. WEGMANN & G. N. DIETSCH. 1987. J. Exp. Med. **166**: 1906-1917.
9. SKIAS, D. D., D.-K. KIM, A. T. REDER et al. 1987. **138**: 3254.

# Immunohistochemical Analysis of Suppressor-Inducer and Helper-Inducer T Cells in Multiple Sclerosis Brain Tissue

RAYMOND A. SOBEL,[a] DAVID A. HAFLER,[b]
EDUARDO E. CASTRO,[a] CHIKAO MORIMOTO,[c] AND
HOWARD L. WEINER[b]

[a]Department of Pathology
Massachusetts General Hospital
Boston, Massachusetts

[b]Center for Neurologic Diseases
Brigham and Women's Hospital
Boston, Massachusetts

[c]Division of Tumor Immunology
Dana-Farber Cancer Institute, and
Harvard Medical School
Boston, Massachusetts

Inflammatory cells in multiple sclerosis (MS) lesions are predominantly activated T cells and macrophages.[1] The T-cell inducer (CD4+) population has been separated into helper-inducer and suppressor-inducer populations on the basis of staining with anti-4B4 and anti-2H4 monoclonal antibodies, respectively.[2,3] There is a decrease of suppressor-inducer cells in the peripheral blood of patients with chronic progressive MS[4] and a loss of functional suppression that correlates with the CD4+2H4+ subset.[5] To further characterize T-cell antigen expression in MS and other central nervous system (CNS) inflammatory diseases and to determine if there is selective accumulation of either suppressor-inducer or helper-inducer T cells in MS lesions, cryostat CNS tissue sections from patients with MS and encephalitis (TABLE 1) were stained with monoclonal antibodies to 2H4, 4B4, CD3, CD4, CD8, and CD25 (interleukin-2 receptor) using immunoperoxidase. The percentage of stained cells in high power fields was counted in encephalitis and MS plaques, plaque edges, and normal-appearing white matter, as already described.[6]

There were more 2H4+ ($p < 0.001$) and CD8+ ($p < 0.01$) cells in viral encephalitis and more 2H4+ cells in paraneoplastic limbic encephalitis ($p < 0.01$) than in any MS compartment (FIG. 1). There were no differences between encephalitis cases and MS plaque edges, where T cells were most numerous, in CD4+, CD3+, CD25+, or 4B4+ cells. There was no staining in control tissues with anti-2H4, -CF4, -CD8, -CD3, or -CD25 antibodies. Anti-4B4 stained most inflammatory cells in MS and encephalitis, and endothelial cells in all cases.

TABLE 1. Central Nervous System Tissues[a]

| Diagnosis | No. of Patients | No. of Tissue Samples |
|---|---|---|
| Multiple sclerosis | 12 | 62 |
| Viral encephalitis | | |
|   Herpes simplex encephalitis | 8 | 8[b] |
|   Subacute sclerosing panencephalitis | 1 | 1 |
| Paraneoplastic limbic encephalitis | 1 | 6 |
| Age-matched normal controls | 5 | 5[c] |

[a] Tissues were obtained from the Massachusetts General Hospital, Brigham and Women's Hospital, Boston, Massachusetts, and from Lynn G. Baird, Boston, Massachusetts, Jack S. Burks, Denver, Colorado, and W. W. Tourtellotte, Los Angeles, California.
[b] Seven biopsies and one autopsy.
[c] One biopsy and four autopsies.

These data indicate a difference in T-cell immune responses between encephalitis and MS. The paucity of 2H4+ cells in MS was not likely due to either postmortem alterations or an inability of these cells to migrate to the brain because numerous 2H4+ cells were found in encephalitis cases at autopsy. Specificity is indicated by nearly identical levels of other T-cell antigens in MS plaque edges and encephalitis. The paucity of 2H4+ cells, persistence of inflammation, and absence of a readily identifiable etiologic agent are also found in tuberculoid leprosy[7] and may indicate analogous immune responses to those in the CNS in MS. The 2H4 antigen is important in inducing suppression *in vitro,*[3,5] and there is likely to be a relationship between decreased suppressor cell function and small numbers of 2H4+ cells in the blood of MS patients.[4] These data suggest that loss of 2H4+ cells is not necessarily due to sequestration in the CNS and that there may be concomitant impaired suppressor-inducer function associated with the paucity of 2H4 antigen expression in the CNS of MS patients, which contributes to ongoing inflammation *in situ.*

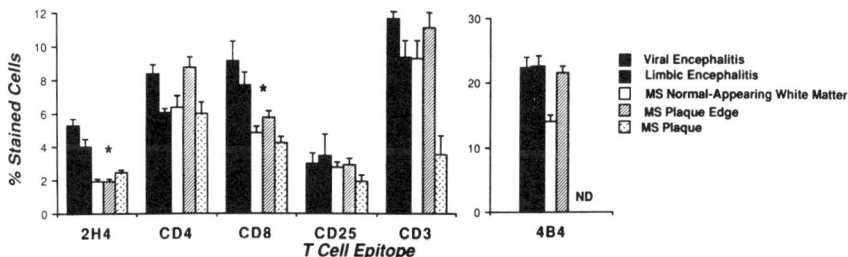

FIGURE 1. T-cell antigens in encephalitis and multiple sclerosis. *Bars* indicate mean percentage of stained cells ± standard error. *Asterisk* indicates epitopes for which all compartments in MS tissues were significantly less than those in viral encephalitis.

## REFERENCES

1. HAUSER, S. L., A. K. BHAN, F. GILLES, M. KEMP, C. KERR & H. L. WEINER. 1986. Ann. Neurol. **19:** 578-587.
2. MORIMOTO, C., N. L. LETVIN, A. W. BOYD, M. HAGAN, H. M. BROWN, M. M. KORNACKI & S. F. SCHLOSSMAN. 1985. J. Immunol. **134:** 3762-3769.
3. MORIMOTO, C., N. L. LETVIN, J. A. DISTASO, W. R. ALDRICH & S. F. SCHLOSSMAN. 1985. J. Immunol. **134:** 1508-1515.
4. MORIMOTO, C., D. A. HAFLER, H. L. WEINER, N. L. LETVIN, M. HAGAN, J. DALEY & S. F. SCHLOSSMAN. 1987. N. Engl. J. Med. **316:** 67-72.
5. CHOFFLON, M. M., H. L. WEINER & D. A. HAFLER. 1987. Neurology **37**(Suppl. 1): 294.
6. SOBEL, R. A., A. B. COLLINS, R. B. COLVIN & A. K. BHAN. 1986. Am. J. Pathol. **125:** 332-338.
7. DEWEESE, N. E., T. SINCHAISRI, T. H. REA & R. L. MODLIN. 1987. J. Clin. Invest. **18:** 484.

# Demonstration of α, β, and γ Interferon in Active Chronic Multiple Sclerosis Lesions[a]

## U. TRAUGOTT[b] AND P. LEBON[c]

[b]Albert Einstein College of Medicine
Bronx, New York

[c]Hôpital Saint Vincent De Paul
Paris, France

By routine morphologic study, active chronic multiple sclerosis (MS) lesions are characterized by a sharply demarcated lesion edge and a zone of inflammation containing mainly lymphocytes and macrophages.[1] Immunocytochemical analysis of inflammatory cells demonstrated densely packed class I (HLA-ABC) and class II (HLA-DR, Ia) major histocompatibility (MHC) antigen-positive macrophages in the center, whereas T cells predominated at the lesion edge. In highly active chronic lesions, CD4+ (helper/inducer) T cells and interleukin-2 receptor(IL-2R)-positive cells penetrated deeply into the normal appearing white matter adjacent to the plaque.[2,3] Class II MHC was detectable on about 10% of endothelial cells and on some astrocytes at the edge of active chronic lesions.[4] Class I MHC was found less consistently on astrocytes than was Class II MHC, and it was mainly present close to lymphocytic and not to macrophage infiltrates.[3,4] Previous studies *in vitro* documented that MHC expression on astroglia can be induced by interferons (IFNs)[5] and that Ia-positive astrocytes can present antigen, such as myelin basic protein, to specifically sensitized T cells.[6] To investigate a possible role of IFNs for lesion pathogenesis in MS, frozen sections of CNS tissue were stained with monoclonal antibodies (mAbs) or polyclonal antisera in combination with the avidin-biotin-peroxidase complex (ABC) technique to demonstrate IFN-α, IFN-β, and IFN-γ. In active chronic MS lesions, all three types of IFN could be detected and showed distinct distribution patterns, whereby IFN-γ was more common than IFN-α and IFN-β. IFN-γ was detectable on a few infiltrating cells, on astrocytes at the lesion edge, and even more frequently in the adjacent normal appearing white matter, thus displaying a distribution similar to that of class II MHC on astroglia. IFN-α was mainly found on macrophages at the edge of the plaque, whereas foamy cells in the lesion center were nonreactive. The presence of IFN-β partially overlapped with that of IFN-α and IFN-γ in that it was demonstrable on some astrocytes and on a few macrophages. IFN-β on astrocytes was most common at the lesion edge, and its distribution was similar to that of class I MHC. In contrast to the intensive labeling of macrophages for IFN-α, staining for IFN-β was cap-like and restricted to areas of contact with other macrophages or astrocytes. In silent chronic MS lesions, IFN-positive cells were rare. These findings indicated

---

[a]This work was supported in part by NMSS RG-1664-B-2; NS 11920, RTC G008000340.

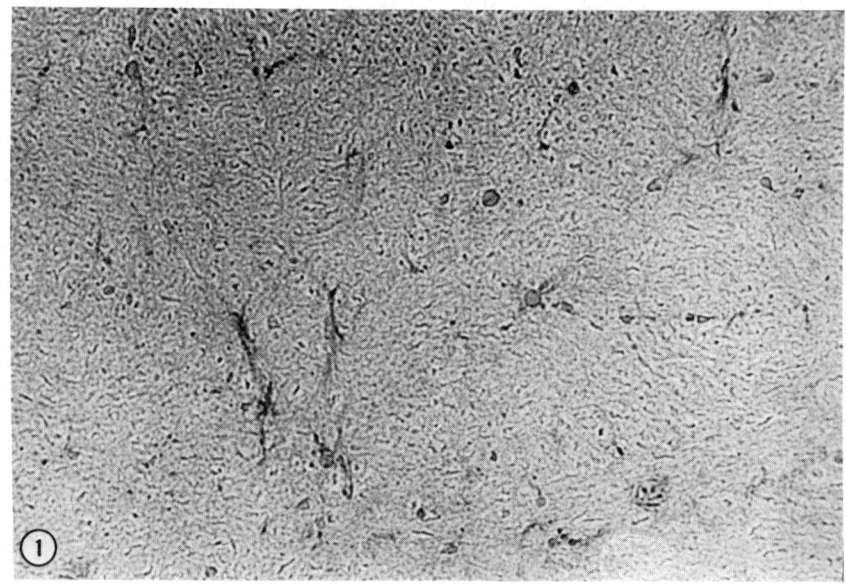

**FIGURE 1.** Active chronic MS, spinal cord; stained with mAb to IFN-$\beta$. Segmental labeling of astrocytes is seen (10 $\mu$m thick frozen sections stained by ABC technique; original magnification $\times$ 320; reduced by 25%).

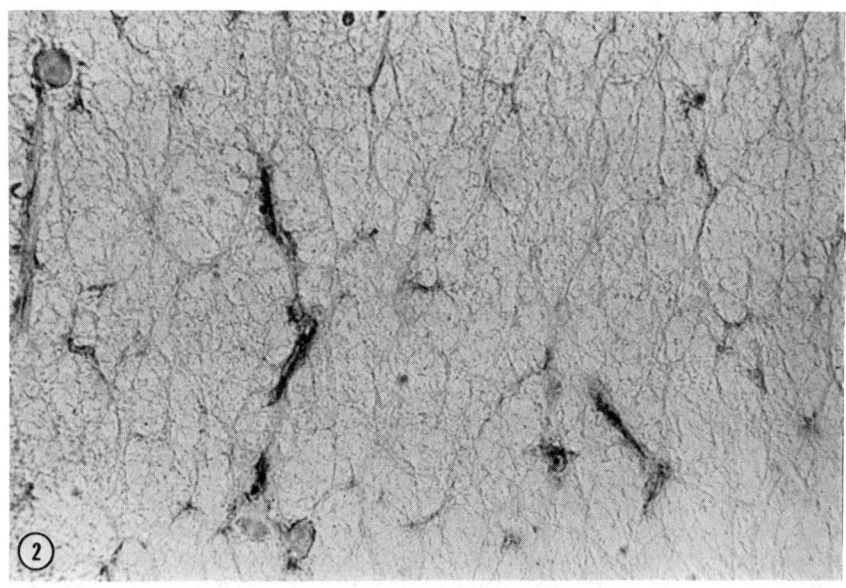

**FIGURE 2.** Active chronic MS, spinal cord; stained with mAb to HLA-ABC. Some astrocytes are labeled in normal appearing white matter. (10 $\mu$m thick frozen sections stained by ABC technique; original magnification $\times$ 320; reduced by 25%).

that similar to the situation *in vitro,* class I and class II MHC expression on astroglia might also be induced *in vivo* by IFN-$\beta$ and IFN-$\gamma$, respectively. Furthermore, they suggest that IFN-$\gamma$ via Ia expression on astrocytes and local antigen presentation might lead to reactivation of the disease process in MS, whereas IFN-$\alpha/\beta$ might be involved in local immunosuppression.

## REFERENCES

1. GREENFIELD, J. G. & R. M. NORMAN. 1971. Demyelinating disease. *In* Greenfield's Neuropathology. W. Blackwood, W. H. McMenemey, A. Meyer, R. M. Norman & D. S. Russell, Eds.: 475-519. Arnold, London.
2. TRAUGOTT, U. & C. S. RAINE. 1984. Further lymphocyte characterization in the central nervous system in multiple sclerosis. *In* Multiple Sclerosis: Experimental and Clinical Aspects. Ann. N.Y. Acad. Sci. **436:** 163-180.
3. TRAUGOTT, U. 1987. Multiple sclerosis: Relevance of class I and class II MHC-expressing cells to lesion development. J. Neuroimmunol. **16:** 203-302.
4. TRAUGOTT, U., L. C. SCHEINBERG & C. S. RAINE. 1985. On the presence of Ia-positive endothelial cells and astrocytes in multiple sclerosis lesions and its relevance to antigen presentation. J. Neuroimmunol. **8:** 1-14.
5. WONG, G. H. W., I. CLARK-LEWIS, A. W. HARRIS & J. W. SCHRADER. 1984. Effect of cloned interferon gamma on expression of H-2 and Ia antigens on cell lines of hemopoietic, lymphoid, epithelial, fibroblastic and neuronal origin. Eur. J. Immunol. **14:** 52-56.
6. FONTANA, A., W. FIERZ & H. WEKERLE. 1984. Astrocytes present myelin basic protein to encephalitogenic T cell lines. Nature **307:** 273-276.

# Immunoglobulin G (IgG) Localization During Acute Autoimmune Demyelination[a]

## G. R. WAYNE MOORE AND CEDRIC S. RAINE

*Departments of Pathology (Neuropathology), Neurology and Neuroscience and the Rose F. Kennedy Center for Research in Mental Retardation and Human Development Albert Einstein College of Medicine Bronx, New York*

Immunoglobulin G (IgG) is found in high concentration in the lesions of multiple sclerosis (MS).[1] The role of IgG in the pathogenesis of this condition is unknown. However, macrophages engaged in myelin breakdown demonstrate capping of IgG.[2] In both MS[3] and its experimental analog, experimental allergic encephalomyelitis (EAE),[4] macrophages can phagocytose myelin by receptor-mediated phagocytosis via clathrin-coated pits. It was postulated that IgG serves as a molecular ligand to bind IgG to an Fc receptor on the macrophage membrane within the clathrin-coated pit[2] before the internalization of myelin within the macrophage.

To further delineate the role of IgG in autoimmune demyelination, we studied lesions of acute EAE by means of immunoelectron microscopy using a post-embedding immunogold technique. Strain 13 guinea pigs were inoculated intracutaneously for acute EAE with an 0.5-ml mixture of bovine white matter and complete Freund's adjuvant. At the first signs of the disease (usually 10-14 days after inoculation), animals were perfused with 4% paraformaldehyde followed by 5% glutaraldehyde. Representative sections of spinal cord and lymph node were post-osmicated, dehydrated in graded alcohols, cleared in propylene oxide, and embedded in Epon 812. Thin sections were mounted on Formvar-coated nickel grids and placed on a 7.5% solution of sodium meta-periodate.[5] The grids were then washed with distilled water followed by a Tris-saline-albumin buffer with Tween at pH 8.2. This procedure was followed by incubations with normal rabbit serum, goat anti-guinea pig Fc fragment of IgG (Cappel, Malvern, Pennsylvania), normal rabbit serum, and rabbit anti-goat IgG coupled to 10 nm colloidal gold (Janssen, Piscataway, New Jersey). Grids were washed with buffer after each step and finally with distilled water. They were then air dried, counterstained with uranyl acetate and lead citrate, and carbon coated. Controls consisted of omission of the primary antiserum or substitution of it with goat IgG, both of which abolished the staining.

In lymph nodes, the technique demonstrated staining of IgG-containing structures such as cisterns of rough endoplasmic reticulum, Golgi apparatus, and secretory vesicles of plasma cells. There was minimal background staining. In acute EAE lesions

---

[a] This work was supported in part by NS 08952, NS 07098, NS 11920, and NMSS 1001-F-6.

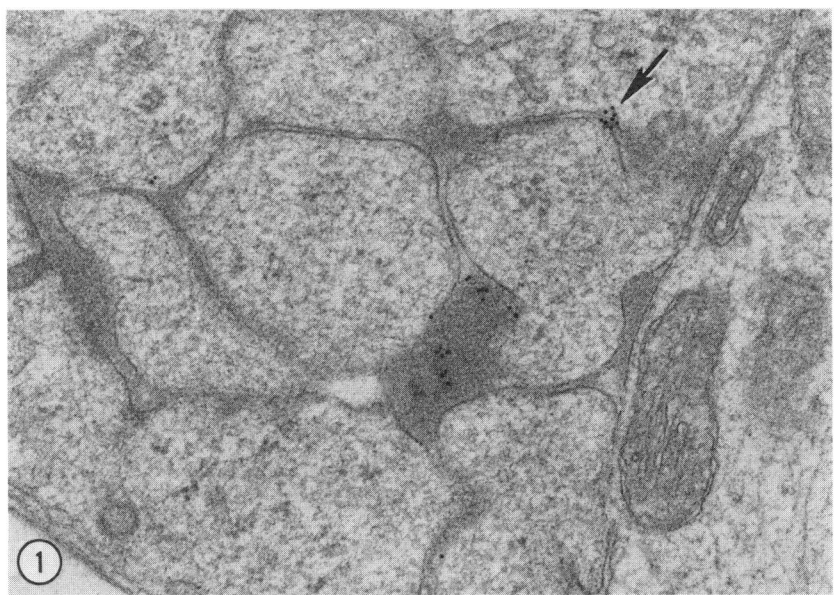

**FIGURE 1.** In this acute EAE lesion stained for IgG, extracellular material resembling fibrin is labeled with 10-nm colloidal gold particles. Focal staining of the macrophage membrane is also evident (*arrow*). (Original magnification × 54,000; reduced by 9%).

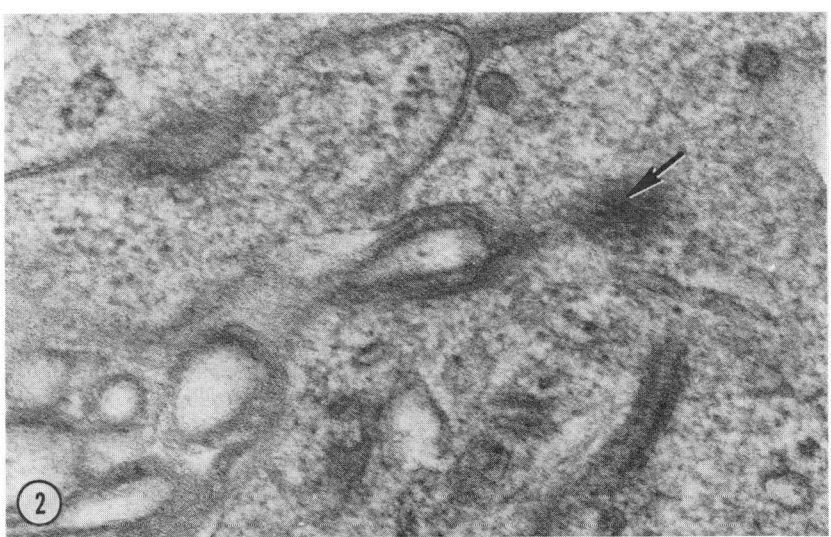

**FIGURE 2.** The crypt between two macrophage processes contains myelin lamellae and terminates in an obliquely sectioned clathrin-coated pit that is labeled for IgG (*arrow*). (Original magnification × 65,800; reduced by 9%).

with active myelin breakdown, there was staining of extracellular electron dense material that resembled fibrin (FIG. 1). Clathrin-coated pits that did not contain phagocytosed material were rarely labeled. Occasionally, clathrin-coated pits attached to myelin being phagocytosed by the macrophage were stained for IgG (FIG. 2). Within macrophages, the tips of whorls of myelin debris within lysosomes were stained, suggesting the location of a point of attachment on the surface of the macrophage before phagocytosis.

In summary, this study shows that IgG can be labeled in glutaraldehyde-fixed osmicated tissue, and our results suggest that IgG serves as the ligand responsible for receptor-mediated phagocytosis of myelin in autoimmune demyelination.

## REFERENCES

1. WALSH, M. J., W. W. TOURTELLOTTE, A. R. POTVIN & J. N. POTVIN. 1983. In Multiple Sclerosis: Pathology, Diagnosis and Management: 275-358. Baltimore, Williams & Wilkins.
2. PRINEAS, J. W. & G. S. GRAHAM. 1981. Ann. Neurol. **10:** 149-158.
3. PRINEAS, J. W. & F. CONNELL. 1978. Neurology **22:** 68-75.
4. EPSTEIN, L. G., J. W. PRINEAS & C. S. RAINE. 1983. J. Neurol. Sci. **61:** 341-348.
5. BENDAYAN, M. & M. ZOLLINGER. 1983. J. Histochem. Cytochem. **31:** 101-109.

# Endothelial Cell Ia Increases Before Inflammatory Cell Infiltration in EAE Induced in Long-tailed Macaques[a]

LYNN M. ROSE,[b] ROSEMARIE PETERSEN,[c] RAJ MEHRA,[c] AND ELLSWORTH C. ALVORD, JR.[c]

*University of Washington
School of Medicine
Departments of Microbiology[b] and Pathology[c]
Seattle, Washington*

Experimental allergic encephalomyelitis (EAE), an autoimmune, inflammatory and demyelinating disease of the central nervous system (CNS), is a model for the human demyelinating disease, multiple sclerosis (MS). In rodent EAE, increased endothelial cell Ia appears to be a pre-inflammatory, target organ-specific alteration that persists during inflammation.[1] This observation suggests that Ia antigens expressed on the endothelial cells might play active immunologic roles in the local antigen presentation to T cells and subsequent development of EAE. This possibility is supported by the fact that EAE can be prevented by anti-Ia monoclonal antibody (mAb).[2]

In this study, we also report an enhanced staining for Ia in the CNS endothelium of long-tailed macaques induced to develop acute EAE by sensitization with monkey myelin basic protein (BP) in complete Freund's adjuvant (CFA). With immuno-peroxidase staining of frozen tissue sections, the frequency of $Ia^+$ cells and vessels was quantitated over time. In early lesions there was no cellular infiltrate and marked staining of the endothelium. In older lesions the endothelium was markedly less positive for Ia, although extensive infiltrates of $Ia^+$ cells persisted in the lesions. These findings suggest that *in vivo* modulation of endothelial Ia expression may play an important role in the progression of EAE.

## METHODS

Experimental allergic encephalomyelitis was induced by intradermal injection of 0.15 ml of a water-in-oil emulsion of CFA containing 7.5 mg of monkey BP and 0.75 mg of heat-killed *Mycobacterium tuberculosis* (H37Ra, Difco) divided among three

---

[a] This work was supported by National Multiple Sclerosis Society Grants RG-1829-A-1 and RG-1708-A-21, and the Regional Primate Research Center NIH Core Grant RRD0166.

sites in the ankle. Control animals were either unsensitized or sensitized with CFA alone. At different times after sensitization, the animals were sacrificed, and blocks of macaque cerebrum or cerebellum containing lesions were frozen. Cryostat sections (5 μm) of frozen tissue were mounted on glass slides and stained with mAb HB10a (anti-HLA-DR class II β chain)[3] or MOPC-21, an irrelevant isotype control, using the indirect immunoperoxidase technique.[4] Sequential sections of tissue were stained with hematoxylin and eosin (H&E) to visualize the cellular infiltrate. The lesions were evaluated for the degree of inflammation and positive Ia staining. Staining patterns were confirmed by two independent observers who studied the coded slides without knowledge of the sensitization or clinical status of the monkey. Ia expression was also studied in normal kidney, liver, and heart tissues from unsensitized, CFA-sensitized, and BP-sensitized animals with acute EAE.

## RESULTS

All animals in this study developed clinical signs of EAE ranging in severity from ± to ++ (TABLE 1). The onset of the acute attack occurred 15-29 days after sensitization with a mean onset of 20 days. None of the CFA-sensitized or unsensitized animals showed neurologic abnormalities, and they had no detectable inflammatory cells in sections stained with H&E or monoclonal antibodies to T cells. Control animals were sacrificed 4 weeks after sensitization with adjuvant. All of the BP-sensitized animals that died or were sacrificed had microscopic evidence of severe acute EAE. Seventy-five percent (12 of 16) had relatively homogeneous continuing processes corresponding to their clinical course of 1-13 days' duration and 25% (4 of 16) had mixtures of acute EAE superimposed on older subacute or healing lesions of 17-29 days' duration. Staining with H&E demonstrated the inflammatory perivascular and parenchymal infiltrates (FIG. 1a).

Control tissues stained with anti-Ia mAb revealed a slight irregular staining of blood vessel endothelium in the CNS and other tissues (FIG. 1b). In BP-sensitized animals the CNS endothelium was heavily stained with anti-Ia mAb before the onset of cellular infiltration and inflammation (FIG. 1c). Ia expression in other tissues did not change. In active lesions large Ia$^+$ cells were numerous and predominated throughout the lesion center. The blood vessel endothelium also stained strongly for class II

TABLE 1. Clinical Signs and Grades of EAE in Long-tailed Macaques

| Severity | Signs |
|---|---|
| ? | Prodromal signs including weight loss, anorexia, yawning, slow response to stimuli, irritability |
| ± | Mild neurologic signs including "headache" (acute distress), "apathy" (indifference), hypokinesia, drooling, clumsiness in using limbs, nystagmus |
| + | Moderate neurologic signs including akinesia, blindness, ataxia, tremor, ptosis, seizures, paresis, incontinence |
| ++ | Severe neurologic signs, including somnolence, quadriplegia |
| +++ | Moribund state with semicoma, coma, decerebration or decortication |
| D | Death |

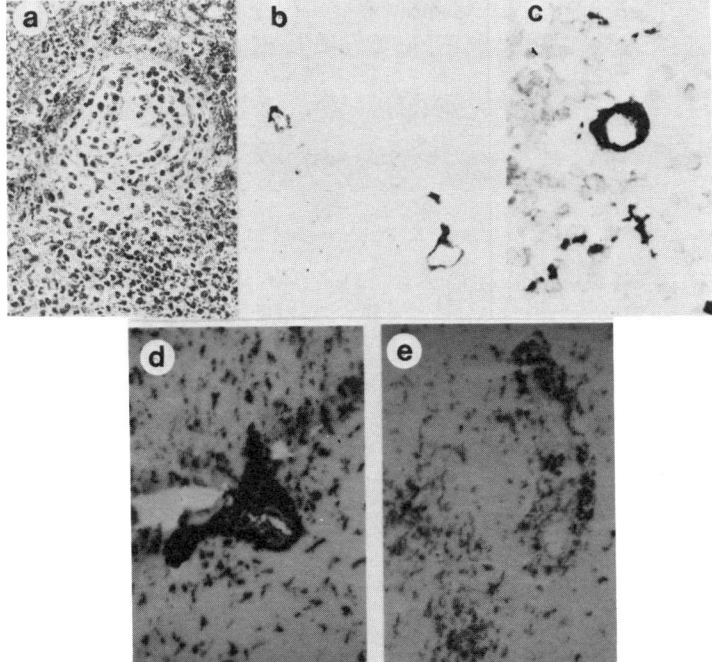

**FIGURE 1.** (a) Frozen section of white matter stained with H&E, showing an exudate extending out from a relatively large mass of exudate in the white matter; (b-e) frozen sections of white matter stained with mAb HB10a to the HLA-DR class II MHC antigen, showing the progression of lesion development; (b) very light endothelial reaction in normal brain; (c) preinflammatory lesion with intense endothelial reaction; (d) active lesion showing increased infiltration of Ia$^+$ cells and decreased Ia on endothelium; and (e) a less active lesion with fewer cells and blood vessels weakly positive for Ia. (Original magnification × 80.)

MHC antigen. The staining of vessel walls appeared to decrease as the inflammation increased (FIG. 1d). In less active, older lesions, Ia$^+$ cells were much less frequent in the lesion center, and blood vessel walls were weakly positive (FIG. 1c). In most animals we found a mixture of lesions, indicating that the induction of new lesions is a continuous, nonsynchronous process.

## CONCLUSIONS

Class II MHC antigen Ia is expressed at low levels on endothelial cells in normal or adjuvant-sensitized animals. In animals induced to develop EAE by sensitization with BP in CFA, the expression of Ia in the CNS increases and is a pre-inflammatory event. We observed a gradual decrease in expression of Ia on the endothelium in active lesions which we interpret as an indication of the age of a lesion. Our study suggests that the expression of Ia is a dynamic event that may play an important role in the progression of EAE.

## REFERENCES

1. SOBEL, R. A., B. W. BLANCHETTE, A. K. BHAN & R. B. COLVIN. 1984. J. Immunol. **132:** 2042-2407.
2. SRIRAM, S. & L. STEINMAN. 1983. J. Exp. Med. **158:** 1362-1367.
3. CLARK, E. A. & I. YOKOCHI. 1984. *In* Leukocyte Typing. B. A. Boumsell, J. Dausset, C. Milstein & S. F. Schlossman, Eds.: 339. Springer Verlag, Berlin.
4. STERNBERGER, L. A. 1979. *In* Immunochemistry.: 104. John Wiley & Sons, New York.

# Occurrence of HLA-DR Reactive Microglia in Alzheimer's Disease

### P. L. McGEER, S. ITAGAKI, H. TAGO, AND E. G. McGEER

*Kinsmen Laboratory of Neurological Research
Faculty of Medicine
Vancouver, B. C. Canada*

Sensitive immunohistochemical procedures were used to detect reactive microglia (macrophages) positive for HLA-DR in postmortem tissue in cases of Alzheimer's disease.[1] In gray matter, these macrophages were concentrated in areas of senile plaque formation (FIG. 1A). They were also found in white matter, such as the anterior commissure, which presumably carries axons of degenerating cortical neurons (FIG. 1B). Double immunostaining with antibodies to HLA-DR and glial fibrillary acidic

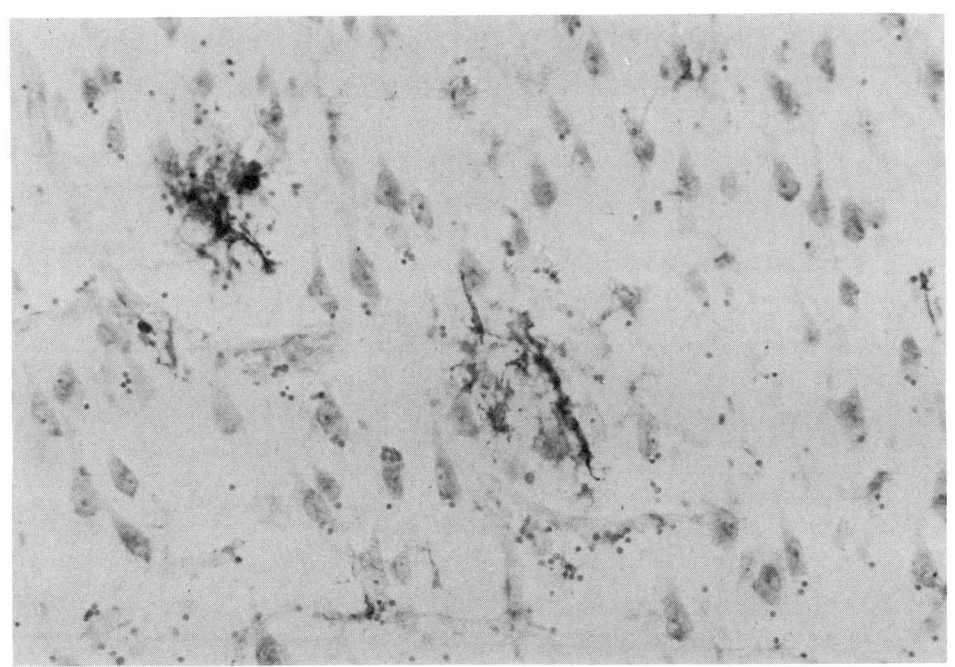

**FIGURE 1A.** HLA-DR stain of Alzheimer hippocampal gray matter, showing reactive microglia (macrophages). (Neutral red counterstain; original magnification × 245.)

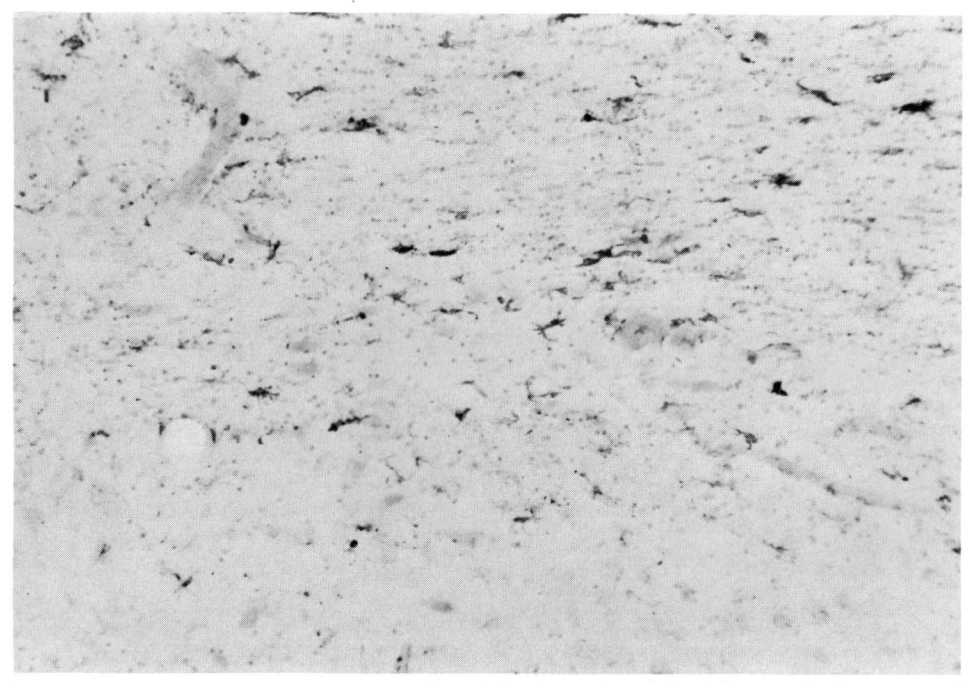

**FIGURE 1B.** HLA-DR stain of white matter of Alzheimer anterior commissure. Many reactive microglia are seen. (Neutral red counterstain; original magnification × 133.)

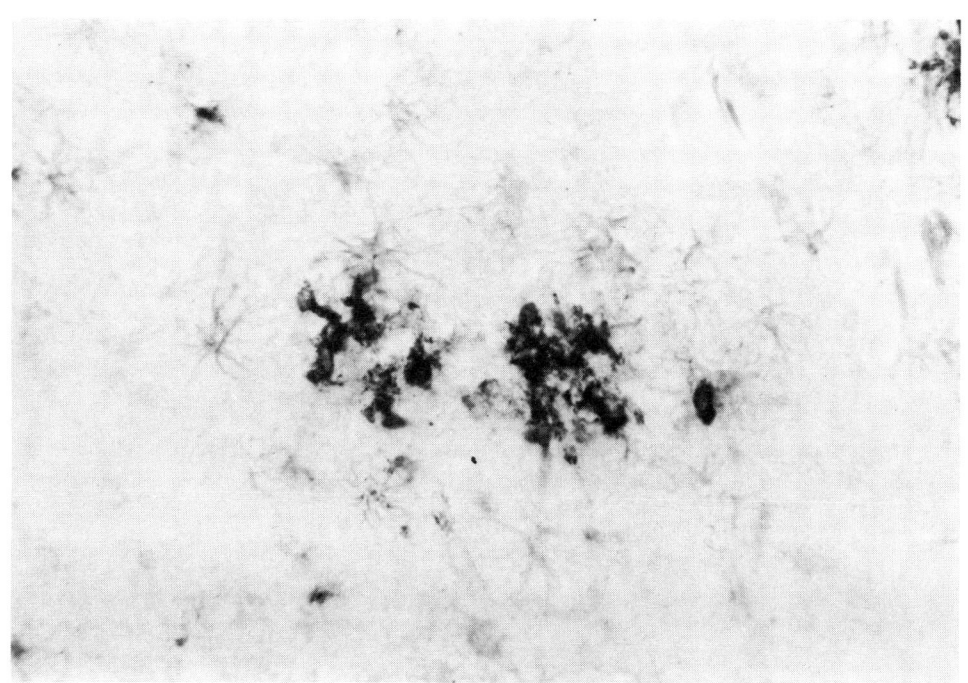

**FIGURE 1C.** Double immunostain for HLA-DR and GFAP in Alzheimer disease hippocampus. HLA-DR-positive reactive microglia (macrophages) surround two senile plaques. Reactive astrocytes are scattered in the matrix (original magnification × 245).

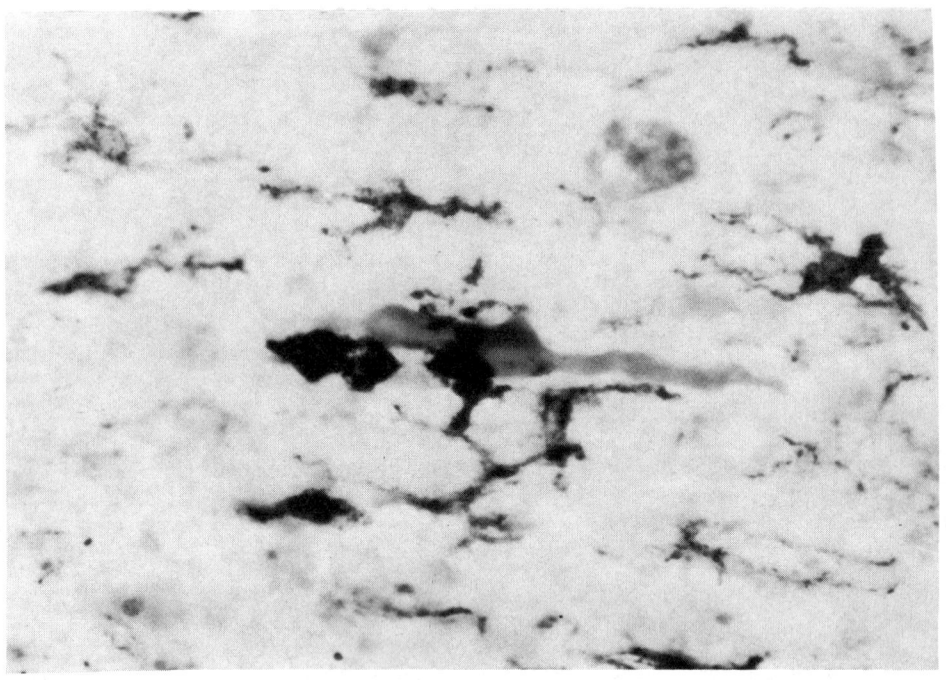

**FIGURE 1D.** Double immunostains for HLA-DR-positive reactive microglia (macrophages) and choline acetyltransferase positive neurons in Alzheimer substantia innominata. HLA-DR positive cells are seen in association with neurons, especially the large neuron with an eccentric nucleus in the center of the picture (original magnification × 490).

TABLE 1. Frequency of HLA-DR-Positive Reactive Microglia and Senile Plaques in Alzheimer's Disease and Control Hippocampus and Cortical Choline Acetyltransferase (ChAT) Levels[a]

| Type | No. of Cases | Age (yr.) | No. of Plaques | No. of HLA-DR-Positive Cells | Average Cortical ChAT[a] |
|---|---|---|---|---|---|
| Alzheimer | 13 | 78 ± 5.7 | 102.7 ± 68.6 (6[b]) | 133.5 ± 43.0 | 0.34 ± 0.25 |
| Control | 12 | 74 ± 11.3 | 8.2 ± 15.7 (5[b]) | 19.2 ± 30.3 | 0.82 ± 0.19 |
| p for group comparison | | Ns | <0.02 | <0.001 | <0.001 |

[a] Average values for ChAT (nmol/100 mg of protein per hour) in seven samples (temporal tip, midtemporal gyrus, precentral gyrus, postcentral gyrus, Broca's area, occipital gyrus, and frontal pole) of each brain were used to calculate the group means. All data are ± SDM.

[b] Number of cases in which plaque counts were done.

protein (GFAP) showed that the HLA-DR-positive microglia were a different population from the GFAP-positive reactive astrocytes that proliferate in areas of neuronal loss (FIG. 1C). Double immunostaining for choline acetyltransferase (ChAT) and HLA-DR in the substantia innominata in cases of Alzheimer's disease demonstrated phagocytosis of degenerating ChAT neurons by HLA-DR-positive reactive microglia (FIG. 1D). The Alzheimer's cases all had reduced ChAT levels as measured biochemically. In the 25 brains studied, the number of hippocampal HLA-DR-positive cells correlated negatively with the average cortical ChAT activity ($r = -0.65$), and in the 11 brains in which complete hippocampal plaque counts were taken the number of hippocampal HLA-DR-positive cells correlated positively with the number of plaques ($r = 0.78$) and negatively with the cortical ChAT activity ($r = -0.76$) (TABLE 1). Significant numbers of round cells staining for leukocyte common antigen (LCA) were also present in diseased Alzheimer's tissue. These presumed lymphocytes could be identified marginated along the walls of capillaries and in the matrix. Moreover, punctate staining with antibody to interleukin-2 receptor (IL-2R) could be seen occasionally in affected areas, especially capillaries. These data are consistent with the existence of a chronic inflammatory process in Alzheimer's disease.

## REFERENCE

1. McGeer, P. L., S. Itagaki, H. Tago & E. G. McGeer. 1987. Reactive microglia in patients with senile dementia of the Alzheimer type are positive for the histocompatibility glycoprotein HLA-DR. Neurosci. Lett. **79**: 195-200.

# Interleukin-2 Blocks Oligodendrocyte Progenitor Proliferation[a]

ROBERT L. KNOBLER,[b] RUSSELL P. SANETO,[c]
AMNON ALTMAN,[d] HOWARD M. JOHNSON,[e] AND
JEAN DE VELLIS[f]

[b]*Department of Neurology*
*Jefferson Medical College*
*Philadelphia, Pennsylvania*

[c]*Department of Neuroscience*
*Oregon Regional Primate Research Center*
*Beaverton, Oregon*

[d]*Department of Immunology*
*Scripps Clinic and Research Foundation*
*La Jolla, California*

[e]*Department of Comparative and Experimental Pathology*
*University of Florida*
*Gainesville, Florida*

[f]*Departments of Anatomy and Psychiatry*
*UCLA School of Medicine*
*Mental Retardation Research Center*
*Laboratory of Biomedical and Environmental Sciences*
*University of California*
*Los Angeles, California*

Remyelination following demyelination is in part dependent on the proliferation of oligodendrocyte progenitor cells. Immune-mediated demyelination is commonly followed by only limited remyelination by oligodendrocytes, suggesting that an immune product may interfere with this process. Activated immune cells present in demyelinated lesions can release a variety of lymphokines. Helper lymphocytes are known to secrete the lymphokine interleukin-2 (IL-2) which interacts with specific IL-2 receptors, recognized by TAC antibody,[1] to induce the proliferation of T lymphocytes. Neonatal rat oligodendrocyte progenitor cells cultured in a serumless, chemically defined medium normally proliferate.[2] However, when exposed to IL-2 at physiologic concentrations (2-5 U/ml), the normal proliferation of these oligodendrocyte pro-

---

[a]This work was supported by research grant RG 1722-A-3 from the National Multiple Sclerosis Society, TIDA K07-NS00961 from the NINCDS, a research award from The Arthur L. Swim Foundation, NIH grants HD06576, CA35299, and AM35411, DOE contract DE-AC03-76-00012, and a Leukemia Society Scholarship to A.A.

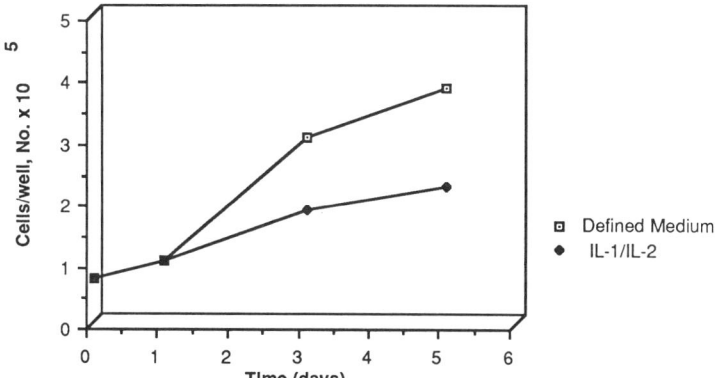

**FIGURE 1.** Growth curve of isolated oligodendrocyte progenitor cells as response to IL-1 combined with IL-2. Progenitor cells were isolated and cultured with IL-1 (3 U/ml) and IL-2 (2 U/ml) (◆) or without these lymphokines (□). Data represent cell numbers per well; values are the mean of six wells.

genitor cells is blocked. Inhibition is documented by reduction in the expected increase in cell number (FIG. 1) and a reduction in the incorporation of tritiated thymidine.[3] Specificity of this activity of IL-2 is demonstrated by blocking this response with antibody to IL-2.[3]

This response depends on the expression of TAC antibody binding (IL-2 receptor) on the oligodendrocyte progenitor cells which can be induced only by the addition

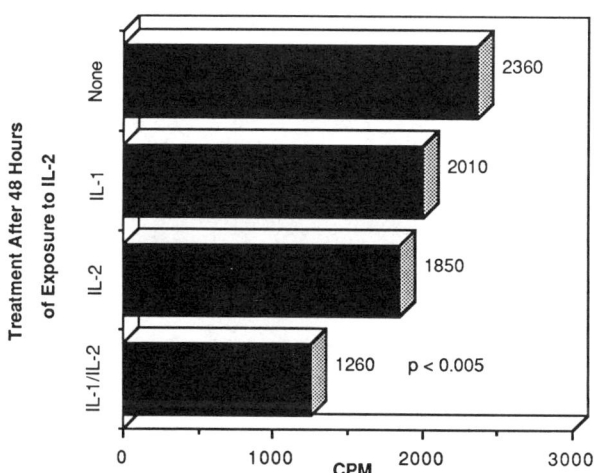

**FIGURE 2.** IL-1 and IL-2 are required for inhibition of $^3$H-thymidine incorporation into oligodendrocyte progenitor cells after exposure to IL-2 for 48 hours or longer. The difference between the IL-1 and IL-2 treatment cultures and those that received none is significant at $p < 0.005$.

of IL-1, at physiologic concentrations (2-5 U/ml), to the serumless, chemically defined medium. In mixed culture, more than 90% of oligodendrocytes present bind TAC antibody; however, oligodendrocytes exposed to IL-2 in serumless medium for 48 hours or longer lose the ability to bind TAC antibody. Therefore, the IL-2 receptor on these oligodendrocytes is down-regulated by IL-2. The addition of IL-1 to the medium leads to the induction of TAC antibody binding and is required to see inhibition of proliferation (FIG. 2). Astrocytes in the mixed glial cell culture are able to produce IL-1[4] and presumably account for the induction of TAC antibody binding activity (IL-2 receptor) on the oligodendrocytes in mixed glial cell cultures. Studies are presently underway to determine if the TAC antibody binding molecule on these cultured rat oligodendrocytes is identical to the receptor molecule on lymphocytes.[5]

These data provide evidence for a potential role of the interleukins in the regulation of oligodendrocyte proliferation, and they suggest that restricted proliferation of oligodendrocyte progenitor cells by the action of lymphokines is a possible mechanism by which impairment of remyelination may occur following immune-mediated demyelination.

## REFERENCES

1. LEONARD, W. L., J. M. DEPPER, T. UCHIYAMA, K. A. SMITH, T. A. WALDMANN & W. C. GREENE. 1982. A monoclonal antibody that appears to recognize the receptor for human T cell growth factor: Partial characterization of the receptor. Nature **300:** 267-269.
2. SANETO, R. P. & J. DE VELLIS. 1985. Characterization of cultured rat oligodendrocytes proliferating in a serum-free chemically defined medium. Proc. Natl. Acad. Sci. USA **82:** 3509-3513.
3. SANETO, R. P., A. ALTMAN, R. L. KNOBLER, H. M. JOHNSON & J. DE VELLIS. 1986. Interleukin 2 mediates the inhibition of oligodendrocyte progenitor cell proliferation in vitro. Proc. Natl. Acad. Sci. USA **83:** 9221-9225.
4. FONTANA, A. B., F. KRISTENSEN, R. DUBS, D. GEMSA & E. WEBER. 1982. Production of prostaglandin E and an interleukin 1-like factor by cultured astrocytes and C6 glioma cells. J. Immunol. **129:** 2413-2419.
5. GREENE, W. C. & W. J. LEONARD. 1986. The human Interleukin 2 receptor. Ann. Rev. Immunol. **4:** 69-95.

# Comparison of Indirect Immunofluorescence and Immunogold-Silver Staining on Cell Surface Antigens of PNS and CNS Cells[a]

CONSTANCE J. DIFIGLIA AND KAY L. FIELDS

*Department of Neurology
Albert Einstein College of Medicine
Bronx, New York 10461*

The immunogold-silver staining method has been applied to the light microscopic visualization of several antigens using monoclonal antibodies 217c (Ran-1), A2B5, and MRC Ox 7 (Thy-1.1). A rat neural tumor cell line, Schwann cells and fibroblasts from the sciatic nerve, and neurons and astrocytes from the cerebellum were stained and good specificity was achieved.

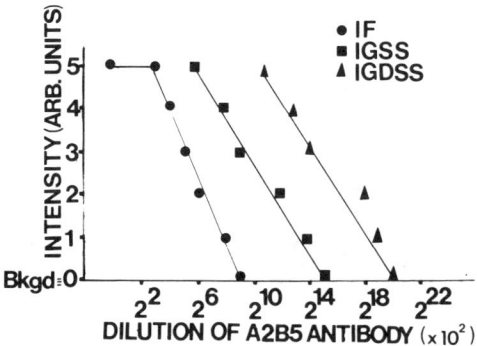

**FIGURE 1.** Comparison of indirect immunofluorescence and immunogold-silver staining for A2B5 on cerebellar neurons in culture. Staining intensity was expressed in arbitrary units from very strong (5 units) to background levels (0). IF = immunofluorescence; IGSS = immunogold-silver staining (one treatment with gelatin-silver reagent); IGDSS = immunogold-double silver staining (two treatments with gelatin-silver reagent).

[a]This work was supported by NIH Grants NS-14580 and NS-07098.

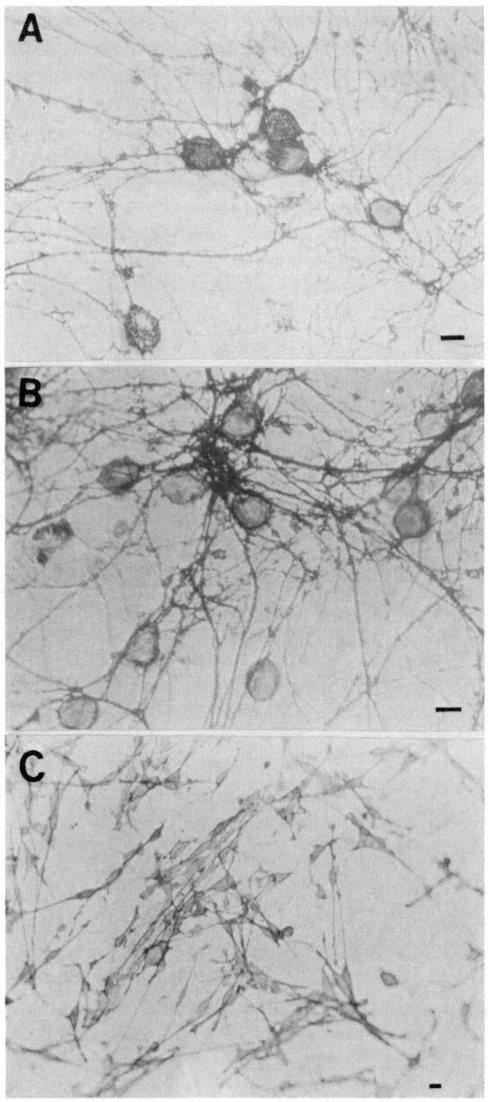

**FIGURE 2.** Immunogold-silver staining with a gelatin-silver reagent. (**A**) A2B5 on cerebellar neurons 21 days *in vitro* using A2B5 ascites (1:1600) and a single silver treatment. (**B**) A2B5 (1:400,000) using two silver treatments. Flat astrocytes lacking A2B5 antigen are present but invisible on bright-field illumination. (**C**) mAb 217c (1:400,000) detecting Ran-1 antigen on Schwann cells, with two silver treatments. Bar = 10 μm.

The method involves four incubation steps: (1) a mouse monoclonal antibody, (2) goat anti-Ig labeled with colloidal gold, (3) fixation, and (4) silver enhancement of colloidal gold by the application of a silver reagent once or twice. For the fourth step, a commercial reagent (Janssen Life Sciences, Intense Kit I) gave good results, but it had the significant disadvantage that the interval between good silver enhancement and high nonspecific deposition of silver was narrow. The kit reagents were also less stable than expected and they deteriorated, giving poor enhancement. A silver reagent containing gelatin was developed with the advantages that silver enhancement could be performed in the light, it could be monitored by color changes of the reagent solution, and the reagent was easy to prepare and economical.

Indirect immunofluorescence was performed on unfixed, live cells grown on glass coverslips in the standard way, and examined at high power magnification using an efficient microscope. For immunogold-silver staining, cells were incubated with primary antibody for 30 minutes, washed, and incubated with colloidal gold-conjugated goat anti-mouse Ig (Auroprobe LM-5 nm, 1:40, Janssen). Cells were then fixed and washed very well, and freshly prepared silver enhancement reagent was applied for 20-25 minutes or until a purple color change occurred in the reagent solution. For greater dilutions of primary antibody ( > 12,800), a first incubation with silver reagent for 15 minutes (or until the reagent solution turned orange) was followed by a stop solution, and then a second (fresh) reagent solution was applied for 20-25 minutes or until the solution turned purple.

With indirect immunofluorescence, moderate intensities were seen for dilutions of the first antibody of 1:1600 or 1:3200. Dilutions of monoclonal antibody up to 100-fold greater than those needed for immunofluorescence were sufficient for the single application of the gelatin-silver reagent (this was the average of five antigen systems). Applying the silver reagent twice, up to a 1,000-fold greater sensitivity than that with fluorescence was obtained (FIG. 1). For example, strong intensity and good cellular detail were obtained on neurons of rat cerebellar cultures labeled with A2B5 diluted 1:1600 (FIG. 2A) and maintained at very high antibody dilution (1:400,000) with two applications of the silver reagent (FIG. 2B). Good intensity was also seen with monoclonal antibody 217c diluted 1:400,000 with two applications of the silver reagent on Schwann cells of rat sciatic nerve, where it detects the Ran-1 antigen (FIG. 2C).

We expect that this method will allow the visualization of surface antigens up to 1,000-fold less abundant than the glycoproteins and glycolipids that can be seen by standard immunofluorescence.

# Loss of Functional Suppression Is Linked to Decreases in Circulating Suppressor-Inducer (CD4+2H4+) T Cells in Multiple Sclerosis

MICHEL CHOFFLON, HOWARD L. WEINER, AND
DAVID A. HAFLER

*Center for Neurologic Diseases
Brigham and Women's Hospital
and
Harvard Medical School
Boston, Massachusetts*

A consistent finding in the peripheral blood of patients with chronic multiple sclerosis (MS) is the loss of functional suppression[1,2] and a low autologous mixed lymphocyte reaction (AMLR).[3,4] Although decreases in the proportion of circulating CD8+ suppressor/cytotoxic T cells in the blood in MS have been observed by some investigators, these decreases have not been linked to losses in functional suppression.[5] A major question in the study of human autoimmune disease is whether abnormalities in immunoregulation and loss of suppression can be attributed to a particular T-cell subset. It has been recognized that the CD4+ inducer population can be separated into helper inducer and suppressor inducer subsets that can be identified by monoclonal antibodies.[6] The suppressor inducer subset has been postulated to interact with CD8+ T cells to induce suppressor effector cells. We recently found decreases in suppressor inducer T cells in progressive MS as measured by two-color immunofluorescence using differentiation markers CD4 and 2H4.[7] In the present study we examined the relationship between functional suppression and circulating CD4+2H4+ T cells using a two-stage assay: (1) T cells were stimulated for 7 days with irradiated non-T cells (AMLR) and harvested. It has been shown that suppressive T cells are generated during the course of the AMLR. (2) The AMLR-generated suppressor T cells were then incubated with mononuclear cells plus pokeweed mitogen and Ig synthesis was measured. There was less AMLR-induced suppression of IgG synthesis in patients with progressive MS (36.7 ± 4.5%) than in the controls (6.9 ± 1.7%) ($p = \leq 0.002$).[8] More importantly, there were significant correlations between decreases in circulating CD4+2H4+ T cells and loss of suppression ($p < 0.0001$) (FIG. 1) and between decreases in circulating CD4+2H4+ T cells and the AMLR ($p = 0.009$, Spearman rank-order coefficient of correlation) (FIG. 2). Thus, decreases in functional suppression and decreases in the AMLR in MS appear tightly linked to CD4+2H4+ cells, and their measurement provides a means to phenotypically monitor suppressor function. Decreases in suppressor inducer T cells may explain in part the immunoregulatory abnormalities observed in MS.

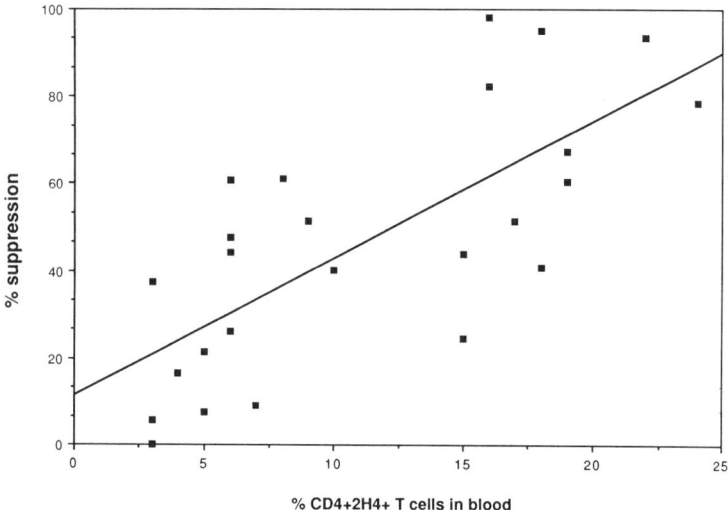

**FIGURE 1.** Functional suppression versus suppressor inducer T cells in multiple sclerosis. The proportion of circulating CD4+2H4+ cells correlated with functional suppression as measured by the inhibition of PWM-induced Ig synthesis by T cells cultured for 7 days with irradiated (5,000 rads) non-T cells (ratio = 1:10, $p < 0.0001$, $r = 0.73$, Spearman rank-order coefficient of correlation).

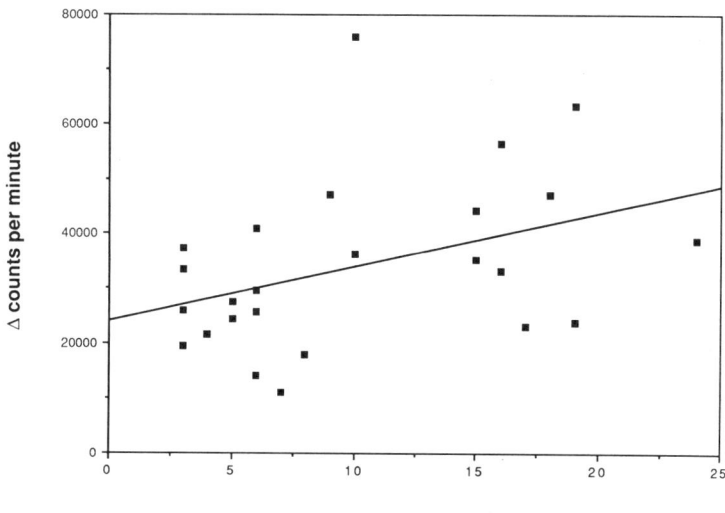

**FIGURE 2.** Autologous mixed lymphocyte reaction (AMLR) versus suppressor inducer cells in multiple sclerosis. To perform the AMLR, $10^5$ T cells were cultured for 7 days with $10^5$ non-T cells (irradiated with 5,000 rads) in 96 well round bottom plates. Two microcuries of [$^3$H] thymidine were added during the last 18 hours of culture, and the AMLR response was calculated by subtracting the counts per minute (cpm) of T cells cultured alone from the cpm of experimental determinants (T+ non-T cells). These values were significantly correlated with the proportion of circulating CD4+2H4+ cells ($p = 0.009$ Spearman rank-order coefficient of correlation) as measured by two-color fluorescence analysis on an Epics C flow cytometer.

## REFERENCES

1. HUDDLESTONE, J. R. & M. B. A. OLDSTONE. 1979. T suppressor lymphocytes fluctuate in parallel with changes in the clinical course of patients with multiple sclerosis. J. Immunol. **123:** 1615.
2. ANTEL, J. P., M. BROWN BANIA, A. REDER & N. CASHMAN. 1986. Activated suppressor cell dysfunction in progressive multiple sclerosis. J. Immunol. **137:** 137.
3. HAFLER, D. A., M. BUCHSBAUM & H. L. WEINER. 1985. Decreased autologous mixed lymphocyte reaction in multiple sclerosis. J. Neuroimmunol. **9:** 339.
4. HIRSCH, R. L. 1986. Defective autologous mixed lymphocyte reactivity in multiple sclerosis. Clin. Exp. Immunol. **64:** 107.
5. OGER, J., L. KASTRUKOFF, M. O'GORMAN & D. W. PATY. 1986. Progressive multiple sclerosis: Abnormal immune functions in vitro and aberrant correlation with enumeration of lymphocyte subpopulations. J. Neuroimmunol. **12:** 37.
6. MORIMOTO, C., N. L. LETVIN, J. DISTASO et al. 1985. The isolation and characterization of the human suppressor inducer T cell subset. J. Immunol. **134:** 1508.
7. MORIMOTO, C., D. A. HAFLER, H. L. WEINER, N. L. LETVIN, M. HAGAN, J. DALEY & S. F. SCHLOSSMAN. 1987. Selective loss of the suppressor/inducer T cell subset in progressive multiple sclerosis. N. Engl. J. Med. **316:** 67.
8. CHOFFLON, M., H. L. WEINER, C. MORIMOTO, D. A. HAFLER. 1988. Loss of functional suppression is linked to decreases in circulating suppressor-inducer T cells in multiple sclerosis. Ann. Neurol. In press.

# A 70-Kd Polypeptide Secreted by Human Peripheral Blood Mononuclear Cells That Suppresses Proliferation of a Human Glioblastoma Cell Line

TIMOTHY J. HEMESATH, DARREL TARASEWICZ,
ALISON O'NEILL, JEFFREY R. GULCHER, AND
KARI STEFANSSON

*Departments of Neurology and Pathology (Neuropathology)*
*University of Chicago*
*Chicago, Illinois 60637*

Activated lymphocytes as well as certain lymphocyte tumor lines have been found to secrete a number of soluble regulatory factors into culture medium.[1] Among these, several factors with antiproliferative activities have been described and in some cases isolated.[2] We set out to isolate and characterize a "suppressor" factor from Concanavalin A (Con A) stimulated human peripheral blood mononuclear cells (PBMNs). This factor reduces the rate of growth of both a human glioblastoma cell line and a human B-cell lymphoma line *in vitro*. It is also secreted by the human T-cell tumor line, MOLT-4. We describe here the influence of this factor on two tumor targets and the isolation procedure that was developed using supernatants from Con-A-stimulated PBMNs as the starting material. This procedure yields a protein from MOLT-4 supernatants that has the same biologic activity and size as the protein from the PBMNs.

## MATERIALS AND METHODS

### Generation of Supernatants

Peripheral blood mononuclear cells were isolated from the blood of health donors by gradient centrifugation through Ficoll-Paque (Pharmacia). Concanavalin A was added to the cells in serum-free medium for a 3-day incubation. MOLT-4 cells were maintained in RPMI 1640 with 10% fetal calf serum and transferred while in log-phase growth to serum-free medium.

## Suppression Assays

The glioblastoma line U-373MG[3] was released from plastic petri dishes by trypsin/EDTA, washed and resuspended in 10% fetal calf serum MEM. The assay was done in round bottom plates with 15,000 cells per well per 100 µl, and 50 µl of supernatant from the Con-A-stimulated PBMNs or 50 µl of medium containing the isolated protein were added to each well. The cells were incubated for 2 days and then pulsed for 5 hours with 1.0 µCi $^3$H-thymidine. Twenty microliters of $10\times$ trypsin were added to each well, the cells were harvested, and isotope incorporation was measured by scintillation counting. Assays using the Daudi cell line[4] as a target were done in flat-bottomed wells at 6,000 cells per well per 100 µl plus 50 µl of supernatants from PBMNs or medium containing the isolated protein. The Daudi cells were incubated for 4 days before pulse and harvest.

## Isolation

Cell-free supernatants were made to 5 mM of EDTA and 1 mM of PMSF before ammonium sulfate precipitation. The precipitation was followed by three liquid chromatography steps. The following columns were run with a Pharmacia FPLC system: a Mono Q (anion exchange), a Mono P (chromatofocusing), and a Superose 6 (gel filtration). The eluate from the gel filtration column, which was the last step in the enrichment process, contained a 70-kd polypeptide in a pure form as evaluated on a silver-stained SDS polyacrylamide gel.

# RESULTS AND DISCUSSION

Supernatants from Con-A-stimulated PBMNs consistently suppressed proliferation of glioblastoma cell line U-373MG. The extent of the suppression varied somewhat among individuals donating the PBMNs. FIGURE 1a shows a typical experiment in which suppression is seen relative to both supernatant from PBMNs without the addition of Con A and to serum-free medium with Con A added. Titration of neat PBMN supernatant (FIG. 1b) shows that suppression falls off with increasing dilution and is no longer evident at 1:100. We have shown that similar suppression can be achieved by adding the PBMN supernatant to B-cell lymphoma Daudi. Conditioned medium from the T-cell tumor line MOLT-4 was also found to suppress proliferation of both U-373MG and Daudi lines. Because MOLT-4 cells maintained in serum-free medium gradually ceased their secretion of suppressor factor, they were grown in 10% fetal calf serum and transferred in log growth to serum-free medium for 3-4 days before harvesting the supernatant. In this way serum-free supernatant was obtained which suppressed nearly as efficiently as fetal calf serum supplemented medium (FIG. 1c).

A purification scheme worked out with PBMN supernatant using column chromatography was successfully applied on a large scale to MOLT-4 supernatant with identical results. The column eluates were evaluated for suppressor activity as were

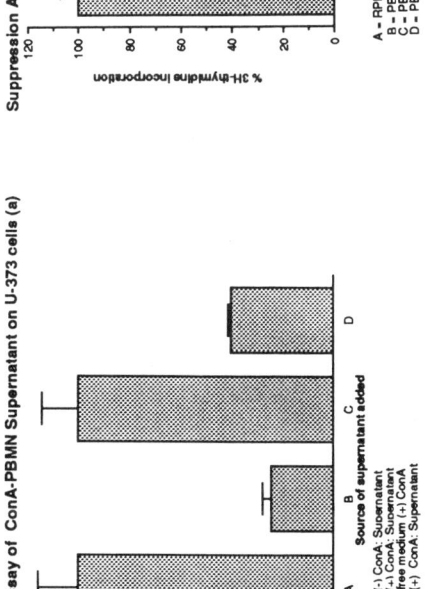
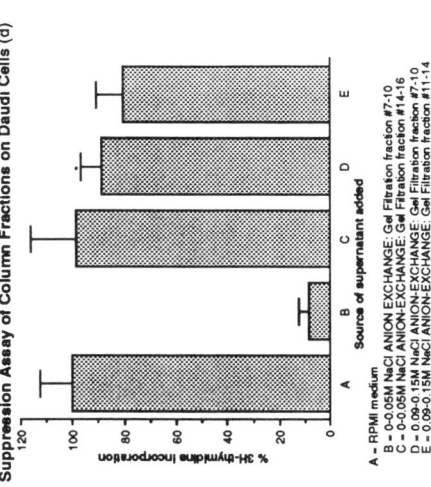
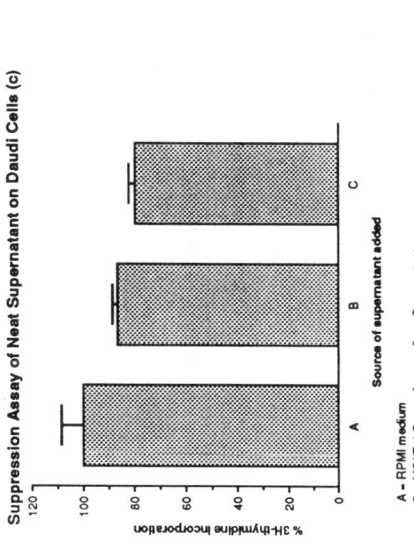

FIGURE 1. Suppression assays performed using the indicated cell lines as described in Materials and Methods. Values are derived from the mean of quadruplicate wells ± standard deviation.

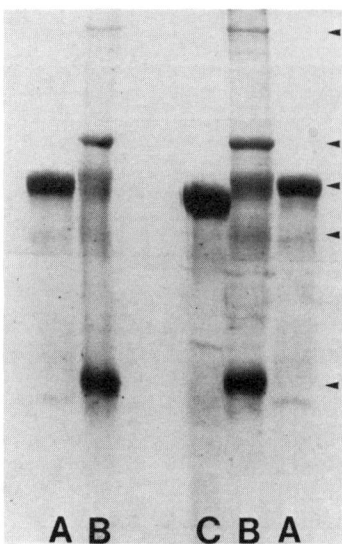

**FIGURE 2.** Silver-stained 7.5% SDS polyacrylamide gel. **Lane A,** Transferrin; **lane B,** molecular weight standards 200, 116, 92, 66, and 45 kd; **lane C,** active peak off final column in purification series (gel filtration).

the neat supernatants. FIGURE 1d shows the results of a typical experiment used to establish the location of suppressor activity. FIGURE 2 shows a silver-stained SDS polyacrylamide gel of the active species selected from the eluate off the final column in the purification series. This ~70-kd polypeptide can be isolated from both PBMN and MOLT-4 supernatants. Hence, we have isolated a polypeptide secreted by PBMNs and a T-cell tumor cell line that suppresses proliferation of certain tumor cell lines *in vitro*. It remains to be seen whether this polypeptide is of importance *in vivo*.

## REFERENCES

1. SANTOLI, D., D. J. TWEARDY, D. FERRERO, B. L. KREIDER & G. ROVERA. 1986. A suppressor lymphokine produced by human T leukemia cell lines. J. Exp. Med. **163:** 18.
2. PENNICA, D., G. E. NEDWIN, J. S. HAYFLICK, P. H. SEEBURG, R. DERYNCK, M. A. PALLADINO, W. J. KOHR, B. B. AGGARWAL & D. V. GOEDDEL. 1984. Human tumor necrosis factor: Precursor structure, expression and homology to lymphotoxin. Nature **312:** 724.
3. BECKMAN, G., L. BECKMAN, J. PONTEN & B. WESTERMARK. 1971. G-6PD and PGM phenotypes of 16 continuous human tumor cell lines. Human Hered. **21:** 238.
4. NILSSON, K., B. C. GIOVANELLS, J. S. STEHLIN & G. KLEIN. 1977. Tumorigenicity of human hematopoietic cell lines in athymic nude mice. Int. J. Cancer **19:** 337.

WORKSHOP 3. LYMPHOCYTE LINES AND DISEASE

# Response of Rat Encephalitogenic T Cells to Synthetic Peptides of Guinea Pig Myelin Basic Protein[a]

ARTHUR A. VANDENBARK,[b,c] GEORGE HASHIM,[d] AND HALINA OFFNER [b,c]

[b]*Neuroimmunology Laboratory*
*VA Medical Center*
*Portland, Oregon*

[c]*Departments of Microbiology and Immunology, and Neurology*
*Oregon Health Sciences University*
*Portland, Oregon*

[d]*St. Luke's Roosevelt Hospital and Columbia University*
*New York, New York*

T-lymphocyte lines and clones selected from Lewis rats immunized with guinea pig basic protein (GP-BP) proliferate and acquire the ability to transfer experimental autoimmune encephalomyelitis (EAE) after activation by the 69-89 peptide of GP-BP in concert with autologous I-A major histocompatibility antigens.[1] To evaluate structural requirements for activation, encephalitogenic T lymphocytes were stimulated with synthetic peptides that comprise overlapping segments of the 69-89 sequence.

T-lymphocyte lines and clones were selected for reactivity to GP-BP or peptides as described previously.[2] Briefly, lymph node cells from rats immunized with GP-BP or S55 (72-84 sequence of GP-BP) were stimulated with GP-BP or peptides for 3 days in culture medium. T cells that proliferated to antigen were expanded in the presence of interleukin-2 (IL-2) until growth slowed. The resting T cells were restimulated with GP-BP presented by irradiated thymic accessory cells and expanded in IL-2 as before. The cyclic stimulation and expansion process was continued until the line was antigen specific. In each cycle, line cells were stimulated in microtiter wells with a range of concentrations of GP-BP or synthetic peptides (0.5-250 μg/ml) representing various regions of the 69-89 region of GP-BP, and the level of proliferation was measured by the uptake of $^3$H-thymidine. In parallel, activated T cells were tested for their ability to transfer clinical EAE to naive rats.

The synthetic peptide representing the 69-89 residues of GP-BP stimulated encephalitogenic T-cell lines over a range of concentrations as well as whole GP-BP (FIG. 1). Peptide sequences 69-84 and 72-84 retained approximately 60% of the activity of GP-BP at the highest peptide concentrations used, and peptide 75-84 was inactive at all concentrations (FIG. 1). This same pattern of reactivity was also observed

---

[a]This work was supported by the National Institutes of Health Grants NS23221, NS23444, and NS21466, and the Veterans Administration.

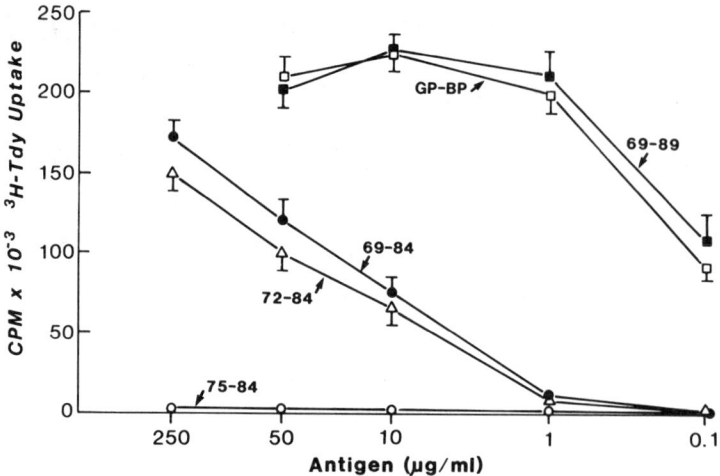

**FIGURE 1.** Proliferation response of an encephalitogenic T-cell line stimulated with GP-BP or synthetic peptides.

**TABLE 1.** Optimal Response of T Cells to GP-BP and Peptides during Process of Selection to Whole GP-BP[a]

| BP/Peptide | BP-17 Line Selection | | |
|---|---|---|---|
| | | CPM × 10⁻³ | |
| | LN | 1st Stimulation | 2nd Stimulation |
| Whole GP-BP | 139 | 231 | 139 |
| 69---------89 | 34 | 120 | 159 |
| 69---------84 | 15 | 38 | 115 |
| 69---------81 | 0 | 0 | 0 |
| 69---------81-mBSA | 0 | 0 | 0 |
| 72---------89 | 17 | 102 | 162 |
| 72---------84 | 15 | 35 | 107 |
| 72---------81 | 0 | 0 | 0 |
| 75---------89 | 12 | 30 | 105 |
| 75---------84 | 0 | 0 | 0 |
| (Leu)$_4$-75---------84 | 3 | 0 | 0 |
| 75---------84-mBSA | 0 | 0 | 0 |
| 75---------81 | 0 | 0 | 0 |
| 80-----89 | 3 | 0 | 0 |
| 69-81 + 75-84 | 0 | 0 | 0 |
| 69-81-mBSA + (Leu)$_4$-75-84 | 0 | 0 | 0 |

[a] The conclusion is that peptide 75-84 contains the minimum sequence required to stimulate encephalitogenic T cells, but it is inactive unless stabilized by residues 72-74 or 85-89.

with other GP-BP-reactive, encephalitogenic T-cell lines and clones, whereas T-cell lines of other specificities were unreactive (data not shown). T-cell lines stimulated with reactive peptide sequences were also able to transfer clinical signs of EAE concomitant with the level of proliferation (data not shown).

After immunization with GP-BP, the response of the developing T-cell line to GP-BP and synthetic peptides was assessed during each selection cycle. As shown in TABLE 1, the response to GP-BP and the 69-89 and 72-89 peptides increased substantially during the first and second stimulations of the line. Responses to peptides 72-84 and 75-89 were less pronounced, although highly significant, and responses to 75-84 were again absent. These data suggested that the 75-84 peptide sequence contained the minimum sequence required to stimulate the encephalitogenic T cells, although no reactivity could be detected unless this sequence was stabilized by residues 72-74 or 85-89. However, no responses were observed to $(Leu)_4$75-84 or 75-84-mBSA, suggesting that at least these other conformations could not produce a similar stabilizing effect (TABLE 1). Additionally, no response to the combination of 69-81 plus 75-84 was observed, suggesting that the relevant determinant needed to be present on a continuous sequence of amino acids.

After immunization with S55 (the 72-84 sequence) a T-cell line selected with S55 responded better to S55 than to whole GP-BP or other peptides, even though this line was still encephalitogenic. These results suggested that T-cell lines that responded preferentially to either whole GP-BP or S55 both retained the capacity to induce clinical EAE. These data support the notion that distinct T-cell subtypes may retain encephalitogenic activity even though their receptors respond optimally to different conformational variants of the encephalitogenic epitope.

## REFERENCES

1. VANDENBARK, A. A., H. OFFNER, T. RESHEF, R. FRITZ, C-H. J. CHOU & I. R. COHEN. 1985. J. Immunol. **135:** 229-235.
2. VANDENBARK, A. A., T. GILL & H. OFFNER. 1985. J. Immunol. **135:** 223-228.

# Analysis of Helper T-Cell Specificity Involved in the Antibody Response to the Acetylcholine Receptor

JOSEPH A. TAMI AND KEITH A. KROLICK

*Department of Microbiology*
*University of Texas Health Science Center*
*San Antonio, Texas 78284*

Myasthenia gravis (MG) is caused by impaired neuromuscular transmission, resulting in weakness and easy fatigability caused by the presence of serum antibodies directed against the muscle receptor for acetylcholine (AChR). An interesting facet of the anti-AChR antibody response is that it depends on regulatory T helper cells ($T_H$). However, the nature of the $T_H$ specificities for AChR is not nearly as well understood as the B-cell specificities; the relationship between $T_H$ responsiveness and ultimate antibody production is unclear.

The goal of this study was to explore the subunit specificities of AChR-reactive T cells. When optimal concentrations (5 μg/ml) of each purified subunit ($\alpha,\beta,\gamma,\delta$) were used to challenge lymph node cells from *rats immunized with native AChR*, it was observed that all four subunits were capable of stimulating proliferative activity (TABLE 1A). Moreover, to gain some insight into potential levels of T-cell cross-reactivity at the subunit level, proliferation cultures were also set up in which lymph node cells from *rats immunized with each of the four subunits* were challenged *in vitro* with each subunit as well as with native AChR. *In vitro* stimulation of subunit-immune T cells with the homologous subunit or any of the other three subunits resulted in proliferative activity. Interestingly, these T cells were only moderately responsive to native AChR.

Next, we examined the influence of T cells with various specificities for AChR subunits with regard to their participation in the anti-AChR antibody response. B cells isolated from AChR-immune lymph nodes were combined *in vitro* with T cells isolated from lymph nodes of rats immunized with either native AChR or purified AChR subunits (TABLE 1B). Results indicted that $T_H$ function can be provided by lymph node cells immune to either native AChR or any of the denatured subunits. Alpha subunit-immune T cells always provided helper function as effectively as did intact AChR in contrast to $\beta$, $\gamma$, or $\delta$ subunit-immune T cells that often induced only 5-20% of the levels of anti-AChR antibody.

Additional information was gained about T-cell specificity against AChR using AChR-specific T-cell hybridomas. A panel of 30 cloned T-cell hybridomas was prepared by fusion of AChR-immune rat lymph node cells with the HAT-sensitive mouse thymoma line BW5147. The resulting rat-mouse hybrid clones were tested for reactivity against AChR and purified subunits by evaluation of antigen-stimulated interleukin-2 secretion, yielding two main observations (TABLE 2). First, most T-cell clones were responsive to the purified $\alpha$ subunit. It is clearly possible that strong B-cell reactivity

TABLE 1. Proliferation and Helper Activities of Polyclonal T Cells with Specificities Restricted to Individual AChR Subunits

A. Proliferative Activity[a]

| In Vivo Priming | Stimulation Index after in Vitro Challenge | | | | |
|---|---|---|---|---|---|
| | AChR | Alpha | Beta | Gamma | Delta |
| AChR | 82 | 32 | 28 | 9 | 10 |
| Alpha subunit | 18 | 31 | 37 | 32 | 20 |
| Beta subunit | 11 | 36 | 18 | 17 | 15 |
| Gamma subunit | 4 | 22 | 17 | 26 | 17 |
| Delta subunit | 2 | 12 | 13 | 6 | 11 |

B. Helper Activity[b]

| B-Cell Specificity | T-Cell Specificity | Anti-AChR Antibody (ng/ml) |
|---|---|---|
| AChR | None | < 10 |
| None | AChR | < 10 |
| AChR | AChR | 498 ± 24 |
| AChR | Alpha | 772 ± 121 |
| AChR | Beta | 114 ± 29 |
| AChR | Gamma | 137 ± 39 |
| AChR | Delta | 116 ± 18 |

[a] T-cell proliferation expressed as stimulation indices calculated by dividing [$^3$H]TdR incorporations of cells stimulated by AChR or subunits, by incorporation into unstimulated cells.

[b] Purified B cells plus T cells of the indicated specificities were cultured for 7 days with native AChR; anti-AChR antibody was determined by radioimmunoassay. Cultures in the absence of antigen challenge yielded no detectable antibody.

TABLE 2. Subunit Reactivities of T-Cell Hybridomas

| Clone | Antigen Reactivity[a] | | | | |
|---|---|---|---|---|---|
| | R | Alpha | Beta | Gamma | Delta |
| A. 1.5 | ++ | ++ | − | − | − |
| 1.17 | + | − | − | + | − |
| B. 2.3 | + | ++ | − | ++ | − |
| 2.4 | + | + | − | − | + |
| 2.6 | ++ | ++ | ++ | − | − |
| 2.25 | + | − | + | + | − |
| 2.30 | ++ | ++ | − | − | + |
| C. 3.1 | ++ | ++ | ++ | + | − |
| 3.7 | ++ | + | − | + | + |
| 3.18 | + | + | − | ++ | ++ |
| 3.20 | ++ | ++ | ++ | ++ | − |
| 3.24 | ++ | + | − | ++ | ++ |
| 3.28 | ++ | + | + | − | ++ |
| 3.32 | ++ | + | − | + | + |
| 3.33 | ++ | ++ | ++ | − | ++ |
| D. 15 Additional clones | ++ | +/++ | +/++ | +/++ | +/++ |

[a]Reactivity pattern of AChR-responsive T-cell hybridomas. Thirty cloned hybrids were challenged with native AChR (indicated as R) or the AChR subunits. Reactivity was evaluated by stimulation of interleukin-2. Panels A, B, C, and D group clones were reactive with AChR plus either 1, 2, 3, or 4 purified subunits, respectively.

against the α subunit observed by others may be a reflection of strong helper signals from nearby α-reactive T cells. Second, most T-cell hybrids examined in this study demonstrated redundant or cross-reactive responsiveness to multiple subunits. Only two clones expressed unique reactivity with a single AChR subunit (α or γ, respectively). The remaining 28 clones were responsive to two (16%), three (27%), or all four (50%) subunits demonstrating antigenic determinants shared among the subunits that are recognized by T cells.

In summary, a predominant T-cell reactivity against AChR was observed to be directed against the α subunit, but frequent cross-reactivity was also observed against two or more other subunits as well. Further refinement of the mapping of T-cell epitopes on AChR awaits the use of low molecular weight AChR peptides.

# Experimental Allergic Encephalomyelitis Mediated by Murine Encephalitogenic T-Cell Lines Specific for Myelin Proteolipid Apoprotein

### JUN-ICHI SATOH, FUMIHIKO KOIKE, AND TAKESHI TABIRA

*The Division of Demyelinating Disease and Aging*
*National Institute of Neuroscience*
*National Center of Neurology and Psychiatry*
*Kodaira, Tokyo, Japan*

Two T-cell lines specific for bovine myelin proteolipid apoprotein (PLP) were established from SJL/J mice and maintained for over 100 days.[1] The long-term cultured line cells bore surface phenotypes of T helper/inducer cells (Lyt-1$^+$, Lyt-2$^-$, and L3T4$^+$) and responded well to bovine, rat, and guinea pig PLP but not to myelin basic protein (BP) (TABLE 1). One line, designated as PL1, responded to major PLP, and another, designated as PL3, responded to both major PLP and DM-20, which are the two major intrinsic membrane proteins of central nervous system (CNS)

TABLE 1. Antigen-Specific Proliferation of the Line Cells

| Antigen or Mitogen (μg/ml) | | PL1 | | PL3 | |
|---|---|---|---|---|---|
| | | ΔCPM ± SD | (SI) | ΔCPM ± SD | (SI) |
| PLP | (10) | 23,917 ± 930 | (55.9) | 20,186 ± 1,472 | (16.8) |
| PLP | (25) | 15,269 ± 889 | (36.0) | 26,672 ± 2,829 | (21.9) |
| Major PLP | (10) | 51,852 ± 3,205 | (119.9) | 20,701 ± 2,328 | (17.2) |
| DM-20 | (10) | 359 ± 392 | (1.8) | 34,326 ± 3,703 | (27.9) |
| RPLP | (10) | 38,575 ± 719 | (91.8) | 32,232 ± 155 | (25.3) |
| GPPLP | (10) | 37,421 ± 3,414 | (86.8) | 34,684 ± 1,662 | (27.2) |
| BBP | (25) | 11 ± 246 | (1.0) | −599 ± 139 | (0.5) |
| GPBP | (25) | −24 ± 185 | (0.9) | −583 ± 122 | (0.5) |
| PPD | (25) | 84 ± 187 | (1.2) | −556 ± 226 | (0.6) |
| Con A | (1) | 21,839 ± 2,730 | (51.1) | 3,580 ± 324 | (3.8) |
| LPS | (10) | −307 ± 118 | (0.3) | −522 ± 152 | (0.6) |

ABBREVIATIONS: PLP - major PLP; DM-20 = of bovine origin; RPLP = rat PLP; GPPLP = guinea pig PLP; BP = basic protein; BBP = bovine BP; GPBP = guinea pig BP.

myelin. Intraperitoneal inoculation of 4 to 30 × $10^6$ PLP-activated line cells followed by injection of pertussis vaccine (2 × $10^7$ organisms) induced acute inflammatory disease of the CNS with typical clinical signs of experimental allergic encephalomyelitis (EAE) mostly in a week in recipient mice that had been treated with low-dose (550 rads) irradiation (TABLE 2). Almost all animals recovered completely, and 2 of 12 animals had a relapse 42 or 75 days after inoculation. The lesions were restricted to the CNS and were characterized by perivascular and parenchymal infiltration of inflammatory cells, fibrin deposit, and primary demyelination. In the severe lesions, axons were also damaged. Encephalitogenicity of PLP has been debated because of the possible contamination with BP. Recently, acute or chronic EAE, or both, has been induced by active challenge with highly purified PLP in some animals;[2,3] however, the possible effect of a minute amount of contaminating BP could not be ruled out completely. Now that PLP-specific effector T cells induce inflammatory demyelination in the CNS, there is no doubt that PLP is a definite encephalitogen. This novel animal

TABLE 2. Experimental Allergic Encephalomyelitis (EAE) Induced by Proteolipid Apoprotein (PLP) in SJL/J Mice

| No. of Cells ($\times 10^{-7}$) | First EAE | | | Second EAE | | Incidence of Histologic EAE |
|---|---|---|---|---|---|---|
| | Incidence | Onset Day | Severity | Incidence | Onset Day | |
| *EAE Induced by PLP-Specific T-Cell Line (PL1)* | | | | | | |
| 3-2 | 4/4 | 6-31 | 4.5 | ... | ... | ... |
| 2-1 | 12/14 | 6-41 | 3.3 | 2/12 | 42, 75 | 11/11 |
| 1- | 3/3 | 7-14 | 2.7 | ... | ... | ... |
| *EAE Induced by Active Challenge with Bovine PLP* | | | | | | |
| ... | 17/19 | 13-21 | 3.8 | 4/11 | 49, 52, 64, 116 | 5/5 |

model is important to our understanding of the pathogenesis of the human demyelinating disease, multiple sclerosis.

## REFERENCES

1. SATOH, J., K. SAKAI, M. ENDOH, F. KOIKE, T. KUNISHITA, T. NAMIKAWA, T. YAMAMURA & T. TABIRA. 1987. Experimental allergic encephalomyelitis mediated by murine encephalitogenic T cell lines specific for myelin proteolipid apoprotein. J. Immunol. **138**: 179.
2. YAMAMURA, T., T. NAMIKAWA, M. ENDOH, T. KUNISHITA & T. TABIRA. 1986. Experimental allergic encephalomyelitis induced by proteolipid protein in Lewis rats. J. Neuroimmunol. **12**: 143.
3. ENDOH, M., T. TABIRA, T. KUNISHITA, K. SAKAI, T. YAMAMURA & T. TAKETOMI. 1986. DM-20, a proteolipid apoprotein, is an encephalitogen of acute and relapsing autoimmune encephalomyelitis in mice. J. Immunol. **137**: 3832.

# Fine Specificities of Myelin Basic Protein-Specific Human T-Cell Clones

## J. R. RICHERT, C. A. REUBEN-BURNSIDE, G. E. DEIBLER, AND M. W. KIES

*Georgetown University Medical Center*
*Washington, DC*
*and*
*The National Institute of Mental Health*
*Bethesda, Maryland*

Myelin basic protein (BP) is a suspected autoimmune target in postviral demyelinating syndromes and in multiple sclerosis (MS). The encephalitogenic portion of the BP molecule varies from species to species and even from strain to strain of experimental animals. Therefore, it cannot be deduced from animal studies which region or regions of the molecule may be targets of a pathogenetic immune response in humans. To identify human T-cell recognition sites on the human BP molecule, we generated a library of BP-specific T-cell clones from the peripheral blood of a patient with MS and examined their patterns of reactivity against fragments of the BP molecule and against a panel of xenogeneic BPs of defined amino acid sequence. The latter are presented in TABLE 1. Fragments of the molecule used in this study are referred to according to the nomenclature in TABLE 1. The rat small BP, from which residues 118-159 are deleted, and the human small BP (deletion of 107-117) were also used.

Thirty of the 40 clones proliferated in response to fragment 99-177 of the human BP molecule; seven reacted with fragment 1-98; three did not proliferate in response to either fragment and presumably recognized epitopes that span the 98-99 cleavage site. Of the three that failed to recognize either fragment, one responded to guinea pig fragment 91-177, thus placing the N-terminus of the epitope that it recognizes between residues 91 and 98. The other two appear to recognize an epitope that spans both 90-91 and 98-99. Four patterns of reactivity were seen with the 30 clones that recognized the C-terminal half of the molecule, and four patterns were also seen with clones reacting with the N-terminal half (TABLE 2). Thus, a minimum of 10 human T-cell recognition sites appear to be present on the BP molecule. Twenty-one clones demonstrated patterns of reactivity that implicated sites encompassing either residues 99-105 or residues 160-177. Patterns that suggested epitopes lying between residues 119 and 150 were seen with nine clones. Of the seven clones reacting with 1-98, at least one recognizes an epitope lying within the first 44 residues of the molecule; the remaining sites have not been narrowed down appreciably.

The data suggest the possibility of an immunodominant site in the C-terminal half of the BP molecule. Studies are currently being planned with synthetic peptide frag-

TABLE 1. Xenogeneic Basic Proteins (BPs) Used in Proliferation Assays

```
                    1                   2                             3
                    0                   0                             0
Hum   A S * Q K R P S Q R H * G S K Y L A T A S T M D H A R H G F L P R H R D T
Bov   A A Q K R P S Q R R | | G S K Y L A T A S T M D H A R H G F L P R H R D T
Rab   A S Q K R P S Q R H | G S K Y L A T A S T M D H A R H G F L P R H R D T
GPig  A S Q K R P S Q R H H G S K Y L A T A S T M D H A R H G F L P R H R D T
Rat   A S Q K R P S Q R H G S K Y L A T A S T M D H A R H G F L P R H R D T
Chic  A S Q K R S * F * H G S K | * M * S T D H A R H G S * L * P R H R D S *

      4                   5                   6                         7
      0                   0                   0                         0
Hum   G I L D S I G R F F G G D R G A P K R G S S G K D A R H P A R T A H Y G
Bov   G I L D S L G R F F G S D R G A P K R G S S G K D D R H A A R T T H Y G
Rab   G I L D S I G R F F G S D R G A P K R G S S G K D | H H | A A R T T H Y G
GPig  G I L D S I G R F F G G D R G A P K R G S S G K D | H H | A A R T T H Y G
Rat   G L L D S L G R F F G G D R | A V P R R G F G K D | H H | A A R A S H V G
Chic  * * * * * * * * * * * * * * * * * * * * * * * * * * * * * * *

                          8                           9
                          0                           0
Hum   S L P Q Q K S R H G R T Q Q D E N P V V H F F K N I V T P R T P P P S Q G
Bov   S L P Q Q K A Q H G R P Q D E N P V V H F F K N I V T P R T P P P S Q G
Rab   S L P Q Q K S Q H G R P Q D E N P V V H F F K N I V T P R T P P P S Q G
GPig  S L P Q Q K S Q | | R S Q D E N P V V H F F K N I V T P R T P P P S Q G
```

```
         1                   2                           3
         0                   0                           0                    4 0
Rat   S  L  P  Q  K  S  Q  —  —  R  T  Q        D  E  N  P  V  V  H  F  F  K  N  I  V  T  P  R  T  P  P  P  S  Q  G
Chic  S  I  P  Q  R  S  Q  H  —  —  R  P (N,D,G,N) P  V  V  H  F  F  K  N  I  V  S  P  R  T  P  P  P  M  Q  A
      *              *        *  *        *              *                       *                          *  *  *

Hum   K  G  R  G  L  S  L  R  F  S  W  G  A  E  G  Q  R  P  G  F  G  Y  G  G  R  A  S  D  Y  K  S  A  H  K
Bov   K  G  R  G  L  S  L  R  F  S  W  G  A  E  G  Q  K  P  G  F  G  Y  G  G  R  A  D  Y  K  S  A  H  K
Rab   K  G  R  G  T  V  L  R  F  S  W  G  A  E  G  Q  K  P  G  F  G  Y  G  G  R  A  A  D  Y  K  S  A  H  K
GPig  K  G  R  G  L  S  L  R  F  S  W  G  A  E  G  Q  K  P  G  F  G  Y  G  G  R  A  —  D  Y  K  S  A  |  K
Rat   K  G  R  G  L  S  L  R  F  S  W  G  A  E  G  Q  K  P  G  F  G  Y  G  G  R  A  S  D  Y  K  S  A  H  K
Chic  K  G  R  G  L  S  L  T  R  F  W  G  G  E  G  H  K  K  G  S  G  Y  G  G  K  F  Y  E  H  K  S  A  H  K
                        *                    *           *           *                 *     *  *

                      5                               6                       7
                      0                               0                       0
Hum   G  F  K  K  G  —  —  V  |  D  A  Q  G  T  L  S  K  I  F  K  K  L  G  G  R  —  —  D  S  R  S  G  S  P  M  A  R  R
Bov   G  L  K  K  G  —  —  |  —  H  A  Q  G  T  L  S  K  I  F  K  K  L  G  G  R  —  —  D  S  R  S  G  S  P  M  A  R  R
Rab   G  L  K  K  G  —  —  A  —  D  A  Q  G  T  L  S  R  L  F  K  K  L  G  G  R  —  —  D  S  R  S  G  S  P  M  A  R  R
GPig  G  F  K  K  G  —  —  A  —  H  D  A  Q  G  T  L  S  K  I  F  K  K  L  G  G  R  —  —  D  S  R  S  G  S  P  M  A  R  R
Rat   G  F  K  K  G  —  —  A  —  D  A  Q  G  T  L  S  K  I  F  K  K  L  G  G  R  —  —  D  S  R  S  G  S  P  M  A  R  R
Chic  G  H  K  G  Y  S  H  Q (G,E,G) T  L  S  K  I  F  K  K  L  G  G  R  P  (S,G,S,G,S)  R  S  G  S  P  V  A  R  R
      *     *     *        *  *                             *                       *                       *
```

NOTE: Amino acid sequences of the myelin basic protein molecules used in this study: human (Hum), bovine (Bov), rabbit (Rab), guinea pig (GPig), rat, and chicken (Chic). The sequences are presented so that homologous residues are placed vertically in relation to one another. Because of various deletions in each of the molecules, this schema results in a total of 177 possible residue sites. The *asterisks across the top* of each segment indicate where human BP differs from any of the other BP molecules. The *asterisks across the bottom* of each segment denote where chicken BP differs from all of the other BP molecules.

TABLE 2. Patterns of Reactivity with Xenogeneic Basic Proteins by Human T-Cell Clones

| Group | No. of Clones | Pattern of Reactivity | | | | |
|---|---|---|---|---|---|---|
| | | Rat (small) | Rabbit | Bovine | Guinea Pig | Chicken |
| 99-177 | | | | | | |
| A | 5 | − | − | − | − | − |
| B | 3 | + | + | + | + | + |
| C | 18 | + | + | + | + | − |
| D | 4 | − | + | + | + | − |
| 1-98 | | | | | | |
| E | 3 | + | + | + | + | + |
| F* | 2 | + | + | + | + | − |
| G | 2 | − | − | − | − | − |

*Preliminary data indicate that one of the two clones in group F reacts with rabbit fragment 1-44, suggesting that group F is subdivided into two subgroups.

ments that will include residues 87-106 and 155-177. Future attempts to specifically suppress the full range of human T-cell responses to BP will most likely require the suppression of multiple T-cell populations expressing a wide range of peptide specificities.

# Alterations in the Pattern of MHC Restriction of T Cells in Relapsing Murine Experimental Allergic Encephalomyelitis

R. M. McCARRON, R. FALLIS, AND D. E. McFARLIN

*Neuroimmunology Branch*
*NINCDS*
*National Institutes of Health*
*Bethesda, Maryland 20892*

In SJL, PL, and SJL × PL (F1) mice, the induction of chronic relapsing murine experimental allergic encephalomyelitis (EAE) by the passive transfer of guinea pig myelin basic protein (GPBP)-immune T cells requires the *in vitro* proliferation of these cells in the presence of GPBP and antigen-presenting cells (APCs).[1,2] Removal of APCs from immune-lymph node cell (LNC) preparations resulted in the loss of both the proliferative response and the concomitant ability to adoptively transfer EAE. The proliferative response of GPBP-immune T-cell populations from F1 mice was reconstituted by the addition of APCs from either SJL, PL, or F1 spleens or lymph nodes. Immune F1 T cells were positively selected to respond to only one of the parental haplotypes by culturing the cells in the presence of either SJL or PL APCs.

TABLE 1. Prior Education of GPBP-Immune F1 T Cells by SJL or PL Macrophages Affects the Proliferative Response of Immune F1 T Cells to GPBP

| Macrophage in Culture | Macrophage in Assay | GPBP ($\mu$g/ml) | | |
|---|---|---|---|---|
| | | 0 | 100 | 10 |
| SJL MO | None | 0.5 | 0.9 | 0.5 |
| SJL MO | SJL MO | 0.9 | 8.7 | 3.4 |
| SJL MO | PL MO | 0.5 | 0.7 | 0.8 |
| PL MO | None | 0.8 | 0.9 | ND |
| PL MO | SJL MO | 1.0 | 1.1 | ND |
| PL MO | PL MO | 1.0 | 17.8 | ND |

NOTE: F1 LNC were harvested 10 days after immunization and were depleted of macrophages (MO) and cultured at $4 \times 10^5$ cells per well with either PL or SJL MO. Exogenous irradiated SJL or PL MO were added at $8 \times 10^5$ cells per well where indicated. Proliferation ($^3$H-TdR incorporation) was measured after 4 days in culture. Data represent the mean ($10^{-3}$) of quadruplicate determinations (SE = 15% mean). ND = not done.

Subsequent cultures of such F1 T cells proliferated to GPBP only in the presence of APCs that exhibited the haplotype of the APCs used in the original selection (TABLE 1). The T cells that displayed haplotype-specific proliferative responses to GPBP-induced chronic relapsing EAE when adoptively transferred into naive F1 mice. Both SJL and PL APCs exhibited the capacity to present GPBP to immune F1 T cells in an encephalitogenic manner. No significant differences in the efficacy of adoptive transfer, the day of onset, or the clinical severity of EAE were observed between animals adoptively transferred with F1 T cells cultured in the presence of SJL or PL APC. All mice adoptively transferred with F1 T cells that were cultured in with either SJL or PL APCs relapsed after approximately 6-7 weeks. Spleen cells (SC) obtained from recipient F1 mice during recovery from a second attack (relapse) proliferated

TABLE 2. Alterations in I-A Restriction of the Proliferative Response to GPBP in Splenic T Cells from Mice with Chronic Relapsing EAE

| Responding Cell | Macrophage in Culture | GPBP ($\mu$g/ml) | | |
|---|---|---|---|---|
| | | 0 | 100 | 10 |
| SC 1 | None | 6.3 | 52.1 | 41.5 |
| T | None | 4.3 | 4.3 | 3.8 |
| T | SJL MO | 5.7 | 27.1 | 21.0 |
| T | PL MO | 6.2 | 18.9 | 15.9 |
| T | F1 MO | 6.0 | 22.5 | 15.9 |
| SC 2 | None | 10.5 | 53.3 | 49.9 |
| T | None | 5.9 | 6.8 | 9.3 |
| T | SJL MO | 7.0 | 13.5 | 10.8 |
| T | PL MO | 6.1 | 29.8 | 26.7 |
| T | F1 MO | 7.6 | 29.8 | 22.9 |

NOTE: F1 T cells from GPBP-immune mice were stimulated with GPBP and exogenous SJL (SC 1) or PL (SC 2) macrophages (MO). After a repeat of this culture and demonstration of a lack of proliferation in the presence of irrelevant exogenous MO, F1 T cells were transferred intravenously to naive F1 mice. Ten weeks following adoptive transfer (2 weeks after recovery from a second attack of EAE), T cells were prepared from recipient spleens and were cultured at $4 \times 10^5$ cells per well in the presence of irradiated SJL or PL MO ($8 \times 10^5$ cells per well) where indicated. Proliferation ($^3$H-TdR incorporation) was measured after 4 days in culture. Data represent the mean ($10^{-3}$) of quadruplicate determinations (SE = 15% mean).

to a wide range of GPBP concentrations. Removal of APCs from these SC cultures resulted in the loss of proliferation to antigen. Purified splenic T-cell populations reconstituted with F1 APCs were able to proliferate to GPBP. The proliferative response to GPBP of these same splenic T-cell preparations could also be reconstituted by culturing these cells in the presence of either SJL or PL APCs. These results were observed irregardless of the haplotype-restriction pattern of the immune F1 T cells originally inoculated into the animal to induce disease. Immune F1 T cells positively selected on either SJL or PL APCs had similar results (TABLE 2). These data suggest that during chronic relapsing EAE, the heterogeneity of relapsed T-cell responses to GPBP is increased to include T cells restricted by additional class II glycoproteins.

Thus, relapses in these animals may be due to the generation of T cells that display additional antigenic specificities and may not be due to the activation of T cells with the same antigenic specificity as those used to induce the disease (acute attack).

## REFERENCES

1. PETTINELLI, C. B. & D. E. MCFARLIN. 1981. Adoptive transfer of experimental allergic encephalomyelitis in SJL/J mice after *in vitro* activation of lymph node cells by myelin basic protein: Requirement for Lyt $1^+$ $2^-$ T lymphocytes. J. Immunol. **127:** 1420-1423.
2. MOKHTARIAN, F., D. E. MCFARLIN & C. S. RAINE. 1984. Adoptive transfer of myelin basic protein-sensitized T cells produces chronic relapsing demyelinating disease in mice. Nature **309:** 356-358.

# Recognition of Intracellular Measles Virus Antigens by HLA Class II Restricted Measles Virus-Specific Cytotoxic T Lymphocytes

STEVEN JACOBSON, RAFICK P. SEKALY,
WILLIAM J. BELLINI, CONNIE L. JOHNSON,
HENRY F. McFARLAND, AND
ERIC O. LONG

*Neuroimmunology Branch*
*National Institutes of Health*
*Bethesda, Maryland 20892*

Measles virus-specific cytotoxic T cells (CTLs) are predominantly T4$^+$ and are restricted by HLA class II determinants.[1] It is not yet known which viral antigens are presented to the CTLs or which antigen presentation pathway is used. HLA class I-restricted CTLs recognize endogenously synthesized proteins on target cells, whereas it has been shown in the influenza system that HLA class II restricted CTLs recognize exogenous proteins that have been endocytosed and processed by the target cell.[2] In establishing a system to answer these questions we generated stable murine DAP.3 fibroblast cell lines transfected with expressible cDNAs for the alpha- and beta-chains of HLA DR1 and HLA DR4. Full-length cDNAs encoding the intracellular nucleocapsid or matrix proteins of measles virus were cloned into expression vectors carrying the hygromycin resistance marker and co-transfected into the HLA-DR expressing murine L cells.

When polyclonal or monoclonal antibodies specific for these measles virus antigens are used, it appears that these cells do not express "native" measles virus proteins. Immunofluorescence or immunoprecipitation of cells pulse-labeled with $^{35}$S-methionine failed to detect viral antigens in these transfectants. Northern blot analysis, however, demonstrated RNA of the appropriate size for measles virus nucleocapsid and matrix genes. Moreover, these transfectants were efficiently lysed by measles virus-specific, T4$^+$ CTLs in an HLA-restricted manner. Therefore, there appears to be no obligate requirement for cell surface expression of viral antigen in this HLA class II restricted CTL response. These experiments demonstrate that the cellular immune response can recognize viral antigens in the apparent absence of "detectable" protein. The only requirement is the genetic information of the appropriate viral gene.

The capacity of measles virus-specific T4$^+$ CTLs to lyse cells transfected with measles virus genes also serves to define the role of the HLA-restricted antigen-presenting cell to CTL. Recent reports suggest that the pathways for HLA class I and class II restricted antigen presentation are different.[3,4] Influenza virus-specific HLA class I restricted CTLs recognize viral antigens that have been degraded in the cell and presented as processed peptides by the HLA class I antigen. This pathway is not inhibited by the lysomotropic inhibitor chloroquine. In contrast, HLA class II restricted CTLs specific for influenza virus recognize peptides that have been derived from exogenous proteins that have been endocytosed and processed by the antigen-presenting cell. This pathway is inhibitable by chloroquine.

Measles virus CTL, unlike the influenza virus, is predominantly HLA class II restricted,[1] and because a defined system for expression of HLA class II and measles virus genes has been developed, this system is ideal to define the pathway involved in HLA class II restricted viral antigen presentation. Chloroquine did not inhibit the lysis of MV-M or MV-N transfectants by measles virus CTLs. In contrast, lysis of these same influenza-virus infected transfectants by influenza virus-specific CTLs that are HLA class II restricted was completely inhibited by chloroquine. These experiments demonstrate that presentation of measles virus antigens by HLA class II antigens does not involve the endocytic pathway. Thus, the antigen presentation pathways for HLA class I and class II determinants may not be entirely separate, and the cytoplasmic processing pathway may be involved in the processing of viral antigens.

## REFERENCES

1. JACOBSON, S., J. R. RICHERT, W. E. BIDDISON, A. SATINSKY, R. J. HARTZMAN & H. F. MCFARLAND. 1984. J. Immunol. **133:** 754.
2. MORRISON, L. A., A. E. LUCKACHER, V. L. BRACIALE, D. FAN & T. J. BRACIALE. 1986. J. Exp. Med. **163:** 903.
3. GERMAIN, R. N. 1986. Nature **322:** 687.
4. TOWNSEND, A. R. M., J. ROTHBARD, F. M. GOTCH, G. BAHADUR, D. WRAITH & A. J. MCMICHAEL. 1986. Cell **44:** 959.

# Blood and Thymic Lymphocyte Responses to Peptide Sequences of the Acetylcholine Receptor in Myasthenia Gravis

G. HARCOURT,[a,b] N. SOMMER,[a] J. ROTHBARD,[c]
D. BEESON,[a] N. WILLCOX,[a] AND
J. NEWSOM-DAVIS[a]

[a]*Department of Neurological Science*
*Royal Free Hospital School of Medicine*
*London, England*

[c]*Imperial Cancer Research Fund*
*Lincolns Inn Fields*
*London, England*

Approximately 60% of anti-acetylcholine receptor (AChR) antibodies found in the serum of patients with myasthenia gravis (MG) recognize a region on the alpha subunit of the AChR known as the main immunogenic region.[1] Recent evidence suggests that most AChR-specific T lymphocytes from MG patients also recognize the alpha subunit.[2] To try and identify the T-cell recognition sites on the AChR, 12 peptides representing sequences of the alpha subunit were tested. They all contain a common four to five amino acid motif thought to be important in T-cell recognition,[3] or they were selected because of the work of Lennon et al.[4]

Peripheral blood lymphocytes (PBLs) from 27 patients with MG and 15 controls, including 11 patients with other neurologic diseases (multiple sclerosis, cerebellar syndrome, peripheral neuropathy, and LEMS) and 4 healthy controls, were assayed for a proliferative response to the 12 peptides. Low density thymus cells from seven patients with MG and lymph node cells from three patients with MG were also tested. The cells were cultured in triplicate wells of microtiter plates at a concentration of 2 × $10^5$ cells per well, and peptides were added to give a final concentration ranging from 1 to 50 µg/ml. Triplicate wells containing purified *Torpedo* AChR (10 µg/ml) were included for each subject. After 72 hours in culture, the cells were pulsed with $^3$H-thymidine, harvested, and counted.

A summary of the proliferative responses of PBL to eight peptides is shown in FIGURE 1. Lymphocytes from a total of 8 of 27 patients with MG and 7 of 15 controls showed a response to peptides 125-143 (disulfide linked or unlinked) and 129-143, some of which are shown in FIGURE 2. Peptide 257-271 induced responses only among

---

[b]Present address: Neuroscience Group, Institute for Molecular Medicine, John Radcliffe Hospital, Headington, Oxford OX3 9DU.

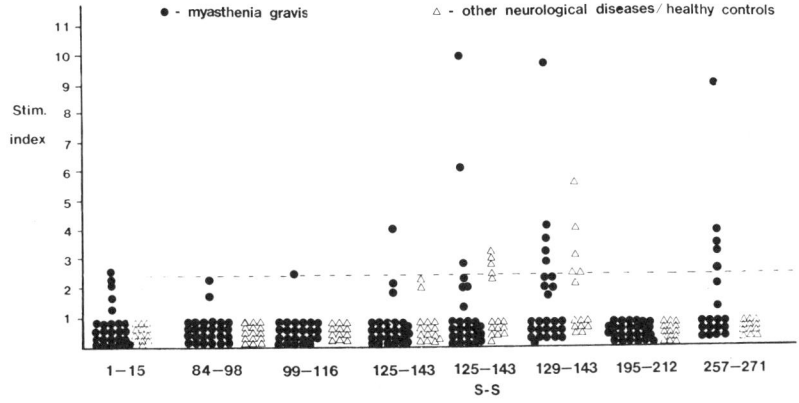

**FIGURE 1.** Responses of peripheral blood mononuclear cells to peptide sequences of the human acetylcholine receptor alpha subunit.

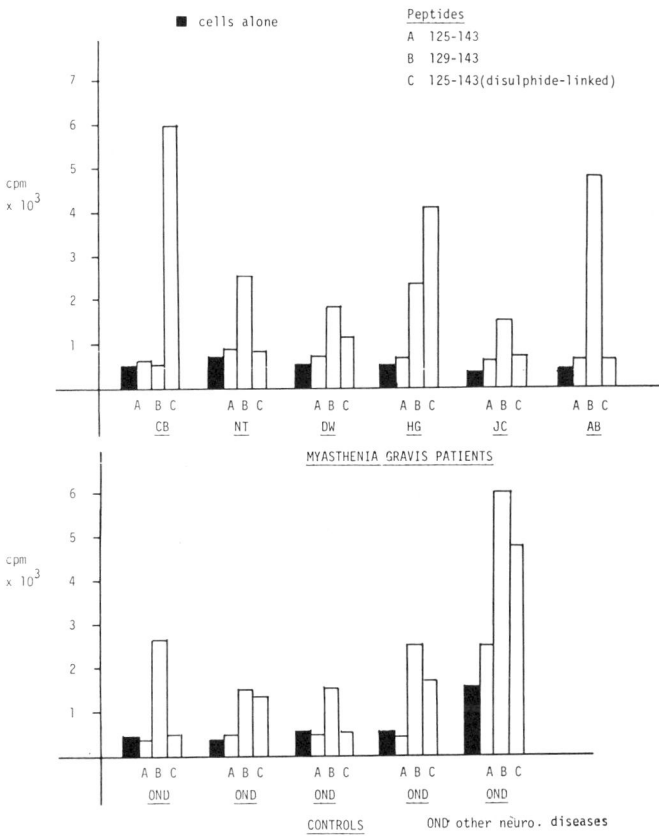

**FIGURE 2.** Proliferative responses of peripheral blood lymphocytes to peptide 125-143, 129-143, and 125-143 (disulfide linked).

patients with MG (5 of 27; SI = 2.8-9.0). Thymic lymphocytes from three of seven patients and lymph node cells from two of three also responded to the three peptides in the region 125-143. None of the other eight peptides tested induced a proliferative response in cells from either patients or controls.

T-lymphocyte lines specifically recognizing *Torpedo* AChR that had previously been isolated from two patients with MG were also assayed for proliferative responses. However, these lines failed to recognize any of the 12 peptides despite an approximately 80% homology between the amino acid sequences of the *Torpedo* and human AChR. Conversely, a line raised against peptide 125-143 (disulfide-linked), which was isolated from a patient with MG, failed to recognize whole *Torpedo* AChR. This lack of recognition in some instances could be due to the effects of single amino acid differences between human peptides and *Torpedo* AChR or to steric interference by adjacent amino acids, both of which are thought to alter the capacity of T lymphocytes to recognize their target.[5]

The stimulation seen in both patients and controls with peptide 125-143 may be the result of cross-reactivity of this peptide sequence with another common antigen or to the presence in all individuals of potential AChR-specific T cells that are normally suppressed in patients without MG. However, because peptide 257-271 induced a response only among patients with MG (18.5%), it may represent one of the T-cell recognition sites on the AChR.

## REFERENCES

1. TZARTOS, S. J. & J. M. LINDSTROM. 1980. Proc. Natl. Acad. Sci. USA **77:** 755-759.
2. HOHLFELD, R. *et al.* 1987. Proc. Natl. Acad. Sci. USA **84:** 5379-5383.
3. ROTHBARD, J. *et al.* 1986. Ann. Inst. Pasteur **137E:** 497-528.
4. LENNON, V. A. *et al.* 1985. Proc. Natl. Acad. Sci. USA **82:** 8805-8809.
5. SETTE, S. *et al.* 1987. Nature **328:** 395-399.

# T-Cell Clones Specific to Acetylcholine Receptor, Its Subunits, and Peptides

## YOSHITAKA FUJII AND JON LINDSTROM

*The Salk Institute for Biological Studies*
*San Diego, California 92138*

Myasthenia gravis (MG) and its animal model, experimental autoimmune MG (EAMG), are antibody-mediated diseases, but the production of antibodies to acetylcholine receptors (AChR) depends on help from T cells.[1] To identify epitopes

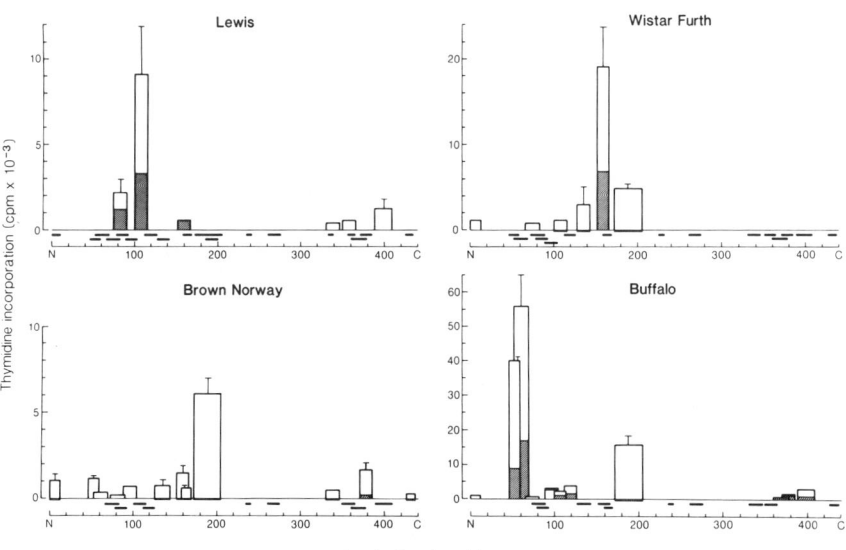

**FIGURE 1.** Different peptides are recognized by AChR-immune T cells in different strains of rats. Lewis, Brown Norway, Wistar Furth, or Buffalo rats were immunized with 30 μg of *Torpedo* AChR, and 4 weeks later nylon wool-passed lymph node cells were tested for their reaction to synthetic peptides from the *Torpedo* AChR α subunit sequence. Proliferation responses to synthetic peptides (mean ± SEM) are indicated by bars above the corresponding positions marked on the base line. *Open* and *hatched* bars indicate responses to $10^{-5}$ and $10^{-6}$M of peptides, respectively. Bars under the baseline indicate negative responses. Responses to α subunit were: Lewis rats = 143,988 cpm, Brown Norway rats = 21,113 cpm, Wistar Furth rats = 140,605 cpm, and Buffalo rats = 145,029 cpm. Note that the scales are different in each panel. Reproduced, with permission, from Fujii and Lindstrom.[2]

recognized by T cells in EAMG rats, we tested native AChR, its subunits, and synthetic peptides covering 62% of the α subunit for their ability to stimulate AChR-primed lymph node cells. AChR-specific long-term T-cell line, and AChR-specific cloned T-cell lines.

Acetylcholine-receptor-primed lymph node cells proliferate in response to all four subunits.[1,2] When these cells were cultured with a panel of synthetic peptides from the α subunit, different sets of peptides were recognized in different strains of rats—Lewis, Brown Norway, Wistar Furth, and Buffalo. For example, [Tyr 100]α100-116 and [Gly 89, Tyr 90]α73-90 stimulated AChR-immune T cells in

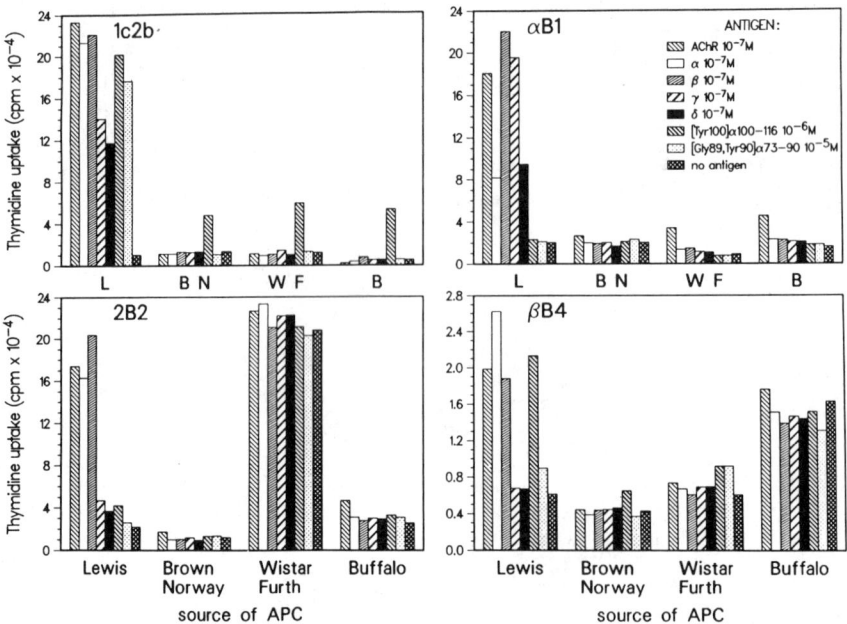

**FIGURE 2.** Responses of AChR-specific T-cell lines to AChR subunits and synthetic peptides are genetically restricted. An AChR-specific long-term T-cell line (1c2b) or cloned cell lines were cultured in the presence of the antigen with irradiated spleen cells from four strains of rats. Thymidine uptake on day 3 of the culture was measured and the mean ± SEM of triplicate cultures are shown. Note alloreactivities of 2B2.

Lewis rats, but not in other strains (FIG. 1), suggesting that peptide specificities of AChR-immune T cells are genetically restricted.

An AChR-specific long-term Lewis rat T-cell line recognized [Tyr 100]α100-116 and [Gly 89, Tyr 90]α73-90, the same peptides that were recognized by the original AChR-immune lymph node cells. Twelve AChR-specific clones were generated by limiting dilution and stimulation with AChR, and four of these clones responded to [Tyr 100]α100-116. These results suggest that the sequence 101-106 of the α subunit is one of the epitopes recognized by T cells in Lewis rats with EAMG. However, the presence of clones that did not react to [Tyr 100]α100-116 indicates that there are other epitopes within the α subunit, or in other subunits, that are recognized by T cells in EAMG.

Unlike lymph node cells as a population, cloned T-cell lines showed unique subunit specificities. However, each clone responded to more than one subunit (FIG. 2). Acetylcholine-receptor-specific clones responded to antigens only when cultured with syngeneic antigen-presenting cells and not with allogeneic cells (FIG. 2).

## REFERENCES

1. DEBAETS, M.C., B. EINARSON, J. LINDSTROM & W. O. WEIGLE. 1982. Lymphocyte activation in experimental autoimmune myasthenia gravis. J. Immunol. **128:** 2228-2235.
2. FUJII, Y. & J. LINDSTROM. 1988. Specificity of the T cell immune response to acetylcholine receptor in experimental autoimmune myasthenia gravis: Response to subunits and synthetic peptides. J. Immunol. **140:** 1830-1837.

# Synergism in the Pathogenesis of EAE Induced by an MBP-Specific T-Cell Line and Monoclonal Antibodies to Galactocerebroside or a Myelin Oligodendroglial Glycoprotein[a]

W. FIERZ,[b] K. HEININGER,[c] B. SCHAEFER,[c]
K. V. TOYKA,[c] C. LININGTON,[d] AND
H. LASSMANN[e]

[b]Section of Clinical Immunology
University Hospital
Zürich, Switzerland

[c]Department of Neurology
University of Düsseldorf
Düsseldorf, Federal Republic of Germany

[d]Department of Medicine
University of Wales
Cardiff, Wales, Great Britain

[e]Department of Neurology
University of Vienna
Vienna, Austria

The fundamental role of T helper cells in the pathogenesis of experimental allergic encephalomyelitis (EAE) was proved in recent years by the establishment of myelin basic protein (MBP)-specific T helper cell lines that induce EAE on transfer to naive recipient animals. In the Lewis rat model, the pathology of this T-cell mediated disease is purely inflammatory without gross demyelination. Conversely, indirect evidence has led for some time to the hypothesis that demyelination is mediated by antibodies. However, intravenous transfer of antimyelin antibodies did not lead to EAE.

In this study we combined two well-defined elements of cellular and humoral autoimmunity to observe synergistic pathogenic effects *in vivo*: a low dose ($10^5$) of MBP-specific T line cells given at day 0 and monoclonal antibodies to a myelin oligodendroglial glycoprotein (MOG)[1] or galactocerebroside (GC)[2] (5 mg) given at

---

[a]This work was supported by the Schweiz. Nationalfonds project no. 3.998-0.86 and the Deutsche Forschungsgemeinschaft SFB 200/B5.

day 5 leads to severe paralytic symptoms, dysfunction of central nervous conduction, and extensive demyelination (FIGS. 1 and 2).

## RESULTS

Antibodies alone:

- no clinical symptoms
- no electrophysiologic changes
- no pathology at all; no lesions even in areas of increased blood-brain barrier permeability (circumventricular)

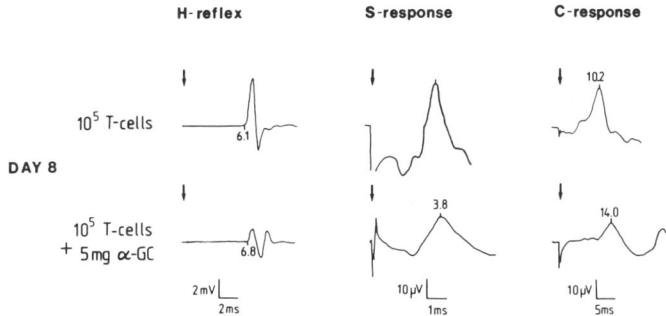

**FIGURE 1.** Slowing of central nervous system conduction. Redrawn original recordings of H-reflexes and lumbar (S-response) and cervical (C-response) somatosensory evoked potentials recorded on day 8 in a Lewis rat injected with $10^5$ MBP-specific T-line cells (day 0) and 5-mg anti-GC monoclonal antibodies (day 5), and in a control rat injected with $10^5$ T cells alone.

Low T-cell dose alone:

- mild paresis of the tail
- minimal electrophysiologic changes
- moderate inflammatory CNS pathology:
  perivenous mononuclear infiltrates
  minimal demyelination

Low T-cell dose + antibodies:

- severe tetraplegia
- slowing of central nervous conduction

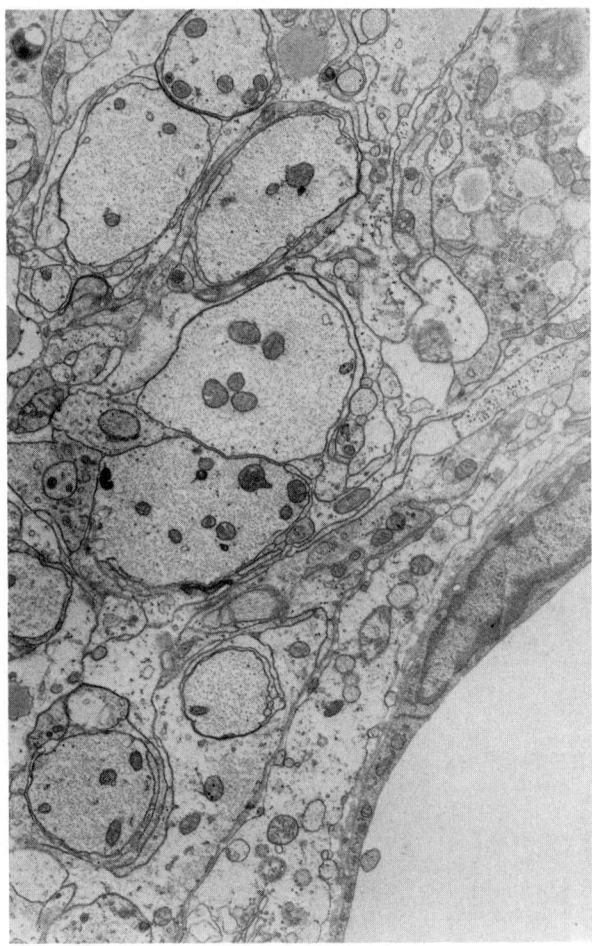

**FIGURE 2.** Demyelinated axons. Electromicrograph from the central nervous system of a Lewis rat 11 days after injection of $10^5$ MBP-specific T-line cells (day 0) and 5-mg anti-GC monoclonal antibodies (day 5) (reduced by 44%).

- moderate increase in CNS inflammation
- vast increase in CNS demyelination
- some axonal degeneration
- remyelination starting 6 days after antibody injection

Difference between anti-MOG and anti-GC:

- GC: lesions predominantly at the root entry zones, frequently vesicular disruption of myelin
- MOG: lesions more perivascular in the depth of the CNS

It is now possible to dissect the complex immunologic mechanisms of the inflammatory and demyelinating form of EAE into cellular and molecular pathogenic components that are amenable to *in vitro* studies as T-cell lines and monoclonal antibodies.

The results show that the recombination of these well-defined immunologic components in a recipient animal synergistically restores the inflammatory and demyelinating pathology and leads to profound CNS dysfunction.

## REFERENCES

1. LININGTON, C. *et al.* 1984. J. Neuroimmunol. **6**: 387.
2. RANSCHT, B. *et al.* 1982. Proc. Natl. Acad. Sci. USA **79**: 2709.

# A Suppressor Cell Line That Prevents the Adoptive Transfer of EAE in Lewis Rats[a]

KAREN ELLERMAN AND STEVEN BROSTOFF

*Department of Neurology*
*Medical University of South Carolina*
*Charleston, South Carolina 29425*

Lewis rats, which spontaneously recover from experimental allergic encephalomyelitis (EAE), are resistant to reinduction of active disease. The observation that effector T-cell lines can be "rescued" from these recovered rats[1] suggests the presence of a suppressor mechanism. Using recovered rats, we succeeded in generating antigen-specific T-cell lines with the characteristics of suppressor cells.

$T_s$ cell lines were generated from the draining lymph nodes of animals immunized 1 month previously with guinea pig myelin basic protein (GP-MBP) in complete Freund's adjuvant. To select for $T_s$ cells rather than $T_h$ cells, the lymph node cells were grown for 7 days in the presence of GP-MBP and cyclosporin A (CsA), an immunosuppressive agent that is believed to inhibit T-cell function. The resulting blasts were purified on ficoll-metrizoate gradients and grown for 1-7 days in the presence of supernatants from concanavalin-A-stimulated cells (CAS) as a source of growth factors. The cells were then maintained in culture by alternate activation with GP-MBP and a source of antigen-presenting cells followed by growth in CAS. As shown in TABLE 1, the $T_s$ cell lines thus generated were specific for GP-MBP, but not for purified protein derivative or bovine $P_2$ protein.

The phenotype of one such mature (15X) line (CsLN-1) was CD4+, CD5+, and negative for both MHC class II I-A and I-E antigens. Approximately 20% of CsLN-1 were CD8+ but only after stimulation with antigen or the lectin concanavalin A; cells grown for 1 week in CAS were not CD8+. Rat CD4+ suppressor T cells are not without precedent. CD4+ T cells have been shown to effect partial[2] or near complete suppression[3] of allograft rejection in two different rat transplantation models.

The cell lines were assayed for suppressive activity by using an adoptive transfer model of EAE.[4] Adoptive transfer of EAE can be achieved with spleen cells taken from GP-MBP sensitized Lewis rats on day 11 or 12 after immunization and activated *in vitro* with antigen. Recipients of $3\text{-}4 \times 10^7$ activated splenocytes develop severe paralytic EAE 4-6 days later. As shown in TABLE 2, recipients of splenocytes mixed with GP-MBP-activated $T_s$, cells during the *in vitro* antigen activation period failed to exhibit clinical evidence of disease after transfer of up to $5 \times 10^7$ cells. Histologic evidence of disease was seen only if the $T_s$ cells were not antigen activated before the 3-day culture period with sensitized spleen cells. This effect was not merely due to

---

[a]The work was supported in part by NIH Grant No. NS 11867.

TABLE 1. Antigen Specificity of the *in Vitro* Proliferation (cpm) of CsLN-1[a]

| | Cycles of Stimulation | | |
|---|---|---|---|
| Antigen | 5× | 8× | 11× |
| None | 24,439 | 19,416 | 448 |
| GP-MBP | 193,894 | 202,413 | 64,938 |
| PPD | 13,374 | 5,428 | NT |
| Concanavalin A | 216,951 | 133,610 | 66,929 |
| $P_2$ | NT | NT | 228 |

NOTE: The *in vitro* proliferation assay was performed as described previously.[4] Results are expressed as counts per minute (cpm) of four replicates. Standard errors were within 20% of the mean and are not shown. GP-MBP, PPD, and $P_2$ were used at 25 µg ml$^{-1}$; concanavalin A was used at 2.5 µg ml$^{-1}$. NT = not tested.
[a] Reproduced, with permission, from Nature 331: 265, 1988.

competition of activated cells for growth factors in the media because an activated $P_2$ T-cell line (O-Lee and Brostoff, unpublished) did not show the same suppressive effect. The result in TABLE 2 clearly demonstrate the ability of these $T_s$ cell lines to prevent the transfer of EAE and as such represents the first isolation of a distinct population of cells with suppressor activity for this model of T-cell activation.

The mechanism of action of these $T_s$ cell lines is unknown, although experimental evidence suggests that the cells may be directed against antigen-specific effector cells. During the generation of these cell lines we noted that direct injection of CsLN-1 cells into recipients resulted in mild clinical disease which decreased in severity with the increased number of cycles of antigenic stimulation until all evidence of clinical disease finally disappeared after 7-8 cycles. The CsLN-1 cells, nevertheless, continued to exhibit a proliferative response from a resting state *in vitro* to irradiated GP-MBP-activated blasts derived from EAE rats in the absence of antigen or antigen-presenting

TABLE 2. Effect of $T_s$ Cell Lines on the Adoptive Transfer of EAE

| | Incidence of EAE | Mean Severity (max = 3.0) | Mean Histology (max = 3.0) |
|---|---|---|---|
| Activated CsLN-1 | 0/12 | 0 | 0.6 (n = 7) |
| Resting CsLN-1 | 1/3 | 0.33 | 1.5 (n = 3) |
| Activated CsLN-4 | 0/3 | 0 | 0 (n = 3) |
| Controls | 15/15 | 2.7 | 2.6 (n = 7) |

NOTE: Adoptive transfer was performed as described previously.[4] To test for suppression, CsLN-1 and CsLN-4 activated *in vitro* for 3 days with GP-MBP and antigen-presenting cells were added to the culture at a ratio of one $T_s$ cell to eight spleen cells. Control animals received 3-4 × 10$^7$ viable spleen cells, whereas test animals received an additional 10$^7$ cells. See reference 4 for grading of clinical severity and histology.

cells. These results suggest that a T suppressor cell directed at a specific determinant on the T effector cell may play a role in regulating EAE in the Lewis rat.

## REFERENCES

1. BEN-NUN, A. & I. R. COHEN. 1982. J. Immunol. **128:** 1450-1457.
2. PADBERG, W. M. *et al.* 1987. J. Immunol. **138:** 3669-3674.
3. HALL, B. *et al.* 1985. J. Exp. Med. **162:** 1683-1694.
4. BROSTOFF, S. W. & D. W. MASON. 1986. J. Neuroimmunol. **10:** 331-340.

# Isolation of Human Lymphocyte Cell Lines Reactive with Whole Human Myelin

## JAMES BURNS AND KIMBERLY LITTLEFIELD

*Department of Neurology*
*University of Utah School of Medicine*
*Salt Lake City, Utah 84132*

Multiple sclerosis may be the result of an autoimmune response directed against CNS myelin. A possible animal model for MS, experimental allergic encephalomyelitis (EAE), may be induced by immunization with purified components of whole myelin including myelin basic protein (MBP), proteolipid protein,[1] and DM-20.[2] T cells reactive with MBP may be isolated from the peripheral blood lymphocytes (PBLs) of human subjects by *in vitro* sensitization with purified MBP.[3] Whether T cells reactive with other myelin antigens may be isolated by similar techniques is unknown. In this study, whole human myelin and delipidated myelin were used for *in vitro* sensitization of PBLs to determine whether lymphocytes recognizing myelin antigens other than MBP may be isolated by this method.

Long-term cell lines reactive with whole human myelin or delipidated myelin were established from the PBL of two normal subjects. Whole human myelin was isolated by the method of Norton and Poduslo.[4] Freshly isolated PBLs were placed in tissue culture with whole human myelin (150 µg/ml) for 7 days. The responding cells were then maintained in culture for up to 2 months by repeated stimulation with whole myelin and antigen-presenting cells. Even though these cells were not exposed to purified MBP, the myelin-reactive cell lines proliferated briskly when cultured with either myelin or MBP. Myelin-reactive cells from each subject were cloned and assayed for responsiveness to myelin and MBP. Six of eight clones from subject 1 responded

TABLE 1. Proliferative Response of Cloned Lymphocytes from Subject 2 to Myelin and Myelin Basic Protein (MBP)[a]

| Clone | Antigen | | |
|---|---|---|---|
| | None | MBP | Myelin |
| 1 | 121 | 372 | 22,990 |
| 3 | 1,387 | 52,994 | 20,150 |
| 7 | 146 | 28,573 | 23,732 |
| 8 | 256 | 63,593 | 27,673 |

[a] Cloned T cells were incubated with irradiated antigen-presenting cells and the antigen indicated (MBP, 50 µg/ml; myelin, 100 µg/ml) for 72 hours. The values shown represent counts per minute (cpm) of tritiated thymidine incorporation.

to both MBP and myelin, suggesting that the cells were sensitized predominantly against MBP during the initial culture with whole myelin. Two clones were poorly reactive with either antigen. Four of five myelin-reactive cloned cells from subject 2 were reactive with MBP as well as myelin. However, clone 1 responded to whole myelin but did not respond to MBP over a wide concentration range (TABLE 1). The myelin antigen recognized by this clone has not been determined.

Thus, following *in vitro* sensitization to whole human myelin, MBP appears to be the major antigen recognized. However, at least one other myelin antigen is also recognized, and lymphocytes reactive with this antigen may be maintained in long-term culture. These results suggest that *in vitro* sensitization to whole myelin may be used to study the human cellular immune response to myelin antigens.

## REFERENCES

1. SOBEL, R. A., R. C. VAN DER VEEN & M. B. LEES. 1986. J. Immunol. **136:** 157.
2. ENDOH, M., T. TABIRA, T. KUNISHITA *et al.* 1986. J. Immunol. **137:** 3832.
3. BURNS, J., A. ROSENZWEIG, B. ZWEIMAN & R. LISAK. 1983. Cell. Immunol. **81:** 435.
4. NORTON, W. T. & S. E. PODUSLO. 1973. J. Neurochem. **21:** 749.

WORKSHOP 4. ANTIBODIES AND COMPLEMENT IN AUTOIMMUNITY

# Voltage-Dependent $Ca^{2+}$ Channels in Small Cell Carcinomas Are Blocked by Autoantibodies from Patients with Lambert-Eaton Myasthenic Syndrome[a]

HENRY J. DE AIZPURUA,[b] GUY E. GRIESMANN,[b] EDWARD H. LAMBERT,[c] AND VANDA A. LENNON[b]

[b] *Neuroimmunology Laboratory*
*Mayo Clinic*
*Rochester, Minnesota 55905*

[c] *Department of Neurology*
*University of Minnesota*
*Minneapolis, Minnesota 55455*

The Lambert-Eaton myasthenic syndrome (LES) is an autoimmune disorder of neuromuscular transmission characterized by muscle weakness, unsteadiness, and in some cases dryness of the eyes and mouth. The physiologic defect is localized presynaptically at the motor endplate where a severe reduction in the number of acetylcholine (ACh) quanta released in response to a nerve stimulus leads to impairment of neuromuscular transmission. There is no evidence of a defect in ACh synthesis or of sensitivity of the postsynaptic membrane to ACh; muscle fiber excitability and conduction are normal. Two striking characteristics of LES are that 65% of patients have small cell lung carcinoma (SCC), and 60% of patients with and without tumor have one or more of a variety of autoantibodies in their sera.[1] LES can be transferred passively to mice by injecting serum IgG from patients with LES.[2]

Voltage-sensitive $Ca^{2+}$ channels have been implicated as the autoantigen of LES. Firstly, the electrophysiologic abnormality in LES is similar to that found when $[Ca^{2+}]$ is reduced in the bathing medium of nerve and muscle. Secondly, membrane particles in the presynaptic active zones (presumptive $Ca^{2+}$ channels) of freeze-fracture replicas of the motor nerve terminals of patients with LES are sparse and frequently disorganized.[3] The same abnormality was demonstrated in nerve terminals of mice injected repeatedly with LES IgG.[4]

It seems plausible that LES may arise as an autoimmune response to antigen(s) common to cholinergic neurons and SCCs. SCCs have been shown to exhibit $Ca^{2+}$ spike electrogenesis in culture,[5] and Roberts *et al.*[6] reported that LES IgG inhibited

---

[a] This work was supported by Grants CA 37343 (VAL) and NS 23691 (EHL) from the National Institutes of Health.

depolarization-dependent uptake of $^{45}Ca^{2+}$ in an SCC line. We found voltage-dependent $Ca^{2+}$ channels in all of eight SCC lines tested, six from patients with and two without LES but not in two non-SCC control cell lines.[7] As illustrated in FIGURE 1, SCC took up $Ca^{2+}$ in response to depolarization regardless of whether or not the patient had LES. $K^+$-stimulated $^{45}Ca^{2+}$ influx was competitively antagonized by $Co^{2+}$ and $Mg^{2+}$ and blocked by nifedipine and nitrendipine in a dose-dependent manner, but not by the $Na^+$ channel blocker tetrodotoxin.

In this study, two SCC lines (one LES and one non-LES) were each exposed to human serum Ig (1 mg/ml) for 3 days before assay. $K^+$-stimulated $^{45}Ca^{2+}$ influx into both lines (1.29 ± 0.04 and 1.64 ± 0.05 nmol/$10^6$ cells) was significantly reduced by Ig from 14 of 19 LES patients (mean ± SE = 0.65 ± 0.06 and 0.76 ± 0.09 nmol/$10^6$ cells [LES and non-LES, respectively], $p < 0.005$), but not by Ig from 53 control subjects (1.33 ± 0.05 and 1.47 ± 0.17 nmol/$10^6$ cells) (FIG. 2). Controls included 13 patients with myasthenia gravis (MG), 5 of whom had thymoma (T), 5 with multiple sclerosis (MS), 8 with paraneoplastic cerebellar degeneration (PCD), 5 with Graves' disease (GR), 5 with pernicious anemia (P) and/or Hashimoto's thyroiditis (H), 11 with SCC without evidence of paraneoplastic syndrome, and 6 normal subjects.

This study confirms that $Ca^{2+}$ channel antagonistic autoantibodies are highly associated with LES. The autoantibodies did not appear to discriminate between SCC from patients with or without LES, and they were found in patients with LES with and without evidence of SCC. It is noteworthy that none of the five patients with

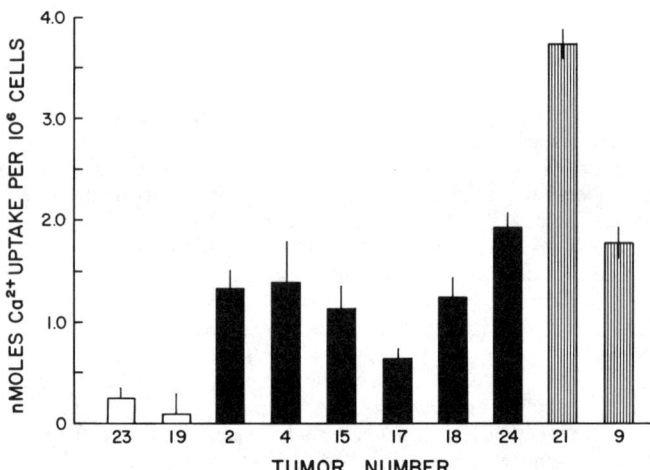

**FIGURE 1.** All tumors except 19 and 23 exhibited significant depolarization-dependent uptake of $Ca^{2+}$. All except 19 and 23 were small cell lung carcinomas (SCCs) and all the SCCs, except 21 and 9, were derived from patients with LES. Tumor 19, an occult cecal adenocarcinoma, was derived from a 69-year-old woman with LES. Tumor 23, an ovarian carcinoma, was derived from a 71-year-old woman with myasthenia gravis. Although the donor of tumor 19 had no evidence of lung cancer, she had a long history of smoking. We previously encountered a patient in whom an occult renal carcinoma (hypernephroma) was found after diagnosis of LES, but in whom a bronchial SCC was found incidentally at autopsy.

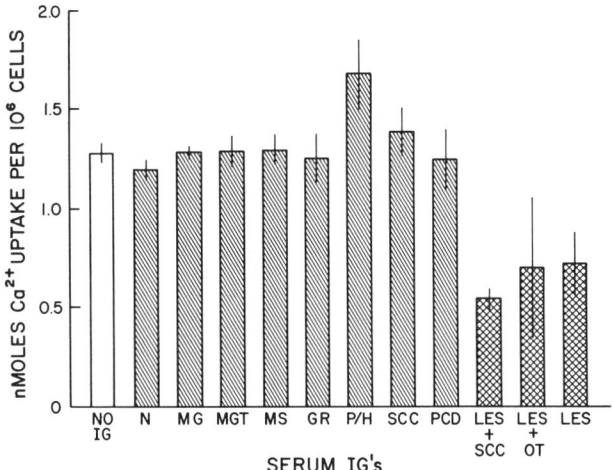

**FIGURE 2.** Small cell lung carcinoma-18 cells (from a patient with LES) were cultured for 3 days with the Ig fraction of serum (1 mg/ml) from 19 patients with LES (8 with SCC, 3 with other tumors [OT], and 8 without evidence of tumor) and 53 control subjects, including 6 normal subjects (N). Similar results were obtained using SCC-9 cells from a patient without LES (data not shown).

LES whose Ig failed to inhibit stimulated $Ca^{2+}$ influx had evidence of SCC. This finding suggests that the patients might have antibodies of a specificity that selectively binds to cholinergic nerve terminals but not to SCC. IgG from patients with LES should prove useful in the identification and purification of an antigen involved in exocytosis of ACh.

## REFERENCES

1. LENNON, V. A. et al. 1982. Muscle Nerve **5:** S21.
2. LANG, B. et al. 1981. Lancet **2:** 224.
3. FUKANAGA, H. et al. 1982. Muscle Nerve **5:** 685.
4. FUKANAGA, H. et al. 1983. Proc. Natl. Acad. Sci. USA **80:** 7636.
5. MCCANN, F. V. et al. 1981. Science **212:** 1155.
6. ROBERTS, A. et al. 1985. Nature **317:** 737.
7. DE AIZPURUA, H. J. et al. 1987. Fed. Proc. **46:** 1380.

# Complement Allotyping Explains MHC Associations in Multiple Sclerosis

## W. J. ZHANG, T. J. COBAIN, R. L. DAWKINS, G. GRIMSLEY, AND I. R. MACKAY

*Departments of Clinical Immunology*
*Royal Perth Hospital*
*Queen Elizabeth II Medical Centre*
*University of Western Australia and the AUSTIMS Study Group*
*Australia*

Previous studies of major histocompatibility complex (MHC) associations with multiple sclerosis (MS) have revealed that numerous alleles may be increased or decreased in frequency.[1,2] To resolve this apparent complexity we undertook complement allotyping in 109 Australian patients included in a study of the effectiveness of interferon and transfer factor. HLA A, B, C, DR, and DQ typing was also undertaken using reagents of workshop standard. Results were compared with those obtained from the Busselton study in Western Australia.

TABLE 1. Supratype: the Most Important Marker of Susceptibility in Multiple Sclerosis

| | MHC Supratype | | | | | Frequency (%) | | | |
|---|---|---|---|---|---|---|---|---|---|
| | | | | | | Controls | MS patients | | |
| A | B | C4A | C4B | Bf | DR | (n = 204) | (n = 109) | CPR | $\chi^2$ Probability[a] |
| | | 3 | 1 | S | | 68.1 | 84.4 | 2.5 | 0.003 |
| | | 3 | 1 | S | 2 | 24.0 | 50.4 | 3.2 | 0.0001 |
| | 7 | 3 | 1 | S | 2 | 14.1 | 34.0 | 3.0 | 0.0004 |
| Total | | | | | 2 | 31.1 | 56.0 | 2.8 | 0.0002 |
| Other[b] | | | | | 2 | 17.0 | 22.0 | 1.4 | ns |
| | | QO | 1 | S | | 33.8 | 29.4 | 0.8 | ns |
| | | QO | 1 | S | 3 | 20.1 | 23.9 | 1.2 | ns |
| | 8 | QO | 1 | S | 3 | 17.6 | 23.9 | 1.5 | ns |
| 1 | 8 | QO | 1 | S | 3 | 12.2 | 22.9 | 2.1 | 0.02 |
| Total | | | | | 3 | 30.9 | 31.2 | 1.0 | ns |
| Other[b] | | | | | 3 | 13.3 | 7.3 | 0.5 | ns |

ABBREVIATIONS: CPR = cross product ratio; ns = not significant.
[a] Probability corrected for number of alleles/antigens examined.
[b] Not included in supratype HLA B7, C4A3, C4B1, BfS, DR2 or B8, C4AQO, C4B1, BfS, DR3.

Analysis of the HLA data revealed increases in alleles previously reported in Caucasians. An alternative approach was provided by C4 allotyping. Table 1 shows that no less than 37 of the 109 patients have the supratype HLA B7, C4A3, C4B1, BfS, DR2 (7,3,1,S,2). This particular supratype accounts for the increases in most of the alleles previously reported. The cross product ratio for the supratype is 3.0 ($p < 0.004$). In contrast, HLA DR2, when not included in the supratype 7,3,1,S,2, is not increased. The HLA A1, B8, C4AQO, C4B1, BfS, DR3 (1,8,3) supratype is slightly increased in patients with MS. These data suggest that the common Caucasian supratype 7,3,1,S,2 carries the gene(s) responsible for susceptibility to MS. The 1,8,3 supratype appears to be only a minor factor, although it has been implicated as a marker of severity.[3]

Because the 7,3,1,S,2 supratype is uncommon and apparently not relevant to MS in oriental populations,[4] similar studies performed on non-Caucasian populations and comparison with the data presented herein may allow localization of the critical gene(s) involved. (8739)

## REFERENCES

1. FRANCIS, D. A., J. R. BATCHELOR, W. I. MCDONALD, I. A. DODI, S. I. HING, J. E. C. HERN & A. W. DOWNIE. 1987. HLA genetic determinants in familial MS. Tissue Antigens **29:** 7-12.
2. BATCHELOR, J. R. & A. COMPSTON. 1978. The significance of the association between HLA and multiple sclerosis. Br. Med. Bull. **34:** 279-284.
3. VAN LAMBALGEN, R., E. A. C. M. SANDERS & J. D'AMARO. 1986. Sex distribution, age of onset and HLA profiles in two types of multiple sclerosis. J. Neurol. Sci. **76:** 13-21.
4. PEI, J., W. Z. XU, S. X. SUN, X. Y. MI, Z. C. HOU, L. H. WANG & B. G. YUE. HLA and Chinese multiple sclerosis. In HLA in Asia-Oceania. Aizawa, M., Ed. Proceedings of the 3rd Asia Oceania Histocompatibility Workshop and Conference. Sapporo, Japan, 1986, pp. 726-729.

# Myelin Vesicles As an *in Vitro* Model to Study Mechanisms of Myelin Damage by Immune Effectors

## PADMAVATHY VANGURI AND MOON L. SHIN

*University of Maryland*
*Department of Pathology*
*Baltimore, Maryland 21201*

An *in vitro* model of myelin vesicles was developed to study myelin damage by immune effectors. Because immune effectors such as complement and cytotoxic lymphocytes produce their effects by target membrane perturbation,[1,2] myelin vesicles that are multilamellar, tightly sealed, maintain a semipermeable membrane barrier, and retain functional enzyme activities and transport systems would be highly suitable.

Myelin was isolated from human spinal cord and purified according to Norton.[3] Resealed myelin vesicles (RMVs) were prepared by incubating myelin (0.8 mg of protein per milliliter) in Hepes buffer, pH 7.4, containing 1.0 mM $MgCl_2$, 100 mM NaCl, and 3 mM Tris for 10 minutes at 37°C. Resealed myelin vesicles were evaluated for a number of physicochemical properties, which are summarized in TABLE 1. Transmission electron microscopy of RMVs showed that most myelin was sealed into vesicles, which ranged from 250 to 1,500 nm in diameter and consisted of one to three lamellae. Resealed myelin vesicles and unsealed myelin were treated with trypsin,

TABLE 1. Properties of Resealed Myelin Vesicles (RMVs)

| | |
|---|---|
| 1. Ultrastructure | Sealed vesicles of 2-6 bilayers (250-1,500 nm) |
| 2. Basic protein hydrolysis by externally added trypsin | Limited proteolysis, indicating vesicles are sealed right side out |
| 3. Fluorescence of Quin-2-loaded RMV on addition of $Ca^{2+}$ | RMVs maintain $Ca^{2+}$-gradient across inner and outer vesicular spaces |
| 4. Basic protein hydrolysis by externally added $Ca^{2+}$ | $Ca^{2+}$-dependent hydrolysis of BP up to 20% with 1.5 mM $Ca^{2+}$ |
| 5. Direct $Ca^{2+}$ binding to RMV and effect of EGTA | RMVs have specific $Ca^{2+}$ binding sites of two different affinities. High affinity $Ca^{2+}$ binding is not removed by EGTA, indicating translocation of $Ca^{2+}$ in membrane |
| 6. $Ca^{2+}$ transport in the presence of added ATP | ATP-dependent $Ca^{2+}$ uptake into RMV, suggesting the presence of $Ca^{2+}$, $Mg^{2+}$-ATPase in myelin |

ABBREVIATIONS: ATP = adenosine triphosphate; BP = basic protein; EGTA = ethyleneglycol tetraacetic acid.

TABLE 2. Use of Resealed Myelin Vesicles (RMVs) to Study Basic Protein Hydrolysis Following Activation of Terminal Complement Proteins

| Experiment | Area under Remaining BP peak | | % Specific BP Hydrolysis by C5b-9 |
|---|---|---|---|
| | C7-Deficient Human Serum[a] | C7-Deficient Human Serum + C7[a] | |
| 1 | 2.81 ± 0.025 | 2.28 ± 0.025 | 18.9 |
| 2 | 12.39 ± 0.72 | 10.32 ± 0.09 | 17.0 |

[a] Resealed myelin vesicles in triplicate were treated with C7-deficient human serum or C7-deficient human serum + C7 in the presence of 0.02 mM $Ca^{2+}$. C-treated RMVs were washed and the remaining intact BP was quantitated by SDS-PAGE and densitometric analysis.

and the hydrolysis of myelin basic protein (BP) was measured by sodium dodecyl sulfate polyacrylamide gel electrophoresis and densitometric analysis of the remaining BP band. Minimal BP hydrolysis occurred in RMVs compared with unsealed myelin, indicating that the vesicles were not permeable to trypsin and sealed right side out in view of the location of BP on the cytoplasmic phase of myelin. $Ca^{2+}$-dependent fluorescence of Quin-2-loaded RMVs was not detected on addition of $Ca^{2+}$ unless ionomycin was also added, indicating that RMVs maintained a $Ca^{2+}$ gradient across the inner aqueous space. Although $Ca^{2+}$ was not transported into RMVs, there was limited hydrolysis of BP which was dependent on $[Ca^{2+}]_o$. This hydrolysis was attributed to the $Ca^{2+}$-binding property of myelin membranes.[4] Resealed myelin vesicles were incubated with a fixed amount of $^{45}Ca$ together with various doses of nonradioactive $CaCl_2$, and the specific amount of $Ca^{2+}$ bound to RMV was measured. Scatchard analysis showed high and low affinity $Ca^{2+}$ binding sites with association constants of $9.5 \times 10^3 \, M^{-1}$ and $1.0 \times 10^2 \, M^{-1}$, respectively. $Ca^{2+}$ bound to RMVs appears to be translocated within the membrane because washing with ethyleneglycol tetraacetic acid (EGTA) did not remove the $Ca^{2+}$ that was bound with higher affinity. $Ca^{2+}$-uptake experiments on RMV indicated that significant increases in $Ca^{2+}$ uptake occurred when adenosine triphosphate (ATP) was added, suggesting that $Ca^{2+}$,$Mg^{2+}$-ATPases are present in myelin and such a mechanism could maintain $[Ca^{2+}]_i$ in vivo.

With this model, the role of terminal complement complexes (TCCs) on BP hydrolysis in RMV that could be mediated by neutral proteases (NP) was investigated. Treatment of RMV with C7-deficient human serum reconstituted with C7 produced significant BP hydrolysis at 0.02 mM $[Ca^{2+}]_o$ (TABLE 2). When purified C5b6-C9 was used to form TCC, similar hydrolysis of BP occurred, indicating the possible activation of NP by TCC.[5] Thus, we believe that the RMV model is suitable for investigation of biochemical consequences of myelin damage by various immune effectors that are involved in demyelination.

## REFERENCES

1. MAYER, M. M. 1982. In Mechanisms of Cell Mediated Cytotoxicity. W. Clark & P. Goldstein, Eds. 193-216. Plenum Press, New York.
2. YOUNG, J. D., Z. A. COHN & E. R. PODACK. 1986. Science 233: 184-190.
3. NORTON, W. T. 1974. Meth. Enzymol. 32: 435-444.
4. HEMMINKI, K. 1974. Biochim. Biophys. Acta 363: 202-210.
5. VANGURI, P. & M. L. SHIN. 1987. Fed Proc. 46: 1196.

# Serum Antibodies to Peripheral Nerve Antigens in Guillain-Barré Syndrome

T. NEGISHI, T. YAMASHITA, K. NOMURA,
T. HOSOKAWA, R. OHNO, K. HAMAGUCHI,
AND K. UYEMURA

*Departments of Neurology and Physiology*
*Saitama Medical School*
*Moroyama, Saitama, Japan*

We previously reported that cellular hypersensitivity to P2 protein (P2) might play an important role in the evolution of experimental allergic neuritis[1] and the Guillain-Barré syndrome (GBS).[2] In the present study, we examined serum antibodies to three different nervous antigens, P2, a synthetic tridecapeptide (SP66-78) corresponding to residues 66-78 of bovine P2, and galactocerebroside (GC), in GBS and other neurologic diseases. Myelin fraction was prepared from bovine peripheral nerve roots, as previously described,[3] and P2 was purified by acid extraction of myelin using the method of Kitamura *et al.*[4] SP66-78 was synthesized in a liquid phase by stepwise elongation according to the method of Suzuki *et al.*[5] Antibody titers were measured by enzyme-linked immunosorbent assay (ELISA) in the sera of 11 patients with GBS,

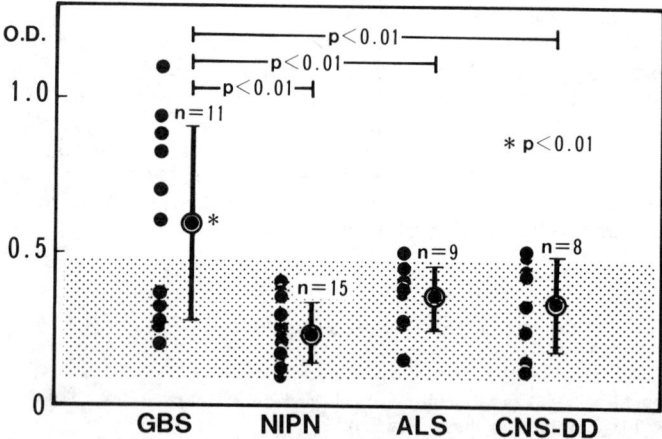

**FIGURE 1.** Anti-P2 antibody titer in various neurologic disorders. The *stippled* area represents the range of 2 standard deviations of the mean value obtained from 24 healthy controls.

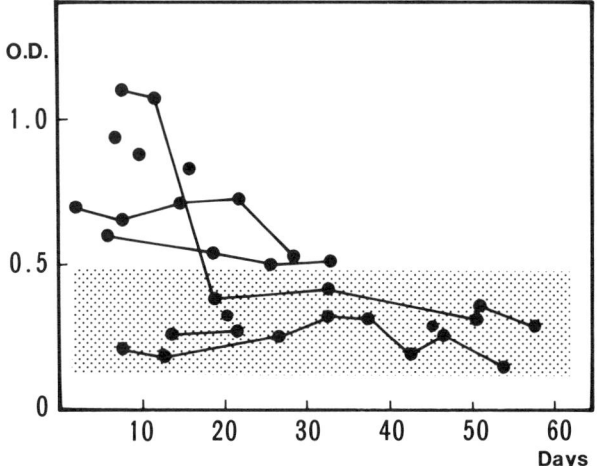

**FIGURE 2.** Correlation between anti-P2 antibody titer and the time course of Guillain-Barré syndrome.

15 patients with noninflammatory peripheral neuropathies (NIPN), 9 with amyotrophic lateral sclerosis (ALS), 8 with degenerative disorders of the central nervous system (CNS-DD), and 24 healthy controls. Peroxidase-conjugated goat antihuman IgG was used for ELISA.

The mean level of anti-P2 antibody titer in 11 patients with GBS on admission was significantly higher than that of patients with NIPN, ALS, and CNS-DD and healthy controls (FIG. 1), and that of anti-SP66-78 antibody titer in GBS was also significantly higher than that in healthy controls. Both anti-P2 antibody and anti-SP66-78 antibody showed approximately 70% absorption on incubation with their reciprocal specific antigen. In GBS, anti-P2 antibody titer was significantly correlated with anti-SP66-78 antibody titer. Most of the anti-P2 antibody in 31 serially examined samples was detected in the early stage of the disease, and in one case it was observed as early as 2 days after the onset of clinical symptoms (FIG. 2). No significant differences, however, were found between GBS and other conditions with regard to anti-GC antibody titers.

It was concluded that the appearance of anti-P2 antibody in GBS might be specific to the disease, suggesting sensitization to P2 or its analogue before the onset of clinical symptoms. Further studies on the possible role of these antibodies are currently in progress.

### REFERENCES

1. NOMURA, K. et al. 1987. J. Neuroimmunol. **15:** 25-35.
2. OHNO, R. et al. 1986. Neurochem. Pathol. **4:** 119-126.
3. UYEMURA, K. et al. 1972. J. Neurochem. **19:** 2607-2614.
4. KITAMURA, K. et al. 1981. Biomed. Res. **2:** 347-363.
5. SUZUKI, M. et al. 1984. In Experimental Allergic Encephalomyelitis: A Useful Model for Multiple Sclerosis. E. C. J. Alvord et al., Eds.: 478-492. Alan R. Liss, New York.

# Neuropathy and Monoclonal IgM M-Protein with Antibody Activity Against Gangliosides

E. NARDELLI,[a] A. J. STECK,[a] M. SCHLUEP,[a]
K. FELGENHAUER,[b] AND F. JERUSALEM [c]

[a] *Service de Neurologie CHUV*
*Lausanne, Switzerland*

[b] *Department of Neurology*
*Göttingen, FRG*

[c] *Department of Neurology*
*Bonn, FRG*

Peripheral neuropathy has been associated with IgM antibody activity against myelin-associated glycoprotein.[1] Recently, attention was directed towards the association of motor neuron syndromes with monoclonal protein.[2,3] We report the study of two cases in which sera with IgM M-protein showed antibody activity against gangliosides.

One patient (Case 1) presented a clinical syndrome with proximal muscle weakness, wasting, fasciculation, and complete sparing of sensory functions, suggesting a diagnosis of a motor neuron disorder. This condition, however, was difficult to separate from a proximal motor neuropathy because electrophysiologic studies as well as pathologic changes in the nerve biopsy were consistent with a disease process also involving the peripheral nerve. The patient's IgM M-protein had antibody activity against gangliosides GM1, GB1b, and asialo-GM1. A peripheral neuropathy in a second patient (Case 2) was associated with antibody activity against GM1 and GD1a.

In both cases preparative and analytic procedures (ELISA in FIG. 1 and TLC plates in FIG. 2, including different blocking reactions and immunoabsorption procedures) with central nervous system (CNS) and peripheral nervous system (PNS) gangliosides as well as single purified gangliosides (GM1, GD1a, GD1b, asialo-GM1, GM2, and GM3) demonstrated the high specificity of the patient's IgM towards the individual ganglioside. The peanut lectin (*Arachis hypogaea*) competitively blocked the antibody activity against GM1 and GD1b in Case 1 but not in Case 2. Immunocytochemistry on human CNS and PNS tissue demonstrated that serum from both cases (dilution 1:500) recognized axons in lumbar roots.

The reactive epitope recognized in Case 1 is the galactosyl (B1-3) *N*-acetylgalactosaminyl moiety shared by gangliosides GM1, GD1b, and asialo-GM1. Several elements of the CNS or PNS are potential targets for these antibodies because glycoconjugates have an important role in the nervous system.[4] The mechanism of nervous tissue injury and the reason for predominant involvement of the CNS in Case 1 or PNS in Case 2 are unknown because the gangliosides recognized by these antibodies are equally distributed in the nervous tissue. The accessibility of these antibodies to the target may be the explanation.

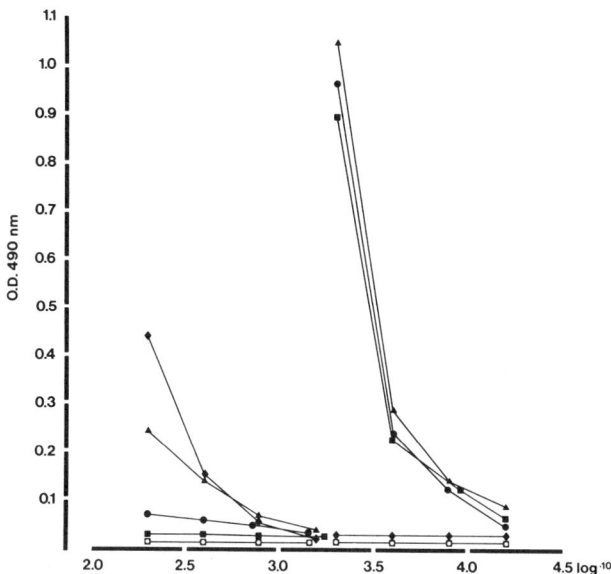

**FIGURE 1.** Binding of patient HA's serum ($\log_{10}$ 3.25-4.5) and that of patient AW ($\log_{10}$ 2.25-3.25) to gangliosides GM1 (▲), GD1a (◆), GD1b (■), asialo-GM1 (●), and GM3 (□) by ELISA.

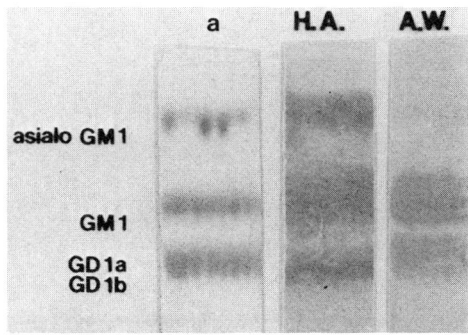

**FIGURE 2.** Gangliosides GM1, GD1b, GD1a, and asialo-GM1 separated by TLC plates with acetic acid, sulfuric acid, and anisaldehyde (50:1:0,3) (a) and immuno-TLC overlays preincubated with serum from patients HA and AW (PAP method).

## REFERENCES

1. STECK, A. J., N. MURRAY, C. MEIER, N. PAGE & G. PERUISSEAU. 1983. Neurology **33:** 19-23.
2. FREDDO, L., R. K. YU, N. LATOV, P. D. DONOFRIO, A. P. HAYS, H. S. GREENBERG, J. W. ALBERS, A. G. ALESSI & D. KEREN. 1986. Neurology **36:** 454-458.
3. SHY, M. E., L. P. ROWLAND, T. SMITH, W. TROJABORG, N. LATOV, W. SHERMAN, M. A. PESCE, R. E. LOVELACE & E. F. OSSERMAN. 1986. Neurology **36:** 1429-1436.
4. FEIZI, T. 1985. Nature **314:** 53-57.

# Mechanism of Arachidonic Acid Release by Terminal Complement Complexes from Rat Oligodendrocyte X C6 Glioma Cell Hybrids

Y. SHIRAZI,[a] F. A. McMORRIS,[b] AND M. L. SHIN [a]

[a] *University of Maryland*
*School of Medicine*
*Baltimore, Maryland 21201*

[b] *The Wistar Institute*
*Philadelphia, Pennsylvania 19104*

Activation of the terminal complement proteins, C5-C9, on target membrane lipid bilayers leads to the insertion of complement peptides and the formation of terminal complement complexes (TCCs). Recently, we showed that rat oligodendrocytes release phospholipid (PLP) and generate arachidonic acid (AA) and leukotriene $B_4$ in response to the complement complex, C5b-9, and maximum leukotriene $B_4$ production is achieved at the C5b-8 stage of TCC assembly.[1]

In the present study, we investigated the biochemical pathways by which TCCs generate AA from clone ROC-1 cells. This clone was produced by fusion of rat oligodendrocytes and $C_6$ glioma cells.[2] Cells were incubated for 18 hours in the presence of $^3$H-AA. They were then sensitized with antibody against hybrid cell stroma and treated for 1 hour with C9-depleted human serum (C9D-HS) or C9D-HS reconstituted with C9. Alternatively, cells were treated with C8D-HS for 15 minutes to prepare cells bearing C5b-7. Cells were then washed and treated with purified C8 plus C9 for 1 hour. The released radiolabeled products were assessed quantitatively by thin layer chromatography and autoradiography. The results showed that the major radiolabeled products following TCC stimulation co-migrated with AA and PLP standards, and the maximum effect was achieved by C5b-9. Pretreatment of cells with pertussis toxin (PT) for 2 hours blocked AA and PLP release by C5b-9 in a dose-dependent manner, with maximum effect observed at 40 ng/ml of the toxin (TABLE 1). In addition, experiments performed to assess the role of extracellular $Ca^{2+}$ in AA release revealed that C5b-9-mediated AA release, but not PLP release, was dependent on extracellular $Ca^{2+}$ (FIG. 1).

Thus, AA generation by C5b-9 from the ROC-1 clone may involve intramembrane interaction of C5b-9 with PT-sensitive G proteins, that could be linked to the activation of $Ca^{2+}$-dependent phospholipases.[3] However, the specific phospholipase activities or the PLP substrates involved in C5b-9-mediated AA release are not known. Nevertheless, we believe that membrane lipid hydrolysis and release of AA-derived inflam-

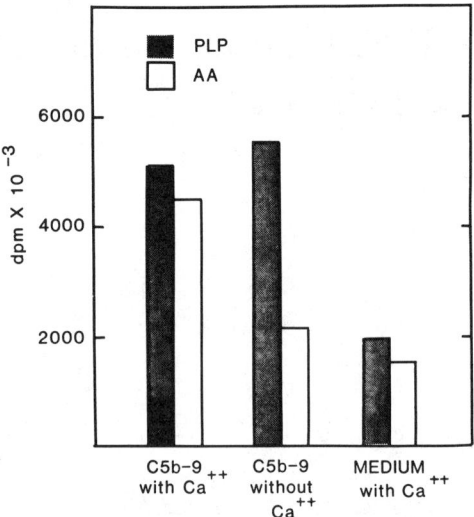

**FIGURE 1.** Effect of extracellular $Ca^{2+}$ on arachidonic acid release by C5b-9. Hybrid cells carrying C5b-7 intermediates were incubated with C8 plus C9 suspended in medium with $Ca^{2+}$ or in medium without $Ca^{2+}$ for 1 hour. The supernatants were extracted and analyzed by thin layer chromatography using isopropyl ether and glacial acetic acid (96:4, V/V) as solvents. As shown here, removal of $Ca^{2+}$ from the medium abolished C5b-9-mediated arachidonic acid release.

**TABLE 1.** Effect of Pertussis Toxin (PT) on Arachidonic Acid (AA) and Phospholipid (PLP) Release from OLG $\times$ C6 Glioma Cell Hybrids by C5b-9

| Treatment | % Release of dpm Incorporated | |
|---|---|---|
| | AA | PLP |
| AB + C9D-HS | 2.65 ± 0.65 | 5.00 ± 0.89 |
| AB + C9D-HS + C9 | 5.10 ± 0.50 | 8.10 ± 0.83 |
| AB + C9D-HS + C9 + 1 µg of PT | 5.20 ± 0.64 | 5.60 ± 0.59 |
| AB + C9D-HS + C9 + 200 ng of PT | 3.30 ± 1.30 | 5.10 ± 0.82 |
| AB + C9D-HS + C9 + 40 ng of PT | 2.50 ± 0.46 | 3.70 ± 1.30 |

NOTE: Pertussis toxin, dose dependently blocked AA, and intact PLP release by C5b-9 with maximum effect observed at 40 ng/ml of the toxin. Experiments not shown here demonstrated that doses less than 40 ng/ml were ineffective in inhibiting AA release. The results are expressed as the percentage of total dpm incorporated, and released as intact PLP and AA. Values are mean ± SD; $n = 4$.

matory mediators as a result of complement activation may be a significant event in inflammatory demyelination occurring in diseases such as multiple sclerosis.

## REFERENCES

1. SHIRAZI, Y., D. K. IMAGAWA & M. L. SHIN. 1987. Release of leukotriene $B_4$ from sublethally injured oligodendrocytes by terminal complement complexes. J. Neurochem. **48:** 271-278.
2. PRESTON, S. L. & F. A. MCMORRIS. 1983. An electric variant of 6-phosphogluconate dehydrogenase in rat and its application in detecting somatic cell hybrids. Biochem. Genet. **21:** 161-165.
3. MAJERUS, P. W., T. M. CONNOLLY, H. DECKMYN, T. S. ROSS, T. E. BROSS, H. ISHII, V. S. BANSAL & D. B. WILSON. 1986. The metabolism of phosphoinositide-derived messenger molecules. Science **234:** 1519-1526.

# Clonal Restriction of Complement-Fixing Antineural Antibodies in the Guillain-Barré Syndrome

## BJÖRN RYBERG

*Department of Neurology*
*University of Lund*
*Lund, Sweden*

The Guillain-Barré syndrome (GBS) is often associated with humoral factors detectable by various immunologic techniques or by effects on peripheral myelin *in vitro* or *in vivo*. Such factors may be involved in the pathogenesis of the disease and provide a rationale for therapeutic plasma exchange.

The complement fixation technique employed in the present study has demonstrated serum antibodies to peripheral nerve tissue in up to 83% and to central nervous tissue in about 50% of the patients during the first weeks of the disease.[1-3] The specificities of these antibodies are largely unknown, but multiple antigens, including lipids, are evidently involved.[2] The antibodies are found in both serum and CSF. Evaluation of their distribution in these media by the antibody index (CSF/serum antibody titer : CSF/serum albumin)[2,4] demonstrates a predominantly extrathecal origin.[2] The presence of complement-fixing antinerve antibodies is significantly correlated with disability, but it does not predict the outcome of plasma exchange.[3]

## MATERIAL AND METHODS

*Serum samples.* Ten GBS sera known to contain complement-fixing antibodies to nerve tissue were studied.

*Antigen preparations.* Fresh homogenates of human lumbar nerve root (1:30, w/v), white matter (1:100, w/v), and gray matter (1:50, w/v) were used as antigens in the complement fixation test.

*Complement fixation test.* This test was performed on a micro scale as described.[1]

*Immunoadsorbents.* Immunoadsorbents specific for human IgM, IgG, kappa light chain, and lambda light chain were prepared by coupling rabbit antisera to CNBr-activated Sepharose 4B. Aliquots of the serum samples were absorbed by passage through these immunoadsorbents and through Protein A-Sepharose CL-4B. The absorbed aliquots were reconcentrated to give levels of unabsorbed proteins close to those in the original sample.

## RESULTS

Immunoadsorbent treatment generally resulted in a depletion of 95% or more of the absorbed constituent. Protein A treatment reduced IgG by 86-97%.

The antineural activity was restricted to IgGκ in four patients and to IgGλ in six. In four of them the antibody activity was not bound to protein A and therefore represents IgG subclass 3. IgM antineural activity was not found in any patient (TABLE 1).

TABLE 1. Characterization of Antineural Antibodies in 10 Guillain-Barré Sera

| Patient | Antigen | Serum Titer | Antibody Characteristics |
|---|---|---|---|
| 1 | Nerve root | 1:4 | IgGλ |
| 2 | Gray matter | 1:16 | IgGλ |
| 3 | Nerve root | 1:8 | IgGκ |
| 4 | Nerve root | 1:8 | IgGλ |
| 5 | Nerve root | 1:32 | IgG3λ |
|   | White matter | 1:32 | IgG3λ |
|   | Gray matter | 1:32 | IgG3λ |
| 6 | White matter | 1:64 | IgG3λ |
|   | Gray matter | 1:64 | IgG3λ |
| 7 | Nerve root | 1:8 | IgG3κ |
|   | White matter | 1:8 | IgG3κ |
|   | Gray matter | 1:8 | IgG3κ |
| 8 | Gray matter | 1:16 | IgGκ |
| 9 | Nerve root | 1:16 | IgGκ |
| 10 | Nerve root | 1:512 | IgG3λ |
|   | White matter | 1:256 | IgG3λ |
|   | Gray matter | 1:512 | IgG3λ |

## DISCUSSION

Contrary to the modified complement fixation technique (C1 fixation and transfer assay) of Koski et al.,[5] which detects IgM antibodies to peripheral myelin in early GBS, our assay detects IgG antibodies to peripheral nerve tissue (including peripheral myelin) and sometimes to central nervous tissue.

The IgG3 subclass restriction of the antineural antibodies in 4 of 10 GBS sera is unexpected in view of the normally low (4-8%) contribution of this subclass to total IgG.

This study reveals a previously unknown clonal restriction of the antineural antibodies associated with GBS.

## REFERENCES

1. RYBERG, B., B. HINDFELT, B. NILSSON & J.-E. OLSSON. 1984. Arch. Neurol. **41:** 1277-1281.
2. RYBERG, B. 1984. Neurology **34:** 1378-1381.
3. OSTERMAN, P. O., J. FAGIUS, B. RYBERG, H. NYLAND & C. A. VEDELER. 1986. Uppsala J. Med. Sci. Suppl. **43:** 65.
4. RYBERG, B. 1980. J. Neurol. Sci. **48:** 1-8.
5. KOSKI, C. L., R. HUMPHREY & M. L. SHIN. 1985. Proc. Natl. Acad. Sci. USA **82:** 905-909.

# Terminal Complement Complexes (SC5b-9) in Cerebrospinal Fluid in Autoimmune Nervous System Diseases

M. E. SANDERS,[a] E. L. ALEXANDER,[b] C. L. KOSKI,[c]
M. L. SHIN,[c] Y. SANO,[c] M. M. FRANK,[a] AND
K. A. JOINER[a]

[a] *National Institutes of Health*
*Bethesda, Maryland*

[b] *Johns Hopkins University*
*Baltimore, Maryland*

[c] *University of Maryland*
*Baltimore, Maryland*

Activation of complement by either classical or alternative pathways leads to cleavage of C5 and subsequent assembly of C5b-9 terminal complement complexes. These complexes consist of one molecule each of C5b, C6, C7, and C8 and a variable number of C9 molecules. Complexes of C5b-9 may be assembled in fluid phase such as in plasma. Such complexes (termed SC5b-9) are rendered water soluble and cytolytically inactive by binding of the regulatory S protein (vitronectin) to the metastable C5b-7 complex. Alternatively, nascent C5b-9 complexes may bind by hydrophobic domains to cell membranes, leading to assembly of potentially cytolytic MC5b-9 complexes. The finding of SC5b-9 complexes in a body fluid implies the potential for tissue-damaging attack by MC5b-9 complexes at sites adjacent to that body fluid.

Dramatic changes in protein conformation accompanying C5b-9 assembly lead to expression of neoantigenic determinants present on assembled complexes, but not present on the unactivated component proteins. One of these neoantigens appears at the step of C9 binding.

We used an ELISA specific for C9 neoantigens[1] to quantitate SC5b-9 in the cerebrospinal fluid (CSF) of patients with a variety of autoimmune nervous system diseases including Guillain-Barré syndrome (GBS),[2] multiple sclerosis (MS), Sjögren's syndrome with focal CNS involvement (SS-CNS),[3] and systemic lupus erythematosus with CNS involvement (SLE-CNS). We detected SC5b-9 in the CSF of 13 of 14 patients with GBS (mean 3.1 µg/ml; range 0-7.1 µg/ml), 16 of 21 patients with MS (1.8; 0-7.5), 14 of 16 patients with SS-CNS (5.4; 0-15.0), and 6 of 7 patients with SLE-CNS (2.1; 0-9.2) (FIG. 1). SC5b-9 was not detected in the CSF of 2 SS and 2 SLE patients without CNS disease. We also quantitated CSF SC5b-9 in 11 patients with noninflammatory CNS diseases including Huntington's disease, hereditary cerebellar degeneration, idiopathic seizures, vestibular neuronitis, and progressive

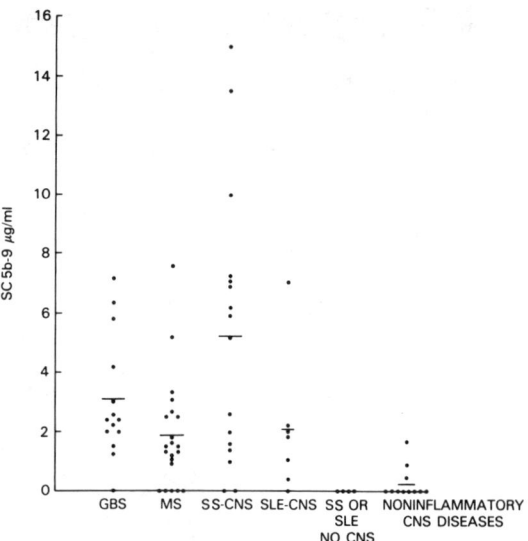

**FIGURE 1.** Cerebrospinal fluid SC5b-9 concentration in µg/ml in patients with Guillain-Barré syndrome (GBS), multiple sclerosis (MS), Sjögren's syndrome with CNS involvement (SS-CNS), systemic lupus erythematosus with CNS involvement (SLE-CNS), SS and SLE patients without CNS involvement (SS or SLE, NO CNS), and patients with a variety of noninflammatory nervous system diseases (see text). *Bars* represent means.

supranuclear palsy, and two patients each with stroke, Parkinson's disease, and pseudotumor cerebri. SC5b-9 was detected in three of these patients (with stroke, pseudotumor, or seizures) at low levels and was not detected in the other eight (mean 0.3 µg/ml; range 0-1.7 µg/ml). By Wilcoxon analysis with correction for multiple comparisons, all four disease categories differed from the noninflammatory disease group with at least $p < 0.05$. Intrathecal activation of terminal complement was indicated by the finding of CSF C5b-9 without concomitant serum C5b-9 in some patients with MS, SS-CNS, and SLE-CNS. Furthermore, in GBS we found a kinetic correlation of serum SC5b-9 levels with antiperipheral nerve myelin antibody titers and have immunohistologically demonstrated C9 neoantigens in diseased peripheral nerves.[4]

These results suggest a role for terminal complement activation in the pathophysiology of GBS, MS, SS-CNS, and SLE-CNS, and raise the possibility that CSF assay for C5b-9 may be clinically useful in selected patients with these diseases.

## REFERENCES

1. SANDERS, M. E., M. A. SCHMETZ, C. H. HAMMER, M. M. FRANK & K. A. JOINER. 1985. Quantitation of activation of the human terminal complement pathway by ELISA. J. Immunol. Methods **85:** 245.
2. SANDERS, M. E., C. L. KOSKI, D. ROBBINS, M. L. SHIN, M. M. FRANK & K. A. JOINER. 1986. Activated terminal complement in cerebrospinal fluid in Guillain-Barre syndrome and multiple sclerosis J. Immunol. **136:** 4456.
3. SANDERS, M. E., E. L. ALEXANDER, C. L. KOSKI, M. M. FRANK & K. A. JOINER. 1987. Detection of activated terminal complement (C5b-9) in cerebrospinal fluid from patients with central nervous system involvement of primary Sjögren's syndrome or systemic lupus erythematosus. J. Immunol. **138:** 2095.
4. KOSKI, C. L., M. E. SANDERS, P. T. SWOVELAND, T. J. LAWLEY, M. L. SHIN, M. M. FRANK & K. A. JOINER. 1987. J. Clin. Invest. **80:** 1492.

WORKSHOP 5. NEURAL CELL MARKERS IN HEALTH AND DISEASE

# Expression of Voltage-Gated Calcium Channels in Tumor Cell Lines of Neuroectodermal or Other Origin

BETHAN LANG, NITA NAGVEKAR,
JASVINDER GILL, ANGELA VINCENT, AND
JOHN NEWSOM-DAVIS

*Department of Neurological Science
Royal Free Hospital School of Medicine
London, England*

The Lambert-Eaton myasthenic syndrome (LEMS) is an autoimmune disorder of the neuromuscular junction characterized by a decrease in the quantal and nonquantal release of acetylcholine from the presynaptic nerve terminal. The disease associates with small (oat) cell lung carcinoma (SCLC) in approximately 60% of cases.[1]

LEMS has an autoimmune etiology in both its cancer-associated and "no cancer detected" forms.[2,3] Electrophysiologic studies in which LEMS IgG was injected into mice indicate a decrease in the number of functional voltage-gated $Ca^{2+}$ channels (VGCC).[4]

We recently showed[5] that a human SCLC line has functionally active VGCCs that exhibit a $K^+$-dependent increase in $^{45}Ca^{2+}$ flux into the cell. This activity can be blocked by the VGCC antagonists nifedipine and methoxyverapamil (D600). $K^+$-stimulated flux can be inhibited by growing the cells in IgG prepared from the plasma of patients with LEMS.

We have investigated the presence of functionally active VGCCs in a variety of cell lines and have also looked for the expression of other markers of neuroectodermal origin such as binding of the monoclonal antibody UJ13A[6] and the presence of "bombesin-like" activity (TABLE 1).

VGCCs have been demonstrated in all the SCLC lines tested. UJ13A binding was found in six of seven lines and bombesin-like activity in three of five lines tested. We were unable to demonstrate the presence of functionally active VGCC or UJ13A binding in any of the non-SCLC lines; two of the large cell carcinomas showed low levels of bombesin-like activity. These results indicate that VGCC may serve as a marker to discriminate SCLC from non-SCLC tumors.

VGCCs were also found in other lines, both human and rodent, which were considered to be neuroectodermal in origin, consistent with the view that SCLC is a tumor originally derived from neuroectodermal tissue.

LEMS IgG blocked $^{45}Ca^{2+}$ flux in all lines (both human and rodent) expressing VGCCs. VGCCs on tumor cells may initiate the autoantibody response in SCLC-

TABLE 1. Functional Voltage-Gated $Ca^{2+}$ Channels in Human and Nonhuman Tumor Cell Lines

| Cell Lines | $K^+$-Stimulated $Ca^{2+}$ Flux | Inhibition by LEMS IgG | UJ13A % Positive | Bombesin-Like Activity |
|---|---|---|---|---|
| A. *Small cell lung carcinoma* | | | | |
| 1. MAR 10 | + | + | 80 | + |
| 2. MAR 10 (adherent) | ++ | + | nd | nd |
| 3. MAR 5 | ++ | + | >90 | nd |
| 4. H128 | +++ | + | 13 | + |
| 5. NIH-82 | ++ | nd | 83 | − |
| 6. UCH-SC1 | ++ | ++ | >90 | − |
| 7. POC | ++ | + | >90 | nd |
| 8. H69 | ++ | nd | >90 | + |
| B. *Non-small cell lung carcinoma* (squamous; large cell and adenocarcinomas) | | | | |
| 9. A427 | − | nr | <10 | − |
| 10. A549 | − | nr | <10 | − |
| 11. JG-HUN | − | nr | 10 | nd |
| 12. JG-CLY | − | nr | <10 | ++ |
| 13. JG-WAR | − | nr | <10 | + |
| C. *Other human cell lines* | | | | |
| 14. K562 Myeloid leukemia | − | nr | nd | − |
| 15. U937 Monoblastic leukemia | − | nr | nd | − |
| 16. HL60 Promyelocyte leukemia | − | nr | 10 | − |
| 17. TE671 Medulloblastoma | − | nr | >90 | − |
| 18. 859 Astrocytoma | − | nr | <10 | − |
| 19. SKN-SH Neuroblastoma | ++ | ++ | 58 | − |
| 20. Kelly neuroblastoma | + | + | >90 | − |
| D. *Nonhuman cell lines* | | | | |
| 21. BC3H1 Mouse glioma | − | nr | nd | nd |
| 22. P3NS1-Ag.1 Mouse myeloma | − | nr | <10 | − |
| 23. PC12 Rat pheochromocytoma | ++ | ++ | <10 | − |
| 24. NG108 Mouse neuroblastoma/rat glioma | ++ | ++ | <10 | − |
| 25. F21D1 Mouse neuroblastoma/human dorsal root ganglia | + | + | <10 | − |

ABBREVIATIONS: nd = not done; nr = not relevant.

associated LEMS. In the remainder, VGCCs on other neuroectodermal cells may be implicated.

## REFERENCES

1. O'NEILL, J. H., N. M. F. MURRAY & J. NEWSOM-DAVIS. 1988. The Lambert-Eaton myasthenic syndrome: A review of 50 cases. Brain, in press.
2. LANG, B., J. NEWSOM-DAVIS, D. WRAY, A. VINCENT & N. MURRAY. 1981. Autoimmune aetiology for myasthenic (Eaton-Lambert) syndrome. Lancet ii: 224-226.
3. LANG, B., J. NEWSOM-DAVIS, C. PRIOR & D. WRAY. 1983. Antibodies to motor nerve terminals: An electrophysiological study of a human myasthenic syndrome transferred to mouse. J. Physiol. (London) 344: 335-345.
4. LANG, B., J. NEWSOM-DAVIS, C. PEERS, C. PRIOR & D. WRAY. 1987. The effect of myasthenic syndrome antibody on presynaptic calcium channels in the mouse. J. Physiol. (London) 390: 257-270.
5. ROBERTS, A., S. PERERA, B. LANG, A. VINCENT & J. NEWSOM-DAVIS. 1985. Paraneoplastic myasthenic syndrome IgG inhibits $^{45}Ca^{2+}$ flux in a human cell carcinoma line. Nature 317: 737-739.
6. ALLAN, P. M., J. GARSON, E. HARPER, V. ASSER, H. COAKHAM, B. BROWNELL & J. KEMPSHEAD. 1983. Biological characterisation and clinical applications of a monoclonal antibody recognising an antigen restricted to neuroectodermal tissues. Int. J. Cancer 31: 591-598.

# Rat Astrocyte Proliferation by Human B-Cell Growth Factors

ETTY N. BENVENISTE,[a,c] JOSEPH L. BUTLER,[b]
DAVID A. GIBBS,[a] ALICE CHEN,[a] AND
JOHN N. WHITAKER[a,c]

*Departments of Neurology,[a] Cell Biology and Anatomy,[c]
and Pediatrics[b]
University of Alabama at Birmingham
Birmingham, Alabama 35294*

The growth of astroglial cells is influenced by a variety of T-cell-derived lymphokines and monokines. These include supernatants derived from mitogen-stimulated human and murine T cells,[1-3] human T- and B-cell lines,[2] HTLV-II transformed human peripheral blood T cells,[3] and purified human interleukin-1 (IL-1).[4]

To determine what specific factor or factors contained within T-cell-derived supernatants are responsible for astrocyte proliferation, we examined the ability of several well-characterized, purified T-cell-derived lymphokines to induce astrocyte proliferation. Although both recombinant interleukin-2 (IL-2)[5] and gamma interferon (IFN-$\gamma$) have no proliferative effect on astrocytes, we discovered that both a 20,000-dalton T-cell-derived B-cell growth factor (BCGF)[6] and a 60,000-dalton B-cell-derived BCGF[7] have stimulatory activity on rat astrocytes. These BCGF-containing supernatants are devoid of IL-1, IL-2, IFN-$\gamma$, and B-cell differentiation factor (BCDF) activity.

## MATERIALS AND METHODS

Primary glial cell cultures were established from neonatal rat cerebra as previously described.[5] After 10 days in primary culture, astrocytes were obtained by trypsinization and plated at $7.5 \times 10^3$ cells/well. Experiments were performed in both the presence and the absence of serum. Dilutions of the test samples were added to the wells at a volume of 0.1 ml/well for a final total volume of 0.2 ml. After various incubation times (48-72 hours), the cells were pulsed with 1 $\mu$Ci $^3$H-thymidine and harvested onto glass filter strips after 17 hours. All experiments are performed in triplicate, and the data are expressed as the mean ± SD.

Human and rat recombinant IFN-$\gamma$ was purchased from Amgen Biologics. The 20,000-dalton BCGF, called 2B11, was generated from 48-hour cultures of T-cell hybridomas ($1 \times 10^6$ cells) in media containing 1% serum,[6] as was the 60,000-dalton BCGF, called Namalva.[7] These supernatants were assayed for IL-1, IL-2, IFN-$\gamma$, and BCDF activity as previously described.

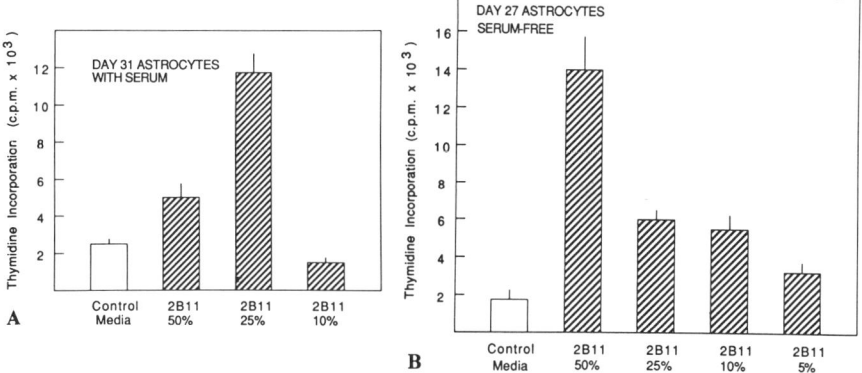
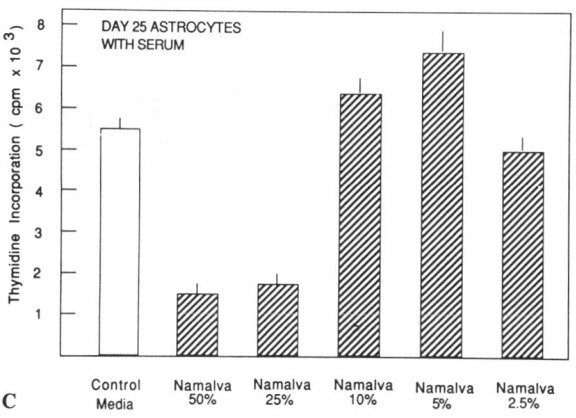
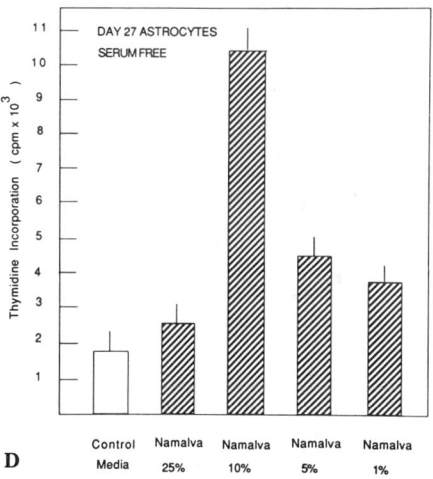

FIGURE 1. B-cell growth factor-induced proliferation of rat astrocytes. Rat astrocytes ($7.5 \times 10^3$/well) were incubated with and without growth factors for 3 days. The cells were then pulsed with 1 $\mu$Ci $^3$H-TdR and harvested onto glass filter strips after 17 hours. (**A**) 2B11-BCGF with 10% serum; (**B**) 2B11-BCGF in serum-free media; (**C**) Namalva-BCGF with 10% serum; and (**D**) Namalva-BCGF in serum-free media.

TABLE 1. Recombinant Rat Gamma-Interferon Inhibits BCGF-Induced Proliferation of Rat Astrocytes

| Stimulant | Time of Addition of IFN-γ, 5 U/ml | $^3$H-TdR Incorporation (cpm ± SD) | % Inhibition |
|---|---|---|---|
| Control media | ... | 6,338 ± 210 | ... |
| | Day 0 | 5,489 ± 691 | |
| 2B11-BCGF 50% v/v | ... | 28,210 ± 1,966 | ... |
| | Day 0 | 18,584 ± 1,978 | 35 |
| | Day 1 | 21,357 ± 2,149 | 25 |
| | Day 2 | 28,215 ± 1,540 | ... |
| 2B11-BCGF 25% v/v | ... | 19,903 ± 676 | ... |
| | Day 0 | 7,203 ± 264 | 64 |
| | Day 1 | 14,343 ± 1,721 | 28 |
| | Day 2 | 18,203 ± 264 | 9 |
| 2B11-BCGF 5% v/v | ... | 11,449 ± 1,728 | ... |
| | Day 0 | 7,398 ± 995 | 36 |
| | Day 1 | 5,909 ± 501 | 49 |
| | Day 2 | 11,416 ± 1,368 | ... |
| Namalva-BCGF 10% v/v | ... | 12,996 ± 477 | ... |
| | Day 0 | 6,417 ± 990 | 51 |
| | Day 1 | 6,166 ± 1,098 | 53 |
| | Day 2 | 12,314 ± 761 | ... |
| Namalva-BCGF 5% v/v | ... | 10,953 ± 152 | ... |
| | Day 0 | 5,489 ± 691 | 50 |
| | Day 1 | 4,863 ± 406 | 56 |
| | Day 2 | nd | |

## RESULTS

As shown in FIGURE 1A and B, 2B11-BCGF significantly stimulated astrocyte proliferation in the presence or absence of serum, whereas Namalva-BCGF was stimulatory only in the absence of serum (FIG. 1C and D). We also demonstrated that IFN-γ inhibits the BCGF-induced proliferation of rat astrocytes in a time-dependent fashion (TABLE 1). In addition to inducing proliferation, 2B11-BCGF appears to induce morphologic changes in these cells. After a 4-day incubation with 2B11-BCGF, the astrocytes appear "more reactive," suggesting some cytoskeletal changes. Lastly, as BCGF was demonstrated to enhance Ia antigen expression on B cells,[8] we were interested in whether BCGF could induce Ia antigen expression on astrocytes. Our preliminary results indicate that neither 2B11 nor Namalva-BCGF can induce Ia antigens on primary rat astrocytes. However, 2B11-BCGF can enhance Ia antigen expression on two human astrocytoma cell lines (U373 and U87), which are both 100% GFAP positive.

Astrocyte hyperproliferation leads to the formation of scar tissue, or "plaques," in the demyelinating disease of multiple sclerosis, which is in part responsible for physical impairment in these patients. BCGF stimulation of astrocyte proliferation may have a role in promoting gliosis associated with inflammatory infiltration of the central nervous system.

## REFERENCES

1. FONTANA, A., A. GRIEDER, S. T. ARRENBRECHT & P. J. GROB. 1980. J. Neurol. Sci. **46:** 55-62.
2. FONTANA, A., U. OTZ, A. L. DE WECK & P. J. GROB. 1982. J. Neuroimmunol. **2:** 73-81.
3. MERRILL, J. E., S. KUTSUNAI, C. MOHLSTROM, F. HOFMAN, J. GROOPMAN & D. W. GOLDE. 1984. Science **224:** 1428-1430.
4. GIULIAN, D. & L. B. LACHMAN. 1985. Science **228:** 497-499.
5. BENVENISTE, E. N. & J. E. MERRILL. 1986. Nature **321:** 610-613.
6. BUTLER, J. L., J. L. AMBRUS, JR. & A. S. FAUCI. 1984. J. Immunol. **133:** 251-255.
7. AMBRUS, J. L. JR., C. H. JURGENSEN, E. J. BROWN & A. S. FAUCI. 1985. J. Exp. Med. **162:** 1319-1335.
8. NOELLE, R., P. H. KRAMMER, J. OHARA, J. W. UHR & E. S. VITETTA. 1984. Proc. Natl. Acad. Sci. USA **81:** 6149-6153.

# EAE Serum Decreases CNPase Activity in Cultures of B104 Cells

R. ELKIN, W. D. LYMAN, C. F. BROSNAN, AND
M. B. BORNSTEIN

*Albert Einstein College of Medicine
Bronx, New York 10461*

There is a need for a rapid and sensitive clinical assay to quantitate the effect of soluble factors associated with primary demyelinating diseases. To date, organotypic cultures of central nervous system (CNS) tissue have proved to be a useful tool for evaluation of myelin changes *in vitro*.[1] However, this method is labor intensive and slow, and the cultures may fail to develop and differentiate to produce myelin.

The B104 cell line, a neuronal cell line derived from rat CNS,[2] expresses a number of neural proteins including 2',3'-cyclic nucleotide 3'-phosphodiesterase (CNPase). CNPase is an oligodendrocyte-associated enzyme whose activity correlates with the amount and integrity of myelin. Activity of this enzyme can be measured using a sensitive fluorometric radioimmunoassay. We have applied this assay system to measure CNPase activity in B104 cell cultures that were exposed to factors known to cause demyelination in organotypic CNS culture.

## MATERIALS AND METHODS

B104 cells (a gift from Dr. R. Ledeen) were grown in RPMI supplemented with 10% fetal calf serum. Cells were dispensed at $1 \times 10^5$ cells/ml in a 24-well tissue culture plate and incubated overnight in 4% $CO_2$ at 37°C. By the following day, semiconfluence was reached, the adherent B104 cells were washed, and 1 ml of RPMI was added to each well. Normal rabbit serum (NRS) or rabbit anti-myelin basic protein (anti-MBP) antiserum, anti-galactocerebroside (anti-GC) antiserum (courtesy of Dr. C. S. Raine), anti-glial fibrillary acidic protein (anti-GFAP) antiserum (a gift from Dr. J. E. Goldman), and anti-white matter (anti-WM) antiserum were added to wells to give final concentrations of 1%, 5%, or 10%, respectively. Cultures were examined by light microscopy (LM) at 3, 6, and 24 hours for morphologic changes and, by fluorometry, for CNPase activity at the same times. For CNPase activity, the cells were washed, 1 ml of trypsin-EDTA was added to each well, the cells were harvested and centrifuged, and the supernatant was aspirated. The cell pellet was lysed and sonicated in 500 µl of distilled water and stored at $-20°C$ until assayed. The fluorometric assay as described by Weissbarth *et al.*[3] was used for CNPase activity in the respective B104 homogenates.

## RESULTS

Monolayers of B104 cells incubated with anti-WM antiserum had marked morphologic changes and a significant decrease in CNPase activity compared with cultures incubated in the presence of medium alone or NRS. These changes were directly proportional to the concentration of anti-WM antiserum added to the test well. Changes in both morphology and CNPase activity could be detected after 30 minutes.

To determine the specificity of these phenomena, rabbit antisera to GC, MBP, and GFAP were used. Anti-GC and anti-MBP antisera had no effect on cell morphology and CNPase activity. However, preliminary data suggest that anti-GFAP antiserum may inhibit CNPase activity in B104 cells without associated morphologic changes.

## DISCUSSION

These preliminary data indicate that B104 cells may provide an assay system for quantitating the demyelinating ability of various soluble factors. Ongoing studies are further examining the specificity and mechanism by which anti-WM and anti-GFAP antisera induce the observed changes. In addition, sera and cerebrospinal fluid from patients with demyelinating diseases will be tested in this assay for the ability to cause changes in B104 cells morphologically and biochemically.

### REFERENCES

1. ROTH, G. A, M. B. BORNSTEIN, M. ROYTTA et al. 1985. J. Neurochem. **44:** 654-657.
2. SCHUBERT, D., S. HEINEMANN, W. CARLISLE et al. 1979. Nature **249:** 224-227.
3. WEISSBARTH, S., H. S. MAKER, G. M. LEHRER et al. 1980. J. Neurochem. **35:** 503-505.

# Antibody for Nerve Growth Factor Detected in Patients with Alzheimer's Disease

BENJAMIN F. ROY, TREY SUNDERLAND, DENNIS
L. MURPHY, AND JOHN M. MORIHISA

*Georgetown University School of Medicine
Laboratory of Clinical Science
National Institute of Mental Health
Washington, D.C. 20007*

The participation of nerve growth factor (NGF) as a trophic factor for cholinergic neurons of the basal forebrain and the selective degeneration of ascending cholinergic projections from the basal forebrain in Alzheimer's disease have led to the hypothesis that reductions in NGF may contribute to the pathogenesis of Alzheimer's disease.[1] The intraventricular administration of antisera for NGF to rats results in histologic degeneration of the septohippocampal projection that is reminiscent of Alzheimer's disease.[2] We report preliminary data of a pilot study using an enzyme-linked immunosorbent assay (ELISA) to detect antibody with reactivity for NGF.

Five patients meeting criteria for primary degenerative dementia (Alzheimer's disease, AD) according to the American Psychiatric Association Diagnostic Statistical Manual, Third Edition 1980 (DSM-III) and age- and sex-matched elderly normal volunteers ($n = 3$) were studied. Subjects were free of chronic medication for at least a 3-week period before the drawing of blood samples. The investigators were blind to diagnoses. The ELISA was performed as previously described.[3]

Antibodies with reactivity for NGF were purified by affinity chromatography from three of five patients with AD (TABLE 1). The purified antibodies of normal volunteers demonstrated minimal reactivity at equivalent IgG concentrations. However, antibody that reacted with NGF at higher concentrations was recovered from normal volunteer 3. Purified anti-NGF IgG from a patient with AD and a normal volunteer immunoprecipitated 50% and 5% of soluble [$^{125}$-I]2.5S NGF, respectively. The binding of F(ab')$_2$ fragment of anti-NGF IgG from a patient with AD was inhibited by 36% by $10^{-9}$ M 2.5S NGF.

The ELISA was modified and employed to detect binding of purified antibodies to rat brain membranes. Anti-NGF IgG from a patient with AD demonstrated 72% greater binding to rat cortex than to rat midbrain-cerebellum (TABLE 2). This binding was reduced 36% by the addition of soluble 2.5S NGF ($5 \times 10^{-9}$ M) to the anti-NGF IgG. A qualitatively similar but quantitatively less reactive anti-NGF IgG recovered from an age-matched normal volunteer demonstrated less binding to rat brain at higher concentrations; its binding to rat cortex was inhibited by 80% following the addition of soluble 2.5S NGF to the antibody.

Theoretically, disordered regulation of an idiotypic network for NGF and its receptor might potentially induce the pathologic and neurochemical alterations in the

TABLE 1. Purification of Antibody for Nerve Growth Factor (NGF)

| Age (yr.) & Sex | | IgG | 2.5S NGF | 7S NGF |
|---|---|---|---|---|
| *Alzheimer's disease* | | | | |
| 1. 42,M | Eluate | 200 | 0.119 | 0.104 |
| | Effluent | 200 | 0.019 | 0.093 |
| 2. 45,F | Eluate | 200 | 0.077 | 0.033 |
| | Effluent | 200 | 0.115 | 0.031 |
| 3. 60,F | Eluate | 200 | 0.029 | 0.888 |
| | Effluent | 200 | 0.027 | 1.071 |
| 4. 62,M | Eluate | 410 | 0.266 | 1.324 |
| | Effluent | 2,343 | 0.001 | 0.094 |
| 5. 72,F | Eluate | 700 | 0.375 | 0.053 |
| | Effluent | 1,400 | 0 | 0.002 |
| *Normal volunteers* | | | | |
| 1. 43,F | Eluate | 1,800 | 0 | 0.015 |
| | Effluent | 1,800 | 0.007 | 0.358 |
| 2. 60,F | Eluate | 1,800 | 0.002 | 0.014 |
| | Effluent | 1,800 | 0.010 | 0.047 |
| 3. 70,F | Eluate | 1,800 | 0.206 | 1.258 |
| | Effluent | 1,800 | 0 | 0.015 |

NOTE: Affinity chromatography was used to isolate anti-nerve growth factor IgG from protein-A-purified IgG samples. Samples were adsorbed to mouse submaxillary gland 7S NGF (Sigma Chemical Co., St. Louis, Missouri) coupled to cyanogen-bromide-activated sepharose 4B (1.0 mg 7S NGF/ml of Sepharose). Elution was performed using 3M potassium thiocyanate followed by 4M guanidine hydrochloride. The concentration of IgG is given as ng/100 $\mu$l. Values reflect the mean of triplicate determinations after the subtraction of background binding to human corticotropin (ACTH).


TABLE 2. Anti-Nerve Growth Factor (NGF) IgG Binding to Rat Brain Membranes[a]

| | IgG | Optical Density at 405 nm | |
|---|---|---|---|
| | | $P_2$ Fraction Rat Brain Membranes | |
| | | Cortex | Cerebellum |
| *Alzheimer's disease* | | | |
| Anti-NGF IgG | 10 ng | 0.629 ± 0.114 | 0.365 ± 0.018 |
| Anti-NGF IgG + NGF[b] | | 0.404 ± 0.006 | 0.329 ± 0.009 |
| *Normal volunteer* | | | |
| Anti-NGF IgG | 32 ng | 0.383 ± 0.001 | 0.298 ± 0.001 |
| Anti-NGF IgG + NGF[b] | | 0.079 ± 0.001 | 0.072 ± 0.001 |

[a] The crude mitochondrial ($P_2$) membrane fraction of rat brain was used for these studies. Preincubation of 0.5 mg of brain protein in 0.5 ml 10 mM $K_2PO_4$, pH 7.4, was carried out for 60 minutes at 26°C. Brain membrane preparations were then washed in 0.1 M Tris-HCl, pH 7.4, and centrifuged at 15,000 rpm. The pellets were rehomogenized and diluted in 0.1 M Tris-HCl, pH 7.4, to a final volume of 5.0 ml. These solutions were allowed to coat an ELISA plate for 2-3 hours at 26°C.
[b] Soluble 2.5S NGF ($5 \times 10^{-9}$ M) was added to anti-NGF IgG 30 minutes before assay.

central cholinergic and somatostatinergic systems observed in AD by an autoimmune mechanism similar to immunosympathectomy in animal experiments. Although these data are insufficient to support this interpretation, further investigation is indicated. It is possible that antibody for NGF is a consequence of the neuropathology of Alzheimer's disease.

## REFERENCES

1. HEFTI, F. & W. WEINER. 1986. Nerve growth factor and Alzheimer's disease. Ann. Neurol. **20:** 275-281.
2. SPRINGER, J. E. & R. LOY. 1985. Intrahippocampal injections of antiserum to nerve growth factor inhibit sympathohippocampal sprouting. Brain Res. Bull. **15:** 629-634.
3. ROY, B. F., J. W. ROSE, H. F. MCFARLAND, D. C. MCFARLIN & D. L. MURPHY. 1986. Anti-$\beta$-endorphin immunoglobulin G in humans. Proc. Natl. Acad. Sci. USA **83:** 8739-8743.

# Cytotoxic Response of Cultured Tumor Infiltrating Lymphocytes to Autologous Human Glioblastoma Cells[a]

M. C. KUPPNER, M. F. HAMOU, AND
N. DE TRIBOLET

*Neurosurgical Service*
*University Hospital*
*Lausanne, Switzerland*

Frozen sections of tumor tissue obtained from patients with malignant gliomas were examined for lymphoid cell infiltrates using a series of monoclonal antibodies to human lymphocytes and an avidin-biotin immunoperoxidase method. The seven glioblastomas studied demonstrated varying degrees of lymphoid cell infiltration. (TABLE 1.)

Analysis of the functional properties of the tumor-infiltrating lymphocytes (TILs) isolated from each biopsy sample was also performed after expansion of the TILs *in vitro* using a microculture system established by Moretta *et al.*,[1] in which the TILs were initially stimulated with phytohemagglutinin and then cultured in the presence of interleukin-2 (IL-2) and feeder cells.

The results show that many of the TIL microcultures obtained in the three cases of glioblastoma with marked to moderate levels of lymphoid cell infiltration, selectively lysed autologous glioblastoma cells *in vitro* but did not lyse a panel of control cells which included allogeneic gliomas, a fresh melanoma target cell line, and NK sensitive line K562.

Phenotypic analysis was performed in several TIL microcultures exhibiting selective autologous tumor killing. The microcultures were found to consist of T lymphocytes ($CD3^+$ cells).

Numerous TIL microcultures obtained from glioblastomas that exhibited marked to slight levels of lymphoid cell infiltration (four cases) lysed both the autologous tumor and the NK target K562.

Low levels of cytotoxicity against allogeneic gliomas and a fresh melanoma target were found to be characteristic of the TILs. In the three remaining cases with rare to negative staining for T cells, most microcultures obtained did not express cytolytic activity against the autologous tumor, and activity against the K562 target was found only in one case.

The peripheral blood lymphocytes (PBLs) of five patients were also cultured and tested in a similar manner to that of the corresponding TILs; however, the level of cytolytic activity achieved by the PBLs against the autologous glioblastoma cells was

---

[a]This work was supported by the Preuss Foundation.

TABLE 1. Lymphoid Cell Subset Infiltration in Human Gliomas

| | Patient | Age (yr.) & Sex | CD2 | CD3 | CD4 | CD8 | CD16 |
|---|---|---|---|---|---|---|---|
| | | | | Immunoperoxidase-Positive Lymphoid Cell Subsets | | | |
| 1. | A.C. | 55, M | - | 3 | 2 | 2 | 3 |
| 2. | M.L. | 60, M | - | 3 | 2 | 3 | 1 |
| 3. | R.P. | 63, M | - | 2 | 0 | 2 | 1 |
| 4. | H.M. | 54, M | - | 1 | R | R | R |
| 5. | G.R. | 71, F | - | R | R | R | R |
| 6. | F.L. | 59, F | - | R | R | R | R |
| 7. | S.J. | 67, F | 1 | 0 | 0 | 0 | 1 |

CODE: 0 = no staining; R = rare positive staining cells; 1 = slight staining (1-5%); 2 = moderate staining (5-10%); 3 = marked intense staining (10-25%).

significantly lower than that obtained by the TILs ($p < 0.001$). *In vitro* sensitization of patients' PBLs with autologous tumor cells did not enhance the cytotoxic response against autologous glioblastoma cells. The present results suggest that there is a degree of sensitization *in vivo* to human glioblastomas because TILs isolated from malignant gliomas that exhibit significant levels of lymphoid cell infiltration selectively lyse autologous glioblastoma cells *in vitro*.

## REFERENCE

1. MORETTA, A., G. PANTALEO, L. MORETTA, J. C. CEROTTINI & M. C. MINGARI. 1983. Direct demonstration of the clonogenic potential of every human peripheral blood T cell. Clonal analysis of HLA-DR expression and cytolytic activity. J. Exp. Med. **157:** 743.

# Phospholipase $A_2$ Activity in Cultured Glial Cells

## Correlation with Appearance of Myelin Markers and Effects of Steroid Hormones

T. BRENNER,[a] S. YEDGAR,[b] J. WEIDENFELD,[a] AND
O. ABRAMSKY[a]

[a]*Department of Neurology*
*Hadassah University Hospital*
*and*
[b]*Department of Biochemistry*
*Hebrew University-Hadassah Medical School*
*Jerusalem, Israel*

Phospholipase $A_2$ ($PLA_2$), which hydrolyzes phospholipid at the sn-2 position to produce fatty acid and lysophospholipid, has been identified in numerous cell types.[1] The activity of this enzyme has been correlated with various cell functions, such as exocytosis, platelet activation, prostaglandin production, and cellular secretion.[1] Glucocorticoids have been shown to cause indirect inhibition of $PLA_2$ by inducing synthesis or release of proteins that possess antiphospholipase properties.[1] Direct inhibition of $PLA_2$ can be achieved by binding to the enzyme of $N$-derivatives of phosphatidylserine.[1,2] In the present study $PLA_2$ activity was determined in cultures of glial

TABLE 1. Phospholipase $A_2$ Activity in Cultured Rat Glial Cells: Correlation with Myelin Markers

| | Days in Culture | | | | |
|---|---|---|---|---|---|
| | 0 | 1 | 2 | 4 | 4+Inh[a] |
| $PLA_2$ (pmol/h/1.5 × $10^6$ cells) | 400 | 1,700 | 2,400 | 5,700 | 3,150 |
| GalC[b] | ND | 10 | 60 | 70 | <10 |
| MBP[b] | ND | <1 | ND | 50 | 50 |
| CNPase[b] | ND | <1 | ND | 50 | ND |
| GFAP[b] | ND | 5 | 5 | 10-15 | 10-15 |

ABBREVIATION: ND = not determined.
[a] Dex-Ps or PsAc (10 nmol) was incubated for 45 minutes and washed, and $C_6$-NBD-PC was added for $PLA_2$ assay or fresh medium for immunofluorescence.
[b] Percentage of cells binding the different antibodies.

cells derived from fetal or adult rats, employing a novel method. The procedure is based on the cellular uptake of phosphatidylcholine (PC) containing a fluorescent-labeled hexanoic acid (C6-NBD) at the second carbon of the phospholipid substrate. This product does not incorporate into other lipids and is not further metabolized. Thus, the produced fluorescent fatty acid is a direct measure of $PLA_2$ activity. Glial cells were isolated from corpus callosum of adult rats by the percoll gradient method.[3] Dissociated brain cells from 16-20-day fetal rats were prepared and cultured as previously described.[4] As indicated in TABLE 1, $PLA_2$ activity exhibited a time-dependent increase over a period of 4 days. In addition, it could be correlated with the appearance of the typical oligodendrocyte myelin markers: galactocerebroside (GalC) myelin basic protein (MBP) and 2'3'-cyclic nucleotide 3' phosphohydrolase (CNPase), but not with the astrocytic marker glial fibrillary acidic protein (GFAP). Furthermore, incubation of the cultures with the specific $PLA_2$ inhibitors,[2] Dex-Ps or PsAc, markedly reduced the percentages of cells binding GalC, whereas the binding of MBP and GFAP was not affected. TABLE 2 shows the effect of 48 hours' pretreatment of cells with various hormonal steroids. Progesterone and testosterone in-

TABLE 2. Effect of Gonadal Steroids and Glucocorticoids on $PLA_2$ Activity in Cultured Rat Glial Cells[a]

|  | $C_6$-NBD-PC Hydrolysed (pmol/h/plate) |
|---|---|
| Control | 1,050 + 47 |
| Progesterone | 470 + 180 |
| Testosterone | 490 + 60 |
| Pregnenolone | 960 + 130 |
| Dexamethasone | 850 + 100 |
| Corticosterone | 850 + 30 |

[a] Cells from 19-day fetal brains were cultured for 2-3 days and then 100 μg of each steroid was added. Twenty-four hours later an additional 100 μg was added (results show the mean of 5-10 assays + SE).

hibited $PLA_2$ activity by 55%, whereas pregnenolone (a biologically inactive steroid precursor) and the glucocorticoids dexamethasone and corticosterone failed to inhibit this enzyme activity.

In conclusion, we provide direct evidence for the presence of $PLA_2$ activity in fetal and adult rat glial cell cultures. This activity increases *in vitro* and is correlated with the appearance of the typical myelin markers, GalC, MBP, and CNPase. Gonadal steroids, but not glucocorticoids, appear to inhibit $PLA_2$ activity in the cultured cells.

### REFERENCES

1. BLACKWELL, G. J. & R. J. FLOWER. 1983. Br. Med. Bull. **39:** 260-264.
2. YEDGAR, S., N. REISFELD & A. DAGAN. 1986. FEBS Lett. **200:** 165-168.
3. HIRAYAMA, M., D. H. SILBERBERG, P. LISAK & D. PLEASURE. 1983. J. Neuropathol. Exp. Neurol. **42:** 16-28.
4. ECCLESTON, P. A. & D. H. SILBERBERG. 1983. Dev. Brain Res. **16:** 1-9.

# Cloning of cDNA for Two Large Polypeptides Found in Myelinating Oligodendrocytes

## JEFFREY R. GULCHER, LINDA S. MARTON, AND KARI STEFANSSON

*Departments of Neurology and Pathology (Neuropathology)*
*University of Chicago*
*Chicago, Illinois 60637*

We previously identified two large glycosylated polypeptides, gp225 and gp150 (225 and 150 kd), in the developing human central nervous system (CNS) having maximal expression during a period roughly corresponding to the time of active myelination.[1] We described the isolation and partial biochemical and immunochemical characterization of these two polypeptides.[2] We showed that although in the normal CNS we only find them in myelinating oligodendrocytes, gp225 appears in reactive astrocytes in and around various kinds of lesions (Gulcher and Stefansson, unpublished data). We recently determined that at a physiologic salt concentration gp225 binds to heparin but gp150 does not (Marton, Gulcher, & Stefansson, unpublished data). Hence, gp225 may bind together cells that have heparin-containing proteoglycans on their surfaces or bridge between such cells and heparin in extracellular matrix.[3]

These two glycosylated polypeptides are immunologically related, sharing both carbohydrate and polypeptide epitopes. Peptide mapping with *Staphylococcus aureus* V8 protease revealed at least one peptide fragment of 20 kd shared by the two proteins (unpublished data). To define the relationship between gp225 and gp150 we set out to clone cDNA, coding for both polypeptides. To do so we used the λgt11 system[4] and isolated the mRNA from the human glioblastoma cell line, U373MG, which produces both polypeptides. We screened the library for antibodies that react with epitopes present on the polypeptide backbones of both gp150 and gp225.

We have so far cloned and analyzed eight distinct positive clones. Six of these eight produced fusion proteins that reacted with our antisera on immunoblots. Restriction maps revealed that the eight clones all overlap with at least one other clone and provide 5 kb of continuous nonoverlapping sequence. The clones fall into two groups on the basis of their restriction maps. Each clone in the two groups overlaps completely with the largest clone in the group. The largest clone in one group measures 5 kb (λ29) and overlaps in a complicated manner with the largest clone in the other group (λ31), which measures 2.9 kb (FIG. 1). The 3' ends of both clones have six restriction sites over 1.5 kb that are identical and the 5' ends have four identical restriction sites over 1 kb. Thus, λ29 and λ31 appear to have identical 3' and 5' ends, but λ29 has an internal 2-kb segment that is not present in λ31. It is of interest that the 2-kb segment, if coding, could account for the size difference between gp150 and gp225. We subcloned this internal segment, unique to λ29, into λgt11 and showed

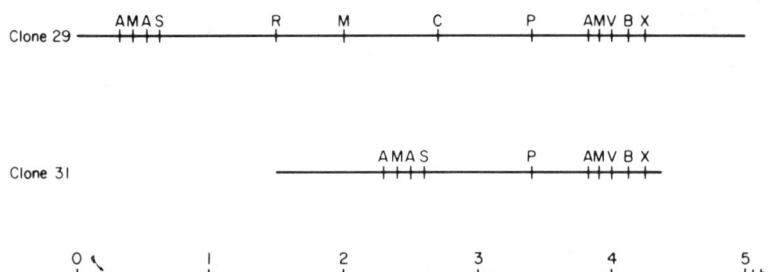

**FIGURE 1.** Restriction maps of the cDNA inserts of the two clones representing the two sets of overlapping clones selected from the library. The larger clone, λ29, represents five positive clones, whereas λ31 represents three positive clones. The left end (tentatively called the 5' end) of each clone contains four identical restriction sites. The 3' end of each clone contains six identical restriction sites. However, the larger clone contains an internal segment of 2 kb that contains three restriction sites not found in the smaller clone. KEY: A-*Apa*I; B-*Bam*HI; C-*Sac*II; M-*Sma*I; P-*Pst*I; R-*Eco*RI; S-*Sst*I; V-*Eco*RV; X-*Xba*I.

that it is indeed coding. Hence it is possible that gp150 and gp225 are derived from alternative splicing of a single transcript from one gene.[5]

## DISCUSSION

Our assumption is that gp225 serves to bind together certain cells that have heparin-containing proteoglycans on their surface and to bind such cells to heparin in the extracellular matrix. As pointed out, gp150 does not bind heparin at physiologic salt concentration. Hence, switching between the expression of gp150 and gp225 may be one mechanism whereby migration (and adhesion) of certain cells are controlled during development and reparative processes. This control appears to be mediated through alternate splicing of one primary message.

### REFERENCES

1. MARTON, L. S. & K. STEFANSSON. 1984. Developmental alterations in molecular weights of proteins in the human central nervous system that react with antibodies against myelin-associated glycoprotein. J. Cell Biol. **99:** 1642-1646.
2. GULCHER, J. R., L. S. MARTON, & K. STEFANSSON. 1986. Two large glycosylated polypeptides found in myelinating oligodendrocytes but not in myelin. Proc. Natl. Acad. Sci. USA **83:** 2118-2122.
3. COLE, G. J. & L. GLASER. 1986. A heparin-binding domain from N-CAM is involved in cell-substratum adhesion. J. Cell Biol. **102:** 403-412.
4. YOUNG, R. A. & R. W. DAVIS. 1983. Efficient isolation of genes by using antibody probes. Proc. Natl. Acad. Sci. USA **80:** 1194-1198.
5. LEFF, S. E., M. G. ROSENFELD & R. M. EVANS. 1986. Complex transcriptional units. Ann. Rev. Biochem. **55:** 1091-1117.

# Neuroleukin Secretion Is Highly Regulated in T Cells But Constitutive in C6 Glioma Cells

GREGORY T. SPEAR AND MARK E. GURNEY

*Department of Pharmacological and Physiological Sciences*
*University of Chicago*
*Chicago, Illinois 60637*

Neuroleukin has been purified, molecularly cloned, and expressed. Recombinant mouse neuroleukin maintains the survival of distinct types of embryonic neurons, is a product of mitogen-stimulated T cells, and induces immunoglobulin secretion by human mononuclear cells. Neuroleukin mRNA is present in brain and in C6 glioma cells, an astrocyte cell line.

We studied the regulation of neuroleukin secretion by a C6 glioma, a T lymphoma (LBRM-33), and a B-cell line (7OZ/3) with a two-site ELISA. The ELISA was performed in microtiter plate wells using the IgG fraction of rabbit anti-rat neuroleukin as the immobilizing antibody and biotinylated IgG from the same antiserum as the detecting antibody. Purified recombinant neuroleukin was used as the standard.

Neuroleukin was detected in supernatants from all three cell lines. Phytohemagglutinin stimulated a five- to tenfold increase in neuroleukin secretion by LBRM-33 cells, but it had no effect on secretion by 7OZ/3 (TABLE 1) or C6 cells (TABLE 2).

Lipopolysaccharide, which stimulates 7OZ/3 cells or phorbol myristate acetate, or gamma interferon had no significant effect on neuroleukin secretion by either the T- or the B-cell line.

LBRM-33 cells secrete interleukin-2 (IL-2) after stimulation with both PHA and IL-1. However, IL-1 had no effect on neuroleukin secretion in either the presence or absence of PHA. Calcium ionophore was also found to induce neuroleukin secretion in LBRM-33 cells at $0.5-1 \times 10^{-6}$M.

TABLE 1. Neuroleukin Secretion Regulated in a T-Cell But Not a B-Cell Line

| Cell Treatment | LBRM-33 (ng NLK/ml) | 7OZ/3 (ng NLK/ml) |
|---|---|---|
| Control | 5.0 | 5.1 |
| LPS | 5.6 | 7.7 |
| TPA | 6.2 | 3.7 |
| IFN | 6.3 | 4.8 |
| PHA | 29.5 | 2.5 |

ABBREVIATIONS: IFN = interferon; LPS = lipopolysaccharide; NLK = neuroleukin; PHA = phytohemagglutinin; TPA = phorbol myristate acetate.

TABLE 2. Induction of Neuroleukin Secretion in C6 Glioma Cells[a]

| Treatment | Neuroleukin (Relative Concentration) |
|---|---|
| None | 8.6 |
| Indomethacin | 6.1 |
| LPS | 12.0 |
| TPA | 13.2 |
| IL-1 | 7.1 |
| PHA | 4.6 |
| IL-2 | 12.2 |
| Monensin | 27.8 |
| Chloroquine | 120.5 |

[a] For abbreviations, see TABLE 1.

C6 gliomas were also found to secrete neuroleukin. Several agents that are known to induce changes in C6 cells were added to cultures, and the amount of neuroleukin was measured (TABLE 2). Of the tested agents, only monensin and chloroquine, two agents that affect intracellular trafficking of secreted proteins, consistently increased neuroleukin secretion. The increase in neuroleukin secretion by the C6 cells was found by 48 hours but not by 24 hours of chloroquine treatment. These results indicate that neuroleukin secretion can be regulated in T lymphocytes but not in B lymphocytes and that glioma cells constitutively secrete neuroleukin.

# A Peanut Agglutinin Binding Glycoprotein in CNS Myelin and Oligodendrocytes

DANIEL D. MIKOL, SARA SZUCHET, AND
KARI STEFANSSON

*Departments of Neurology and Pathology (Neuropathology)*
*University of Chicago*
*Chicago, Illinois 60637*

In our studies of lectin-binding polypeptides in the developing human central nervous system (CNS), we used immunoblots containing electrophoresed polypeptides from homogenates of CNS tissues from individuals of various ages. Through these studies we identified a 120-kd peanut agglutinin (PNA) binding polypeptide (120 kdpp), which is in greater concentration in white than gray matter (FIG. 1). It is present among electrophoresed polypeptides from human CNS myelin as isolated by the method of Norton and Poduslo,[1] and it appears to be the only PNA-binding polypeptide in CNS myelin. It is not in peripheral nervous system myelin or in the peripheral nervous system in general as judged by PNA binding to immunoblots.

Most of this polypeptide appears to be bound to membranes and can be released from the membranes with phosphatidylinositol (PI)-specific phospholipase C (PLC) but not with phosphatidylcholine-specific PLC. The enzymatically released polypeptide has the molecular weight of 105 kd. Hence the 120 kdpp is probably linked to membranes through a PI linkage as is Thy-1, acetylcholinesterase, the 120-kd form of the neuronal cell adhesion molecule and several other proteins.[2] To our knowledge this makes the 120 kdpp the first myelin protein known to be linked to membranes in this manner.

To isolate 120 kdpp, we used as the first step the release of the polypeptide from membranes with PI-specific PLC followed by two runs over a PNA-affinity column. The eluate from the second run over the affinity column contained the 120 kdpp in a pure form, as evaluated both on silver-stained polyacrylamide gels and from sequence analysis on a gas-phase sequenator (see below).

The isolated 105 kdpp was subjected to enzymatic treatment to assess its carbohydrate composition. Neuraminidase cleavage of sialic acids resulted in a 95-kd polypeptide and treatment, with endoglycosidase H or endoglycosidase F yielded polypeptides of 90 or 80 kd, respectively. Endoglycosidase H cleaves only high-mannose N-linked glycans,[3] and endoglycosidase F cleaves both high-mannose and complex N-linked glycans.[4] The PNA binding to the 120 kdpp was unaffected by treatment with these three enzymes, which suggested the presence of an O-linked carbohydrate. When cleavage with endoglycosidase F was followed by incubation with neuraminidase and finally with O-glycanase, a 75-kd polypeptide was obtained that did not bind PNA. Using a gas-phase sequenator we determined the N-terminal 28 amino acid residues of 120 kdpp as follows (uncertain identifications are given in parentheses):

I-C-P-L-Q--(H)-I-(H)-T-E--R-H-R-H-V--D-C-S-G-R--D-L-S-T-(L)--P-P-G
　　　　5　　　　　　10　　　　　15　　　　　20　　　　　25

We used affinity-purified polyclonal antibodies from antiserum raised in Lewis rats against the 120 kdpp for immunohistochemical staining and on immunoblots. On immunoblots containing polypeptides from adult human CNS, these antibodies bind only to the 120 kdpp. The immunohistochemical staining obtained is not very clean when these antibodies are applied to adult human autopsy tissues (FIG. 2A and B). However, the myelin sheaths are the only structures that obviously stain, and at higher magnification it appears that the mesaxons stain, but the compact myelin does not.

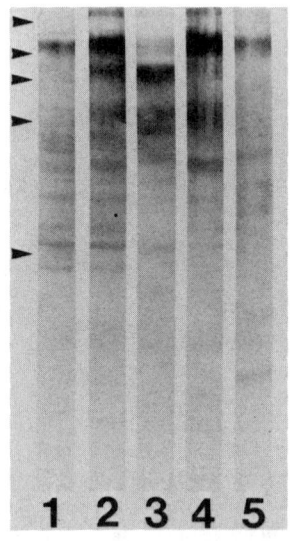

FIGURE 1. Peanut agglutinin staining to electrophoresed CNS tissue fractions. Equal amounts of total protein from (1) crude gray matter, (2) crude white matter, (3) the 100,000 × g supernatant, or (4) the 100,000 × g pellet of white matter, and (5) isolated myelin were separated on 10% Laemmli gel.[5] The 120 kdpp is present in greater amount in white matter than in gray matter and in greater amount in white matter pellet than in myelin.

We looked for the 120 kdpp in ovine oligodendrocytes after we had demonstrated the polypeptide in ovine myelin. We used cultures of ovine oligodendrocytes that are over 98% pure. Immunofluorescent staining using the aforementioned affinity-purified antibodies showed that the 120 kdpp is on the surface of the oligodendrocytes (FIG. 2C). Immunoblots containing polypeptides from the oligodendrocytes showed that the antibodies only bound to polypeptides of molecular weights corresponding to the 120 kdpp and that expression of the 120 kdpp increased with increasing time in culture (FIG. 2D). In addition, the 105 kdpp could be extracted from the culture supernatants by PNA affinity chromatography, suggesting endogenous phospholipase activity. Hence, we have isolated and characterized somewhat a novel glycoprotein that is found in both isolated oligodendrocytes and CNS myelin. It is not present in peripheral nervous system myelin. This protein is the only PNA-binding glycoprotein in CNS myelin.

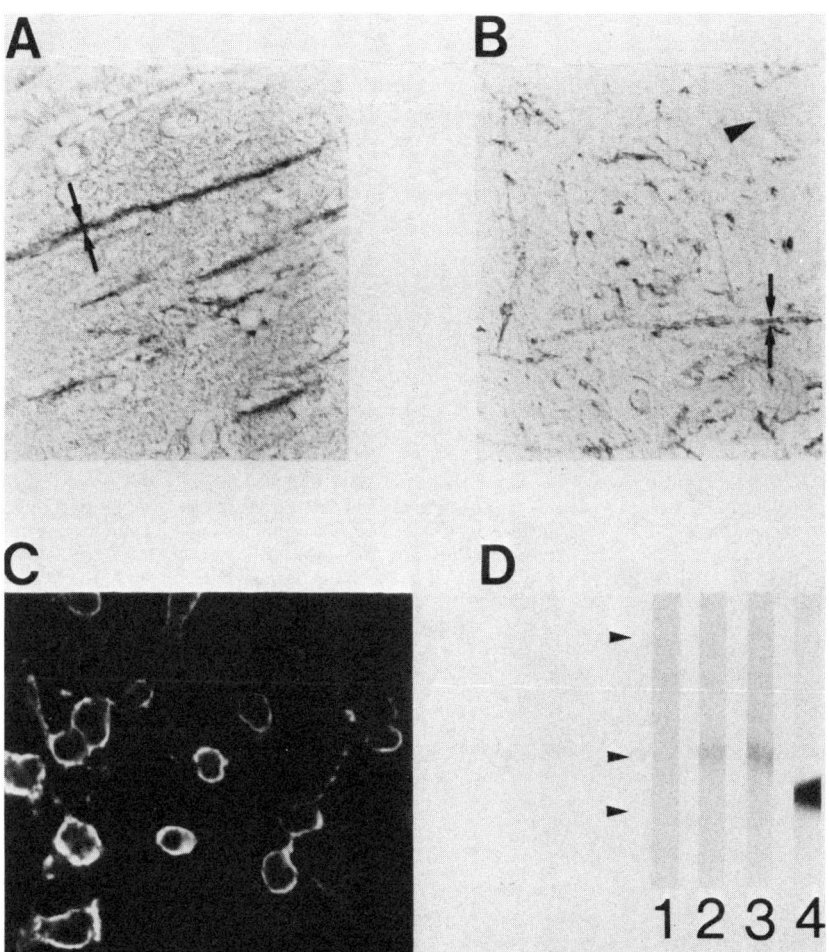

**FIGURE 2.** Localization of 120 kdpp using polyclonal antibodies. (**A** and **B**) PAP staining of formalin-fixed paraffin-embedded sections of the human spinal cord with polyclonal rat antisera (1:50) against 120 kdpp as visualized using Nomarski optics. Myelin sheaths are intensely stained (*arrows* in **A** and **B**), whereas a neuron (*arrowhead* in **B**) is unstained. (**C**) Immunofluorescent staining of an ovine oligodendrocyte culture after 2 weeks' attachment with antibodies specific to the 120 kdpp. (**D**) After varying times in culture (5, 25, and 75 days; *lanes 1 through 3*), cells were washed, and the same amount of protein was added per lane for immunoblotting on a 7.5% Laemmli gel. The supernatant from the cells in C was collected, clarified by centrifugation, and the 105 kdpp extracted by PNA affinity chromatography (*lane 4*). Hence, expression of 120 kdpp increases with increasing time in culture, and the 105 kdpp can be harvested from the supernatants.

## SUMMARY

We isolated and characterized a 120-kd PNA-binding polypeptide from the human CNS. This polypeptide is linked to membranes through a PI linkage. After release from membranes by PLC it measures 105 kd, 30 kd of which appear to be contributed by N-linked carbohydrates. We isolated the polypeptide by the use of PLC and PNA affinity chromatography and used it to raise polyclonal antibodies and to determine the N-terminal sequence. Immunohistochemical and immunochemical studies using these antibodies showed that 120 kdpp is present in both myelin and oligodendrocytes.

## REFERENCES

1. NORTON, W. T. & S. E. PODUSLO. 1973. Myelination in the rat brain: Method of myelin isolation. J. Neurochem. **21:** 749-757.
2. LOW, M. G. 1987. Biochemistry of the glycosylphosphatidylinositol membrane protein anchors. Biochem. J. **244:** 1-13.
3. TARENTINO, A. L. & F. MALEY. 1974. Purification and properties of an endo-$\beta$-N-acetylglucosaminidase from *Streptomyces griseus*. J. Biol. Chem. **249:** 811-817.
4. ELDER, J.H. & S. ALEXANDER. 1982. Endo-$\beta$-N-acetylglucosaminidase F: Endoglycosidase from *Flavobacterium meningosepticum* that cleaves both high-mannose and complex glycoproteins. Proc. Natl. Acad. Sci. USA **79:** 4540-4544.
5. LAEMMLI, U. D. 1970. Cleavage of structural proteins during the assembly of the head of bacteriophage T4. Nature (London) **227:** 680-685.

# Cells Proliferating *in Vitro* to Local Brain Injury Are Primarily of Hematic Origin and Differ from Those Associated with Anterograde Degeneration

## I. R. KATZ, L. IACOVITTI, AND D. J. REIS

*Division of Neurobiology*
*Cornell University Medical College*
*New York, New York 10021*

It has long been known that brain injury elicits local cellular proliferation. However, it is still uncertain whether the proliferating cells are of central neural or hematic origin.[1,2] In the past, uncertainties have arisen in part because of limitations inherent in *in vivo* methodology. In the present study, we developed an *in vitro* technique to establish: (a) the time course and magnitude of the local cellular proliferation in response to a lesion of the caudate nucleus (CN) produced by the excitotoxin ibotenic acid; (b) the phenotype of the responding cells; and (c) whether the character of the proliferating response (PR) in the damaged CN is comparable to cellular changes observed in the ipsilateral substantia nigra (SN), the site of termination of projections from a direct striatonigral pathway.

Ibotenic acid was stereotaxically injected in three sites (4 μg/0.4 μl) of one CN in anesthetized adult rats. Rats were decapitated between 1 and 60 days after the lesion. Controls either received vehicle injections or were unoperated. The tissues analyzed included the ipsilateral ($CN_I$) and contralateral CN ($CN_C$) and ipsilateral ($SN_I$) and contralateral SN ($SN_C$), and, as sites remote from the lesion, the hypothalamus and cerebral cortex. Tissue was dissected, dissociated, plated, and incubated in cultures for 3-4 days. At that time, $^3$H-thymidine incorporation (0.2 μCi, 6.7 Ci/mmol) was measured in four replicate cultures.

In cells from $CN_I$ (FIG. 1) there was a 2.4-fold increase in the PR by 1 day after the lesion. Interestingly, the PR also increased in the $CN_C$ cells. Peak PR was reached by day 9 after the lesion ($CN_I$: 1153%; $CN_C$: 214% of control). While the response declined, it remained significantly elevated through day 60. A PR was also seen in the $SN_I$ which peaked earlier (day 3) and lasted only for 2-3 weeks. Maximum response was 365% of control. No PR was seen in $SN_C$, hypothalamus, or cortex. To determine the phenotype of reacting cells, cultures were immunocytochemically labeled with monoclonal antibodies to cell surface markers of lymphocytes, monocytes, and macrophages (w3/25),[4] fibroblasts (Thy 1.1), and a polyclonal antibody to intermediate filaments of astrocytes (GFAP).[5] Proliferating cells in the $CN_I$ and $CN_C$ at peak consisted of 75% blood monocytes, macrophages, and T helper lymphocytes (w3/25-positive cells), the remainder being GFAP-positive astrocytes and Thy 1.1-

positive fibroblasts (TABLE 1). Preliminary autoradiographic and immunocytochemical double labeling experiments confirmed that most proliferating cells in CN belong to the w3/25 phenotype. To verify that a significant amount of the PR was indeed due to the presence of blood-borne lymphocytes and monocytes, we used a cytolytic antibody, 0X35 (IgG2a), that recognizes another determinant on the w3/25 molecule. In the presence of complement, 50% of cultured cells derived from both $CN_I$ and $CN_C$ were eliminated in a proliferative assay. In the $SN_I$ the phenotypic response was different in that at peak response only 30% of the proliferating cells were of hematic origin, the remainder being glia.

## SUMMARY

(a) The PR elicited by excitotoxic destruction of intrinsic neurons in the CN has a rapid onset, peaks within 2 weeks, and persists indefinitely; (b) the majority of the proliferating cells are not intrinsic to the CNS but are of hematic origin; (c) a small

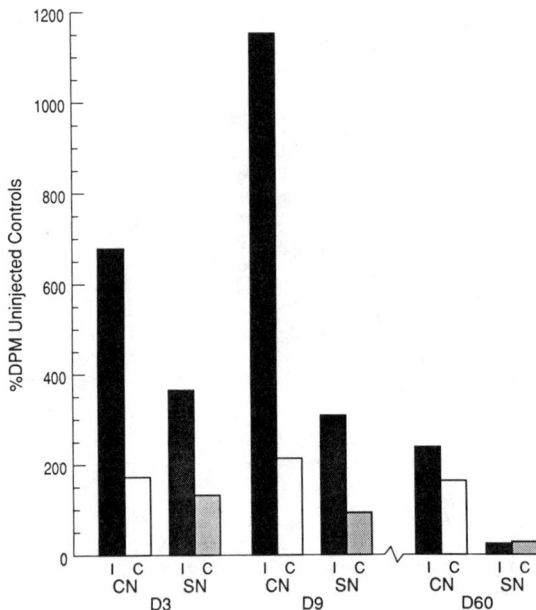

**FIGURE 1.** Proliferative responses at different times postlesion. Rats were killed at various days after ibotenic acid injections, and their brains were dissected and dissociated. $CN_I$ and $CN_C$ or $SN_I$ and $SN_C$-derived cells were plated and incubated in 3-4-day cultures. $^3$H-thymidine incorporation was measured in four replicate wells. The *in vitro* proliferating cells included about 70% adherent populations, consisting of glia and blood-derived monocytes-macrophages. The remainder consisted of cells in supernatant that were blood derived only (data not shown). Results are expressed as % DPM of uninjected controls ($n = 2$-5 experiments). DPM CN controls: 2,276 ± 459; DPM SN controls: 2,492 ± 767; $n = 2$-8 experiments.

TABLE 1. Proportion of Phenotypes in Culture Following Increased Survival Time after the Lesion[a]

| | Time after the Lesion | | | | | | | | |
|---|---|---|---|---|---|---|---|---|---|
| | Day −1 (% Total) | | | Day 9 (% Total) | | | Day 60 (% Total) | | |
| Cell Origin | w 3/25 | GF AP | Thy 1.1 | w 3/25 | GF AP | Thy 1.1 | w 3/25 | FG AP | Thy 1.1 |
| Uninjected CN | 5 | 15 | 80 | ... | ... | ... | ... | ... | ... |
| Ibotenic-acid-lesioned CN | ... | ... | ... | 70 | 15 | 15 | 40 | 30 | 30 |
| Contralateral CN | ... | ... | ... | 50 | 25 | 25 | 35 | 25 | 40 |
| Sham-lesioned CN[b] | ... | ... | ... | 30 | 15 | 55 | ... | ... | ... |
| Sham-contralateral CN[b] | ... | ... | ... | 20 | 15 | 65 | ... | ... | ... |

[a] Each injection day represents an average of 3-5 experiments. Cells were cultured for 6-9 days after injection.

[a] Sham-operated rats were injected with 0.4 μl of 0.1 M phosphate buffer into three sites of one caudate nucleus (CN).

NOTE: In the ipsilateral SN, at peak time after the lesion (day 3), 70% of proliferating cells were Thy 1.1$^+$ fibroblasts or GFAP$^+$ astrocytes and only 30% belonged to the w3/25 blood-borne phenotype.

mirror-image response is seen in the contralateral CN; (d) the proliferating response in anterogradely degenerating terminals in SN differs in time course, magnitude, and phenotypically from that initiated by direct neuronal loss. We conclude that the majority of proliferating cells at the site of selective neuronal injury in brain are of hematic origin in contrast to that initiated during anterograde degeneration, which consists primarily of intrinsic cells of brain (glia).

## REFERENCES

1. KONIGSMARK, B. W. & R. L. SIDMAN. 1963. Origin of brain macrophages in the mouse. J. Neuropathol. Exp. Neurol. **22:** 643-676.
2. CAVANAGH, J. B. 1970. The proliferation of astrocytes around a needle wound in the rat brain. J. Anat. **106:** 471-487.
3. SAJI, M. & D. J. REIS. 1987. Delayed transneuronal death of substantia nigra neurons prevented by gamma-aminobutyric acid agonist. Science **235:** 66-69.
4. JEFFERIES, W. A., J. R. GREEN & A. F. WILLIAMS. 1985. Authentic T helper CD4 (w3/25) antigen on rat peritoneal macrophages. J. Exp. Med. **162:** 117-127.
5. BIGNAMI, A. & D. DAHL. 1974. Astrocyte-specific protein and neuroglial differentiation. An immunofluorescence study with antibodies to the glial fibrillary acidic protein. J. Comp. Neurol. **153:** 27-38.

WORKSHOP 6. GLIA-NEURON INTERACTIONS

# Interactions of Astroglia-Derived Factors with Hippocampal Neurons[a]

### H. P. MATTHIESSEN, C. SCHMALENBACH, AND H. W. MÜLLER

*Molecular Neurobiology Laboratory*
*Department of Neurology*
*University of Düsseldorf*
*Düsseldorf, FRG*

Serum-free conditioned media (CM) from highly enriched cultures of neonatal cerebral astrocytes (less than 5% nonglial cells) contain neurite-promoting activity (NPA, percentage of viable cells bearing processes >2 cell diameters) when tested in a quantitative cell culture bioassay using neurons from embryonic (E18) rat hippocampus.

Conditioned media of various neural and nonneural cell lines also show this neurite-promoting activity, and it has been suggested that laminin (LN) or a complex of LN with some heparan sulfate proteoglycan or both are the almost exclusive components in CM with NPA.[1,2] Recently, part of the NPA produced by primary astroglial cultures was identified as immunoreactive for LN.[3] In addition, it was shown that astrocytes in culture synthesize and secrete fibronectin (FN).[4] We are presenting evidence that in CM produced in serum-free primary culture of neonatal astroglia from rat cerebrum, both FN and LN are neurite-growth-promoting components for hippocampal neurons from embryonic rats.

Astroglial CM, which was concentrated by ultrafiltration on YM 10 membranes (Amicon) in the presence of protease inhibitors, dialyzed, and lyophilized (retentate >10 kd) showed an NPA (7-12 µg of protein gave half-maximal neuritic growth) that was 1-2 orders of magnitude less than that of purified extracellular matrix proteins LN and FN. Conditioned media contain immunoreactivity for LN (predominantly the β-chain) and FN as shown by Western blotting of SDS-PAGE gels on nitrocellulose and by ELISA. The FN concentration (1.1 ± 0.3 µg/ml) in fresh CM reached 15-fold the amount of LN (0.07 ± 0.02 µg/ml) and it increased while astrocytes were in culture. Expression of LN and FN by cultured astrocytes could also be shown by immunofluorescence microscopy. FPLC separation of astroglial CM by gel filtration on Superose 6 (optimal fractionation range 5-5000 kd) recovered most of the biologic activity in fractions containing either LN or FN or both (FIG. 1). This was also true for the void volume (40,000 kd) of the column. By anion exchange chromatography, two main peaks of activity could be distinguished (FIG. 2). Most of the activity was eluted at 800-1000 mM NaCl and correlated with the highest peak of anti-LN immunoreactivity. This peak possibly consists of a complex of LN with a highly negatively charged heparan sulfate proteoglycan. This possibility is supported by gel filtration

---

[a] This work was supported in part by the Deutsche Forschungsgemeinschaft (Mu 630/3-1) and Bayer AG (Wuppertal). C. Schmalenbach is the recipient of a fellowship from BMFT.

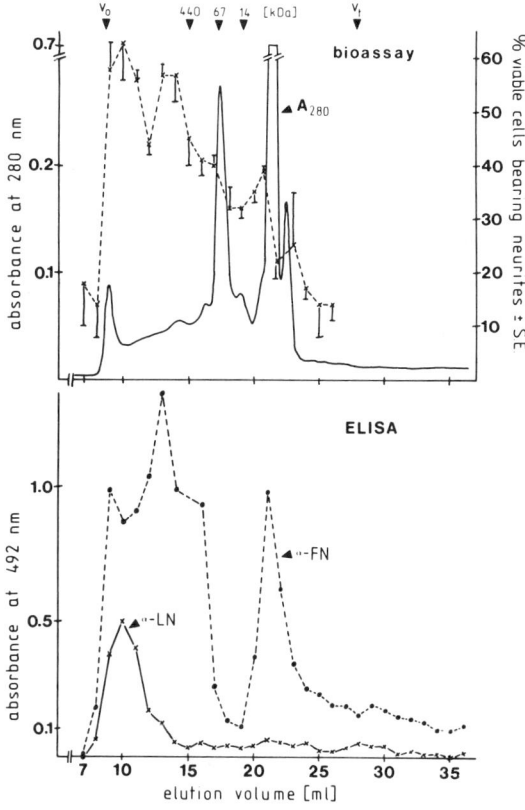

**FIGURE 1.** Separation of astroglial conditioned media (CM) by gel filtration on Superose 6 (FPLC). Separation of 4.2 mg of astroglial conditioned medium (ACM) in 200 $\mu$l of 50 mM Tris/HCL-buffer (pH 7.4, 100 mM NaCl) was achieved by gel filtration on Superose 6 (Pharmacia, FPLC) with the same buffer as eluent. Protein concentration was determined with Coomassie Blue G-250 according to Bradford. The laminin (LN) and fibronectin (FN) concentration was measured by ELISA: 40 $\mu$l of the fractions were bound to flat bottom microtiter plates in carbonate buffer of pH 9.6 at 4°C overnight. Unspecific binding was reduced by blocking plastic sites with 1% BSA in carbonate buffer of pH 9.6. Anti-mouse LN (rabbit, Bethesda Research Laboratories) and anti-human FN (rabbit, Collaborative Research) were diluted 1:1000 in PBS (0.05% Tween 20, 1% BSA) and filled into the microplate for 30 minutes at 37°C. The washed plates were incubated with peroxidase-conjugated anti-rabbit IgG (goat, Cappel), diluted 1:1000 in PBS-Tween (4% BSA) for 15 minutes at 37°C. As substrate, we used a solution of 50 mg of o-phenylene-diamine in 100 ml of 25 mM citric acid and 50 mM of hydrogenphosphate containing 0.05% $H_2O_2$. The enzymatic reaction was stopped with 2 M $H_2SO_4$, and the absorption at 492 nm was measured. For determination of the neurite-promoting activity (NPA; 1 U is defined as that amount of CM in micrograms of protein that induces half-maximal neuritic growth), glass coverslips precoated with poly-L-lysine (0.1 mg/ml) were incubated with 500 $\mu$l of column fractions overnight at 37°C. Then, $3 \times 10^4$ embryonal (E18) neurons from rat hippocampus were added to coverslips in serum-free hormone supplemented (5 $\mu$g/ml of insulin, 1 $\mu$/ml of transferrin, 20 nmol/l of hydrocortisone, 0.3 nmol/l of triiodothyronine) N2 medium. After 18 hours of incubation at 37°C and 10% $CO_2$, the number of viable cells bearing neurites greater than 2 cell diameters was determined.

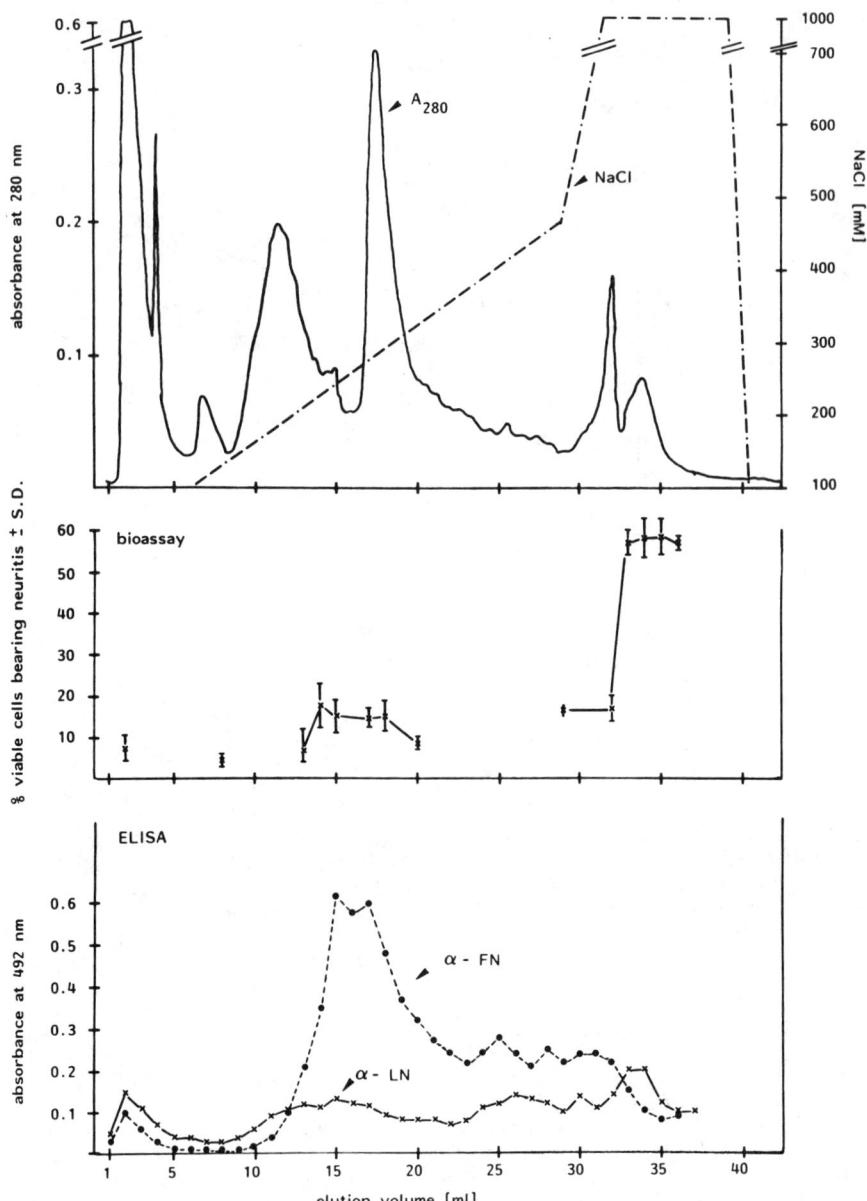

**FIGURE 2.** Separation of astroglial CM by anion exchange chromatography on Mono Q (FPLC). Separation of 5.2 mg of astroglial conditioned medium in 500 μl of 50 mM Tris/HCl buffer (pH 7.4, 100 mM NaCl) was achieved by anion exchange chromatography on Mono Q (Pharmacia, FPLC). The bound material was eluted with a linear gradient ranging from 100-1,000 mM NaCl in the buffer described. Laminin and fibronectin concentrations and the neurite-promoting activity were determined as described in the legend for Figure 1.

of these fractions on Superose 6 which resulted in immunoreactivity for LN in the void volume and by separation of $^{35}$S-sulfate-labeled astroglial CM components on this column which gave a peak of $\beta$-activity in the same column fractions. A smaller peak of NPA was eluted at 200-300 mM NaCl which corresponded to the peak fractions of anti-FN immunoreactivity for free FN as shown by ELISA and Western blotting. These fractions also contained small amounts of free LN ($\frac{1}{20}$ compared to FN). By comparison with a dose response curve of pure mouse LN in the bioassay, however, the concentration of free LN in these fractions was too low to account for the observed NPA. We conclude that NPA in astroglial CM is associated with both LN, possibly bound in a heparan sulfate proteoglycan complex, and FN.

## REFERENCES

1. LANDER, A. D., D. K. FUJII & L. F. REICHARDT. 1985. Proc. Natl. Acad. Sci. USA **82**: 2183.
2. DAVIS, G. E., M. MANTHORPE, E. ENGVALL & S. VARON. 1985. J. Neurosci. **5**: 2662.
3. BECKH, S., H. W. MÜLLER & W. SEIFERT. 1987. In Glial-Neuronal Communication in Development and Regeneration. H. H. Althaus & W. Seifert, Eds. NATO ASI Series H: Cell Biology, Vol. 2:385. Springer Verlag, Heidelberg.
4. PRICE, J. & O. HYNES. 1985. J. Neuroscience **5**: 2205.

# Changes in Astrocyte Extracellular Matrix with Differentiation and after Contact with Neurites[a]

## MARCH D. ARD[b] AND RICHARD P. BUNGE

*Department of Anatomy and Neurobiology*
*Washington University School of Medicine*
*St. Louis, Missouri 63110*

The state of differentiation of astrocytes may be a key determinant of their capacity to participate in cell-cell interactions. Specifically, mature astrocytes may be less able than immature astrocytes to support axonal growth. We wished to test whether changes in extracellular matrix production were related to changes in neurite-astrocyte interactions, because extracellular matrix is known to promote the growth of some types of neurites[1] and astrocytes have been shown to produce extracellular matrix.[2,3] To test this hypothesis in tissue culture, we used the method of McCarthy and de Vellis[4] to prepare neonatal rat cortical astrocytes. Differentiation of the cells in culture, as *in vivo*, is marked by reduced proliferative activity as well as stellate morphologic development. Immunocytochemical labeling with antiserum to glial fibrillary acidic protein identified the cells as astrocytes[5] and demonstrated their morphologic characteristics.

We found that the presence of extracellular matrix on the astrocyte surface correlated with an immature stage of differentiation in which the astrocytes were flat in shape and rapidly growing. In short-term (5 days to 2 weeks) cultures grown in serum-containing medium, light microscopic immunostaining of living cells showed both laminin and heparan sulfate proteoglycan (HSPG) immunoreactivity in a patchy, fibrillar pattern. A loosely organized and patchy extracellular matrix was visible also by electron microscopy (FIG. 1).

In contrast, extracellular matrix was much reduced in conditions in which differentiated astrocytes exhibited a stellate morphology and slower population growth. Differentiation occurred in short-term cultures in defined medium and in long-term (4-6 weeks) cultures in serum-containing medium. Both light microscopic immunostaining of living cultures and electron microscopy demonstrated this pattern of extracellular matrix expression.

Neurites from co-cultured rat dorsal root ganglion were grown on astrocyte monolayers. Immunostaining for HSPG and laminin was greatly reduced wherever neurites contacted astrocytes. Nevertheless, neurites contacted and extended on astrocyte sur-

---

[a] This work was supported by NIH Grant NS09923; M. D. Ard is a fellow of the National Multiple Sclerosis Society.

[b] Current address: Department of Anatomy, University of Mississippi Medical Center, Jackson, Mississippi 39216.

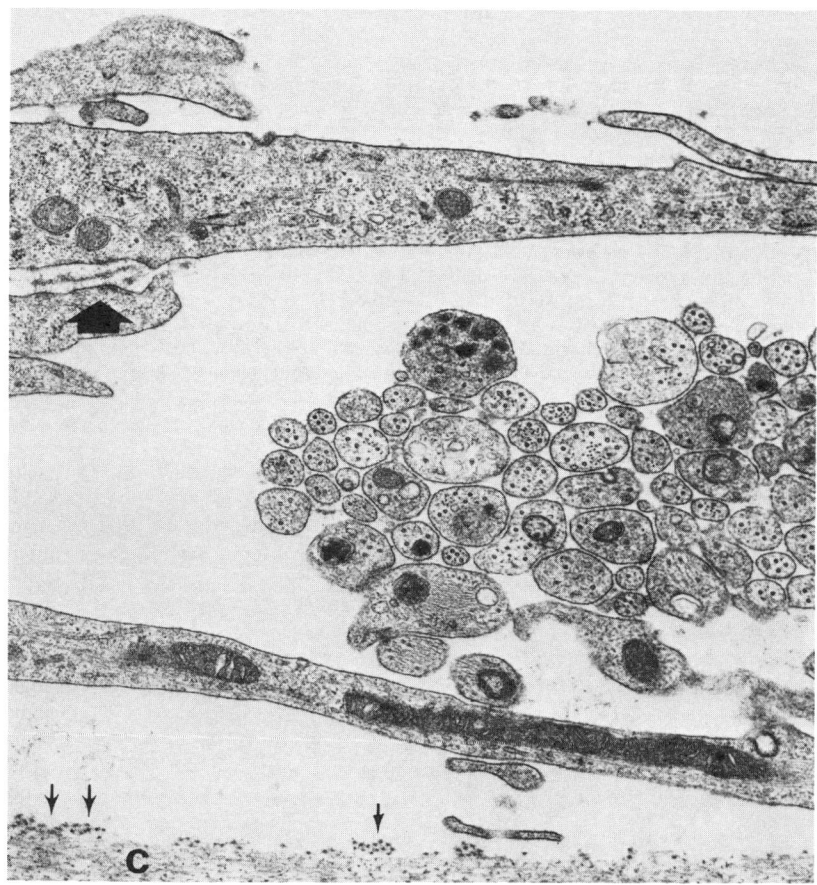

**FIGURE 1.** A bundle of dorsal root ganglion neurites, identifiable by their orderly arrays of cross-sectioned microtubules, is enclosed in the wide intercellular space between astrocyte processes. Occasional astrocyte processes, marked by an accumulation of glial filaments, travel with the bundle of neurites. Two forms of astrocytic extracellular matrix are present: a patch of basal lamina-like material (*thick arrow*) attached to membrane densities near the upper left of the electron micrograph, and small, dense granules (*thin arrows*) deposited on the collagen substratum (c) at the bottom of the field. The neurites are not in contact with either of these deposits. (Original magnification × 10,000.)

faces in preference to the collagen substratum in all conditions studied, regardless of the presence or absence of extracellular matrix or the level of morphologic differentiation of the astrocytes.

These observations indicate that production of extracellular matrix by astrocytes varies with their state of differentiation, and that the expression of HSPG and laminin on the astrocyte surface is not required for interaction with growing neurites of sensory ganglion cells. The present results are described in detail elsewhere.[6]

## REFERENCES

1. ARD, M. D., R. P. BUNGE & M. B. BUNGE. 1987. A comparison of the Schwann cell surface and Schwann cell extracellular matrix as promoters of neurite growth. J. Neurocytol. **16:** 539-555.
2. LIESI, P., D. DAHL & A. VAHERI. 1983. Laminin is produced by early rat astrocytes in primary culture. J. Cell Biol. **96:** 920-924.
3. LIESI, P., T. KIRKWOOD & A. VAHERI. 1986. Fibronectin is expressed by astrocytes cultured from embryonic and early postnatal rat brain. Exp. Cell Res. **163:** 175-185.
4. MCCARTHY, K. & J. DE VELLIS. 1980. Preparation of separate astroglial and oligodendroglial cell cultures from rat cerebral tissue. J. Cell Biol. **85:** 890-902.
5. BIGNAMI, A., L. F. ENG, D. DAHL & C. T. UYEDA. 1972. Localization of the glial fibrillary acidic protein in astrocytes by immunofluorescence. Brain Res. **43:** 429-435.
6. ARD, M. D. & R. P. BUNGE. 1988. Heparan sulfate proteoglycan and laminin immunoreactivity on cultured astrocytes: Relationship to differentiation and to neurite growth. J. Neurosci., in press.

# Antisera to an Axolemma-Enriched Fraction Have Antiaxon and Antimyelin Effects *in Vitro*[a]

DENNIS N. BOURDETTE,[b] FREDRICK J. SEIL,[b]
CHARLES K. MESHUL,[b] JOHN W. BIGBEE,[c] GEORGE
H. DeVRIES,[c] AND HARISH C. AGRAWAL[d]

[b]*Neurology Research*
*Veterans Administration Medical Center and Department of*
*Neurology*
*Oregon Health Sciences University*
*Portland, Oregon*

[c]*Department of Biochemistry*
*Medical College of Virginia*
*Richmond, Virginia*

[d]*Departments of Pediatrics and Neurology*
*Washington University School of Medicine*
*and*
*Division of Pediatric Research*
*St. Louis Children's Hospital*
*St. Louis, Missouri*

Antibodies to axons might be involved in the pathogenesis of some inflammatory and degenerative diseases of the nervous system. Antiaxon antibodies might be capable of destroying axons, preventing regeneration of damaged axons, and interfering with the interactions between axons and oligodendrocytes or Schwann cells needed for remyelination. To investigate the pathogenetic potential of antiaxon antibodies, we studied the effects of antisera to an axolemma-enriched fraction (AEF) on spinal cord-dorsal root ganglia (SC-DRG) explant cultures.

Antisera were prepared by immunization of rabbits with rat brain AEF.[1,2] The antisera to AEF contained antibodies that bound several axolemmal proteins and immunohistochemically stained nodal and internodal axolemma in the peripheral nervous system.[1] To test for antiaxon and antimyelin effects, the antisera were applied to SC-DRG explant cultures prepared from 14-day fetal Swiss-Webster mice by established procedures.[3] The antisera were tested for their ability to prevent axonal development and myelination by growing the SC-DRG for 15-18 days in medium containing test sera. The antisera were tested for their ability to destroy mature axons and cause demyelination by applying test sera to SC-DRG cultures after 18 days of

---

[a]This work was supported by the Veterans Administration (D.N.B., F.J.S., and C.K.M.), NIH-NS 10821 and 15408 (G.H.D.), and NIH-NS 13464 and 19414 (H.C.A.).

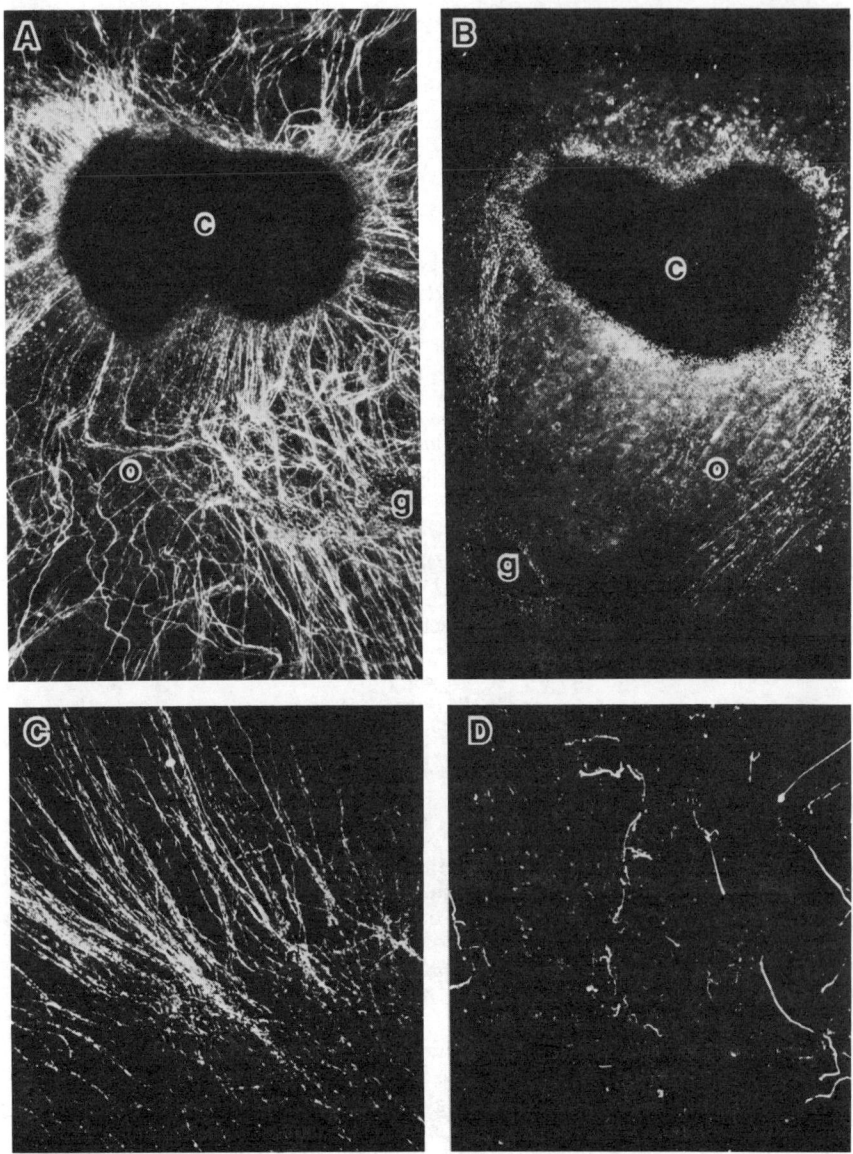

**FIGURE 1.** Silver-impregnated, whole-mount fixed cultures were photographed under darkfield conditions. (**A**) Normal spinal cord (SC) (c) and dorsal root ganglia (DRG) (g) explants after 18 days *in vitro* (DIV). The outgrowth (o) zone contains a large number of axons. (**B**) SC (c) and DRG (g) explants (18 DIV) after exposure to an antiserum to axolemma-enriched fraction (AEF) for 14 days, revealing few axons in the outgrowth (o) region. (**C**) Normal axons in the outgrowth zone of a culture grown for 22 days in normal medium. (**D**) Outgrowth zone in a culture (22 DIV) grown in normal medium for 18 days and then exposed to an antiserum to AEF for 4 days before fixation. No normal axons remain, and there are several fragments of axons.

growth in normal medium. Inhibition of axonal outgrowth and myelination inhibiting and demyelinating activities were determined as previously described.[2,4] Controls consisted of cultures maintained in normal medium and cultures exposed to preimmune sera and to a rabbit antiserum to the chloroform-methanol insoluble protein (CMIP) fraction of myelin.[4]

All four antisera to AEF profoundly inhibited axonal outgrowth from the SC and DRG explants, but they did not affect axons within the SC explants (FIG. 1). All four antisera were capable of destroying mature axons in the outgrowth zone, but they did not destroy axons restricted to the SC explants (FIG. 1). Dorsal root ganglia and ventral horn neurons exposed to the antisera had light and electron microscopic changes consistent with a severe axotomy reaction. Three of four antisera inhibited

TABLE 1. Antimyelin Effects of Antisera to Axolemma-Enriched Fraction (AEF)[a]

|  | Cultures Myelinated (fraction) | Myelination Inhibition | Cultures Demyelinated (fraction) | Demyelination |
|---|---|---|---|---|
| Preimmune sera |  |  |  |  |
| 1 | 5/6 | — | 0/8 | — |
| 2 | 5/7 | — | 0/6 | — |
| 3 | 5/7 | — | 0/6 | — |
| 4 | 6/6 | — | 0/8 | — |
| 5 | 6/6 | — | 0/8 | — |
| Antiserum to CMIP[b] |  |  |  |  |
|  | 2/7 | + | 5/7 | + |
| Antisera to AEF |  |  |  |  |
| 001[c] | 0/5 | + | 0/8 | — |
| 002[c] | 0/6 | + | 0/8 | — |
| T[c] | 0/8 | + | 0/6 | — |
| G | 7/8 | — | 0/7 | — |

[a] Sera were tested for myelination inhibition and demyelination activities as previously described.[4]

[b] The antiserum to chloroform-methanol insoluble protein (CMIP) served as a positive control and had antimyelin activity as previously described.[4]

[c] Reacted with galactocerebroside using an enzyme-linked immunosorbent assay.

myelination, but none of the antisera to AEF caused central demyelination (TABLE 1). The three antisera that caused myelination inhibition contained antibodies to galactocerebroside, whereas the antiserum that did not cause myelination inhibition did not react with galactocerebroside. The preimmune sera did not have antiaxon or antimyelin activity. The antiserum to CMIP did not have antiaxon activity, but it did have both myelination inhibiting and demyelinating activities.

Antisera to AEF destroy axons and inhibit axonal outgrowth *in vitro,* and some antisera inhibit myelination. The axonal antigens responsible for the antiaxon activity of these antisera are not known. The myelination-inhibiting activity of antisera to AEF may be mediated by antibodies to galactocerebroside. These studies on the antiaxon and antimyelin effects of antisera to AEF provide an impetus for investigating the role of autoimmune reactions to axolemma in inflammatory and neurodegenerative diseases in humans.

## REFERENCES

1. BIGBEE, J. W., V. P. CALABRESE & G. W. DEVRIES. 1985. J. Neuroimmunol. **7:** 221-229.
2. BOURDETTE, D. N., F. J. SEIL, J. W. BIGBEE, G. H. DEVRIES, M. M. GARWOOD, & H. C. AGRAWAL. 1986. Brain Res. **366:** 333-337.
3. PETERSON, E. R., S. M. CRAIN & M. R. MURRAY. 1965. Z. Zellforsch. **66:** 130-154.
4. SEIL, F. J., M. M. GARWOOD, H. B. CLARK & H. C. AGRAWAL. 1983. Brain Res. **288:** 384-388.

# Substance P Stimulates Release of Arachidonic Acid Cyclooxygenation Products from Primary Culture Rat Astrocytes

HANS-PETER HARTUNG, KURT HEININGER,
BÄRBEL SCHÄFER, AND KLAUS V. TOYKA

*Department of Neurology*
*University of Düsseldorf*
*Düsseldorf, FRG*

There is growing evidence that the neuropeptide substance P (SP), through stimulation of leukocytes, is involved in inflammatory responses. The recent demonstration that SP specifically binds to and activates both T lymphocytes and macrophages further suggests a role of this undecapeptide in immunoregulation.[1-3] Astrocytes, which constitute key cellular components of immunoinflammatory responses within the central nervous system, express SP receptors on their surface.[4] We examined the possible effects of SP on arachidonic acid metabolism in astrocytes.

## METHODS

Astrocytes were prepared from neonatal Lewis rats.[5] Cells were used after 2-3 weeks when monolayers had grown confluent. Ninety-four percent were glial fibrillary acidic protein (GFAP) positive. Cultures were exposed to various concentrations of SP, the peptide fragments SP(1-4), SP(2-11), and SP(5-11), or medium (Dulbecco's minimal essential medium [DMEM] containing 5% fetal calf serum) alone. Controls included incubates of astrocytes challenged with SP in the presence of the cyclooxygenase blocker indomethacin or the joint cyclooxygenase and lipoxygenase inhibitor BW755c. Astrocytes were cultured for up to 48 hours when supernatants were collected and stored until radioimmunoassay was performed for prostaglandin E (PGE), thromboxane $B_2$ ($TBX_2$), 6-keto-prostaglandin $F_1$, and leukotriene $C_4$.[2] Endotoxin contamination of reagents or culture media was excluded by the limulus amebocyte lysate assay.

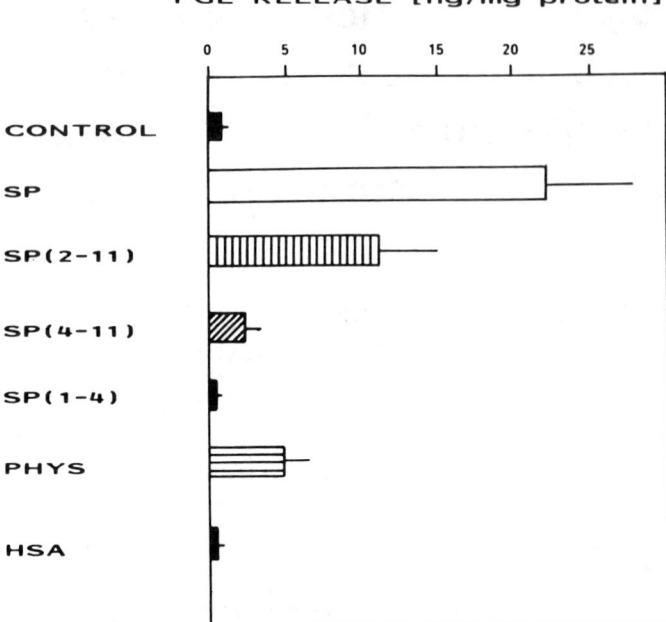

**FIGURE 1.** Dose-related stimulation of prostaglandin E (PGE) release from astrocytes. Primary culture rat astrocytes were challenged with indicated concentrations of substance P (SP), SP fragments, or the tachykinin physalaemin (PHYS), or were incubated in medium alone. Culture supernates were collected after 48 hours and examined for release of PGE by radioimmunoassay. Results are related to protein content of culture dishes.

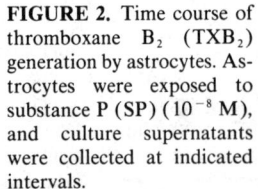
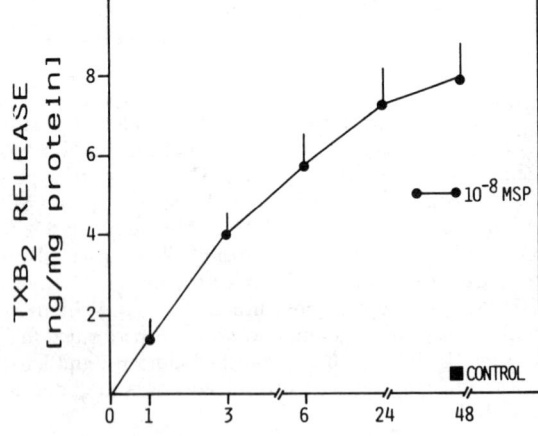

**FIGURE 2.** Time course of thromboxane $B_2$ ($TXB_2$) generation by astrocytes. Astrocytes were exposed to substance P (SP) ($10^{-8}$ M), and culture supernatants were collected at indicated intervals.

## RESULTS AND DISCUSSION

Substance P at nano- to micromolar concentrations evoked a noncytotoxic release of PGE and $TXB_2$ in a dose-dependent manner (FIG. 1). Kinetic studies indicated that release was maximal within 6 hours of adding SP (FIG. 2). To study the peptide structural requirements for this novel action of SP, cultures were exposed to the N-terminal tetrapeptide SP(1-4) or the carboxyterminals SP(2-11) and SP(5-11). As shown in FIGURE 1, the stimulatory properties reside in its carboxyterminal sequence. The addition of indomethacin or BW755c (both at $10^{-6}$ M concentrations) abrogated prostanoid formation. We demonstrated that binding of SP to its receptor on cultured astrocytes induces the conversion of arachidonic acid into the cyclooxygenase products PGE and $TXB_2$. These prostanoids exert proinflammatory actions and can act on immunocompetent cells, leading to either up- or down-regulation of immune responses. In view of the role attributed to astrocytes in the initiation of immune responses within the CNS, their release of arachidonic acid cyclooxygenation products may be important in the pathogenesis of immunoinflammatory diseases affecting the brain.

### REFERENCES

1. McGILLIS, D. G., M. L. ORGANIST & D. G. PAYAN. 1987. Substance P and immunoregulation. Fed. Proc. **46:** 196.
2. HARTUNG, H. P., K. WOLTERS & K. V. TOYKA. 1986. Substance P: Binding properties and studies on cellular responses in guinea pig macrophages. J. Immunol. **136:** 3856.
3. HARTUNG, H. P. & K. V. TOYKA. 1988. Substance P, the immune system and inflammation. Int. Rev. Immunol. in press.
4. TORRENS Y., J. C. BEAUJOUAN, M. SAFFROY, M. C. DAQUET DE MONTETY, L. BERGSTRÖM & J. GLOWINSKI. 1986. Substance P receptors in primary cultures of cortical astrocytes from the mouse. Proc. Natl. Acad. Sci. USA **83:** 9216.
5. FIERZ, W., B. ENDLER, K. RESKE, H. WEKERLE & A. FONTANA. 1985. Astrocytes as antigen-presenting cells. I. Induction of Ia antigen expression on astrocytes by T cells via immune interferon and its effects on antigen presentation. J. Immunol. **134:** 3785.

# Insulin-Like Growth Factor-I Stimulates Regeneration of Oligodendrocytes *in Vitro*[a]

ROBIN L. MOZELL AND F. ARTHUR McMORRIS

*The Wistar Institute of Anatomy and Biology*
*Philadelphia, Pennsylvania 19104*

Insulin-like growth factor-I (IGF-I) induces a 60-fold increase in the number of oligodendrocytes that appear in developing rat brain cell cultures.[1] Insulin-like growth factors are known to promote growth-related processes, such as protein and DNA synthesis, and cell proliferation, as well as to stimulate cell differentiation in many cell types.[2-4] Two IGFs have been described: IGF-I, also known as somatomedin-C, and IGF-II.

Because multiple sclerosis is an episodic disease whose primary target is myelin, it was of interest to investigate if IGF-I could stimulate oligodendrocyte development and remyelination after a demyelinating episode. Two different culture systems were used for this study: (1) a monolayer system established from dissociated cerebral hemispheres of 1-day-old rats,[1] and (2) an aggregate culture system initiated from dissociated brains of 16-day-old rat fetuses[5,6] (i.e., 6 days prenatal). We developed an *in vitro* complement-mediated cytotoxicity procedure, using antibody against galactocerebroside (GC), a surface marker for oligodendrocytes, in conjunction with rabbit complement (C') to specifically kill oligodendrocytes in the cultures. This procedure was performed when the cultures were approximately the same developmental age (13 days *in vitro* [DIV] for monolayer cultures, 20 DIV for aggregate cultures). After removal of complement and antibody and after at least a 24-hour recovery period, cultures were harvested for immunohistochemical analysis. Initially, the number of oligodendrocytes in cultures treated with antibody and C' was reduced 80% as compared with those in control cultures, whereas other cells in the cultures (astrocytes and neurons) appeared unaffected by the treatment. With time, the number of oligodendrocytes present in the cultures increased, with the greatest increase, as well as the fastest rate of recovery, being observed in monolayer cultures (FIGS. 1 and 2) and aggregate cultures (data not shown) supplemented with 100 ng/ml of IGF-I after antibody and complement treatment.

These data suggest the presence of an oligodendrocyte precursor (GC-negative cell) that is capable of reestablishing the oligodendrocyte population in these cultures after a complement-mediated cytotoxic event. These putative precursors are apparently stimulated by IGF-I to produce more oligodendrocytes. It remains to be determined if the increase in the number of oligodendrocytes is due to increased proliferation of the precursors, enhanced differentiation into oligodendrocytes, or both.

---

[a] This work was supported by National Multiple Sclerosis Society Grant #1767-A-1, NINCDS Grant #NS11036, and NSF Grant #BNS-8518023.

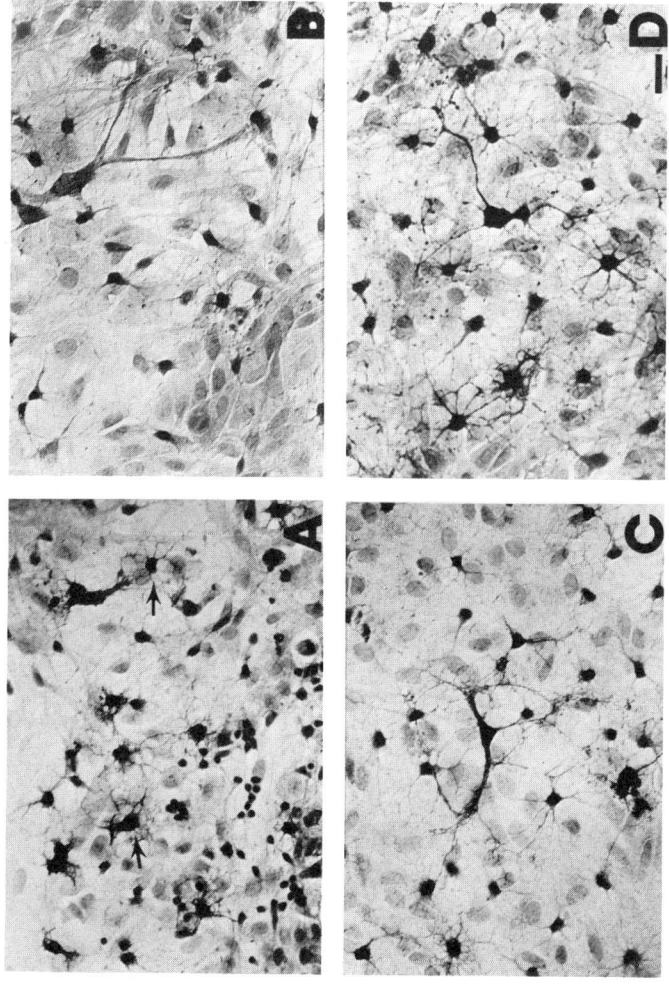

FIGURE 1. Reappearance of oligodendrocytes in monolayer culture after a 1-hour treatment with C′ and antibody against galactocerebroside (GC) at 13 days in vitro (DIV). Cells were stained by the avidin-biotin complex method using antibody against 2′3′ cyclic nucleotide 3′ phosphohydrolase (CNP) which is specific for oligodendrocytes. Arrows point to representative immunoperoxidase-stained oligodendrocytes, which are visible against a background of hematoxylin-stained nuclei of CNP-negative cells. (A) Untreated control culture 14 DIV. (B-D) Cultures treated with C′ and anti-GC: (B) 14 DIV; (C) 22 DIV; (D) 22 DIV, supplemented with 100 ng/ml of IGF-I starting at 13 DIV. Bar represents 20 μm.

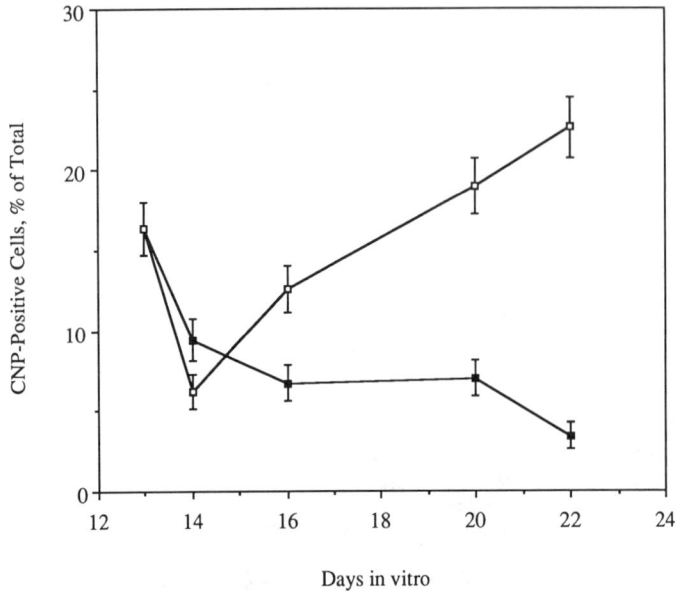

**FIGURE 2.** Effect of insulin-like growth factor-I (IGF-I) on the number of oligodendrocytes in monolayer cultures at various time points after a 1-hour treatment with C' and antibody against galactocerebroside at 13 days *in vitro*. The number of oligodendrocytes (CNP-positive cells, expressed as percentage of total cell number ± SEM) was determined at the time points indicated. For each point, at least 500 cells were scored. *Closed squares:* cultures not given IGF-I after C' and antibody treatment. *Open squares:* cultures supplemented with 100 ng/ml of IGF-I after treatment.

The complement-mediated cytotoxicity procedure using the aggregate culture system provides a useful means to study factors affecting the regeneration of oligodendrocytes and remyelination *in vitro*. Results using this technique clearly show that IGF-I plays an important role in the regeneration of oligodendrocytes after experimental demyelination.

## REFERENCES

1. McMorris, F. A., T. M. Smith, S. DeSalvo, & R. Furlanetto. 1986. Proc. Natl. Acad. Sci. USA **83:** 822-826.
2. Froesch, E. R., C. Schmid, J. Schwander & J. Zapf. 1985. Ann. Rev. Physiol. **47:** 443-467.
3. Phillips, L. S. & R. Vassilopoulou-Sellin. 1980. N. Engl. J. Med. **302:** 371-380.
4. Phillips, L. S. & R. Vassilopoulou-Sellin. 1980. N. Engl. J. Med. **302:** 438-446.
5. Matthieu, J.-M., P. Honegger, P. Favrod, E. Gautier, & M. Dolivo. 1979. J. Neurochem. **32:** 869-881.
6. Matthieu, J.-M., P. Honegger, B. D. Trapp, S. R. Cohen, & H. deF. Webster, 1978. Neuroscience **3:** 565-572.

# Intracellular Messengers

## Influence of Oligodendrocyte Substratum Adhesion[a]

TIMOTHY VARTANIAN, GLYN DAWSON, AND
SARA SZUCHET

*Departments of Biochemistry and Molecular
Biology, Pediatrics and Neurology
The University of Chicago and
The Brain Research Institute
Chicago, Illinois 60637*

Adhesion of oligodendrocytes (OLGs), isolated from ovine white matter, to a polylysine substratum induces the synthesis of myelin components[1,2] and ultimately results in the formation of membranous structures that resemble myelin morphologically and biochemically.[3] We have investigated the early events associated with OLG-substratum adhesion in order to define the nature of the signal(s) involved in myelinogenesis. In previous work we showed that subsequent to OLG-substratum attachment, two OLG/myelin proteins are phosphorylated: myelin basic protein (MBP) and 2', 3', cyclic nucleotide 3' phosphohydrolase (CNPase). The phosphorylation of both proteins could be stimulated by diacylglycerol (DAG) or tumor-promoting phorbol esters (TPA), indicating that protein kinase C (PKC) was the mediator. Activation of protein kinase A (PKA) with forskolin (an effector of adenylate cyclase) led to the inhibition and stimulation, respectively, of MBP[4,5] and CNPase phosphorylations, showing that MBP is a substrate for only PKC, whereas CNPase is a substrate for both PKC and PKA.

We studied the effect of OLG-substratum adhesion on the generation of the second messengers, DAG and cAMP. Isolated OLGs kept in suspension culture have 2 pmol/mg of protein of cAMP and show a two- to threefold increase when stimulated with either prostaglandin $E_1$ ($PGE_1$), forskolin, or vasoactive intestinal polypeptide (VIP), but they do not respond to isoproterenol (a $\beta$-adrenergic agonist). In contrast, parallel cultures allowed to attach for 24 hours have 4 pmol/mg of protein of cAMP and respond with a sixfold increase to $PGE_1$, forskolin, and isoproterenol, but not to VIP (Fig. 1A).

The generation of DAG, as assessed by 1-[$^{14}$C]-arachidonate incorporation and resolution of lipids by thin layer chromatography, was twofold elevated in attached than nonattached OLG (Fig. 1B).

Receptor-mediated generation of cAMP and DAG provides a mechanism of control of PKC and PKA and thus of the state of OLG/myelin protein phosphorylations.

---

[a]This work was supported by Grants RG-1223-D5 from the National Multiple Sclerosis Society and HD-04583 from the National Institutes of Health.

**FIGURE 1.** Positive and negative effectors of protein kinases in oligodendrocytes (OLGs). (**A**) Effect of OLG-substratum adhesion on the generation of cAMP. Unattached (*solid bars*) and 24-hour attached (*hatched bars*) OLG cultures were incubated for 30 minutes in the presence of isobutylmethylxanthine (a phosphodiesterase inhibitor) and the agonist indicated: control solution (HOH), forskolin ($1 \times 10^{-6}$M), prostaglandin $E_1$ ($PGE_1$) ($1 \times 10^{-6}$M), isoproterenol ($1 \times 10^{-6}$M), and vasoactive intestinal polypeptide (VIP) ($1 \times 10^{-6}$M). Reactions were terminated, cAMP was quantitated by radioimmunoassay, and results were normalized to protein content (by the method of Lowry). (**B**) Influence of OLG-substratum adhesion on 1-[$^{14}$C] arachidonate incorporation into DAG. Cultures of OLGs, differing only by 24 hours of attachment, were labeled with 2.5 μCi of 1-[$^{14}$C] arachidonic acid in serum-free Dulbecco's modified Eagle's medium (DMEM) for 60 minutes. Reactions were terminated by the addition of ice cold 10% trichloroacetic acid (TCA) and lipids extracted with acidified chloroform/methanol. DAG, resolved by high-performance thin-layer chromatography and identified by autoradiography, was quantitated by liquid scintillation spectrophotometry. Results are presented as the cpm normalized to protein (BioRad assay). OLG(F) = floating OLG; OLG(A) = attached OLG. (**C**) Effect of psychosine on myelin basic protein (MBP) phosphorylation in OLGs. Cultures of OLGs after 21 days of attachment were labeled with 100 μCi of $^{32}PO_4^{3-}$ in phosphate-free DMEM for 30 minutes in the presence (*lane 2*) or absence (*lane 1*) of 50 μM of psychosine. Reactions were terminated by the addition of ice cold 15% TCA, and MBP was immunoprecipitated with a polyclonal rabbit antibovine MBP serum (gift from Dr. A. T. Campagnoni) and resolved by 12% SDS-PAGE as previously described.[4] The autoradiograph of the dried gel is shown.

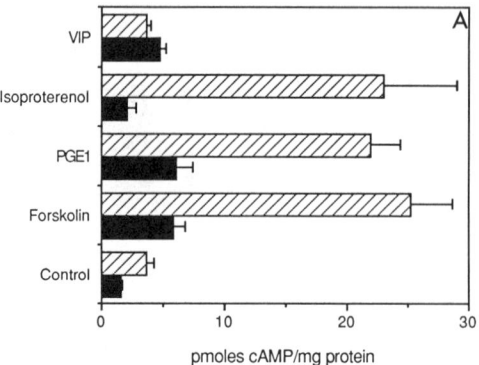

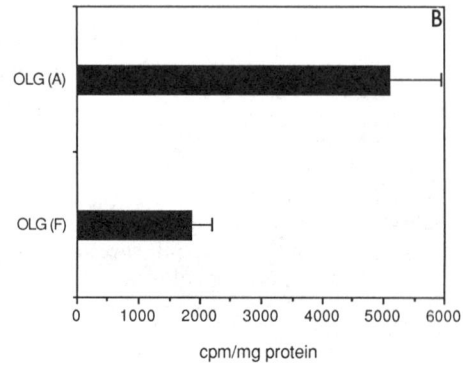

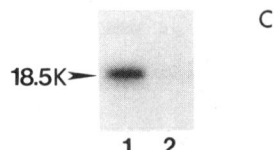

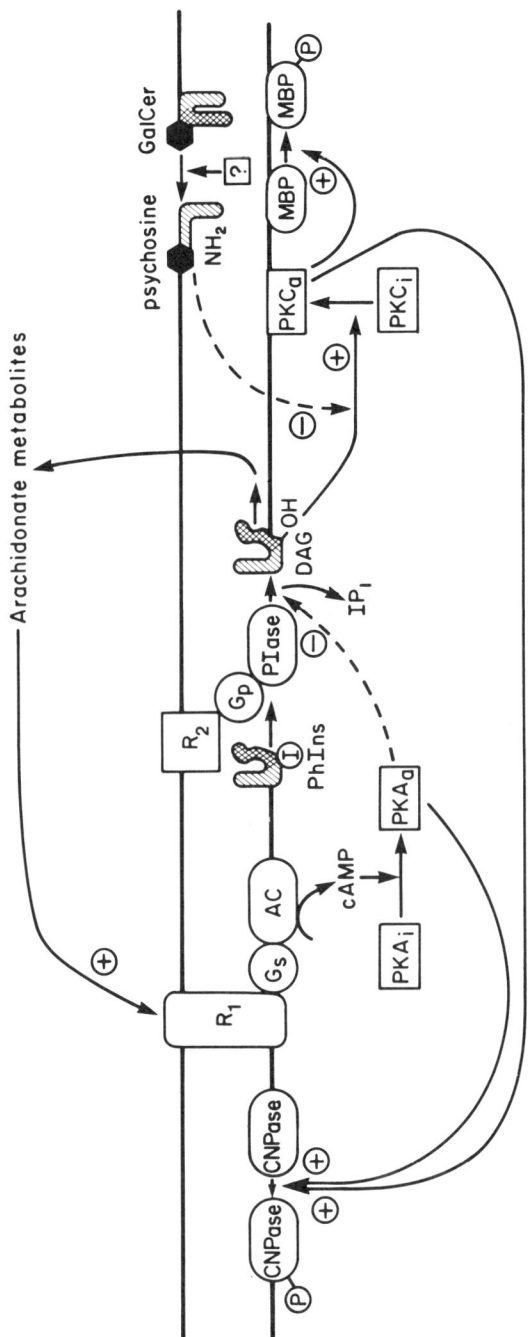

**FIGURE 2.** Schematic diagram of the events postulated to be occurring at the oligodendrocyte (OLG) plasma membrane following OLG adhesion to a polylysine substratum. Adenylate-cyclase-linked receptors ($R_1$) switch from vasoactive intestinal polypeptide (VIP) and prostaglandin $E_1$ ($PGE_1$) in floating OLG to a β-adrenergic receptor and $PGE_1$ in attached OLG. Attachment results in the generation of DAG from phosphatidylinositol, translocation of protein kinase C (PKC) from the cytosol to the membrane with its concurrent activation, and the phosphorylation of PKC substrates such as myelin basic protein (MBP) and CNPase. DAG is a source for arachidonate, the precursor of prostaglandins, thromboxanes, and leukotrienes. Production of cAMP and subsequent activation of protein kinase A (PKA) potentiates the phosphorylation of CNPase while inhibiting the phosphorylation of MBP. Cyclic AMP-mediated inhibition of MBP phosphorylation appears to result from diminished release of DAG. Inhibition of PKC can also be accomplished by the addition of exogenous psychosine, a lysosphingolipid, and this may occur *in situ* by N-deacylation of sphingolipids (abundant in OLG plasma membrane).

Another pathway that could yield metabolites to control PKC activity may be the N-deacylation of OLG glycosphingolipids. Psychosine was shown to be an inhibitor of PKC.[6] Accordingly, FIGURE 1C shows that psychosine causes an inhibition of MBP phosphorylation that is reversed by TPA. It is interesting that psychosine treatment of OLG cultures has a profound degenerative effect on OLG processes, implicating PKC in process extension and perhaps in myelinogenesis. FIGURE 2 presents a speculative model of our current views of the events that follow OLG attachment to a substratum. This model implicates DAG and cAMP in signaling myelinogenesis and proposes phosphorylation/dephosphorylation of MBP and CNPase as key events in this process.

## REFERENCES

1. SZUCHET, S., S. H. YIM & S. MONSMA. 1983. Proc. Natl. Acad. Sci. USA **80:** 7019-7023.
2. YIM, S. H., S. SZUCHET & P. POLAK. 1986. J. Biol. Chem. **261:** 11808-11815.
3. SZUCHET, S., P. E. POLAK & S. H. YIM. 1986. Dev. Neurosci. **8:** 208-221.
4. VARTANIAN, T., S. SZUCHET, G. DAWSON & A. T. CAMPAGNONI. 1986. Science **234:** 1395-1398.
5. ULMER, J. B., A. M. EDWARDS, F. A. MCMORRIS & P. E. BRAUN. 1987. J. Biol. Chem. **262:** 1748-1755.
6. HANNUN, Y. A. & R. M. BELL. 1987. Science **235:** 670-674.

# Glioblastoma-Cell-Derived T-Cell Suppressor Factor (G-TsF)

## Sequence Analysis and Biologic Mechanism of G-TsF

C. SIEPL,[a] S. BODMER,[a] E. HOFER,[b] M. WRANN,[b]
K. FREI,[a] AND A. FONTANA[a]

[a]*Section of Clinical Immunology and
Department of Neurosurgery
University Hospital
Zürich, Switzerland*

[b]*Sandoz Forschungsinstitut
Vienna, Austria*

Patients with glioblastoma show impaired cell-mediated immunity as manifested by cutaneous anergy to a variety of antigens and a decrease in T-cell blastogenic responsiveness *in vitro*.[1-3] In addition, T cells infiltrating glioblastoma tissue are unresponsive to mitogenic stimulation.[4] In tumor cyst fluid of patients with glioblastoma[5] and in the patients' serum, nondialyzable factors that inhibit lymphocyte proliferation can be detected before but not after tumor removal.[1]

Recently, we demonstrated that human glioblastoma cell line 308 releases a factor into the culture medium—termed "glioblastoma-derived T-cell suppressor factor" (G-TsF)—that inhibits T-cell proliferation *in vitro*.[6] Purified to homogeneity the factor was identified as a protein with a molecular weight of 12.5 kd. Aminoterminal sequence

TABLE 1. N-Terminal 25 Amino Acids of Human G-TsF[a]

| | 1 | | | | | | | | | 10 | | | | | | | | | 20 | | | | | | |
|---|---|---|---|---|---|---|---|---|---|---|---|---|---|---|---|---|---|---|---|---|---|---|---|---|---|
| h.G-TsF | A | L | D | A | A | Y | C | F | R | N | V | Q | D | N | C | C | L | R | P | L | Y | I | D | F | K |
| b.CIF-B | A | L | D | A | A | Y | C | F | R | N | V | Q | D | N | C | C | L | R | P | L | Y | I | D | F | K |
| h.TGFβ2 | A | L | D | A | A | Y | C | F | R | N | V | Q | D | N | C | C | L | R | P | L | Y | I | D | F | K |
| h.TGFβ1 | A | L | D | T | N | Y | C | F | S | S | T | E | K | N | C | C | V | R | Q | L | Y | I | D | F | R |

[a] The data of the N-terminal amino acid sequence of human G-TsF are compared to the sequences of bovine CIF-B[9], human TGF$_{β1}$,[8] and TGF$_{β2}$.[10]

TABLE 2. G-TsF-Mediated Inhibition of Antigen and IL-2-Induced Growth of T Cells

| Cultures | Additions G-TsF | Additions Control | OVA-7 T-Cell Proliferation (cpm ± SD) |
|---|---|---|---|
| *Experiment I*[a] | | | |
| OVA-7 T | − | − | 705 ± 11.4 |
| + OVA | − | − | 599 ± 9.1 |
| + APC | − | + | 72,260 ± 4,905.2 |
| + APC | + | − | 25,827 ± 1,314.9 |
| *Experiment II*[b] | | | |
| OVA-7 T | − | − | 279 ± 38 |
| OVA-7 T + IL-2 | − | + | 215,015 ± 7,298 |
| OVA-7 T + IL-2 | + | − | 16,831 ± 1,571 |

[a]*Experiment I.* OVA-7 T cells (H-2$^b$, 2 × 10$^4$) were cultured in 200 μl of serum-free Iscove's medium complete (Behring), supplemented with 2-mercaptoethanol (0.05 mM) and l-glutamine (0.3 mg/ml), for 72 hours in the presence of antigen (ovalbumin [OVA], 2.3 μM) and irradiated antigen-presenting cells (APC: 1 × 10$^6$ thymocytes, H-2$^b$). Purified G-TsF was added at a concentration of 4 × 10$^{-11}$M; the G-TsF control consisted of 0.1% TFA in 2-propanol (25% v/v) used for elution of G-TsF from the final Pro-RPC column.
[b]*Experiment II.* OVA-7 T cells (1 × 10$^4$) were cultured as just described in the presence of IL-2 (50 U/ml) with purified G-TsF at a concentration of 1.6 × 10$^{-11}$M.
Fourteen hours before harvest, 1 μCi $^3$H-thymidine per well was added.

analysis of G-TsF[7] demonstrated that 15 of 25 amino acids are identical to human transforming growth factor-$\beta$ (TGF$\beta$).[8] Identical sequences have been obtained independently for bone-derived bovine cartilage-inducing factor B (CIF-B)[9] and TG-$\beta$2 being purified from human platelets[10] (TABLE 1). When tested at a concentration of 4 × 10$^{-11}$M on a T-helper cell line (OVA-7 T), purified G-TsF inhibited the growth of OVA-7 T cells being activated with antigen and in the presence of thymocytes as antigen-presenting cells (TABLE 2, Experiment I). In addition, G-TsF was found to directly interfere with the growth-promoting effect of interleukin-2 on OVA-7 T cells (TABLE 2, Experiment II).

If released *in vivo*, G-TsF may contribute to impaired immunosurveillance and to the cellular immunodeficiency state detected in patients with glioblastoma.

## REFERENCES

1. BROOKS, W. H., M. G. NETSKY, D. E. NORMANSELL & D. A. HORWITZ. 1972. J. Exp. Med. **136:** 1631-1647.
2. THOMAS, D. G. T., C. B. LANNIGAN & P. O. BEHAN. 1975. Lancet **1:** 1389-1390.
3. ROSZMAN, T. L., W. H. BROOKS & L. H. ELLIOTT. 1982. Cancer **50:** 1273-1279.
4. MIESCHER, S., T. L. WHITESIDE, ST. CARREL & V. VON FLIEDNER. 1986. J. Immunol. **136:** 1899-1907.
5. KIKUCHI, K. & E. A. NEUWELT. 1983. J. Neurosurg. **59:** 790-799.
6. FONTANA, A., H. HENGARTNER, N. DE TRIBOLET & E. WEBER. 1984. J. Immunol. **132:** 1837-1844.

7. WRANN, M., S. BODMER, R. DE MARTIN, C. SIEPL, R. HOFER-WARBINEK, K. FREI, E. HOFER & A. FONTANA. 1987. EMBO **6:** 1633-1636.
8. DERYNCK, R., J. A. JARRETT, E. Y. CHEN, D. H. EATON, J. R. BELL, R. K. ASSOIAN, A. B. ROBERTS, M. B. SPORN & D. V. GOEDDEL. 1985. Nature **316:** 701-705.
9. SEYEDIN, S. M., P. R. SEGARINI, D. M. ROSEN, A. Y. THOMPSON, H. BENTZ & J. GRAYCAR. 1987. J. Biol. Chem. **262:** 1946-1949.
10. IKEDA, T., M. N. LIOUBIN & H. MARQUARDT. 1987. Biochemistry **26:** 2406-2410.

WORKSHOP 7. CROSS-RECOGNITION BETWEEN NERVOUS AND IMMUNE SYSTEM ANTIGEN

# Antineuronal Autoantibodies in Neurologic Paraneoplastic Syndromes

## NEIL E. ANDERSON AND JEROME B. POSNER

*Department of Neurology*
*Memorial Sloan-Kettering Cancer Center*
*New York, New York 10021*

The identification of antineuronal autoantibodies in some patients with neurologic paraneoplastic syndromes suggests that autoimmune mechanisms may play a role in the pathogenesis of some of these diseases. To answer some of the unresolved questions about these antibodies, we reviewed the clinical and immunologic findings in 135 patients with a clinically suspected neurologic paraneoplastic syndrome. Sera from these patients were tested for antineuronal antibodies by immunohistochemical methods and by testing with Western blots of Purkinje and cerebral cortex neurons. Control sera were obtained from patients with other neurologic diseases associated with cancer (135), other neurologic diseases without cancer (151), cancer without neurologic symptoms (168), and normal individuals (32).

Several different antineuronal autoantibodies were identified (TABLES 1 and 2). The most common was an antibody against 34-38 and 62-64 kd proteins in the cytoplasm of Purkinje cells. This antibody produced coarse, granular staining of the cytoplasm of Purkinje cells. It was found in 18 women with cancer, usually ovarian or breast carcinoma, and a stereotypic clinical syndrome of severe subacute pancerebellar dysfunction that usually preceded diagnosis of the tumor. Atypical anti-Purkinje cell antibodies, which stained Purkinje cell cytoplasm diffusely, were found in two other patients with paraneoplastic cerebellar degeneration and colon and lung

TABLE 1. Antibody and Antigen Characteristics

| | n | Antibody Titer | Antigen Distribution | Antigen Mr (kd) | "False Positives" |
|---|---|---|---|---|---|
| Anti-Purkinje cell antibody | 18 | 1:1000-1:40,000 | Purkinje cell cytoplasm; "Nissl staining" | 34-38, 62-64 | 1 |
| Atypical anti-Purkinje cell antibody | 2 | 1:1000, 1:4000 | Purkinje cell cytoplasm; "diffuse staining" | Not known | 0 |
| Antineuronal nuclear antibody I (anti-Hu) | 13 | 1:800-1:40,000 | All neuronal nuclei | 35-38 | 0 |
| Antineuronal nuclear antibody II | 3 | 1:200-1:1000 | All neuronal nuclei | 53-61, 79-84 | 0 |

TABLE 2. Clinical Correlations

|  | n | Sex (M:F) | Tumor | Neurologic Syndrome |
|---|---|---|---|---|
| Anti-Purkinje cell antibody | 18 | 0:18 | Ovary, 9; Breast, 6; Unknown, 3 | Subacute cerebellar degeneration |
| Atypical anti-Purkinje cell antibody | 2 | 1:1 | Lung, 1; Colon, 1 | Subacute cerebellar degeneration |
| Antineuronal nuclear antibody I (anti-Hu) | 13 | 5:8 | Lung (small cell), 13 | Subacute sensory neuronopathy; Encephalomyelitis; Autonomic neuropathy; Cerebellar ataxia |
| Antineuronal nuclear antibody II | 3 | 0:3 | Breast | Truncal ataxia; variable associated signs |

adenocarcinomas. An antibody reactive with 35-38 kd nucleoproteins in central nervous system and dorsal root and trigeminal ganglion neurons was identified in 13 patients with small cell lung carcinoma and neurologic disease. The dominant clinical syndrome in these patients was usually a subacute sensory neuronopathy, but in some of them encephalomyelitis, autonomic failure, and cerebellar ataxia dominated the clinical picture. A different antineuronal nuclear antibody that recognized 53-61 and 79-84 kd antigens was found in three patients with breast cancer and cerebellar ataxia. With one possible exception, these antineuronal autoantibodies were not identified in sera from controls. Therefore, antineuronal autoantibodies are highly specific markers for neurologic paraneoplastic syndromes. Their detection in a patient without known cancer should prompt a careful search for a tumor at a site appropriate to the type of antibody identified. Identification of autoantibodies in patients with neurologic paraneoplastic syndromes suggests that some of these diseases may have an autoimmune etiology, but conclusive proof of their role in the pathogenesis of neurologic diseases is not yet available.

# Antibodies to Sulfated Glucuronic Acid Containing Glycosphingolipids in Neuropathy Associated with Anti-Mag Antibodies and in Normal Individuals

SCOTT McGINNIS, TATSUO KOHRIYAMA, ROBERT K. YU, MICHAEL A. PESCE, AND NORMAN LATOV

*Departments of Neurology*
*Columbia University*
*New York, New York*
*and*
*Yale University*
*New Haven, Connecticut*

In approximately 50% of patients with neuropathy and IgM monoclonal gammopathy, the monoclonal antibodies (M-proteins) bind to a carbohydrate epitope shared by the myelin-associated glycoprotein (MAG), and by several other glycoproteins and two glycolipids in peripheral nerve.[1] The reactive glycolipids were identified as sulfated glucuronic acid containing paragloboside (SGPG) and sulfated glucuronic acid containing lactosaminyl paragloboside (SGLPG).[2,3]

The occurrence of IgM antibodies to the major cross-reactive glycolipid, SGPG,

TABLE 1. Antibodies to Sulfated Glucuronic Acid Containing Paragloboside (SGPG) in Normal Subjects and in Patients with Neurologic and Rheumatologic Diseases without Monoclonal Gammopathy

| Diagnosis | Total No. of Patients Tested | Total No. of Reactive Sera | Antibody Titer |
|---|---|---|---|
| Motor neuron disease | 14 | 4 | 1:25, 1:50, 1:100, 1:400 |
| Parkinson's disease | 9 | 0 | |
| Multiple sclerosis | 6 | 1 | 1:200 |
| Systemic lupus erythematosus and rheumatoid arthritis | 8 | 5 | 1:25, 1:25, 1:50, 1:100, 1:100 |
| Peripheral neuropathy | 19 | 3 | 1:25, 1:100, 1:12, 800 |
| Other neurologic diseases | 10 | 3 | 1:25, 1:50, 1:100 |
| Normal subjects | 14 | 4 | 1:100, 1:100, 1:200, 1:200 |
| Total | 80 | 20 | |

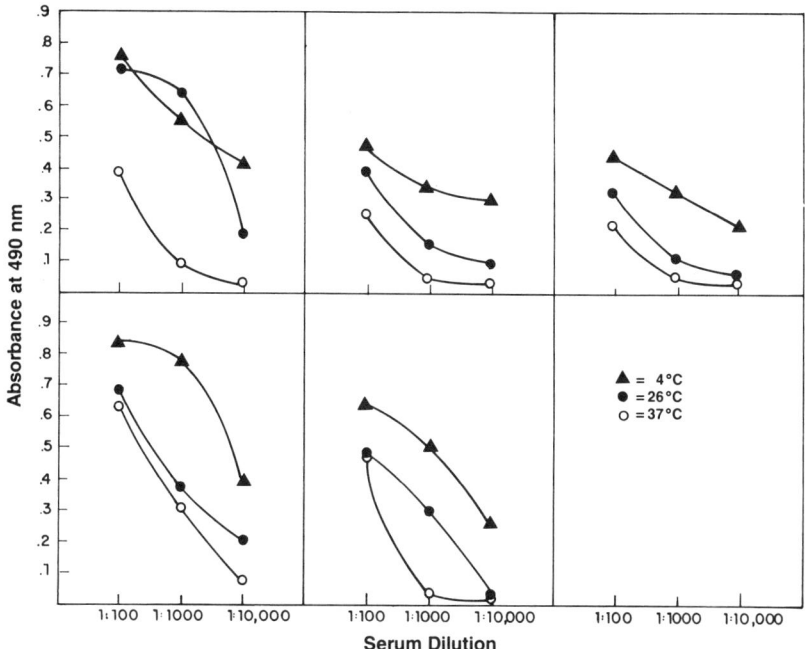

**FIGURE 1.** Binding of serum IgM from patients with neuropathy and anti-MAG M-proteins to sulfated glucuronic acid containing paragloboside by ELISA. Binding was measured at increasing serum dilutions and determined at three temperatures: 37°C, 26°C, and 4°C.

was investigated in patients with neuropathy and in control subjects, using a sensitive ELISA system. In five patients with neuropathy and anti-MAG M-proteins, antibody titers were detectable at serum dilutions greater than 1:10,000, and binding was strongest at 4°C (FIG. 1). Low levels of IgM binding to the glycolipid were also detected in sera of patients with other neurologic or rheumatologic diseases and in normal subjects (TABLE 1). Binding activity was present in 25% of the sera tested, and titers ranged between 1:25 and 1:400. One patient with peripheral neuropathy and vasculitis had a measurable titer of 1:12,800 in the absence of monoclonal gammopathy.

The data suggest that cold-reactive anti-SGPG IgM antibodies are frequent constituents of the normal human antibody repertoire. Monoclonal anti-SGPG or anti-MAG antibodies may then result from the abnormal proliferation of individual B-cell clones with the same specificity. In some cases, the resting B cells may be polyclonally activated to secrete anti-SGPG antibodies in the absence of monoclonal gammopathy.

## REFERENCES

1. CHOU, D. K. H., A. A. ILYAS, J. E. EVANS, C. COSTELLO, R. H. QUARLES & F. B. JANGALWALA. 1986. Structure of sulfated glycuronyl glycolipids in the nervous system reacting with HNK-1 antibody and some IgM paraproteins in neuropathy. J. Biol. Chem. **261:** 11717-11725.

2. ARIGA, T., T. KOHRIYAMA, L. FREDDO, N. LATOV, M. SAITO, K. KOW, S. ANDO, M. SUZUKI, M. HEMLING, K. L. RINEHYART, S. KUSUNOKI & R. K. YU. 1987. Characterization of sulfated glucuronic acid containing glycolipids reacting with IgM M-proteins in patients with neuropathy. J. Biol. Chem. **262:** 848-853.
3. LATOV, N. 1987. Peripheral neuropathy and IgM monoclonal gammopathy. *In* Clinical Neuroimmunology. P. O. Behan & J. Aarli, Eds. Blackwell Publication, London.

# Mammalian Reovirus Receptor Expression by Oligodendrocytes

JEFFREY A. COHEN,[a] ROBERT C. SERGOTT,[a] HERBERT M. GELLER,[b] MARK J. BROWN,[a] AND MARK I. GREENE[c]

[a]*Department of Neurology*
*University of Pennsylvania School of Medicine*
*Philadelphia, Pennsylvania*

[b]*Department of Pharmacology*
*UMDNJ—the Robert Wood Johnson Medical School at Rutgers*
*Piscataway, New Jersey*

[c]*Department of Pathology*
*University of Pennsylvania School of Medicine*
*Philadelphia, Pennsylvania*

A serotype-specific cell surface receptor for the mammalian reovirus type 3 is defined by the mouse monoclonal anti-receptor antibody 87.92.6[1] and the xenogeneic rabbit antiserum anti-ID3,[2] both directed against an idiotope of the 9B.G5 anti-reovirus type 3 hemagglutinin antibody. The reovirus receptor and the $\beta_2$-adrenergic receptor have similar tissue distributions and biochemical features.[3] However, the catecholamine and virus binding sites appear to be distinct. Whereas the binding of beta agonists typically leads to activation of adenylate cyclase and the accumulation of intracellular cyclic AMP, the binding of intact reovirus type 3, purified hemagglutinin, and anti-reovirus receptor antibodies inhibit DNA synthesis and cell growth of mouse L fibroblasts, mouse R1.1 thymoma cells, and rat B104 neuroblastoma cells (reference 4 and unpublished data). Recent studies demonstrated that immunoreactive reovirus receptor is expressed by mature oligodendrocytes and both type 1 and type 2 astrocytes.[5] The present studies were undertaken to determine the timing and cellular specificity of expression of immunoreactive reovirus receptor during glial development and to determine the effects of antibody binding on oligodendrocytes or myelin *in vivo*.

## METHODS

Developing glia were isolated from neonatal rat optic nerves and cultured on poly-L-lysine-coated coverslips in N2 medium.[6] The cellular specificity of reovirus receptor expression was determined by immunofluorescence microscopy after double labeling of the cells with anti-reovirus receptor antibody, anti-ID3, and antibodies specific for glial differentiation markers,[7] A2B5, 04, galactocerebroside (GalC), myelin basic protein (MBP), and glial fibrillary acidic protein (GFAP). To determine the timing of expression, cultures were examined sequentially over 4 days. Each coverslip was examined in its entirety (400-450 cells), and the cells expressing each marker were enumerated. The total number of cells in the cultures did not appear to change substantially over this time period.

To study the effects of anti-receptor antibody *in vivo*, 15 to 35 µl of test solution containing 50-150 ng of antibody were injected into the optic nerves of adult male Hartley guinea pigs. After intervals of 4-24 hours the nerves were fixed *in situ*, excised, processed, and examined by transmission electron microscopy.

## RESULTS

In the glial cultures, the relative proportion and absolute number of 0-2A progenitor cells, defined as round cells with short processes and the A2B5(+) 04(±), GalC(−), GFAP(−) phenotype, decreased over time (TABLE 1). Only a small fraction, mainly process-bearing cells staining faintly for A2B5, expressed reovirus receptor. Approximately half the immature oligodendrocytes, cells with multiple branching proceses and the surface phenotype A2B5(±) 04(+) GalC(−), expressed the receptor, which appeared coincident with or just following 04. The number of mature oligodendrocytes, defined as cells with extensive arborizations expressing GalC and later MBP, increased over time. Virtually all of these cells expressed reovirus receptor. The numbers of type 1 astrocytes, flat cells with the A2B5(−) GFAP(+) phenotype, and of type 2 astrocytes, process-bearing cells with the A2B5(±) GFAP(+) phenotype, and the proportions expressing reovirus receptor increased progressively during the culture period.

The appearance of the reovirus receptor in a stage-specific manner during glial differentiation and the similarity of the virus receptor to the β-adrenergic receptor suggest that ligand binding to this molecule may have functional effects on glial cells. Microinjection of antibody into guinea pig optic nerves was undertaken to look for such effects *in vivo*. Within 4 hours after injection of 50-150 ng of purified 87.92.6 anti-reovirus receptor antibody, myelin vesiculation and separation of myelin lamellae

TABLE 1. Reovirus Receptor Expression by Developing Glia Isolated from Neonatal Rat Optic Nerves

| Day of Culture | Proportion of Cells Expressing Reovirus Receptor Among: | | | | |
|---|---|---|---|---|---|
| | A2B5(+) | 04(+) | GalC(+) | MBP(+) | GFAP(+) |
| 1 | 8/92 | 34/51 | 17/19 | 1/3 | 11/102 |
| 2 | 6/27 | 59/128 | 19/23 | 1/1 | 97/147 |
| 3 | 23/123 | 55/99 | 63/71 | 24/24 | Not done |
| 4 | 15/24 | 69/97 | 85/99 | 37/41 | 209/289 |

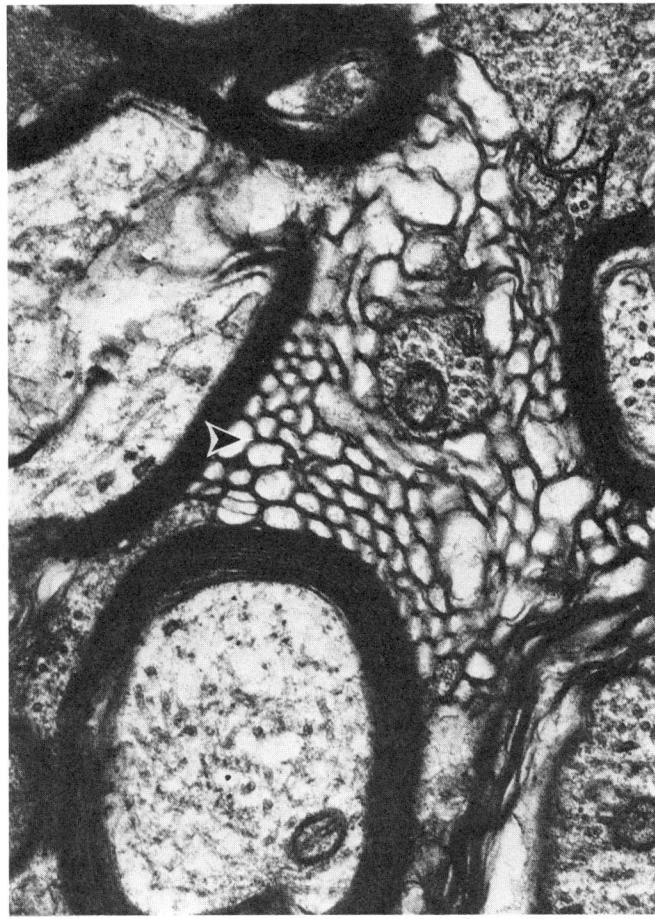

**FIGURE 1.** Changes in myelin morphology induced by anti-reovirus receptor antibody *in vivo*. The photomicrograph demonstrates myelin vesiculation (▶) 24 hours after the injection of approximately 50 ng of purified monoclonal anti-reovirus receptor antibody, 87.92.6, into a guinea pig optic nerve. The involved axon and surrounding myelinated fibers are normal in appearance. Original magnification × 67,800; reduced by 30%.

were observed in the absence of a prominent inflammatory cell infiltrate or altered axonal morphology. More widespread changes were seen 24 hours after injection (FIG. 1). Injection of anti-ID3 produced similar changes. Injection of PBS alone, pre-immune rabbit serum, and H022.1, an isotype-matched (IgMk) control antibody purified in a manner identical to that of the anti-receptor antibodies, produced no effects on myelin morphology. In contrast to antibody directed against GalC,[8] anti-reovirus receptor antibody did not require the addition of exogenous complement proteins to produce ultrastructural changes.

## DISCUSSION

Neonatal rat optic nerve cultures provide a useful model system with which to study the regulation of expression of the reovirus receptor during glial cell maturation. The reovirus receptor is expressed on mature astrocytes and oligodendrocytes and appears in a stage-specific manner during oligodendrocyte differentiation. Anti-reovirus receptor antibodies are capable of producing changes in myelin morphology *in vivo*. The lack of a requirement for exogenous complement proteins and of a significant inflammatory cell infiltrate suggests that this effect results directly from the interaction of antibody with the receptor and does not require additional humoral or cellular immune mechanisms. Autoreactive anti-receptor antibodies (anti-idiotypes) generated during normal immune responses to viral infection may similarly alter oligodendrocyte development or function.

### REFERENCES

1. NOSEWORTHY, J. H., B. N. FIELDS, M. A. DICHTER, C. SOBOTKA, E. PIZER, L. L. PERRY, J. T. NEPOM & M. I. GREENE. 1983. J. Immunol. **131:** 2533.
2. NEPOM, J. T., H. L. WEINER, M. A. DICHTER, M. TARDIEU, D. R. SPRIGGS, C. F. GRAMM, M. L. POWERS, B. N. FIELDS & M. I. GREENE. 1982. J. Exp. Med. **155:** 155.
3. CO, M. S., G. N. GAULTON, A. TOMINAGA, C. J. HOMCY, B. N. FIELDS & M. I. GREENE. 1985. Proc. Natl. Acad. Sci. USA **82:** 5315.
4. SHARPE, A. H. & B. N. FIELDS. 1981. J. Virol. **38:** 389.
5. VENTIMIGLIA, R., M. I. GREENE & H. M. GELLER. 1987. Proc. Natl. Acad. Sci. USA **84:** 5073.
6. RAFF, M. C., R. H. MILLER & M. NOBLE. 1983. Nature **303:** 390.
7. KENNEDY, P. G. E. 1982. J. Neuroimmunol. **2:** 35.
8. SERGOTT, R. C., M. J. BROWN, D. H. SILBERBERG & R. P. LISAK. 1984. J. Neurol. Sci. **64:** 297.

# Isolation and Characterization of *Borrelia Burgdorferi*-Specific and Autoreactive T-Cell Lines from the Cerebrospinal Fluid of Patients with Lyme Meningoradiculomyelitis[a]

ROLAND MARTIN,[b] JOHANNES ORTLAUF,[b]
VERONIKA STICHT-GROH,[c] AND
HANS GEORG MERTENS[b]

[b]*Department of Neurology*
*University of Würzburg*
*Würzburg, FRG*

[c]*Institute of Hygiene and Microbiology*
*University of Würzburg*
*Würzburg, FRG*

Lyme disease, a tick-borne spirochetal illness, may involve different organs such as joints, heart, skin, and the central and peripheral nervous system (CNS and PNS). Neurologic manifestations include meningoradiculitis or even radiculomyelitis, encephalomyelitis, and encephalopathy. Apart from *Borrelia burgdorferi* (Bb)-specific humoral immune reactions including the production of Bb-specific oligoclonal IgG bands within the cerebrospinal fluid (CSF), the finding of Bb-specific T lymphocytes in the peripheral blood and the CSF has been reported.[1]

To analyze CSF T cells in more detail, 505 T-cell lines (TCLs) were directly expanded from the CSF of three patients with Lyme radiculomyelitis using the limiting dilution technique.[2] Following expansion, cells were characterized for phenotype, proliferative responses to a panel of CNS and PNS autoantigens, and for natural killer (NK)-like cytotoxicity in $^{51}$Cr release assays using the myeloid cell line, K562, as target. The vast majority of TCLs were positive for CD3, CD4, and HLA class II antigens, but not for CD8. Proliferative assays ($^3$H-thymidine incorporation) gave the following results: 33 TCLs responded on stimulation with Bb antigen, 16 with myelin basic protein (MBP), 16 with whole peripheral myelin (PM), two with galactocerebrosides (Gal), 1 with P2 protein, a basic myelin component of the peripheral nerve, and 1 with cardiolipin which is found in mitochondrial membranes and bacterial cell walls. A sample of Bb-specific and MBP-specific TCLs is shown in TABLE 1. The proliferative response of specific TCLs tested was restricted by HLA class II antigens (TABLE 2). Ten percent of the TCLs mediated NK-like cytotoxicity shown by lysis

---

[a]This work was supported by grant Sti 63/4-1 of the Deutsche Forschungsgemeinschaft.

TABLE 1. Proliferative Responses of a Sample of Bb-Specific and MBP-Specific TCLs Isolated from the CSF of Patients with Chronic Lyme Radiculomyelitis[a]

| | $^3$H-Thymidine Incorporation in the Presence of: | | |
|---|---|---|---|
| TCL No. | Bb Antigen | Medium | IL-2 |
| E6/10B | 119,810 ± 5,450 | 1,090 ± 280 | 13,020 ± 340 |
| D2/60 | 15,180 ± 5,500 | 1,120 ± 340 | 1,600 ± 120 |
| H10/10B | 15,630 ± 560 | 1,070 ± 90 | 1,920 ± 620 |
| D2/180A | 4,080 ± 510 | 340 ± 90 | 3,510 ± 10 |
| TCL No. | MBP | Medium | IL-2 |
| B4/180 | 2,900 ± 550 | 180 ± 140 | 1,340 ± 50 |
| H11/180A | 1,840 ± 580 | 100 ± 40 | 1,510 ± 50 |
| C2/180 | 14,870 ± 2,870 | 50 ± 40 | 21,510 ± 5,760 |
| B9/90 | 13,430 ± 5,130 | 710 ± 210 | 6,010 ± 1,820 |

ABBREVIATIONS: Bb = *Borrelia burgdorferi;* IL-2 = interleukin-2; MBP = myelin basic protein; TCL = T-cell lines.

[a] Cells were tested in the presence of autologous antigen presenting cells and results expressed as counts per minute (cpm).

TABLE 2. HLA Class II Restriction of the Proliferative Response on Stimulation with *Borrelia burgdorferi* (Bb) Antigen of Two Bb-Specific T-Cell Lines (TCLs)[a]

| | $^3$H-Thymidine Incorporation in the Presence of: | | | | |
|---|---|---|---|---|---|
| TCL No. | Auto. APC + Bb Antigen | Allo. APC + Bb Antigen | Auto. APC + Med. | Allo. APC + Med. | Allo. APC + PHA |
| E3/30B | 28,120 ± 1,210 | 250 ± 40 | 980 −230 | nd[b] | 980 ± 290 |
| D3/30A | 69,930 ± 10,410 | 29,400 ± 5,510 | 7,020 ± 2,550 | 5,930 ± 2,180 | 22,520 ± 710 |

[a] HLA class II of autologous (auto.) APC: DRw6/DRw11; DQw1/DQw3. HLA class II of allogeneic (allo.) APC: DR3/DR7; DQw2/DQw2.
[b] nd = not done.

of K562 myeloid cells. Some of the cell lines were kept in culture for longer periods of time and later analyzed for helper function. One Bb-specific TCL exhibited helper function for specific IgG when it was co-cultivated with autologous B cells in the presence of antigen.

These data show that in patients with chronic nervous system manifestations of Lyme disease, not only Bb-specific T cells, but also those responding to CNS or PNS autoantigens can be found in the CSF. Analysis of the specificity and function of these cells only became possible by their expansion as oligoclonal TCLs or T-cell clones. Whether the autoreactive T cells that had been induced by *B. burgdorferi* are of pathogenetic significance remains to be determined.

## REFERENCES

1. PACHNER, A. R., A. C. STEERE, L. H. SIGAL & C. J. JOHNSON. 1985. Antigen-specific proliferation of CSF lymphocytes in Lyme disease. Neurology **35:** 1642-1644.
2. MORETTA, A., G. PANTALEO, L. MORETTA, J. C. CEROTTINI & M. C. MINGARI. 1983. Direct demonstration of the clonogenic potential of every human peripheral blood T cell. J. Exp. Med. **157:** 743-754.

# Monoclonal Antibodies Against the P2 Protein of Peripheral Myelin and d18 Protein of PC 12 Cells Bind to Antigen-Presenting Cells and Inhibit T-Cell Activation[a]

DONARD S. DWYER,[b] F. PIERRE VANDERVEGT,[c]
JOACHIM BARTELS, AND GEORGE B. BROWN

[b]Neuropsychiatry Research Program
Department of Psychiatry
and
[c]Medical Genetics Laboratory
University of Alabama at Birmingham
Birmingham, Alabama 35294

The P2 protein is a major structural component of peripheral myelin, although its precise function is not known. Immunization of animals with peripheral nerve or the P2 protein can lead to demyelination and accompanying paralysis that is reminiscent of the Guillain-Barré syndrome in humans. Monoclonal antibodies (mAbs) have been produced against P2 protein and the neuronal-like cell line PC 12. The antibodies against P2 were co-incubated with T-cell lines specific for P2 in the presence or absence of antigen. Other studies in our laboratory demonstrated that the addition of mAbs against the acetylcholine receptor (AChR) to AChR-specific T cells and antigen leads to enhanced activation of the T cells.[1] Surprisingly, one of the anti-P2 mAbs, BC 18, inhibited T-cell activation rather than enhancing it. In addition, a second mAb, PC 11, which reacts with a cell surface antigen on PC 12 cells, inhibited T-cell activation to a similar extent. It seemed possible that the antibodies might inhibit T-cell activation by binding to the P2 protein and competing with the T cells for recognition of antigen. However, this argument is ruled out by two pieces of evidence: (1) PC 11 does not bind to P2 protein, and (2) these antibodies also interfered with T-cell activation of lines specific for other antigens (data not shown).

Data in FIGURE 1 summarize the results obtained with BC 18 and PC 11 in inhibiting T-cell activation in response to various types of stimulation. As just discussed, these antibodies potently inhibited T-cell activation by various antigens. When higher concentrations of antibody than those shown are used, an 80-90% reduction in proliferation can be achieved. In addition, the antibodies inhibited T-cell activation by the mitogen concanavalin A. However, as seen in FIGURE 1, alloreactivity (C57B1/

---

[a]This work is supported by a grant (RG 1734-A-1) from the National Multiple Sclerosis Society.

6 cells versus irradiated BALB/c stimulator cells) was not effected by BC 18 or PC 11. In fact, in every experiment there has actually been a slight enhancement in alloreactivity in the presence of these antibodies.

To determine the site of action of the mAbs, various cell populations were stained for immunofluorescence. Both PC 11 and BC 18 stained the PC 12 cell line. Although not shown here, PC 11 also inhibits neurite outgrowth from PC 12 cells in response to nerve growth factor. This finding may provide a clue about the mode of action of these antibodies. T cells and B-cell hybridomas were not stained by BC 18 or PC 11, whereas antigen-presenting cell populations (APCs) that included macrophages and dendritic cells were positive.[2] These findings indicate that the mAbs are somehow interfering with antigen presentation at the level of the presenting cell, thereby dis-

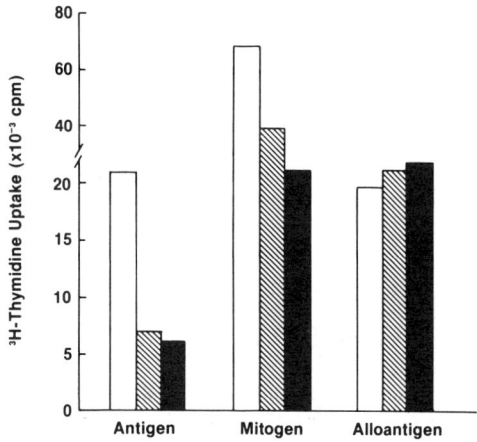

**FIGURE 1.** Inhibition of T-cell activation by monoclonal antibodies (mAbs). The P2-specific T-cell line, SA, was incubated ($1 \times 10^5$ cells/ml) with irradiated spleen cells ($4\text{-}5 \times 10^5$/ml) in round-bottomed wells with or without antigen and in the presence or absence of mAb. After 48 hours, tritiated thymidine was added, and after an additional 15 hours, the cells were harvested and the filters counted. For these studies, 25 μl of supernatant containing mAb were used. Antigen (P2 protein) was added at a concentration of 2 μg/ml and mitogen (Con A) at 2.5 μg/ml. Alloreactivity was measured in a similar fashion by reacting C57B1/6 lymph node cells with irradiated BALB/c antigen-presenting cells (APCs). The *open bar* represents a control mAb supernatant, the *cross-hatched bar*, BC18, and the *solid bar*, PC 11.

turbing T-cell activation. We have analyzed PC 12 cells and APCs by Western blotting to determine the nature of the antigen recognized by BC 18 and PC 11. The mAbs reacted with two bands on the nitrocellulose blot that had estimated molecular weights of 18,000 and 36,000 daltons.[2] The 18-kd band is similar in size to the P2 protein, and we consider the larger band to be a dimer.

Finally, we examined the effects of adding the inhibitory antibodies at various times after initiation of the T-cell culture. The results are shown in FIGURE 2. T-cell proliferation was reduced by about 25% when the antibodies were added at the same time or within 15 minutes after the initiation of T-cell culture with antigen. There was a 40% reduction when the antibody was added after 30 minutes and an increase

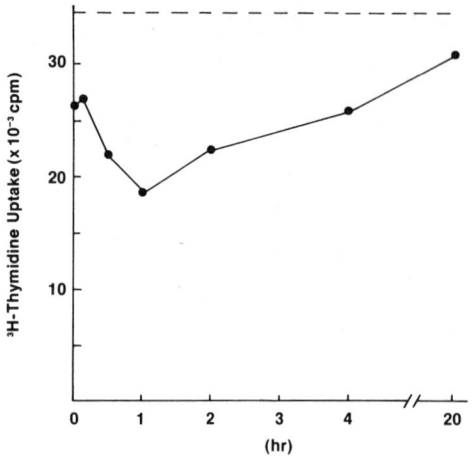

**FIGURE 2.** The effect of delaying administration of inhibitory monoclonal antibodies (mAbs). Antigen-specific T-cell activation was set up as described in FIGURE 1. The BC18 mAb was added either at the initiation of culture with antigen or after various delays. T-cell proliferation was measured for all cultures at the same time (after 48 hours). The data represent $^3$H-thymidine uptake measured after a 15-hour incubation with label.

to nearly 50% inhibition of activation with a 1-hour delay. If the mAbs were added after longer delays, there was less inhibition, until with a 20-hour delay there was only a 12% reduction. These data suggest that there is a critical stage in antigen presentation occurring about 1 hour after the addition of antigen that is particularly sensitive to the action of the mAbs.

On the basis of amino acid sequence homology, the P2 protein has been assigned to a family of lipid-binding proteins.[3] We suggest that the P2-like protein of APCs and PC12 cells is a member of this family. Antibodies against this protein may interfere with antigen presentation by inhibiting the transport or attachment of lipids or by effecting the production of lipid-derived second messengers.

## REFERENCES

1. SCHALKE, B. C. G., W. E. F. KLINKERT, H. WEKERLE & D. S. DWYER. 1985. J. Immunol. **134:** 3643–3648.
2. DWYER, D. S., F. P. VANDERVEGT, J. BARTELS & G. B. BROWN. 1987. J. Immunol. Submitted for publication.
3. TAKAHASKI, K., S. ODANI & T. ONO. 1982. Biochem. Biophys. Res. Comm. **106:** 1099–1105.

# Expression of Leukocyte Antigens on an Oligodendroglial Cell Line[a]

LYNN M. ROSE,[b] SUSANNE L. JACKEVICIUS,[b] AND
EDWARD A. CLARK [b,c]

[b]Department of Microbiology
and
[c]Regional Primate Research Center
University of Washington School of Medicine
Seattle, Washington

The KG-1 human oligodendroglial cell line was established from a mixed glioma.[1] Morphologically, the KG-1 cells have a perinuclear halo, dichotomous branching, and a tendency to aggregate and float in culture. In small aggregates, most cells are bipolar. The cells synthesize the S-100 protein specific to neural tissue and express galactocerebroside on their surface. We are using these cells to study the expression of surface antigens and the ability of cytokines to induce proliferation and/or differentiation of oligodendrocytes *in vitro*. We report here the results of flow cytometric analysis of KG-1 cells using monoclonal antibodies to surface antigens expressed by leukocytes. In addition, we report the ability of B-cell stimulatory factor-2 (BSF-2) to induce the expression of a surface molecule recognized by anti-CD4 monoclonal antibody.

## METHOD

The KG-1 oligodendroglial cell line is maintained in phenol-red free Eagle's minimum essential medium containing 10% fetal bovine serum, amino acids, and antibiotics. Cells are removed from flasks by washing twice to remove serum proteins and then treating them with Versene buffer (0.6 mM EDTA in phosphate-buffered saline solution) for 4 minutes at 37°C. Cells are dislodged by striking the side of the flask. Cell surface antigens are detected by indirect immunofluorescence; $5 \times 10^5$ cells in 0.05 ml are incubated for 30 minutes with monoclonal antibody (mAb), washed twice, and then incubated with R-phycoerythrin(PE)-conjugated goat anti-mouse IgG (Biomeda). Positive fluorescence is measured on a FACStar Flow Cytometer (Becton-Dickinson).

Changes in the expression of surface molecules following exposure to T-cell or macrophage-derived growth factors are also being studied. The differentiative effect

---

[a]This work was supported by National Multiple Sclerosis Society Grant RG-1829-A-1 (L.M.R.) and Regional Primate Research Center NIH Core Grant RR00166.

of one cytokine, B-cell stimulatory factor-2 (BSF-2),[2] on KG-1 is described. Expression of the CD4 molecule on KG-1 cells was measured after culturing $2.0 \times 10^6$ cells for 2 days with BSF-2 (3.0 U/ml) or medium, and then staining the cells, as just described, with monoclonal antibody to human CD4 and other leukocyte surface antigens.

## RESULTS

One color flow cytometric analysis of KG-1 cells indicates that these cells are expressing the oligodendrocyte-specific antigen galactocerebroside (not shown). In addition, these cells are expressing antigens that are recognized by monoclonal antibodies to the Ia class II major histocompatibility antigen, the common leukocyte antigen T200, and the natural killer (NK) cell-associated HNK-1 surface antigen (FIG. 1A-D). When KG-1 oligodendroglial cells were cultured 48 hours with medium (FIG. 2, upper panel) or BSF-2 (FIG. 2, lower panel) and then stained with the OKT4a mAb followed by PE-conjugated goat anti-mouse IgG, there is an 18% increase in the frequency of putative $CD4^+$ KG-1 cells exposed to the BSF-2 differentiation factor. Studies are in progress to biochemically analyze these surface structures.

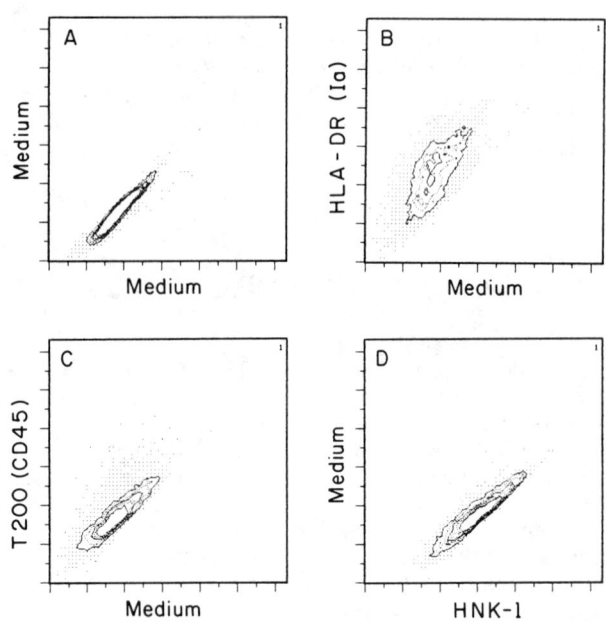

**FIGURE 1.** One-color analysis of the KG-1 oligodendrocyte cell line. (**A**) Cells stained with medium alone. Analysis indicates that these cells are expressing antigens recognized by monoclonal antibodies to (**B**) the HLA-DR class II MHC antigen (detected with PE-HLA-DR mAb, Becton-Dickinson); (**C**) the T200 common leukocyte antigen (detected with mAb 13.2 and PE-goat anti-mouse IgG (Biomeda), the 13.2 mAb was kindly provided by Dr. Walter Newman; and (**D**) the HNK-1 antigen (detected with FITC-HNK-1 mAb).

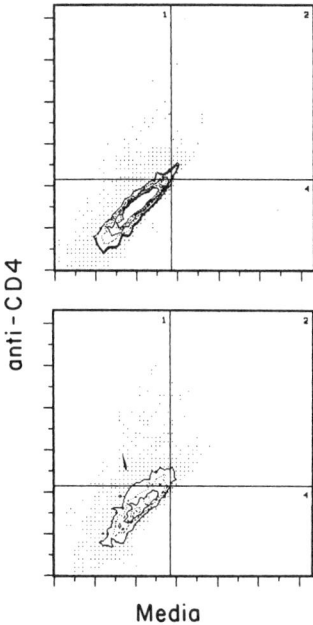

FIGURE 2. KG-1 oligodendrocytes were cultured 48 hours with media (*upper panel*) or BSF-2 (*lower panel*) and then stained with PE-OKT4a. After 48 hours there is an 18% increase in the frequency of CD4$^+$ cells exposed to the BSF-2 growth factor.

## CONCLUSIONS

Several studies have indicated that surface antigens previously thought to be expressed exclusively on cells of hematopoietic lineage may also be expressed in the brain. We demonstrated that mAb to the common leukocyte antigen T200 (CD45) recognizes a structure on human oligodendrocytes. Monoclonal antibodies to Ia antigen and to the HNK-1 antigen also recognize structures on normal human oligodendrocytes.[3,4] Whether these molecules are identical or serve similar functions in the brain as in the immune system is not known. Analysis of the structure and function of these molecules has been difficult, owing in part to the difficulty in obtaining homogeneous populations of oligodendrocytes to work with. There are several advantages to using the KG-1 cell line for these studies. KG-1 cells express many of the same antigens as do normal oligodendrocytes and can be grown in large amounts necessary for biochemical analysis of surface antigens and for analysis of specific mRNAs. In addition, they are easy to examine by flow cytometry and being homogeneous, provide a unique opportunity to study the effects of specific growth factors *in vitro*. Initial experiments with BSF-2, a B-cell differentiation factor that is produced by T cells,[2] and astrocytoma lines (T. Hirano, personal communication) induce the apparent expression of low levels of CD4 on the surface of KG-1 cells.

## REFERENCES

1. MIYAKE, E. 1979. Acta Neuropathol. (Berl.) **46:** 51-55.
2. HIRANO, T. *et al.* 1986. Nature **324:** 73-76.
3. KIM, S. U., G. MORETTO & D. H. SHIN. 1985. J. Neuroimmunol **10:** 141-149.
4. MCGARRY, R. C., R. H. HELFAND, R. H. QUARLES & J. C. RODER. 1983. Nature **306:** 376-378.

# Characterization and *in Vitro* Use of a Monoclonal Anti-Idiotypic Antibody Against HNK-1

## M. SCHLUEP, N. PAGE, G. PERRUISSEAU, AND A. J. STECK

*Laboratory of Neurobiology*
*Department of Neurology*
*Lausanne, Switzerland*

A mouse monoclonal IgM antibody, HNK-1, produced against a membrane antigen from the cultured T-cell line, HSB-2, reacts with a specific antigen on human natural killer cells and with myelin-associated glycoprotein (MAG), a component of both peripheral and central myelin, which is thought to play a role in cell-cell interactions within the nervous system.

HNK-1 was used as an immunogen to obtain mouse monoclonal anti-idiotypic antibodies. Supernatants from hybridoma colonies were screened for antibody activity against HNK-1 using radioimmunoassay. Monoclonal G6D9 was selected, affinity purified, and characterized as an $IgG_1$ kappa. G6D9 reacted specifically with an epitope of HNK-1 and inhibited in a dose-dependent manner the binding of HNK-1 to its specific antigen MAG.

With an indirect immunofluorescence technique, G6D9 showed both cytoplasmic and surface staining on HNK-1 antibody-secreting cells (FIG. 1).

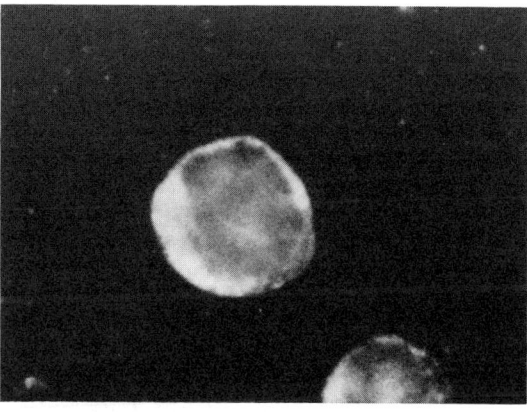

**FIGURE 1.** HNK-1-producing hybridomas were reacted with G6D9 followed by fluorescent anti-mouse IgG(Fc specific).

Complement-mediated cytotoxic tests were carried out as follows, and cell lysis was estimated by trypan blue dye exclusion. Cells were incubated sequentially with G6D9, rabbit anti-mouse IgG(Fc), and rabbit complement. In this system, G6D9 caused 42% lysis of HNK-1-producing cells (background lysis without G6D9 was 11%). $^{51}$Cr release assays carried out in parallel gave an overall similar pattern of results but with lower values for lysis.

G6D9, being an anti-idiotypic antibody, will be a useful tool to study specific cytotoxicity and immunoregulation *in vivo*. Furthermore, such antibodies will be a good model for autoimmune diseases in humans.

# Lesion-Induced Changes of Astrocyte Morphology and Protein Expression in Rat Optic Nerve

GUIDO STOLL AND HANS-WERNER MUELLER

*Molecular Neurobiology and Neuroimmunology Laboratory*
*Department of Neurology*
*University of Düsseldorf*
*Düsseldorf, FRG*

The identity of the cell type(s) in the central nervous system (CNS) responsible for myelin phagocytosis and degradation during Wallerian degeneration is still controversial. It has been suggested that hematogenous macrophages, astrocytes, and/or microglia could be involved. Immunologic markers are now available to specifically identify distinct cell types in the CNS such as antibodies to glial fibrillary acid protein (GFAP) for astrocytes and ED1 antibodies for macrophages.[1] Apolipoprotein E (apoE), a serum protein known to be involved in both transport and metabolism of phospholipids and cholesterol, was shown to be synthesized at elevated rates following injury of mature peripheral and central nerves.[2,3] After peripheral nerve injury ED1-positive macrophages enter the distal stump and express large amounts of apoE.[4] In the normal adult optic nerve, GFAP-positive astrocytes possess significant concentrations of apoE.

Here we report on the fate of astrocytes and the origin of phagocytic cells in the rat optic nerve after crush by immunocytochemical methods using marker antibodies. Crushing rat optic nerve (ON) induces a sequence of distinct changes in astroglial morphology and in the expression of specific proteins. At the molecular level, one of the most prominent effects following ON injury was the rapid disappearance of apoE from astroglial cell bodies within 3 days.[4] Simultaneously, typical reactive astrocyte morphology was expressed and maintained for several weeks in degenerating ON. However, 6-8 weeks after the lesion the morphology of GFAP-positive astrocytes was markedly altered by retraction of processes and rounding of the cell body, now resembling large phagocytic cells (FIG. 1). These GFAP-positive phagocytes are further characterized by the expression of the established macrophage marker ED1, but they do not contain apoE. Only occasionally did ED1/apoE-positive hematogenous macrophages occur in the injured ON.

The lesion-induced response of astrocytes reported here includes a rapid change at the molecular level (reorganization of apoE) as well as slow alterations in morphology. Here we provide two lines of evidence to suggest that phagocytic activity in the ON is mainly delivered by altered astrocytes: (1) phagocytic cells in ON commonly express astrocyte- and macrophage-marker proteins GFAP and ED1, respectively, and (2) these cells can clearly be distinguished from ED1-positive macrophages coexpressing apoE which infiltrate the peripheral nervous system after injury.[4] Our results

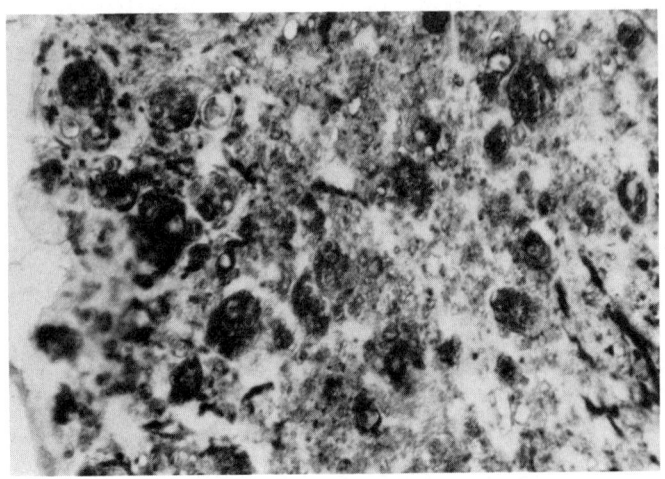

**FIGURE 1.** Optic nerve 6 weeks after crush. GFAP-positive astrocytes are rounded, now resembling large phagocytic cells. In addition, typical astroglial processes are stained.

demonstrate molecular and structural properties shared by astrocytes in the injured ON and macrophages of the immune system, indicating significant astroglial plasticity in response to CNS injury.

## REFERENCES

1. DIJKSTRA, C. D. *et al.* 1985. Immunology **54:** 589.
2. MUELLER, H.-W. *et al.* 1985. Science **228:** 499.
3. IGNATIUS, M. J. *et al.* 1986. Proc. Natl. Acad. Sci. USA **83:** 1125.
4. STOLL, G. & H.-W. MUELLER. 1986. Neurosci. Lett. **72:** 223.

# Glia Cells as Immunoregulatory Elements

## Up- and Down-Regulatory Activities of Astrocyte Clones

DEMING SUN, RICHARD MEYERMANN, AND
HARTMUT WEKERLE

*Max-Planck-Society
Clinical Research Unit for Multiple Sclerosis
Würzburg, FRG*

Astrocytes are pivotal cell components in the central nervous system (CNS) where they provide functional and structural support for neurons and retain their ability to divide and grow in response to neural damage. That astrocytes are potential antigen-presenting cells points to the possibility that they are an important cell component in immune responses of the CNS.

We isolated a series of astrocyte clones which enabled us to document functional heterogeneity of astrocytes on the clonal level. Our results demonstrated that some astrocyte clones (represented by F10) are potent antigen-presenting cells. They can be induced readily by exogenous gamma-interferon (IFN-γ) to express major histocompatibility complex (MHC) class II antigens on their membranes to function as accessory cells in both antigen-specific and lectin-mediated T-cell proliferation assays. Other clones (e.g., clone B10) had distinctive suppressive activity on T-cell function. (FIG.1) The suppressive activities of astrocyte clones were found to be radiosensitive, but resistant to indomethacin treatment. The concanavalin A response of thymocytes was much more sensitive to the suppressive activity of astrocytes than the interleukin-2 (IL-2) dependent T-cell proliferation.

The possible role of the suppressive activity of the local glial cells *in vivo* was studied in a passively induced experimental allergic encephalomyelitis (EAE) model. The recipient Lewis rats were first irradiated with a lethal dose (750 R) and then transferred with encephalitogenic, MBP-specific T-line cells (S1) to induce EAE. As shown in FIGURE 2a and b, both nonirradiated and irradiated animals treated with the same dose of activated encephalitogenic T cells developed EAE. The course of the disease was practically identical—a self-limited disease course that began on day 5 and demonstrated spontaneous remission on days 7 and 8. However, when the animals were rechallenged with a second dose of encephalitogenic T cells on day 20, only the nonirradiated animals showed resistance to the autoaggressive T cells. Reconstitution of the irradiated recipients with normal spleen cells restored the capacity to develop resistance to the challenge of the encephalitogenic T cells (FIG. 2c).

The findings that transferred EAE in irradiated rats is self-limited and is inde-

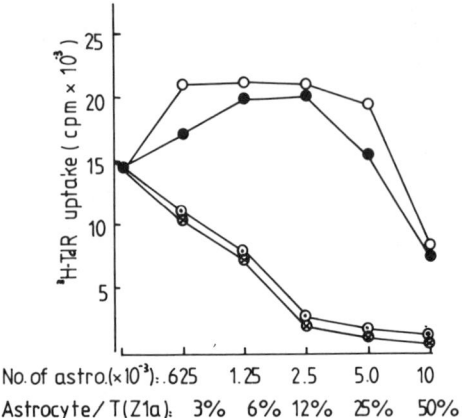

**FIGURE 1.** Immunodownregulatory effect of astrocyte clones. Myelin basic protein (MBP)-specific T-line cells (Z.Ia) were activated in cultures by irradiated syngeneic thymus cells (as antigen-presenting cells) and MBP. Clonal astrocytes were incubated in IFN-γ-containing medium for 48 hours, irradiated (4,000 R), and added in graded numbers to the cultures to evaluate their downregulatory potential. Clones B5 (⊙) and B10 (⊗) were downregulatory, whereas F10 (○) and C12 (●) were not.

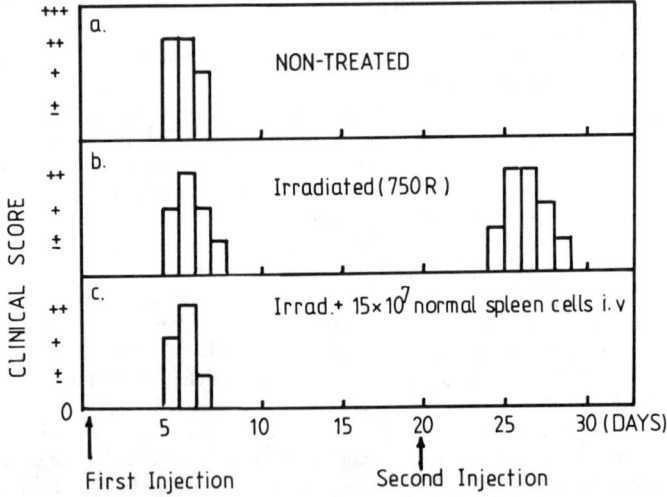

**FIGURE 2.** Transferred experimental allergic encephalomyelitis (EAE) in irradiated rats. Lewis rats were pretreated as indicated and were transferred with $2 \times 10^6$ myelin basic protein-specific encephalitogenic T cells for inducing and reinducing EAE. Lethally irradiated (750 R) Lewis rats failed to develop acquired resistance to the reinduction of transferred EAE, but their ability to recover from transferred EAE is maintained.

pendent from the acquired *resistance* which depends on immune cells suggest that nonimmune cells, probably elements of the CNS microenvironment, are responsible for the *recovery* from induced EAE in the Lewis rat. In the context of the *in vitro* demonstration that some but not all astrocytes can suppress activation of T cells, it is reasonable to believe that the suppressive activity of the local glial cells contributes to the recovery of Lewis rats from induced EAE.

# Autoantibody Reactive Integral Membrane Antigens of Thymocytes and Brain

## A. NARENDRAN AND S. A. HOFFMAN

*Department of Botany and Microbiology*
*Arizona State University*
*Tempe, Arizona 85287*

It is becoming increasingly apparent that many diseases with central nervous system (CNS) involvement have an immune pathogenesis. The current study is part of ongoing investigations to better understand the role of brain reactive autoantibodies in mediating CNS disorders in systemic lupus erythematosus (SLE).

Two murine models of SLE, NZB/W and MRL/lpr, were used to study the diversity of brain reactive autoantibodies and the cross-reactivity between autoantibody reactive brain and thymocyte integral membrane antigens.

Integral membrane proteins were prepared from brain and thymus of 4-week-old MRL/mp animals. Briefly, preparation entailed the solubilization of cell membranes of dissociated brain and thymus in a nonionic detergent (Triton X114) solution and the subsequent extraction of the integral membrane proteins by phase separation. These proteins were then separated on SDS-polyacrylamide gels under nonreducing conditions and transferred to nitrocellulose membranes. These membranes were then probed with sera from 6-month-old NZB/W and MRL/lpr mice followed by enzyme-labeled anti-mouse antibodies.

Results obtained indicate the following: (1) A diversity of brain reactive autoantibodies are displayed in the sera of NZB/W and MRL/lpr mice. Some of these antibodies are common to all (or most) of the animals within a strain; many are unique to individual animals. (2) A high percentage of the autoantibodies showed binding to antigens that were cross-reactive between brain and thymocytes. This was particularly true of the NZB/W strain, whereas the MRL/lpr mice showed a much lower percentage of such antibodies. (3) Those antibodies that bound to cross-reactive antigens appeared to be of the IgM isotype.

These results indicate the need to characterize the types of brain reactive autoantibodies found in autoimmune-mediated CNS disorders. They also raise the possibility that brain reactive autoantibodies of the IgM isotype may not be clinically significant in producing neuropsychiatric manifestations as they are more likely to be adsorbed out *in vivo* (an idea that would have to be further investigated).

# A Monoclonal Antibody with Anti-Lipomodulin Activity Reverses a β-Adrenergic Response[a]

### NINA L. PAUL,[b,c] CURTIS A. WILLIAMS,[c] AND NICOLE SCHUPF [d]

*[c] SUNY College at Purchase*
*Purchase, New York 10577*

*[d] Manhattanville College*
*Purchase, New York 10577*

To understand the role of autoantibodies in neuropsychiatric disorders, we have adapted *in vivo* assays to relate antigen molecules or cells to neurochemically coded behaviors. The test used here is the action of epinephrine (EPI) via β-adrenergic receptors in the lateral hypothalamus (LH) to suppress eating in rats deprived of food for 18 hours.

Lipomodulin, an inhibitor of phospholipase $A_2$ ($PLA_2$), is induced by glucocorticoids. $PLA_2$ converts membrane phospholipids to arachidonic acid, a precursor of prostaglandins (PGs) and other mediators of inflammation. Interactions between PGs and adrenergic receptor systems, especially beta systems, are reported in many tissues. Patients with systemic lupus erythematosus have circulating antibody with anti-lipomodulin (ALM) activity,[1] and they frequently display neuropsychiatric dysfunction. We predicted that ALM in the lateral hypothalamus would disrupt β-adrenergic function, possibly by the disinhibition of $PLA_2$ and increased production of PGs.

## METHODS

Cannulas to the lateral hypothalamus were implanted in 10 Charles River CD male rats. Animals were housed individually, with food and water freely available except on experimental days. Eighteen hours before the measured food intake period, food was removed from the cages. Phosphate-buffered saline solution (PBS) or 60 pmol of ALM (MAB.4-4C3,[2] supplied by M. Nirenberg) in 1.5 µl was injected at 0700 hours; PBS or 100 nmol of EPI in 1 µl was injected at 1200 hours, after which food intake was measured.

---

[a]This work was supported by National Institutes of Health Grant NS17168.

[b]Current address: Department of Epidemiology and Public Health, Yale University School of Medicine, New Haven, Connecticut 06510.

## RESULTS

Epinephrine significantly reduced food intake compared to PBS in both the 0-15 and 15-30 minute intervals (paired $t$ tests: $p < 0.01$; FIG. 1). ALM appears to reverse this effect, but this is not statistically significant. ALM (20 pmol) alone at 0.5, 1, and 5 hours before testing had no effect on food intake.

The animals could be separated into two groups on the basis of their response to EPI (ANOVA: $p < 0.001$; FIG. 2). In the responders, ALM completely reversed the suppression of eating by EPI (paired $t$ test: $p < 0.01$), but it had no effect in the nonresponders. An explanation for the differences in response to EPI was sought through histologic analysis of the cannula implantation site. The reaction site of the nonresponders was 0.3 mm posterior to that of the responders.

## CONCLUSION

Anti-lipomodulin reversed the effect of EPI on food intake by fasted rats. Although the results reported here are consistent with our initial hypothesis, the antibody (MAB.4-4C3) was later shown to react with other antigens in the brain;[3] therefore, the mechanism by which it decreased the $\beta$-adrenergic activity is unclear. It may be possible to test our hypothesis more convincingly with a carefully screened antibody

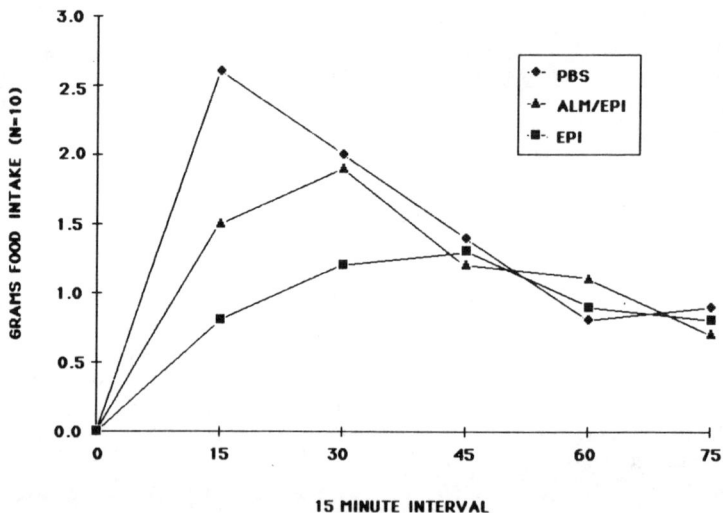

**FIGURE 1.** Epinephrine (EPI) inhibits food intake of fasted rats, and this inhibition is partially reversed by anti-lipomodulin (ALM). Food intake was measured at five consecutive 15-minute periods.

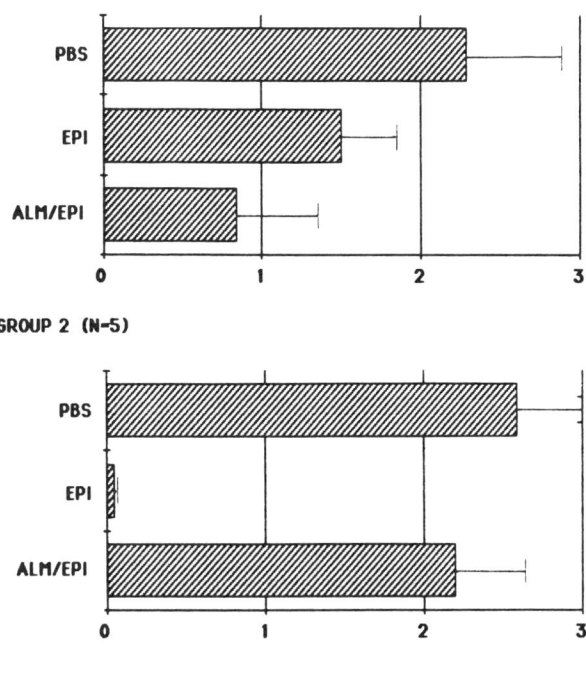

**FIGURE 2.** The animals responded as two groups to epinephrine (EPI) and anti-lipomodulin (ALM) plus EPI. The amount of food eaten during the first 15 minutes of testing is shown in the nonresponsive (group I) and responsive (group II) rats. PBS = phosphate-buffered saline solution.

to recombinant lipomodulin (lipocortin[4]). Our general conclusion, nevertheless, is that thoughtful selection of CNS sites and neurochemical systems can help to define a role for autoantibodies in CNS dysfunctions.

## REFERENCES

1. HIRATA, F., R. DEL CARMINE, C. A. NELSON, J. AXELROD, E. SCHIFFMANN, A. WARABI, A. L. DE BLAS, M. NIRENBERG, V. MANGANIELLO, M. VAUGHAN, S. KUMAGAI, I. GREEN, J. L. DECKER & A. D. STEINBERG. 1981. Proc. Natl. Acad. Sci. (USA) **78:** 3190-3193.
2. DE BLAS, A. L., N. A. BUSIS & M. NIRENBERG. 1981. *In* Monoclonal Antibodies to Neural Antigens: 181-191. Cold Spring Harbor Laboratory, New York.
3. DE BLAS, A. L., R. O. KULJIS & H. M. CHERWINSKI. 1984. Brain Res. **322:** 277-287.
4. WALLNER, B. P., R. J. MATTALIANO, C. HESSION, R. L. CATE, R. TIZARD, L. K. SINCLAIR, C. FOELLER, E. P. CHOW, J. L. BROWNING, K. L. RAMACHANDRAN & R. B. PEPINSKY. 1986. Nature **320:** 77-81.

# Antibody Cross-Reactivity Between Myelin Basic Protein and CD3 Antigen of T Cells

## Implications for Autoimmunity

W. WEBER,[a] Z. JINGWU,[b] J. BORST,[c]
AND W. BUURMAN [d]

[a]*Departments of Neurology and* [d]*General Surgery*
*Academic Hospital Maastricht*
*Maastricht, The Netherlands*

[b]*Dr. L. Willemsinstitute*
*Diepenbeek, Belgium*

[c]*Netherlands Cancer Institute*
*Amsterdam, The Netherlands*

This report describes the cross-reactivity between two biologically important human cell surface molecules, namely, myelin basic protein (MBP) and CD3 antigen of T cells, as recognized by murine monoclonal antibody (mAb) WW.B1. Myelin basic protein, a protein essential to signal conduction in the central nervous system, is a well-known target antigen for immune processes leading to autoimmune encephalomyelitis in humans and experimental animals. CD3, non-covalently linked to the specific T-cell receptor for antigen, is an essential signal transducer in human T-lymphocyte activation.

The hybridoma cell line secreting the WW.B1 mAb, which was originally raised against purified human MBP (as shown by enzyme-linked immunosorbent assay, radioimmunoassay, and immunoblotting), was subcloned three times and malignant ascites was produced. Mononoclonality of the ascites was assessed by isoelectric focusing. The WW.B1 mAb appeared to react with 70% of normal human peripheral blood T lymphocytes in Fluorescence-Activated Cell Sorter (FACS) analysis, an observation that was confirmed in experiments with cells of 24 healthy blood donors. Additional studies demonstrated that anti-MBP mAb WW.B1 was able to modulate the CD3 molecule off the surface of normal human T lymphocytes. Cross-absorption experiments indicated that the apparent anti-CD3 reactivity and the anti-MBP reactivity resided in one and the same antibody.

The WW.B1 antibody appeared to influence human T-lymphocyte functions in a mode similar to that of known anti-CD3 mAbs: it was highly mitogenic for normal human peripheral blood T lymphocytes and could block the specific cytolytic function of normal human cytolytic T-cell populations.

Immunoprecipitation studies with iodinated normal human peripheral blood mono-

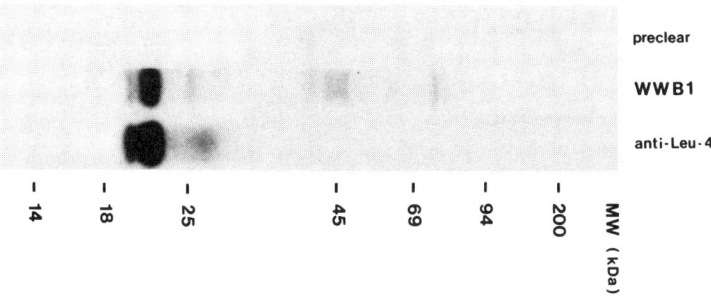

**FIGURE 1.** Immunoprecipitation of WW.B1 target antigen on T cells. $100 \times 10^6$ PBMC were surface labeled with 1 mCi of Na$^{125}$I (Amersham, U.K.) using 1,3,4,6-tetrachloro-3α,6α-diphenylglycoluril (Iodogen, Pierce Chemical Co., Rockford, IL) as a catalyst. Cells were lysed with 1% Nonidet P-40 in 0.01 M triethanolamine-HCl, pH 7.8, 0.125 M NaCl, 1 mM phenylmethylsulfonylfluoride, and 0.02 mg/ml trypsin inhibitor. Nuclear debris was removed by centrifugation, and immunoprecipitation was performed using protein A-CL4B sepharose beads (Pharmacia, Uppsala, Sweden) coated with mAbs, as described.[20] SDS-polyacrylamide electrophoresis was performed according to a modification of the Laemmli procedure, using a 10-15% gradient gel. For autoradiography, Kodak-XAR-5 film was used in combination with intensifier screens (Cronex Lighting Plus, Dupont, Newton, CT).

nuclear cells proved that WW.B1 reacted with the same 20-kd T-cell surface structure as did known anti-CD3 mAbs OKT3 and anti-Leu 4 (FIG. 1).

Since we found that mAb WW.B1 induced lysis of MBP-bearing cells by nonspecific cytolytic T-cell populations, possibly by cross-linking of MBP to CD3, the aforedescribed antibody cross-reactivity between MBP and CD3 may be an important mechanism in immune disorders involving the central nervous system.

Inflammatory processes within the brain compartment, leading to the formation of anti-MBP antibodies (as reported in diseases such as multiple sclerosis), may thus give rise, in certain individuals, to antibodies similar in reactivity to WW.B1. Such antibodies, also reacting with CD3, could influence T-cell functions *in vivo:* particularly, T cells could be induced to proliferate and perform nonspecific lysis of MBP-expressing cells, thus amplifying nonspecifically an ongoing inflammatory process leading to brain tissue damage. Conversely, the emergence of such anti-CD3 antibodies within the brain compartment might lead, by nonspecific suppression of T-cell function, to a relative immunodeficient state in the brain, thus enabling (slow) viruses to proliferate. Whether such mechanisms play a role in human disorders such as multiple sclerosis is currently under investigation in our laboratory.

# Expression of Class II Antigens on Peripheral Nerve Allografts

L. T. YU, W. F. HICKEY, W. S. SILVERS, D. LAROSSA, AND A. M. ROSTAMI

*University of Pennsylvania*
*Philadelphia, Pennsylvania*

Cellular major histocompatibility complex (MHC) antigen expression has been identified in demyelinating neuropathies[1] and the organ transplant rejection phenomenon.[2,3] To further investigate the expression of these antigens by cells in the peripheral nervous system, we studied the *in vivo* expression of MHC class I and class II antigens using a model of peripheral nerve allotransplantation.

## MATERIALS AND METHODS

A 4.25-cm peripheral nerve allograft (from Lewis [LE] rats) or isograft (from Brown Norway [BN] rats) was transplanted into a peroneal nerve gap surgically created in separate groups of recipient BN rats ($n = 15$). The grafts were resected and cryostat sections prepared at 4, 8, 15, 30, and 60 days after transplantation. Expression of MHC antigens was examined by immunohistochemical methods with the following monoclonal antibodies: OX-6 (recognizes LE and BN class II antigens), OX-3 (recognizes only LE class II antigens), OX-18 (recognizes LE and BN class I antigens), and I-169 (recognizes only LE class I antigens). T-cell subsets and macrophages were identified using appropriate monoclonal antibodies.[4] Donor (LE) or recipient (BN) origin of MHC antigens could be identified by comparing immunoperoxidase positive cells using these primary antibodies on serial sections of each graft specimen. All recipient animals were later skin grafted with LE skin to evaluate sensitization to LE transplantation antigens.

## RESULTS

The normal peripheral nerve expressed low levels of MHC class I and class II antigens (FIG. 1): class I on endothelial cells and class II on interstitial cells (Schwann cells or fibroblasts). After transplantation, LE nerve allografts expressed donor-derived (LE) class II antigens on the endothelial cells within the nerve (FIG. 2). Peak expression occurred 8 days after transplantation and was distinguished from isograft en-

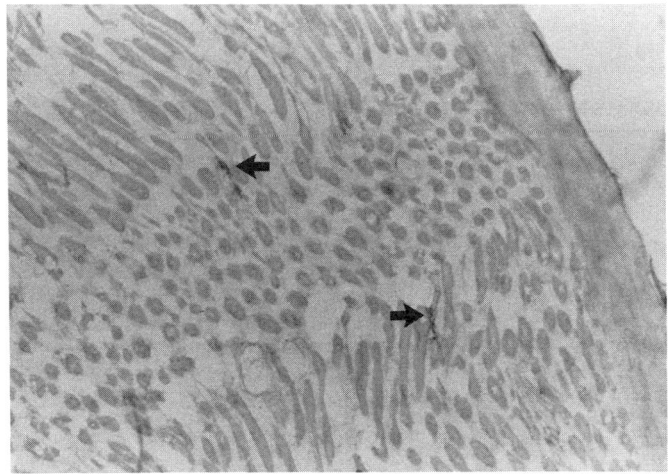

**FIGURE 1.** Normal peripheral nerve stained with OX-3, identifying baseline LE class II positive interstitial cells.

dothelial cells which remained class II antigen negative. Both iso- and allografts expressed high levels of donor-specific class I and class II antigens on interstitial cells between 8 and 15 days after transplantation. Maximal inflammation occurred on day 15. Although no donor antigens could be detected in allografts at 30 days, recipient T cells and macrophage infiltrates were evident in the nerve up to day 60. All nerve allografted recipients later rejected LE skin grafts in an accelerated fashion ( < 7 days).

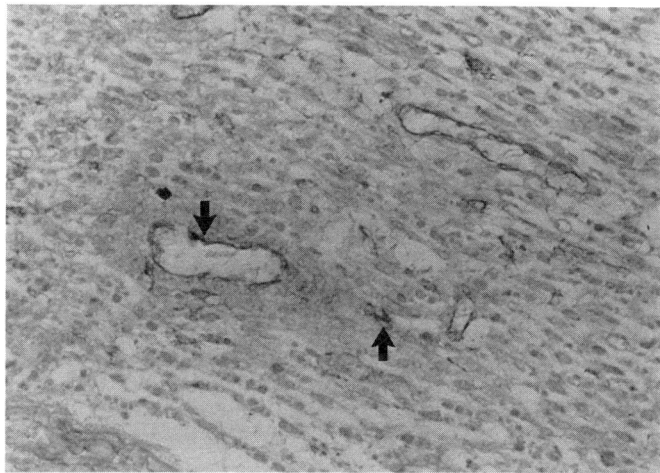

**FIGURE 2.** LE nerve graft 15 days after transplantation stained with OX-3, demonstrating stimulated expression of LE class II positivity on graft endothelial and interstitial cells.

## CONCLUSIONS

These studies demonstrate that: (1) Both MHC class I and II antigens are constitutively expressed at low levels in the normal peripheral nerve—class I on endothelial cells and class II on interstitial cells (Schwann cells or fibroblasts). (2) Graft cell expression of donor-derived MHC antigens can be up-regulated or induced by the *in vivo* allograft transplantation model in a pattern that can be distinguished from the nonspecific stimulation seen in isograft transplants. Endothelial cell expression of donor class II antigens is unique to the allograft phenomenon. Peak expression of all donor antigens occurs 8-15 days after transplantation and cannot be detected after 30 days, suggesting that the allograft rejection response has eliminated these cells. (3) The cells contained in the allograft are capable of sensitizing the recipient animal to donor transplantation antigens. Studies are in progress to characterize these cells and to determine their role in antigen presentation.

### REFERENCES

1. POLLARD, J. D. *et al.* 1987. Ann. Neurol. **21:** 337.
2. BARCLAY, A. N. & D. W. MASON. 1983. Nature **303:** 832.
3. STEINIGER, B. *et al.* 1985. Transplantation **40:** 234.
4. HICKEY, W. F. *et al.* 1983. J. Immunol. **131:** 6.

# Down-Regulation of Gamma-Interferon-Induced Class II Expression of Human Glioma Cells by Recombinant Beta-Interferon

JEYMOHAN JOSEPH, CONCETTA D'IMPERIO, ROBERT L. KNOBLER, AND FRED D. LUBLIN

*Jefferson Medical College
Philadelphia, Pennsylvania 19107*

Recombinant beta-interferon has been used in the treatment of glioblastoma multiforme[1] and more recently in the treatment of multiple sclerosis. We were interested in examining the role of beta-interferon in modulating class II antigen expression on central nervous system tissues, because of the role of this molecule in modulating antitumor immune response as well as autoimmune antigen presentation in multiple sclerosis. We used primary cultures derived from surgically resected glioblastoma multiforme tissue. Astrocytic identity of these cells was determined by immunofluorescence staining for glial fibrillary acidic protein. The influence of human recombinant interferon (Betaseron, Triton Biosciences, Alameda, California) on class II antigen expression on glioblastoma-multiforme-derived cells was examined.

The cultures were treated with varying doses of beta- and gamma-interferon (10, 100, 1,000, and 10,000 U/ml) for 72 hours, and class II (HLA-DR) antigen expression

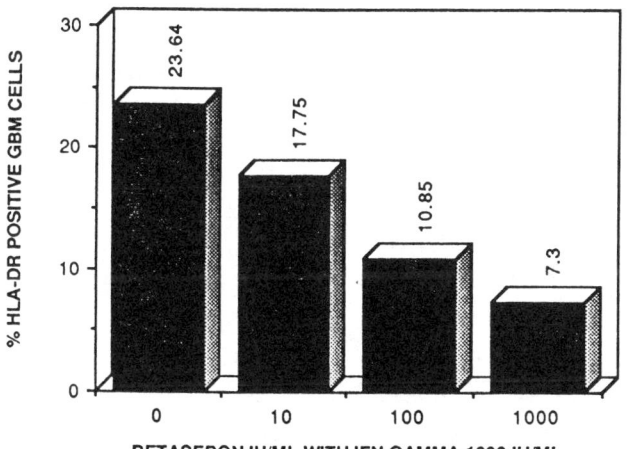

**FIGURE 1.** Interferon beta serine effects of gamma-interferon-induced HLA-DR when administered simultaneously. Cells were treated with 1,000 U/ml of gamma-interferon and varying doses of interferon beta serine (10, 100, and 1,000 U/ml).

was assessed by flow cytometry (Epics C, Coulter Diagnostics, Hialeah, Florida). Class II antigens were not constitutively expressed on these cells and were not induced by beta-interferon. However, recombinant gamma-interferon (Immuneron, Biogen, Cambridge, Massachusetts) increased class II expression on these cells in a dose-dependent manner. When increasing doses of beta-interferon are added simultaneously with an optimal dose of gamma-interferon, a dose-dependent decrease in class II expression is seen (FIG. 1). Such down-regulation of gamma-interferon-induced class II expression by beta-interferon was reported in murine macrophages.[2,3]

The timing of treatment of beta- and gamma-interferon appears to be crucial. With concurrent treatment using 100 U/ml of beta- and gamma-interferon, an 18% reduction in cells expressing class II antigen occurred (TABLE 1). Pretreatment of cultures for 72 hours with beta-interferon, followed by concurrent dosing with beta- and gamma-interferon, yielded a 90% reduction in class II expression compared with that of cells treated with gamma-interferon alone.

TABLE 1. Treatment Profile of Beta- and Gamma-Interferon (100 U/ml each)

| Treatment Profile | Percentage of HLA-DR-Positive Cells |
|---|---|
| Untreated | 2.13 |
| Gamma-interferon treatment for 72 hours | 47.59 |
| No pretreatment; beta- and gamma-interferon administered simultaneously for 72 hours | 37.13 |
| Beta-interferon pretreatment for 72 hours followed by combined treatment of beta- + gamma-interferon for 72 hours | 5.53 |
| Beta-interferon pretreatment for 72 hours followed by additional treatment with beta-interferon for 72 hours | 2.26 |

These findings suggest that beta-interferon can both down-regulate class II expression and block its induction on a human glioma cell culture, and that repeated treatment with beta-interferon is more effective in this regard than is a single dose.

## REFERENCES

1. DUFF, T. A., E. BORDEN, J. BAY, J. PIEPMEIR & K. SIELAFF. 1986. Phase II trial of interferon-beta for treatment of recurrent glioblastoma multiforme. J. Neurosurg. **64:** 408.
2. LING, P. D., M. K. WARREN & S. N. VOGEL. 1985. Antagonistic effect of interferon beta on interferon gamma induced expression of IA antigen in murine macrophages. J. Immunol. **135:** 1857.
3. INABA, K., M. KITAURA, T. KATO, Y. WATANABE, Y. KAWADE & S. MURAMATSU. 1986. Contrasting effects of alpha/beta and gamma interferons on expression of macrophage Ia antigens. J. Exp. Med. **163:** 1030.

# Neurotransmitter Modulation of the Human Class II Gene DRα on Multiforme Glioblastoma Cell Lines

## A Molecular Analysis

### J. TING, P. SHERMAN, S. YOKOTA, T. MOORE, AND P. BASTA

*Department of Microbiology*
*University of North Carolina*
*Chapel Hill, North Carolina*

Class II major histocompatibility (MHC) antigens are cell surface proteins that regulate the overall immune response by mediating interactions among various immunocompetent cells.[1] We are interested in class II antigen expression in the brain. It was shown in our laboratory and in others that a small population of cells in the brain express or can be induced to express class II antigens.[2-4] Expression of these antigens in the brain has been implicated in autoimmune-like diseases of the central nervous system.

In this study, we examined the ability of neurotransmitters to alter class II antigen

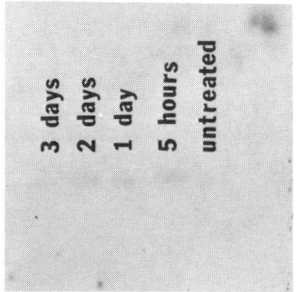 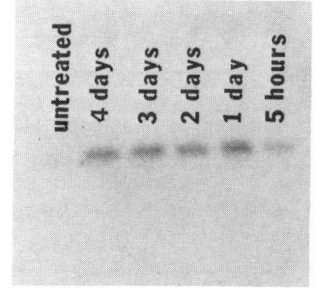

**FIGURE 1.** Northern analysis of untreated, isoproterenol-treated, and DBcAMP-treated U-373-MG. Total cellular RNA from untreated control, isoproterenol-treated (*panel A*), or DBcAMP-treated (*panel B*) cells was denatured and blotted onto nitrocellulose filters. The blot was hybridized to the DRα-specific probe, pp34-RI-3.[5] Seven and a half micrograms of RNA were used per lane; quantitative determinations were made by optical density and by hybridization to an rRNA-specific probe. Fresh isoproterenol was added each day at a concentration of $5 \times 10^{-6}$ M, according to time course specifications. DBcAMP (1 mm) was added once, at the start of each time point.

and mRNA expression. As a model system, we examined the expression of the human class II gene, DRα, in multiforme glioblastoma cells.[5] We showed that isoproterenol, a β-adrenergic agonist, increases both the RNA (FIG. 1) and the protein products (data not shown) of DRα. To determine if the DRα induction observed with this agonist was due to an increase in intracellular cAMP, we treated U-373-MG with the cAMP analog, 3':5'-cyclic monophosphate (DBcAMP), to artificially increase cAMP levels. RNA levels from cells treated with DBcAMP mimicked the response seen with isoproterenol (FIG. 1). To determine if this induction was transcriptionally regulated, we performed nuclear run-on experiments to measure newly synthesized transcripts (FIG. 2). The increase seen in newly synthesized DRα-specific transcripts in DBcAMP treated versus untreated groups correlated with the increase in steady state RNA, indicating transcriptional control. We have also begun to analyze the gene for regulatory sequences that are responsive to DBcAMP treatment, using the technique of DNA-mediated gene transfer. Preliminary evidence indicates that region −178 to −119 bp of the DRα gene is important in this regulation (data not shown).

In conclusion, isoproterenol causes the induction of both RNA and protein levels

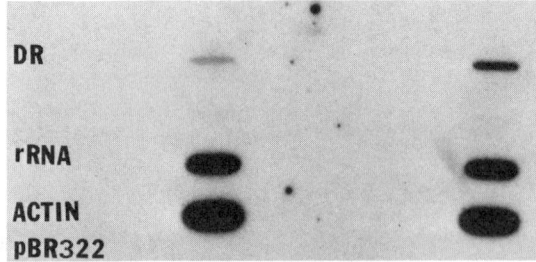

**FIGURE 2.** Nuclear run-on of untreated and DBcAMP-treated U-373-MG. Nuclei were prepared from both DBcAMP-treated and untreated U-373-MG cells, and 32P-labeled nascent transcripts were prepared, isolated, and used as probes for DNA immobilized on nitrocellulose, according to the method of Yuan and Tucker.[6]

of the human class II gene, DRα. The kinetics and level of this induced response indicate that it may be due to increased levels of cAMP. In addition, we have shown that the cAMP-mediated induction is transcriptionally regulated, and the DNA region required for this induction may be located within 178 base pairs of upstream DRα sequence.

## REFERENCES

1. BENACERAF, B. 1981. Science **212**: 1229.
2. TING, J. *et al.* 1981. Proc. Natl. Acad. Sci. USA **78**: 3170.
3. HAUSER, S. *et al.* 1983. J. Neuroimmunol. **5**: 197.
4. FONTANA, A. 1984. Nature **307**: 273.
5. BASTA, P. *et al.* 1986. J. Immunol. **138**: 1275.
6. YUAN, D. & P. TUCKER. 1984. J. Exp. Med. **160**: 564.

# Functional Implications of Class I MHC Modulation in Neural Tissue

LOIS A. LAMPSON,[a] JAMES P. WHELAN, AND
GABRIELA SIEGEL

*Departments of Anatomy and Neurology*
*University of Pennsylvania School of Medicine*
*and*
*Children's Cancer Research Center*
*Joseph Stokes Jr. Research Institute*
*Children's Hospital of Philadelphia*
*Philadelphia, Pennsylvania*

Although most normal neural cells lack major histocompatibility complex (MHC) products, greater expression can be seen in pathologic or experimental situations.[1] Whether these molecules serve an immunologic or a nonimmunologic role in cell differentiation or homeostasis is not known. We have focused on class I molecules. Previous work confirms that class I proteins with the appropriate mRNA, structure (1- and 2-D gels), and polymorphic specificity can be produced by human neural cell lines.[2] Here, we asked whether class I plays a role in the development or homeostasis of neural cells.

## MATERIALS AND METHODS

Beta$_2$-microglobulin (b2-m) is the invariant light chain of all class I molecules. A rabbit antiserum to murine b2-m was used as a broad probe for class I proteins in the mouse. The serum was used to examine frozen or formaldehyde-fixed, paraffin-embedded tissues in the avidin-biotin-complex (ABC) assay as described.[3] A rabbit serum to human b2-m, and a panel of monoclonal antibodies to b2-m and other class I determinants were used in the ABC assay to analyze frozen biopsy specimens of human tissue.[1] In all assays, well-characterized class-I-positive cells served as internal positive controls.

---

[a] Address for correspondence: Center for Neurologic Diseases, Biosciences Research Building, Brigham and Women's Hospital, Boston, MA 02115.

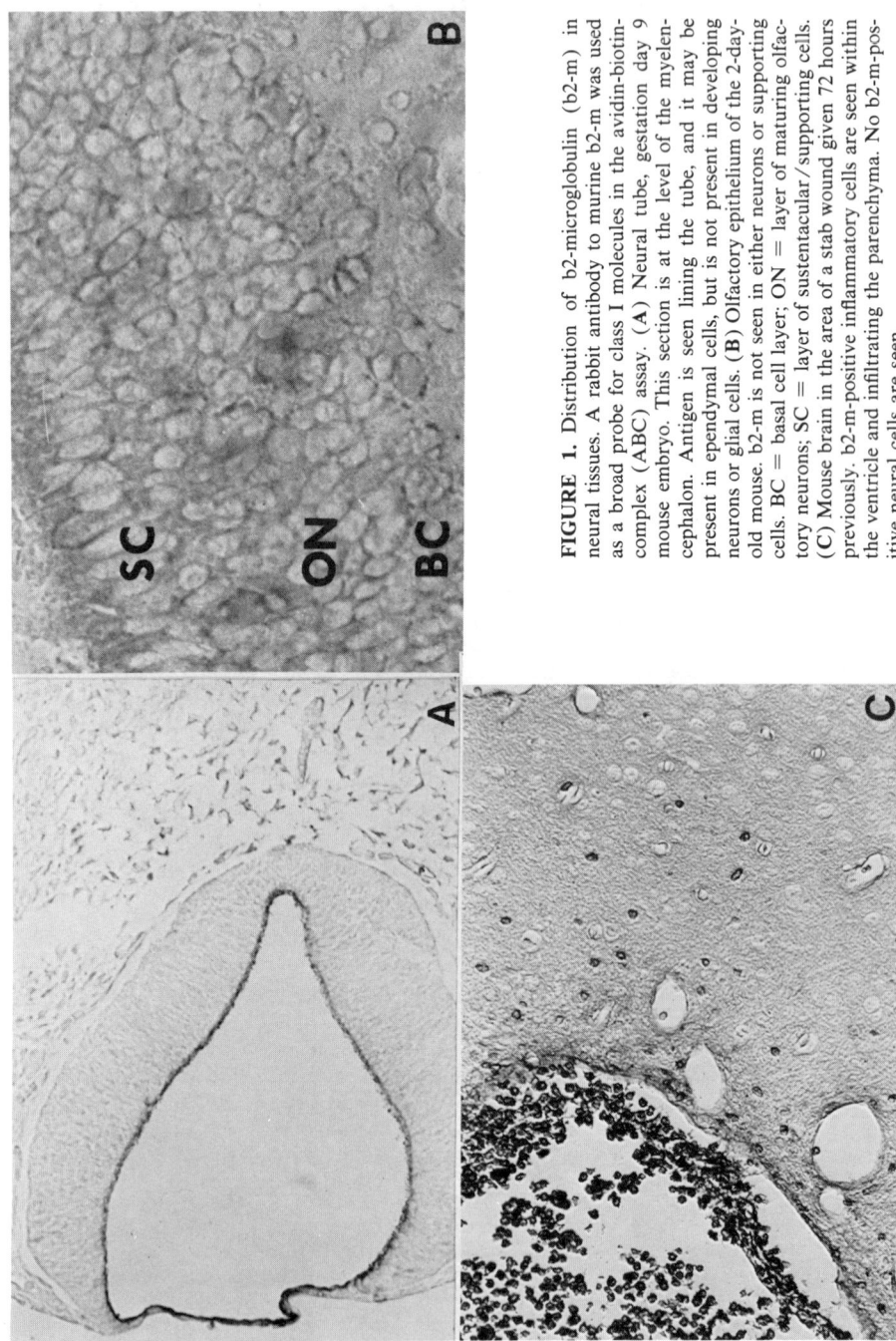

FIGURE 1. Distribution of b2-microglobulin (b2-m) in neural tissues. A rabbit antibody to murine b2-m was used as a broad probe for class I molecules in the avidin-biotin-complex (ABC) assay. (**A**) Neural tube, gestation day 9 mouse embryo. This section is at the level of the myelencephalon. Antigen is seen lining the tube, and it may be present in ependymal cells, but is not present in developing neurons or glial cells. (**B**) Olfactory epithelium of the 2-day-old mouse. b2-m is not seen in either neurons or supporting cells. BC = basal cell layer; ON = layer of maturing olfactory neurons; SC = layer of sustentacular/supporting cells. (**C**) Mouse brain in the area of a stab wound given 72 hours previously. b2-m-positive inflammatory cells are seen within the ventricle and infiltrating the parenchyma. No b2-m-positive neural cells are seen.

## RESULTS

In normal adult neural tissue, either human or murine, class I is detected only in blood vessel walls.[1] To examine developing tissue, mouse embryos at 7-14 days of gestation were studied in serial sections. b2-m was seen in nonneural cells, serving as an internal positive control. Yet b2-m was not detected on any neural cell type. The tissues examined included the neural tube, neural crest, spinal ganglia, and day-14 head[4] (FIG. IA).

The olfactory epithelium of the 2-day-old mouse was used as a model for regenerating neural tissue. b2-m-positive cells were seen in nonneural tissue, such as respiratory epithelium, but not in any neural cell (FIG. 1B). In addition to the olfactory epithelium, the vomeronasal organ, the olfactory bulb, and the rest of the day-2 head were also examined. No b2-m antigen was seen in neural cells.[5]

Much neural tissue is sequestered from blood-borne elements by a blood-tissue barrier. We asked whether class I modulation would be observed when neural cells are exposed to blood-borne modulators or to the external environment. The tissues examined included the area postrema, a barrier-free region of normal mouse brain; human neuroblastoma, a peripheral tumor; and human CNS gliomas, where the blood-brain barrier may be disrupted. Class I antigen was not seen in neural cells of the area postrema[3] or in most tumor cells.[1] The olfactory nerve endings were also negative.[5] In all cases, positive nonneural cell types were seen in the same sections.

To determine if class I expression would be increased in response to trauma, mouse brain was examined in the area of a stab wound. Reactive astrocytes in the wound area were strongly glial fibrillary acidic protein (GFAP) positive. b2-m was detected on infiltrating leukocytes, but not on the reactive astrocytes or on any other neural cell[6] (FIG. 1C).

## DISCUSSION

The accumulated evidence argues against a role for class I molecules in normal growth, differentiation, maintenance, or repair of neural cells, and against class I modulation as a nonspecific response to injury. These studies provide a background for interpreting the class I modulation that is seen in specific clinical situations.

## REFERENCES

1. LAMPSON, L. A. 1987. Molecular bases of the immune response to neural antigens. Trends in Neurosci. **10:** 211-216.
2. LAMPSON, L. A. & D. L. GEORGE. 1986. IFN-mediated induction of class I MHC products in human neuronal cell lines: Analysis of HLA and b2-m RNA and HLA-A and HLA-B proteins and polymorphic specificities. J. Interferon Res. **6:** 257-265.
3. WHELAN, J. P., U. ERICKSSON, & L. A. LAMPSON. 1986. Expression of mouse b2-microglobulin in frozen and formaldehyde-fixed central nervous tissue: Comparison of tissue behind the blood-brain barrier and tissue in a barrier-free region. J. Immunol. **137** 2561-2566.

4. LAMPSON, L. A. & J. P. WHELAN. 1987. A role for the major histocompatibility complex in normal differentiation of non-lymphoid tissues. Proceedings of the 19th Miami Winter Symposium. Advances in Gene Technology: Molecular Biology of Development. ICSU Short Reports **7:** 125.
5. WHELAN, J. P., C. J. WYSOCKI & L. A. LAMPSON. 1986. Distribution of b2-microglobulin in olfactory epithelium: A proliferating neuroepithelium not protected by a blood-tissue barrier. J. Immunol. **137:** 2567-2571.
6. LAMPSON, L. A. & G. SIEGEL. 1987. Defining the mechanisms that govern immune acceptance or rejection of neural tissue. Prog. Brain Res., in press.

# West Nile Virus Infection Modulates the Expression of Class I and Class II MHC Antigens on Astrocytes *in Vitro*

Y. LIU, N. KING, A. KESSON, R. V. BLANDEN, AND
A. MÜLLBACHER

*Department of Microbiology
John Curtin School of Medical Research
Australian National University
Canberra, Australia*

The major histocompatibility complex (MHC) antigens make an essential contribution to the antigen epitopes recognized by T lymphocytes, and the cell surface concentration of MHC antigen is an important variable in determining induction and effector function of T-cell-mediated immune responses. Therefore, the effect of viral infection on host MHC antigen expression may be an important mechanism modulating the immune response to certain viral infections.

Flaviviruses are a group of viruses that cause neurologic diseases. We have chosen the West Nile virus (WNV) as representative of the group for the study of the pathogenesis of infection in the central nervous system. We investigated the effect of WNV infection on the expression of class I and class II MHC antigens on astrocytes prepared from CBA/H ($H-2^k$) mouse neonates.

West Nile virus productively infects astrocytes and concomitantly induces interferon production. West Nile virus infection up-regulates class I and class II MHC antigen expression on the cell surface as detected by flow cytometry using monoclonal antibodies specific for $H-2K^k$, $H-2D^k$, and $H-2I-A^k$ (FIG. 1). Poly I:C, a synthetic interferon inducer, up-regulates class I MHC antigen expression to an extent similar to that obtained with WNV infection, but does not change class II MHC expression (FIG. 1c and f). These data suggest that up-regulation of class I MHC antigens may be interferon dependent.

West Nile virus infection enhances T-cell recognition of astrocytes. Astrocytes infected with influenza virus are not lysed by influenza virus immune cytotoxic T cells. However, astrocytes infected with WNV for 48 hours before influenza virus infection are susceptible to influenza virus immune cytotoxic T cells. Similarly, WNV-infected CBA/H ($H-2^k$) astrocytes stimulate an $H-2I^k$-specific alloreactive T-cell line, as measured by T-cell proliferation and interleukin-2 production, much more efficiently than do uninfected astrocytes. The stimulation can be blocked by $H-2I-A^k$-specific monoclonal antibody (FIG. 2).

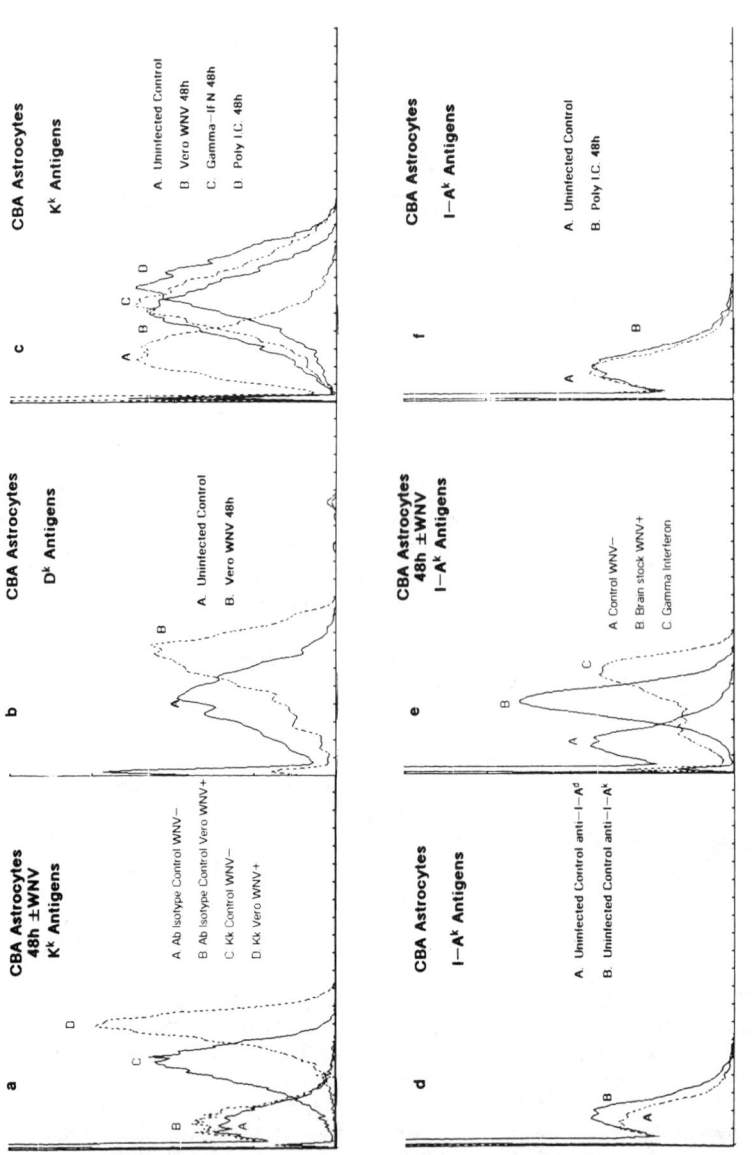

**FIGURE 1.** Expression of cell surface MHC antigens on astrocytes as determined by flow cytometry with monoclonal antibodies specific for MHC subregions.

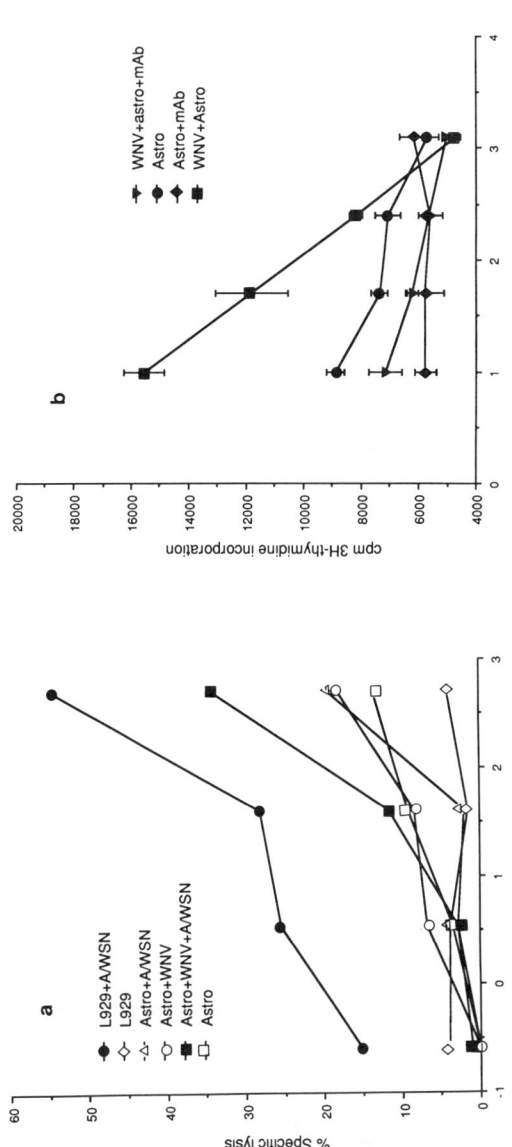

FIGURE 2. T-cell recognition of astrocytes. **a**, cytotoxicity of influenza virus A/WSN immune cytotoxic T cell, secondary culture; **b**, interleukin-2 release of H-2I$^k$-specific T-cell line, passage 11.

# Measles Virus Infection Causes Expression of Class I and Class II MHC Antigens in Rat Brain

T. OLSSON, J. MAEHLEN, A. LÖVE, L. KLARESKOG,
E. NORRBY, AND K. KRISTENSSON

*Department of Pathology and Neurology*
*Huddinge University Hospital*
*Department of Virology, SBL,*
*Karolinska Institute*
*Stockholm, Sweden*
*and*
*Department of Med. Phys. Chem.*
*Uppsala University*
*Uppsala, Sweden*

An important factor in the outcome of a viral infection is the occurrence of cells expressing major histocompatibility (MHC) class I and class II antigens, because activation and the effects or functions of T cells depend on recognition of the virus antigen in the context of MHC antigens. Under normal conditions, the nervous system has low levels of MHC antigen expression.[1] However, enhanced expression of both class I and class II MHC antigens occurs during certain circumstances. Among others, gamma-interferon and coronavirus infections induce both class I and class II antigen expression on neural cells *in vitro*.[2-5] We studied the extent to which these antigens can be induced during fatal or nonfatal measles virus encephalitis in the rat as well as the occurrence of immunocompetent cells in infected rat brains, as detected by immunostaining.[6]

Lewis rats (age 3-14 days) were injected intracerebrally with a hamster neurotropic strain (HNT) of measles virus. Controls received a similar suspension without virus. The animals were killed between day 4 and day 48 after inoculation, and the brains were dissected and frozen. Coronal sections were cut, fixed, and subjected to immunohistochemistry. Monoclonal antibodies to viral antigen, class I and II MHC antigen, and antibodies for T cells and T-cell subsets were used (TABLE 1), and the binding was visualized by a modified peroxidase antiperoxidase method.

In controls, anti-class I immunoreactivity was detected in intracerebral vessels, but not in brain parenchyma, and anti-class II immunoreactivity was absent within the brains of uninfected rats. In both young rats with fatal disease and older rats with a milder course of the infection, a marked induction of both class I and class II MHC antigens was detected (TABLE 1). The anti-class I immunoreactivity was distributed diffusely, probably involving most types of cells in the brain, whereas anti-class II immunoreactivity occurred mostly on cells around intracerebral vessels and in small foci in the brain parenchyma. The distribution of class I antigen was not limited to inflammatory cells or areas of the brain where viral antigens were demonstrated. This may suggest induction by some soluble signal substance released during the early phases of the viral infection. In 14-day-old rats with nonfatal infection, there was marked infiltration of T lymphocytes of cytotoxic/suppressor phenotype in the brain parenchyma, whereas T helper cell phenotypes were mainly located perivascularly. In brains from newborn rats with fatal injection none or only a few lymphocytes were detected.

In conclusion, our study emphasizes that the levels of class I and class II transplantation antigens can readily be enhanced in the brain during a viral infection, providing the necessary elements for lymphocyte activation and function.

TABLE 1. Detection of Different Antigen-Containing Cells by Use of a Panel of Monoclonal Antibodies and Immunoperoxidase Staining

| Infected Day Postpartum | Killed Day after Inoculation | 16AC5 Virus Nucleocapsid | Ox 18 Class I Antigen | Ox 6 Class II Antigen | W3/13 Pan T Cells | Ox 8 T Cytotoxic Suppressor | W3/25 T Helper |
|---|---|---|---|---|---|---|---|
| 3 | 9 | ++ | +++ | ++ | + | + | + |
| 14 | 9 | ++ | +++ | ++ | ++ | +++ | ++ |
| 14 | 49 | + | + | + | − | − | + |
| Controls | 4-49 | − | −[a] | − | − | − | − |

NOTE: Each row shows observations in 2-4 animals. The results are expressed as the average number of cells per visual field as evaluated on whole sections of the brains ( − = none; + = 1-2; ++ = 3-4; +++ = >5 labeled cells). For diffuse anti-class I immunoreactivity, reaction intensity and extension were graded.

[a] Brain parenchyma was unstained, whereas endothelial, choroid plexus, and ependymal cells showed anti-class I immunoreactivity.

## REFERENCES

1. VITETTA, E. S. & D. CAPRA. 1978. The protein products of the murine 17th chromosome: Genetics and structure. Adv. Immunol. 26: 147.
2. LAMPSON, L. A. & C. A. FISHER. 1984. Weak HLA b2-microglobulin expression of neuronal cell lines can be modulated by interferon. Proc. Natl. Acad. Sci. USA 81: 6476.
3. WONG, G. H. W., P. BARTLETT, I. CLARK-LEWIS, F. BATTYE & J. W. SCHRADER. 1984. Inducible expression of H-2 and Ia antigens on brain cells. Nature 310: 688.
4. FIERZ, W., B. ENDLER, K. RESE, H. WEKERLE & A. FONTANA. 1985. Astrocytes as antigen-presenting cells. I. Induction of Ia antigen expression on astrocytes by T cells via immune interferon and its effect on antigen presentation. J. Immunol. 134: 3785.
5. SUZUMURA, A., E. LAVI, S. R. WEISS & D. H. SILBERBERG. 1986. Coronavirus infection induces H-2-antigen expression on oligodendrocytes and astrocytes. Science 232: 991.
6. OLSSON, T., J. MAEHLEN, A. LÖVE, L. KLARESKOG, E. NORRBY & K. KRISTENSSON. 1987. Induction of class I and class II transplantation antigens in rat brain during fatal and non-fatal measles virus infection. J. Neuroimmunol. 16: 215.
7. MASSA, P. T., R. DÖRRIES & V. TER MEULEN. 1986. Viral particles induce Ia antigen expression on astrocytes. Nature 320: 543.

# Tumor Necrosis Factor Induces Expression of MHC Class I Antigens on Mouse Astrocytes

E. LAVI, A. SUZUMURA, D. M. MURASKO,
E. M. MURRAY, D. H. SILBERBERG, AND
S. R. WEISS

*Departments of Microbiology and Neurology
University of Pennsylvania School of Medicine
Philadelphia, Pennsylvania 19104*

Neural cells do not express major histocompatibility complex (MHC) antigens on their surface.[1] Nevertheless, under certain conditions, cells of the CNS may be subjected to immune-mediated reactions. To understand the pathogenesis of neurologic diseases with putative immune-mediated mechanism, it is necessary to identify factors that enhance MHC antigen expression on neural cells. Such expression, along with lymphocytic infiltration of the brain, is a prerequisite for cell-mediated immune reaction against CNS cells.[2] In vascular endothelial cells and dermal fibroblasts, tumor necrosis factor[3] (TNF) has been shown to modulate MHC class I antigen expression.[4] Therefore, we tested the effect of TNF on CNS cells.

## EFFECT OF TNF ON MHC ANTIGEN EXPRESSION

Astrocyte-enriched cultures (from C57BL/6 or BALB/c mice) treated with TNF showed significantly higher binding in radioimmunoassay than did untreated cultures when haplotype-specific anti-class I antibodies (anti-H-2D$^b$, K$^b$) were used, but not with nonhaplotype-specific anti-class I antibodies (anti-H-2D$^k$, K$^k$) (TABLE 1). Astrocyte-enriched cultures did not exhibit binding to anti-class II antibodies (anti-Ia$^b$) after TNF treatment. Oligodendrocyte-enriched cultures showed low background binding similar to that of negative controls with or without treatment with TNF. When graded concentrations of classical TNF were used, induction could be seen at $\geq 100$ U/ml but not at 10 U/ml (TABLE 2). Both mouse TNF[5] (classical TNF) and macrophage TNF[5] induced MHC class I expression on astrocytes (TABLE 2).

## CELL TYPE SPECIFICITY OF MHC EXPRESSION

Double immunofluorescence staining was used with anti-H-2 and cell specific markers. GFAP-positive cells (astrocytes) showed positive staining for MHC class I

TABLE 1. MHC Antigen Expression on C57BL/6 Mouse Glial Cells: Radioimmunoassay*

| Cells | Treatment | $H-2D^b,K^b$ | $I-A^b$ | SP2/0 | $H-2D^k,K^k$ |
|---|---|---|---|---|---|
| Astrocytes | - | 1,116 ± 92 | 1,009 ± 82 | 1,117 ± 80 | NT |
|  | TNF | 2,043 ± 136† | 1,182 ± 158 | 1,216 ± 30 | 1,182 ± 60 |
|  | TNF+anti-TNF | 1,129 ± 52 | 1,122 ± 129 | 1,267 ± 161 | 1,174 ± 20 |
| Oligodendrocytes | - | 624 ± 79 | 622 ± 26 | 689 ± 95 | 560 ± 23 |
|  | TNF | 639 ± 97 | 579 ± 65 | 555 ± 60 | 613 ± 57 |

*Data represent mean cpm ± standard deviation of triplicate coverslips.
†$p < 0.001$ when compared with negative controls.

antigens, but were negative for class II. Normal mouse serum, SP2/0 supernatant, and monoclonal antibodies against noncorresponding H-2 class I or class II did not stain these positive cells. GalC-positive cells (oligodendrocytes) did not show staining for either class I or class II antigens.

## SPECIFICITY OF TNF INDUCTION

When classical TNF was incubated with anti-TNF antibodies, H-2 antigen induction on astrocytes was blocked (TABLES 1 and 2). The anti-TNF antibodies that

TABLE 2. MHC Class I Antigen Expression in Mixed Glial Cultures after Various Treatments

| Treatment | H-2 Class I[a] |
|---|---|
| Classical TNF (U/ml) |  |
| 5,000 | + |
| 500 | − |
| 50 | − |
| Macrophage TNF (U/ml) |  |
| 1,000 | + |
| 100 | + |
| 10 | − |
| Macrophage TNF 100 U/ml + rabbit-anti-TNF 80 nu/ml | − |
| Macrophage TNF 100 U/ml + normal rabbit serum | + |
| Classical TNF 5,000 U/ml + rabbit-anti-TNF 80 nu/ml | − |
| IFN-γ 10 U/ml | + |
| IFN-γ 10 U/ml + rabbit-anti-mouse IFN-γ 100 nu/ml | − |
| IFN-γ 10 U/ml + normal rabbit serum | + |
| Classical TNF 5,000 U/ml + rabbit anti-IFN-γ 500 nu/ml | + |
| Classical TNF 5,000 U/ml + normal rabbit serum | + |
| Classical TNF 5,000 U/ml + sheep-anti-IFN-α/β 2,000 nu/ml | + |
| Classical TNF 5,000 U/ml + normal sheep serum | + |
| DME + 10% fetal calf serum | − |

[a]H-2 induction was assessed by indirect immunofluorescence on duplicate coverslips and read by two observers against a negative control consisting of similar cultures treated with SP2/0 medium supplemented with 100 μg/ml of an irrelevant IgG.

were prepared against classical TNF blocked H-2 induction on astrocytes treated with either classical TNF or macrophage TNF (TABLE 2). To rule out the possibility that interferon (IFN) in the TNF preparation could account for the induction of MHC antigens, the level of IFN in the classical TNF preparation was measured and was found to be 20 U/ml. However, when TNF was incubated with at least 10 times excess anti-IFN antibodies (either $\alpha/\beta$ or $\gamma$) before incubation with the cultures, induction of MHC class I antigens on astrocytes was not abolished (TABLE 2).

## CONCLUSION

The effect of TNF on expression of MHC antigens was examined in mouse glial cells *in vitro*. TNF induced MHC class I, but not class II, antigen expression on the surface of astrocytes but not on oligodendrocytes. Glial cells do not normally express detectable amounts of MHC antigens. Therefore, TNF may play a role in the immunopathogenesis of neurologic diseases that involve MHC class I restricted reactions.

### REFERENCES

1. LAMPSON, L. A. & W. F. HICKEY. 1986. Monoclonal antibody analysis of MHC expression in human brain biopsies: Tissue ranging from "histologically normal" to that showing different levels of glial tumor involvement. J. Immunol. **136:** 4054-4062.
2. BENACERRAF, B. 1981. Role of MHC gene products in immune regulation. Science **212:** 1229-1238.
3. BEUTLER, B. & A. CERAMI. 1986. Cachectin and tumor necrosis factor as two sides of the same biological coin. Nature **320:** 584-588.
4. COLLINS, T., L. A. LAPIERRE, W. FIERZ, J. L. STROMINGER & J. S. POBER. 1986. Recombinant human tumor necrosis factor increases mRNA levels and surface expression of HLA-A,B antigens in vascular endothelial cells and dermal fibroblasts in vitro. Proc. Natl. Acad. Sci. USA **83:** 446-450.
5. FLICK, D. A. & G. E. GIFFORD. 1986. Production of tumor necrosis factor in unprimed mice: Mechanism of endotoxin mediated tumor necrosis. Immunobiology **171:** 320.

# Characterization of B Cells and IA Expression in Sindbis Virus Encephalitis

## W. R. TYOR, T. R. MOENCH, AND D. E. GRIFFIN

*Departments of Medicine and Neurology*
*The Johns Hopkins University School of Medicine*
*Baltimore, Maryland 21205*

Sindbis virus (SV) is an alphavirus closely related to Western equine encephalitis virus that causes an acute, nonfatal meningoencephalitis in immunologically normal and athymic mice when injected intracerebrally. The inflammatory response is characterized by subependymal and perivascular mononuclear infiltrates. These mononuclear cells include helper and suppressor T cells, B cells, and macrophages. Early in encephalitis the majority of cells are helper T cells. Initially, B cells comprise a small percentage of the total inflammatory cells, but this percentage steadily increases during the course of encephalitis. The role of T cells in recruiting B cells into the central nervous system (CNS) has not been defined. In addition, the stage of differentiation and antigen specificity of these B cells are unknown.

To better characterize B cells entering the CNS and compare them with B cells in the periphery, antibodies against B cells and mouse immunoglobulin isotypes were used to immunocytochemically identify all B cells bearing these markers in the inflammatory cuffs, spleens, and peripheral blood of mice with SV encephalitis. In conjunction with our studies of B cells we examined the expression of IA antigen in the CNS of normal and athymic mice during this acute viral encephalitis.

Sindbis virus encephalitis is characterized initially by B cells that express IgM or IgM/IgD (day 3 after SV inoculation). These cells for the most part are replaced later in the encephalitis (day 10-14) by B cells with IgG1, IgG2a, and IgG2b on their surfaces. This process is reflected in the spleen. Normally, B cells in the spleen express IgM and IgD, with much smaller percentages bearing the IgG and IgA isotypes. During SV encephalitis IgM-labeled B cells decrease in the spleen, and IgG2a- and IgG2b-labeled B cells increase.

The demonstration in athymic nude mice of markedly decreased numbers and percentages of B cells in perivascular inflammatory cuffs suggests that T cells are required for the subsequent infiltration of B cells during SV encephalitis. The B cells that do enter continue to express primarily IgM, indicating a lack of maturation to the more "mature" isotypes.

IA is initially expressed by perivascular mononuclear cells in the brain on day 2 after SV inoculation. Later, it is also expressed by stellate parenchymal cells and perivascular endothelial cells and/or pericytes. In nude mice the expression of IA in all of these cell types is markedly blunted, suggesting that T cells are required for the full expression of IA in the brain.

## REFERENCES

1. MOENCH, T. R. & D. E. GRIFFIN. 1984. Immunocytochemical identification and quantitation of the mononuclear cells in the cerebrospinal fluid, meninges, and brain during acute viral meningoencephalitis. J. Exp. Med. **159:** 77.
2. ABNEY, E. R. *et al.* 1978. Sequential expression of immunoglobulin on developing mouse B lymphocytes: A systematic survey that suggests a model for the generation of immunoglobulin isotype diversity. J. Immunol. **120:** 2041.
3. RODRIGUEZ, M. *et al.* 1987. Immune response gene products (Ia antigens) on glial and endothelial cells in virus-induced demyelination. J. Immunol. **138:** 3438.

# MHC-Dependent Neural Allograft Rejection

### K. RAO,[a] H. W. KUNZ,[b] T. J. GILL, III,[b] AND R. D. LUND [a]

[a]*Department of Neurobiology,
Anatomy and Cell Science*
*and*
[b]*Department of Pathology
University of Pittsburgh School of Medicine
Pittsburgh, Pennsylvania 15261*

Previous work in this laboratory investigated the viability of retinas transplanted from embryonic CD-1 mouse embryos into the brains of newborn Sprague-Dawley rats. Sixty-three percent of these retinas survive and make substantial connections with appropriate regions of the host brains. However, when CD-1 mouse skin is grafted onto the host rat subsequent to neural transplantation, 96% of the retinal transplants are rejected. We have extended this experimental approach, using genetically defined inbred and congeneic rat strains to determine the extent of involvement of (1) antigens associated with the major histocompatibility complex (MHC) (RTI) and (2) the non-MHC antigens.

Retinas taken from fetal (DA) ($RT1^a$) rats of a gestational age of 14-15 days were transferred to the cerebral aqueduct of neonatal (BN) ($RT1^n$) rats. One month later, the host was challenged with skin grafts from animals that differed from the recipients at (1) both MHC and non-MHC loci (DA), (2) MHC loci only (BN.1A), and (3) non-MHC loci only (DA.1N) (TABLE 1). Serum samples taken from the recipient animals before and after skin grafting were analyzed for antibodies against RT1 and non-MHC antigens. This analysis was performed to study the response of the host immune system to both the neural grafts as well as the subsequently placed skin grafts.

Animals were sacrificed 6-14 days after skin grafting. Frozen sections (30 $\mu$m) of the brain were cut, and adjacent series of sections were stained by various techniques in order to study the cellular organization and the degree of lymphocytic infiltration of the retinal transplants.

TABLE 1. Genetic Disparity Between Donor Strains of Congeneic Rats and BN Recipients

| Donor Strain | RT1 Haplotype | At MHC Loci | At Non-MHC Loci |
|---|---|---|---|
| DA | a | Different | Different |
| BN.1A | a | Different | Identical |
| DA.1N | n | Identical | Different |
| BN | n | Identical | Identical |

From the results that are available so far, it appears that the rejection of allografts is dependent on both MHC and non-MHC antigens. The time taken for the onset (as evidenced by the presence of lymphocytes around the blood vessels within the transplant) and the progress of the rejection process seems to be different in these two cases. The retinal transplants in the brains of animals receiving no skin grafts survived at least 3.5 months. Antibody levels indicate that in 4 of 24 animals studied, the host immune system had been sensitized by the neural allograft. These animals were excluded from further investigation. In the control group comprised of BN animals that had been transplanted with BN retinas as newborns, no evidence of host sensitization was found.

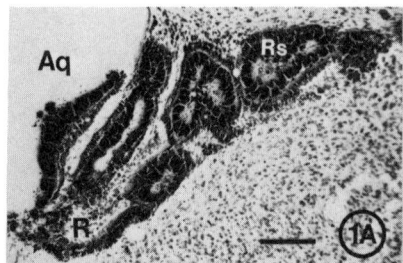
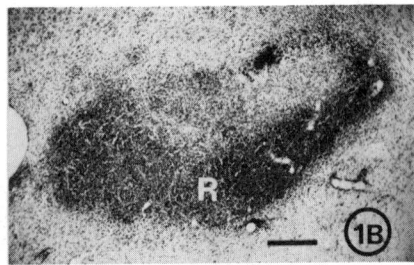

**FIGURE 1.** (A) Nissl-stained coronal section of a rat midbrain, showing a retinal transplant (R) adjacent to the cerebral aqueduct (Aq). The retina was allowed to survive for 4 weeks. The retinal xenograft was taken from an embryonic mouse and placed in a rat 1 day after birth. It has differentiated into the normal retinal layers seen here in the form of rosettes (Rs). Bar signifies 150 $\mu$m. (B) Nissl-stained coronal section of a rat midbrain, showing a rat retinal allograft (R) undergoing rejection. The retina was taken from an embryonic DA rat and placed in a newborn BN rat. One month later, skin from a BN.1A rat was grafted onto the flank of the host rat. The lack of clear definition of the layers is the result of lymphocytic infiltration. Bar signifies 150 $\mu$m.

## REFERENCES

1. RAO, K., R. D. LUND, H. W. KUNZ & T. J. GILL, III. Immunological implications of xenogeneic and allogeneic transplantation to neonatal rats. *In* Progress in Brain Research. D. M. Gash & J. R. Sladek, Jr., Eds. Elsevier, New York. In press.
2. LUND, R. D., K. RAO, M. H. HANKIN, H. W. KUNZ & T. J. GILL, III. 1987. Transplantation of retina and visual cortex to rat brains of different ages: Maturation, connection patterns and immunological consequences. Ann. N. Y. Acad. Sci. **495**: 227-241.
3. KUNZ, H. W. & T. J. GILL, III. 1974. Genetic studies in inbred rats. 1. Two new histocompatibility alleles. J. Immunogen. **1**: 413-420.

# MHC Antigen Expression on Glial Cells

AKIO SUZUMURA AND DONALD H. SILBERBERG

*Department of Neurology*
*University of Pennsylvania*
*Philadelphia, Pennsylvania*

We have shown that lymphokines, especially gamma-interferon ($\gamma$-IFN), induce major histocompatibility complex (MHC) class I antigen expression on oligodendrocytes and astrocytes.[1,2] More recently, we demonstrated that $\gamma$-IFN induces MHC class II antigen expression on isolated macrophage-microglia.[3] MHC class II antigen expression on astrocytes is reportedly inducible by $\gamma$-IFN[4] or viral infection.[5] In the previous study, we found that infection of the central nervous system with MHV-A59, a neurotropic coronavirus, induces class I, but not class II, MHC antigen expression on oligodendrocytes and astrocytes.[6] We sometimes found Ia antigen expression on $\gamma$-IFN-treated astrocytes by indirect immunofluorescence; however, this finding could not be confirmed by radioimmunoassay.

In this study, we examined more precisely the expression of MHC antigen on glial cells by indirect immunofluorescence (IF), radioimmunoassay (RIA), and $^{51}$Cr release assay. Oligodendrocyte-enriched (Oligo), astrocyte-enriched (Ast) cultures and isolated macrophage-microglia (Mi) were stimulated with $\gamma$-IFN (50 U/ml for 2 days). They were then examined for the expression of MHC antigens.

Unstimulated Oligo and Ast did not express either class I (H-2) or class II (Ia) antigen on their surface. $\gamma$-IFN induces H-2 antigen expression on both Oligo and Ast. Although Ia antigen was sometimes detected on $\gamma$-IFN-treated astrocytes (FIG. 1), most Ast usually remained Ia negative even after $\gamma$-IFN treatment.

Radioimmunoassay confirmed the induction of H-2 antigen, but not Ia antigen, on Oligo and Ast (TABLE 1). By $^{51}$Cr release assay using the same monoclonal anti-MHC antibodies plus complement, we detected H-2 antigen expression on unstimulated Mi, and both H-2 and Ia antigen on $\gamma$-IFN-treated Mi. However, we could not detect Ia antigen on $\gamma$-IFN-treated Ast under the same assay conditions (TABLE 2).

This study confirmed the induction of class I MHC antigen expression on Oligo and Ast by three different assays. We could detect Ia antigen on $\gamma$-IFN-treated Mi. However, we could not confirm Ia antigen expression on $\gamma$-IFN-treated astrocytes by

TABLE 1. MHC Antigen Expression: Radioimmunoassay[a]

| AKR | H-2D$^k$K$^k$ | I-A$^k$ | I-E/C$^k$ | MEM | H-2D$^b$K$^b$ | I-A$^b$ |
|---|---|---|---|---|---|---|
| Oligo | 1,264 ± 89[b] | 546 ± 102 | 571 ± 46 | 653 ± 49 | 601 ± 74 | 556 ± 93 |
| Ast | 3,437 ± 362[b] | 1,086 ± 70 | 1,026 ± 27 | 1,182 ± 173 | 1,127 ± 188 | 1,252 ± 183 |

[a]Each culture was treated with 50 U/ml of $\gamma$-IFN for 2 days before assay.
[b]$p < 0.001$.

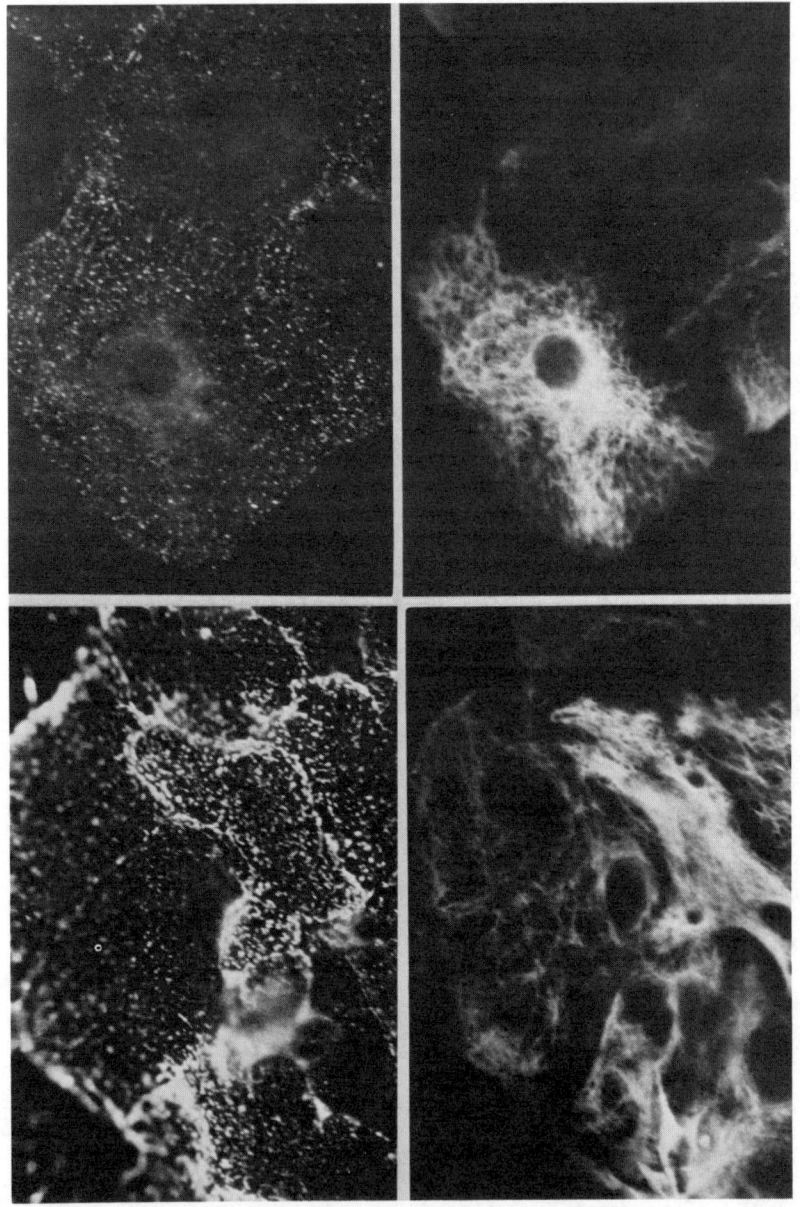

**FIGURE 1.** Induction of H-2 antigen expression (*left*) and Ia antigen (*right*) on GFAP-positive astrocytes by γ-IFN.

TABLE 2. MHC Antigen Expression: $^{51}$Cr Release Assay[a]

|  |  | H-2D$^k$K$^k$ | I-A$^k$ | I-E/C$^k$ | MEM | H-2D$^b$K$^b$ | I-A$^b$ |
|---|---|---|---|---|---|---|---|
| Mi | (−) | 31.2 ± 10.9[b] | 14.9 ± 1.0 | 15.5 ± 6.1 | 13.7 ± 2.5 | 14.8 ± 2.2 | 16.8 ± 4.2 |
|  | γ-IFN | 47.3 ± 5.0[b] | 39.5 ± 6.7[b] | 28.7 ± 9.0[b] | 15.5 ± 4.2 | 14.5 ± 6.2 | 16.4 ± 4.2 |
| Ast | (−) | 10.3 ± 1.9 | 12.2 ± 2.8 | NT | 11.4 ± 2.0 | 10.0 ± 1.0 | 10.1 ± 4.9 |
|  | γ-IFN | 34.4 ± 3.2[b] | 12.8 ± 2.2 | 13.2 ± 3.7 | 12.4 ± 1.9 | 11.2 ± 3.3 | 10.8 ± 0.7 |

[a]Each value represents mean ± standard deviation of individual % $^{51}$Cr release ($n = 9$).
[b]$p < 0.001$.

means of RIA and $^{51}$Cr release assay. These observations, along with the fact that Mi have very similar properties as peripheral blood macrophages,[3] suggest a possible immunoregulatory function of Mi as is characteristic of the cells of monocyte lineage.

## REFERENCES

1. SUZUMURA, A. & D. H. SILBERBERG. 1985. Brain Res. **336:** 171-175.
2. SUZUMURA, A. et al. 1986. J. Neuroimmunol. **11:** 179-190.
3. SUZUMURA, A. et al. 1987. J. Neuroimmunol. **15:** 263-278.
4. WONG, G. H. W. et al. 1984. Nature **310:** 688-691.
5. MASSA, P. T. et al. 1986. Nature **320:** 543-546.
6. SUZUMURA, A. et al. 1986. Science **232:** 991-993.

# Accessory Cell Competence of Human Glial Cells in Mitogenic Activation of Resting Peripheral T Cells

N. CASHMAN,[a] S. BOULET,[a] L. CRAGG,[a]
L. BAMBRIDGE,[b] AND J. ANTEL[a]

*Departments of Neurology [a] and Biochemistry [b]
McGill University
Montreal, Quebec, Canada*

We previously demonstrated that highly purified sheep oligodendrocytes exhibit accessory-cell activity in mitogenic activation of human peripheral T cells with OKT3[1] and Concanavalin A (Con A),[2] but we were unable to determine if cross-species interactions, including possible sheep T11 receptor binding, contributed to T-cell activation. We now demonstrate that human glial cells also exhibit accessory cell function.

Glial cells were isolated from surgically resected white matter obtained by trypsin dissociation, Percol gradient centrifugation, and differential substrate adherence, using the method of Kim et al.,[3] and were cultured 5 to 30 days before use. Astrocyte-enriched (lobar white matter) and oligodendrocyte-enriched (corpus callosum) cultures were 80-95% glial fibrillary acidic protein (GFAP) or galactocerebroside (GC) immunoreactive, respectively. The majority of unstained cells in preparations were fusiform, probably fibroblasts. In two experiments, no cell stained for OKM-1, a monocyte marker. We had no microglial-specific stain. Double staining with major histocompatibility complex (MHC) monoclonal antibodies and GFAP or GC antibodies established that some astrocytes and oligodendrocytes expressed class I and class II MHC antigens.

T cells were purified by sequential sheep RBC rosetting, plastic adherence, nylon wool fractionation, and leucine methyl ester treatment. Thereafter, 10-20K potential accessory cells (astrocytes, oligodendrocytes, skin fibroblasts, or peripheral E$^-$ cells) were irradiated with 6-10K rads and co-cultured in RPMI + 10% fetal calf serum with 100K autologous or allogenic T cells in microtiter wells, in the presence and absence of mitogens. At 3 days, cultures were pulsed with $^3$(H)-thymidine, harvested, and counted.

Purified human T cells were not stimulated by OKT3 in the absence of accessory cells (FIG. 1). T cells also were not significantly stimulated in 3-day co-cultures with glial cells, skin fibroblasts, or autologous or allogenic E$^-$ cells in the absence of OKT3 (FIG. 1, TABLE 1). Mitogenic stimulation was observed (FIG. 1, TABLE 1) when T cells were co-cultured with E$^-$ cells (SI range 7.0-859), astrocytes (SI 12.3-330), and oligodendrocytes (SI 13.6-2922) in the presence of OKT3; skin fibroblasts provided no accessory function. T-cell preparations, devoid of stimulation when cultured

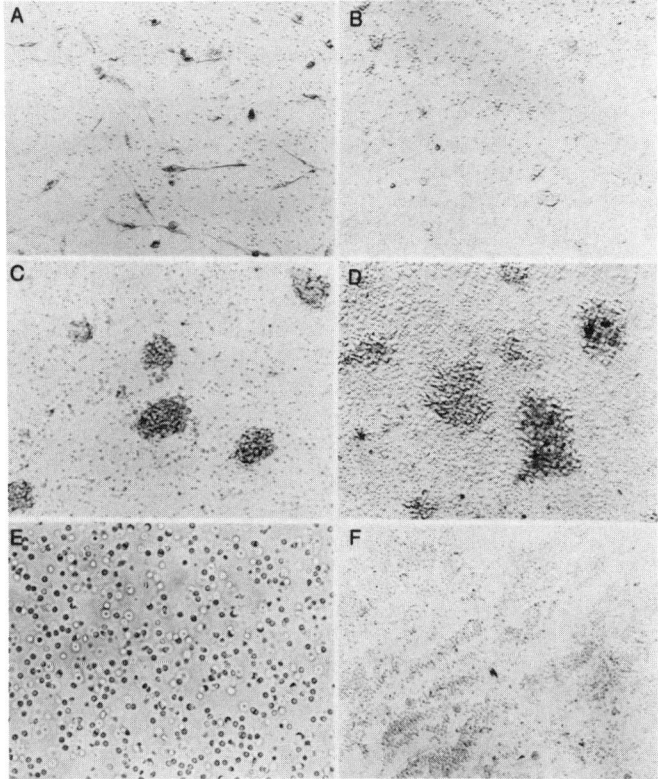

**FIGURE 1.** Glial cultures provide accessory cell function in mitogenic activation of purified human T cells by OKT3. A and B, No blastogenic response to T cells co-cultured for 3 days with astrocyte-enriched (A) or oligodendrocyte-enriched (B) glial cultures. C and D, Blastogenic transformation of T cells induced by the addition of OKT3 10 ng/ml to sister cultures of A and B. E, No OKT3 activation of T cells in the absence of accessory cells. F, No OKT3 activation of T cells co-cultured with human fibroblasts.

TABLE 1. Accessory Cell-Mediated OKT3 Mitogenesis[a]

| Culture Conditions | T Cells + E⁻ Cells | T Cells + Astrocytes | T Cells + Oligodendrocytes |
|---|---|---|---|
| No antibody | 331 ± 106 | 1,184 ± 958 | 424 ± 221 |
|  | ($n = 5$) | ($n = 4$) | ($n = 4$) |
| + OKT3 | 106,184 ± 72,214 | 65,794 ± 45,944 | 55,996 ± 32,215 |
|  | ($n = 4$) | ($n = 4$) | ($n = 4$) |

[a] One hundred thousand purified human T cells were co-cultured with 50,000 E⁻ cells or 10-20,000 astrocyte-enriched or oligodendrocyte-enriched human glial cells in the presence or absence of OKT3 10 ng/ml. Results are expressed in ³(H)-thymidine cpm ± SEM.

with Con A (SI <2), also exhibited proliferation when co-cultured with accessory E⁻ cells, astrocytes, and oligodendrocytes.

Our data indicate that human glial cells can serve as accessory cells for OKT3-induced and Con-A-induced activation of both autologous and allogenic T cells. Accessory cell-mediated OKT3 activation requires membrane Fc receptors and secretion of a soluble second signal.[4] Although we were able to exclude contaminating monocytes in our glial preparations, we were unable to achieve absolute purity of astrocytic and oligodendrocytic preparations. Thus, a nonmonocytic Fc receptor-bearing cell was present in our glial cultures, which was also capable of secreting a second signal for T-cell activation. The competence of glial cells to provide accessory function for T-cell mitogenesis suggests a model for brain lymphocyte activation in inflammatory neurologic diseases.

## REFERENCES

1. CASHMAN, N. R. & A. NORONHA. 1986. J. Immunol. **136:** 4460-4463.
2. CASHMAN, N. R., A. B. C. NORONHA, K. E. BRIGHT & M. A. JENSEN. 1986. Ann. Neurol. **20:** 169.
3. KIM, S. U. 1985. J. Neuroimmunol. **8:** 255-282.
4. HARA, T. & S. M. FU. 1985. J. Exp. Med. **161:** 641-656.

# Microglia Express MHC Class II in Normal and Demyelinating Human White Matter

G. M. HAYES, M. N. WOODROOFE, AND
M. L. CUZNER

*Multiple Sclerosis Society Laboratory
Department of Neurochemistry
Institute of Neurology
London, England*

In this study we reexamined the potential for antigen presentation in the brain by detailed analysis of major histocompatibility complex (MHC) class II expression in white matter from the normal control brain and that of patients with multiple sclerosis (MS).[1-3] Tissue blocks were analyzed immunohistochemically with two anti-MHC class II antibodies directed against the extracellular domain and the cytoplasmic tail of the HLA-DR molecule, respectively, in conjunction with markers for microglia and astrocytes.

## METHODS

*CNS Tissue:* (a) Normal-appearing white matter was dissected postmortem from the brain and spinal cord of seven patients with MS, three active and four chronic. (b) Normal and neurologic (OND) control tissue was obtained at postmortem examination in eight and five patients, respectively, with an age range of 33-64 years.

*Immunocytochemistry:* Ten-micron frozen sections were fixed in acetone at 4°C for 10 minutes. The avidin-biotin peroxidase complex method was used to visualize the antigens. The monoclonal antibodies used in this study included EBM/11, a macrophage/microglia marker supplied as a supernatant from Dakopatts (High Wycombe, Bucks, UK), TAL 1B5 specific for the HLA-DR determinant of MHC class II, a purified antibody at a protein concentration of 2 mg/ml (Dr. P. Beverley, UCH, London), and VIC-Y1, an undiluted monoclonal supernatant specific for the cytoplasmic invariant chain of class II MHC (Dr. W. Knapp, Vienna).

## RESULTS

Antibody titration curves for TAL 1B5 (FIG. 1) and EBM/11 were similar. At all antibody dilutions, the number and staining intensity of positive cells were greater in MS tissue than in control brain (FIG. 2). On hematoxylin counterstaining the MS group had the greatest mean cellularity (1,227 ± 238). The two control groups were similar (normal, 803 ± 244; OND 915 ± 291). When the numbers of EBM/11-positive and TAL 1B5-positive cells were plotted against each other, the ratio was 1:1 in all three groups. The active MS cases had the largest number of positive cells (up to 320 positive cells/mm$^2$) when compared with those of any other group (80-160 positive cells/mm$^2$). The morphologic characteristics and distribution of the EBM/11-positive and TAL 1B5-positive cells were similar and did not resemble those of GFAP-positive cells.

## DISCUSSION

In normal human white matter the predominant cell type expressing MHC class II is the microglia. This population of cells reacts with the pan macrophage marker, EBM/11, and constitutes about 13% of the glial cell population. The intensity of staining was enhanced and the absolute number of class II positive microglia increased in normal-appearing white matter from the brain of patients with MS.[4] As T-cell activation in MS may occur in the brain, the up-regulation of MHC class II microglia may reflect their function as antigen-presenting cells in the development of inflammatory lesions.

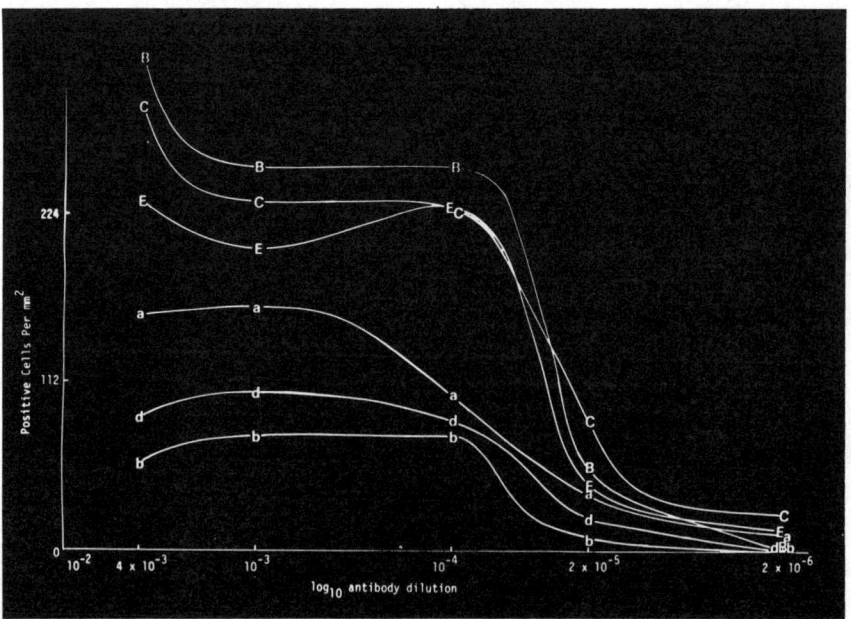

**FIGURE 1.** The effect of antibody dilution on the quantitation of TAL IB5-positive cells in control (**a, b, and d**) and MS (**B, C, and E**) white matter.

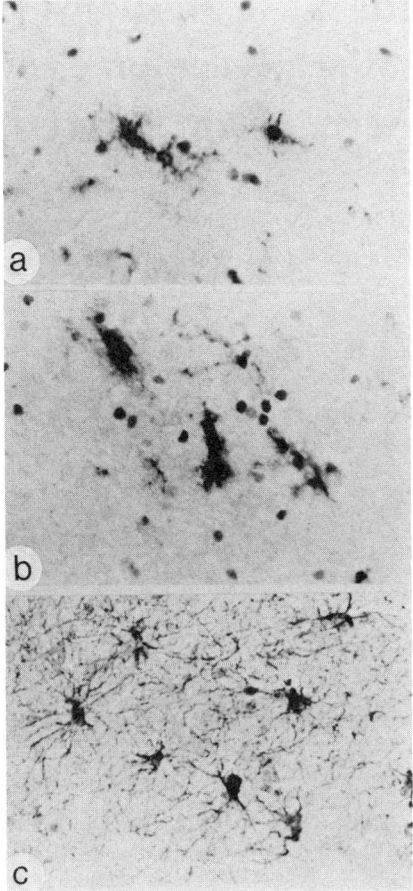

**FIGURE 2.** Frozen sections of white matter from (**a**) control and (**b**) MS brain stained by the "ABC" peroxidase method for MHC class II with monoclonal antibody TAL IB5 (diluted 1:1000). Panel **c** is MS white matter stained with anti-GFAP for astrocytes (diluted 1:5000) (magnification × 600).

## REFERENCES

1. TRAUGOTT, U., C. SCHEINBERG & C. S. RAINE. 1985. J. Neuroimmunol. **8:** 1-14.
2. LAMPSON, L. A. & W. F. HICKEY. 1986. J. Immunol. **136:** 4054-4062.
3. WOODROOFE, M. N., A. S. BELLAMY, M. FELDMAN, A. N. DAVISON & M. L. CUZNER. 1986. J. Neurol. Sci. **74:** 135-152.
4. HAYES, G. M., M. N. WOODROOFE & M. L. CUZNER. 1987. J. Neurol. Sci. **80:** 25-37.

WORKSHOP 9. MONOCLONAL ANTIBODIES IN AChR EPITOPES

# Proliferative Responses to Acetylcholine Receptor Peptides in Myasthenia Gravis

S. BERRIH-AKNIN,[a] S. COHEN-KAMINSKY,[a]
D. NEUMANN,[b] J. F. BACH,[c] AND S. FUCHS[b]

[a]CNRS UA 04-1159
Centre Chirurgical Marie-Lannelongue
92350 Le Plessis-Robinson, France

[b]Department of Chemical Immunology
Weizmann Institute
Israel

[c]INSERM U25
Hôpital Necker
75730 Paris, France

Myasthenia gravis (MG) is an autoimmune disorder of neuromuscular transmission. Antibodies directed against acetylcholine receptor (AChR) are detected in more than 85% of patients' sera.[1,2]

The recent availability of the entire AChR sequence makes it possible to use a synthetic peptide approach to analyze the distribution of antigenic determinants. The cholinergic binding site has been localized in the 185-196 fragment of the α-subunit, and one of the phosphorylation sites in AChR has been located in the large cytoplasmic domain of the α-subunit.[3,4] A highly immunogenic region was also described at the 351-368 region.[5] The peptide α-125-147 can induce experimental allergic myasthenia gravis and anti-AChR antibody production which cause antigenic modulation.[6]

We employed synthetic peptides corresponding to selected domains of the α-subunit of human (H) or torpedo (T) AChR in a proliferation assay using peripheral blood lymphocytes from 34 patients with MG and 17 healthy volunteers. The specific aims of this study were first to define some epitopes of the AChR involved in MG autoimmune response and second, by comparing the responses to H and T peptides, to identify species-specific epitopes. Eight peptides prepared as previously described[7] were used: three H peptides (169-181, 185-196, and 351-368) and the corresponding T peptides as well as T 330-340 and T 394-409 peptides were also investigated. Responses were considered positive when higher than the mean of the controls + 2.6 SD for each peptide.

Several conclusions were drawn: (1) H peptide 169-181 located nearby the α-bungarotoxin (α-Bgt) binding site induced a proliferative response in 8 of 34 patients with MG. The corresponding T peptide was positive in only two patients included in the eight patients responding to the H peptide. (2) Peptide 185-196, which included part of the α-Bgt binding site, gave negative responses whether it was from the human or the torpedo sequence. (3) Peptide 351-368, corresponding to a highly immunogenic region, induced a positive response in 5 of 34 cases with the human sequence. With the torpedo equivalent, only two patients (among the five patients with a positive response) responded. (4) Torpedo peptides T 330-340 and T 394-409 induced a positive response in three cases for each of the two peptides, but only in patients with a positive response to either the H 169-181 or the H 351-368 peptide. (5) Patients responding to the peptides generally presented with IIb grade severity and a high anti-AChR antibody titer. (6) There was no positive response with an unrelated peptide control. Furthermore, no positive response was observed in the healthy controls.

It should be noted that a proliferative response was obtained against a cytoplasmic site (351-368 peptide), thus being independent of α-subunit conformation. This result is consistent with those of Fuchs and Lindstrom,[5,8] demonstrating that this region is highly immunogenic as reflected by the presence of antibodies to this portion after immunizing animals with denatured AChR. To explain the autoreactivity against a cytoplasmic part of the AChR, one could hypothesize that cytoplasmic epitopes become accessible after degradation of AChR sites by antibodies[9-11] and after processing by antigen-presenting cells. Finally, it should be underlined that although most positive responses were obtained with the human sequence, there is a partial cross-reactivity between human and torpedo peptides, namely for the 169-181 and 351-368 domains.

Taken altogether, our results indicate that in MG, autoreactive clones specific to defined domains of the AChR α-subunit can be stimulated by the corresponding synthetic peptides. These domains might be involved in MG autoimmune anti-AChR response. The current study provides direct evidence for the involvement of sequences 169-181 and 351-368 of the α-subunit of AChR in the autoimmune response occurring in patients with MG.

## REFERENCES

1. LINDSTROM, H. M., M. L. SEYBOLD, V. A. LENNON, S. WHITTINGHAM & D. D. DUANE. 1976. Neurology (Minneap.) **26:** 1054-1059.
2. COMPSTON, D. A. S., A. VINCENT, J. NEWSOM-DAVIS & J. R. BATCHELOR. 1980. Brain **103:** 579-601.
3. NEUMANN, D., D. BARCHAN, M. FRIDKIN & S. FUCHS. 1986. Proc. Natl. Acad. Sci. USA **83:** 9250-9253.
4. SAFRAN, A., D. NEUMANN & S. FUCHS. 1986. Embo. J. **5:** 3175-3178.
5. SOUROUJON, M. C., D. NEUMANN, S. PIZZIGHELLA, A. SAFRAN & S. FUCHS. 1986. Biochem. Biophys. Commun. **135:** 82-89.
6. LENNON, A. V., D. J. MCCORMICK, E. H. LAMBERT, G. E. GRIESMANN & Z. ATASSI. 1985. Proc. Natl. Acad. Sci. USA **82:** 8805-8809.
7. NEUMANN, D., J. M. GERSITONI, M. FRIDKIN & S. FUCHS. 1985. Proc. Natl. Acad. Sci. USA **82:** 3490-3493.
8. LINDSTROM, 1986. J. Trends Neurosci. **9:** 401-407.
9. DRACHMAN, D. B., R. N. ADAMS, L. F. JOSIFEK, A. PESTRONK & E. F. STANDLEY. 1981. Ann. N.Y. Acad. Sci. **377:** 175-187.
10. ENGEL, A. G., K. SAHASHI & G. FUMAGALLI. 1981. Ann. N.Y. Acad. Sci. **377:** 158-174.
11. LENNON, V. A., M. E. SEYBOLD, J. LINDSTROM, C. COCHRANE & R. J. YULEVITCH. 1977. Exp. Med. **147:** 973.

# Responsiveness of Myasthenia Gravis Lymphocytes to Recombinant Interleukin-2

S. COHEN-KAMINSKY, S. BERRIH-AKNIN,
AND D. SAFAR

*CNRS UA 04-1159*
*Centre Chirurgical Marie-Lannelongue*
*92350 Le Plessis-Robinson, France*

Myasthenia gravis (MG) is an autoimmune disorder of neuromuscular transmission characterized by the presence of autoantibodies directed against acetylcholine receptor (AChR).[1] Although thymectomy leads to clinical improvement, the anti-AChR antibody titers do not decrease significantly after surgery,[2] indicating that other mechanisms are probably implicated in the pathogenesis of MG. In addition, several arguments reviewed in reference 3 suggest a close relation between disease pathogenesis and thymic function. Thus, we examined if cellular mechanisms could be involved, and we investigated the activation status of thymic and peripheral blood lymphocytes in MG by testing their ability to respond to recombinant interleukin-2 (r-IL-2) without previous stimulation.

Peripheral blood lymphocytes (PBLs) in MG and hyperplastic thymuses from thymectomized patients were collected at Marie-Lannelongue hospital. Controls were healthy blood volunteers and fragments of thymus from subjects undergoing cardiac surgery. Proliferative response to r-Il-2 of PBLs was significantly higher in patients with MG ($n = 124$) than in controls ($n = 46$) (TABLE 1). Correlations established about clinical features revealed a higher PBL response to r-IL-2 in young patients with a high anti-AChR antibody titer and a IIB grade severity and in patients before thymectomy. Furthermore, the response decreased with delay after thymectomy. The group studied before thymectomy ($n = 30$) was significantly different from the group studied at least 6 months after surgery ($n = 94$) ($p < 0.05$). No correlation was observed between r-IL-2 response and sex, T4/T8 ratio and corticosteroid treatment. Thymic lymphocytes gave similar results for kinetics of the response and optimal r-IL-2 dose. However, the magnitude of the response was generally higher compared with that of blood lymphocytes. The MG group ($n = 24$) was significantly different from the control group ($n = 17$) (TABLE 1).

The response to r-IL-2 of PBLs or thymocytes was time- and dose-dependent of r-IL-2 (optimal at 6-day treatment with 20-50 U/ml of r-IL-2) and could be inhibited by a blocking anti-IL-2 receptor antibody (anti-TAC), which supports the specificity of the response and proves that the proliferation observed is mediated by the binding of IL-2 to its receptor. The high proliferative response of MG lymphocytes was well correlated with an increase in TAC-positive cells during the culture with r-IL-2 as evaluated by flow cytometry analysis. In cultures of thymocytes, the TAC-positive cells were found to be T cells totally CD37 negative and CD2 positive, CD1 negative, mostly CD3 positive, and partially DR positive. In the blood, occasionally few TAC-positive cells were found CD37 positive.

Taken altogether, these data suggest that in MG a high proportion of T lymphocytes, namely, those from the thymus, show functional signs of preactivation, which is reflected by a hyperreactivity to r-IL-2 of MG lymphocytes without previous stimulation. Because this hyperreactivity is found mainly in MG thymic cells or in PBLs of patients only before thymectomy, it is suggested that the responsible cells could originate in the thymus. They could result from a primary autosensitization against an AChR-like molecule previously demonstrated in the thymus.[4] After thymectomy, these cells could decrease in the periphery. The subsequent disappearance of hyperreactivity to r-IL-2 in PBLs of most patients with MG 1 year after surgery, associated with a general clinical improvement after thymectomy,[5] supports this hypothesis. Finally, these lymphocytes could represent autoreactive cells involved in the pathogenesis of MG through a T-cell mechanism. However, it should be pointed out that phenotypic signs of activated T cells (namely, IL-2 receptor expression) could not be detected on freshly extracted cells. Therefore, our results raise the possibility of a

TABLE 1. Correlations between Clinical Data and Lymphocyte Proliferation to r-IL-2[a]

| Cells | Group | Patient Number | $\Delta$cpm ± SEM | $p$ Value versus Controls |
|---|---|---|---|---|
| PBL | Controls | 46 | 15,408 ± 1,345 | — |
|  | MG | 124 | 23,265 ± 1,822 | <0.02 |
| Thymocytes | Controls | 17 | 27,147 ± 2,793 | — |
|  | MG | 24 | 59,154 ± 6,545 | <0.001 |

[a] The proliferation of PBLs or thymocytes to 6-day treatment with 20 U/ml of r-IL-2 is expressed as $\Delta$cpm (cpm with r-IL-2 − cpm without r-IL-2).

different IL-2-receptor regulation and/or expression on MG T cells, as described in multiple sclerosis.[6] Alternatively, MG T lymphocytes could have receptor dysfunction related to the expression of an abnormal IL-2-receptor molecule as demonstrated in T-cell leukemia.[7] Establishing the validity of these nonmutually exclusive theories deserves further investigation.

**REFERENCES**

1. LINDSTROM, J. M., M. L. SEYBOLD, V. A. LENNON, S. WHITTINGHAM & D. D. DUANE. 1976. Neurology (Minneap.) **26:** 1054-1059.
2. ENGEL, A. G. 1984. Ann. Neurol. **16:** 519-534.
3. BERRIH-AKNIN, S., E. MOREL, F. RAIMOND, S. SAFAR, C. GAUD, J. P. BINET, P. LEVASSEUR & J. F. BACH. Ann. N.Y. Acad. Sci. **505:** 50-70.
4. RAIMOND, F., E. MOREL & J. F. BACH. 1984. J. Neuroimmunol. **6:** 31-34.
5. LE BRIGAND, H., P. LEVASSEUR, A. R. MIRANDA, C. GAUD & I. WOJAKOWSKI. 1980. Ann. Chir. **34:** 169-172.
6. DE FREITAS, E. C. S. SANDBERG-WOLLHEIM, K. SCHONELY, M. BOUFAL & H. KOPROWSKY. 1986. Proc. Natl. Acad. Sci. (USA) **83:** 2637-2641.
7. YODOI, J. & T. UCHIYAMA. 1986. Immunol. Rev. **92:** 135-156.

# Monoclonal Antibodies as Probes for Acetylcholine Receptor Epitopes in Thymuses and Thymic Epithelial Tumors of Patients with Myasthenia Gravis and Nonmyasthenic Controls

THOMAS KIRCHNER,[a] SOCRATES TZARTOS,[b]
FLORIAN HOPPE,[a] BERTHOLD SCHALKE,[c]
HARTMUT WEKERLE,[d] AND HANS KONRAD
MÜLLER-HERMELINK [a]

[a]*Institute of Pathology*
*University of Würzburg*
*Würzburg, FRG*

[b]*Hellenic Pasteur Institute*
*Athens, Greece*

[c]*Department of Neurology*
*University of Würzburg*
*Würzburg, FRG*

[d]*Max-Planck-Society*
*Clinical Research Unit for Multiple Sclerosis*
*Würzburg, FRG*

Myasthenia gravis (MG) is associated with heterogeneous thymus changes. Thymitis with lymphoid follicular hyperplasia (LFH) is found in 60-80% and thymoma in 10% of the patients. These divergent morphologic findings correspond to different clinical groups of patients with MG and might be related to various mechanisms of tolerance breakdown. A possible link between them could be the expression of acetylcholine receptors (AChRs) or AChR-like epitopes (Eps) in both tumor-free thymuses and thymic epithelial tumors of patients with MG. Previously α-bungarotoxin (α-Bgt) binding sites were demonstrated on thymic myoid cells (MyCs)[1] and epithelial cells (ECs),[2] and recently a cobrotoxin binding protein was isolated from MG-associated thymomas.[3] However, α-Bgt binding may not sufficiently prove the presence of complete AChRs.[4] Therefore, we applied monoclonal antibodies (mAbs) for an *in situ* demonstration of AChR Eps on thymic cells.

Normal thymuses of 10 nonmyasthenic persons (age 2 days-57 years), thymitis with LFH in 13 patients with MG (age 8-45 years), thymic epithelial tumors of 8 patients with MG (age 36-72 years), and 6 patients without MG (age 47-72 years) were studied by immunohistochemistry on cryostat section. MAbs 152, 153, and 155[5] to the cytoplasmic site of the α-AChR subunit, as well as mAbs 195, 202, 203, and 207[6] to the extracellular main immunogenic region (MIR) of the α-AChR subunit were used with comparable final concentrations (0.3-1.0 μg/ml). These mAbs labeled human motor endplates, but only showed few minor cross-reactions with some skeletal muscle fibers, nerve fibers, and fat cells in extrathymic human tissues. Thymic cells with AChR Eps were characterized by double immunostaining (indirect immunoperoxidase technique for the first antigen and alkaline phosphatase technique for the second antigen) using mAbs to AChR Eps and mAbs to cytokeratin for ECs, vimentin for mesenchymal cells, and desmin for MyCs. Results were compared with the intrathymic binding of the FITC-labeled α-Bgt that was shown to be inhibited by preincubation with unlabeled α-Bgt.

In all tumor-free thymuses of MG and nonmyasthenic patients, mAbs to the cytoplasmic site of α-AChR subunit and FITC-α-Bgt bound to MyCs and a subset of ECs at Hassall's corpuscles (FIG. 1a). Epithelial cells were not labeled by mAbs

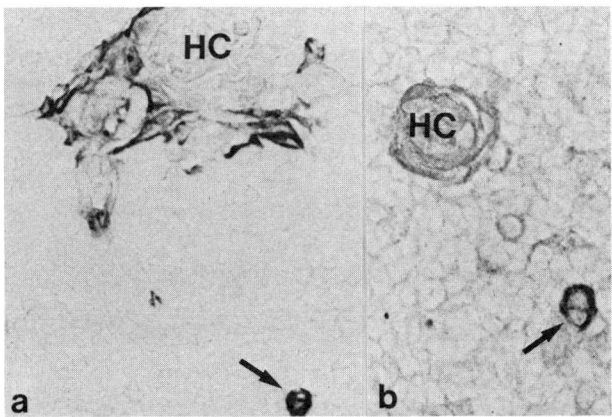

**FIGURE 1.** Acetylcholine receptor epitopes in tumor-free thymus. (**a**) MAb 155 to the cytoplasmic site of the α-subunit labels some epithelial cells at a Hassall's corpuscle (HC) and a round myoid cell (*arrow*); magnification × 308. (**b**) MAb 207 to the extracellular main immunogenic region only binds to a round myoid cell; magnification × 480.

to the extracellular MIR of AChRs. However, a minority of MyCs also expressed MIR Eps (FIG. 1b). They were found to be less common in patients with MG (MIR-positive MyCs in 4 of 13 thymuses) than in nonmyasthenic controls (MIR-positive MyCs in 5 of 10 thymuses).

In thymic epithelial tumors, mAbs to the cytoplasmic site of α-AChR subunit and FITC-α-Bgt labeled neoplastic ECs (FIG. 2). Binding was seen only in some tumors, and significantly correlated with the presence of MG. All 8 tumors in patients with MG, but only 2 of 6 tumors in patients without MG showed positive neoplastic ECs. There was no expression of MIR Eps within the neoplasms. Myoid cells were detected only in tumor-free thymic remnants, but not inside the tumors.

We assume that MyCs might express complete AChRs including the MIR, whereas non-neoplastic and neoplastic thymic ECs probably contain only incomplete AChRs or receptor-like molecules that must still be further defined. Generally, intrathymic

AChR Eps are not MG specific, because they also occur in nonmyasthenic persons. However, a correlation between the expression of AChR epitopes and the presence of MG is found for thymic epithelial tumors. Additional studies have to prove if the different expression of AChR Eps in tumor-free thymuses and thymic epithelial tumors is related to heterogeneous region specificities of serum AChR antibodies in patients with MG.

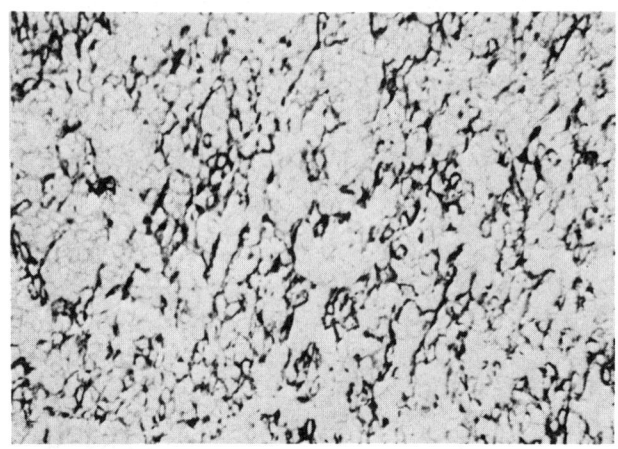

**FIGURE 2.** Acetylcholine receptor epitopes in thymoma. MAb 155 to the cytoplasmic site of the α-subunit strongly labels neoplastic epithelial cells; magnification × 240.

## REFERENCES

1. KAO, I. & D. B. DRACHMAN. 1977. Science **195:** 74-75.
2. ENGEL, W. K. *et al.* 1977. Lancet **I:** 1310-1311.
3. KAWANAMI, S. *et al.* 1987. J. Neurol. **234:** 207-210.
4. WHITING, P. J. *et al.* 1987. Nature **327:** 515-518.
5. TZARTOS, S. *et al.* 1986. J. Neuroimmunol. **10:** 235-253.
6. TZARTOS, S. *et al.* 1983. FEBS Letters **158:** 116-118.

# Stimulation of Autoimmune Helper T Lymphocytes from Patients with Myasthenia Gravis with Synthetic Peptides of the Acetylcholine Receptor Alpha Subunit[a]

REINHARD HOHLFELD,[b] KLAUS V. TOYKA,[b]
LUCINDA L. MINER,[c] AND
BIANCA M. CONTI-TRONCONI [c]

[b]*Department of Neurology*
*University of Düsseldorf*
*Düsseldorf, FRG*

[c]*Department of Biochemistry*
*University of Minnesota*
*St. Paul, Minnesota*

What do the autoimmune T helper cells that regulate autoantibody production in myasthenia gravis "see" on the acetylcholine receptor (AChR) molecule? At one extreme, the T-cell autoimmune response could be monoclonal, which would immediately suggest specific immunotherapy of myasthenia. At the other extreme, the T-cell response could be so heterogeneous that it might be impossible to define any immunodominant T-cell epitopes on the AChR. We have studied this problem by selecting AChR-reactive human T-cell lines using AChR from *Torpedo californica* and by attempting to define stepwise the epitope specificity of these cells. First, we established that the AChR-specific helper T cells do not distinguish between native and denatured AChR. Next, we used isolated (denatured) AChR subunits to show that these T cells react preferentially to alpha subunit determinants.[1] These results prompted us to use synthetic peptides corresponding to human alpha subunit sequences to further probe the T-cell repertoire.

To find candidate "T cell sites" on the alpha subunit, the primary sequence of the human AChR alpha subunit was analyzed for periodic hydrophobicity with a computer program called AMPHI.[2] (The analysis was kindly performed by Drs. J. Cornette, H. Margalit, C. DeLisi, and J. A. Berzofsky.) The rationale behind this approach is the assumption that T-cell antigenic sites have a propensity to form amphipathic alpha helices.[2]

From a library of synthetic peptides that represents almost the entire human alpha subunit, we chose the peptides that correspond best to the sequences with the highest

---

[a]This study was supported by the Muscular Dystrophy Association and by the Deutsche Forschungsgemeinschaft (DFG; Grant SFB 200, B5). R.H. is a Heisenberg Fellow of the DFG.

amphipathic score values. These peptides were used to (a) stimulate unselected peripheral blood cells (PBL) from myasthenic patients, and (b) to stimulate preselected AChR-specific T cells.

Peripheral blood cells from 12 patients were tested for reactivity with peptide 1 (1-14), 2 (7-22), and 3 (19-34). In addition, PBLs from 8 patients were also tested with peptide 10 (118-137), 17 (304-322), 18 (320-337), 22 (364-380), and 23 (376-393). The stimulating peptide concentration was 0.5 $\mu$M. A stimulation index greater than 2 was observed with peptide 1, 2 and/or 3 in 3 of 12 patients, with peptide 17 and/or 18 in 2 patients, and with peptide 10 in 1 patient. None of the patients reacted to peptide 23.

AChR-reactive T-cell lines were selected from two patients with Torpedo AChR. These cells were tested for reactivity with peptides 1-3 that correspond to the alpha subunit sequence with the highest amphipathic score in both human and torpedo AChR. The peptides elicited 10-30% of the response induced with intact AChR. Different peptides were recognized by the T cells of the two patients.[3]

We conclude from these results that the aminoterminal region of the AChR alpha-chain contains T-cell-stimulating determinants that have a propensity to form an amphipathic alpha helix. However, because the T-cell response to the candidate synthetic peptides was much smaller than that to intact AChR, it is likely that other T-cell-stimulating epitopes exist on the alpha subunit. Our findings suggest further that there is both intra- and interindividual heterogeneity of the T-cell autoimmune reaction in myasthenia gravis.

## REFERENCES

1. HOHLFELD, R., K. V. TOYKA, S. J. TZARTOS, W. CARSON & B. M. CONTI-TRONCONI. 1987. Human T-helper lymphocytes in myasthenia gravis recognize the nicotinic receptor alpha subunit. Proc. Natl. Acad. Sci. USA **84:** 5379-5383.
2. MARGALIT, H., J. SPOUGE, J. CORNETTE, K. CEASE, C. DELISI & J. A. BERZOFSKY. Prediction of immunodominant helper T cell antigenic sites from the primary sequence. J. Immunol. **138:** 2213-2229.
3. HOHLFELD, R., K. V. TOYKA, L. L. MINER, S. L. WALGRAVE & B. M. CONTI-TRONCONI. 1988. Amphipathic segment of the nicotinic receptor alpha subunit contains epitopes recognized by T lymphocytes in myesthenia gravis. J. Clin. Invest. **81:** 657-660.

# MHC Association Between Antistriational Antibody-Negative Myasthenia Gravis in the Chinese

W. GIN, B. R. HAWKINS, W. J. ZHANG, V. WONG,
Y. L. YU, AND R. L. DAWKINS

*Departments of Clinical Immunology*
*Royal Perth Hospital and*
*QEII Medical Centre*
*Perth, Western Australia*
*and*
*Department of Pathology*
*University of Hong Kong*
*Queen Mary Hospital Compound*
*Hong Kong*

Immunogenetic factors are known to be important in the development of at least one form of adult onset myasthenia gravis (MG), that is, generalized MG with thymic hyperplasia is associated with A1 B8 DR3 (1,8,3) in adult caucasoids.[1] The same major histocompatibility complex genes are negatively associated with antistriational antibodies (anti-Str) and thymoma.[1] Complement allotyping has shown that patients with A1 B8 DR3 also have DQ2 and the BfS, C4AQ0, C4B1 complotype, indicating that the susceptibility gene(s) is located between HLA B and DQ. An equivalent marker in other races has not been identified. In the Chinese, studies show increases in HLA Bw46[2] and also in DRw9,[3] but complement allotypes have not been examined. To address this, complement allotypes were determined in 166 Hong Kong Chinese patients with previous HLA typing, using high voltage agarose gel electrophoresis and immunofixation.[4]

The BfS, C4A4, C4B2 complotype was found to be frequent (FIG. 1); 67 patients (40.4%) had the complete Bw46, BfS, C4A4, C4B2, DRw9 (46,S,4,2,9) supratype. 46,S,4,2,9 was particularly frequent among the younger patients (FIG. 2) and those with absent or low titers of antiacetylcholine receptor antibodies (anti-AChR) irrespective of age. By contrast, anti-AChR was elevated in almost all of the 20 patients with anti-Str, all but one of whom were older than 21 years of age. There was a negative association between anti-Str and 46,S,4,2,9.

These results show that 1,8,3 in caucasoid patients and 46,S,4,2,9 in Chinese are similar in that they are negatively associated with anti-Str. However, 1,8,3 and 46,S,4,2,9 differ in that the former is associated with higher titers of anti-AChR, whereas the latter is associated with a younger age of onset. In keeping with these differences, comparison of 1,8,3 and 46,S,4,2,9 using pulsed field gel electrophoresis and Southern blotting has revealed multiple differences. The 1,8,3 supratype contains at least four major deletions, whereas 46,S,4,2,9 has an insertion.[5] Despite these results,

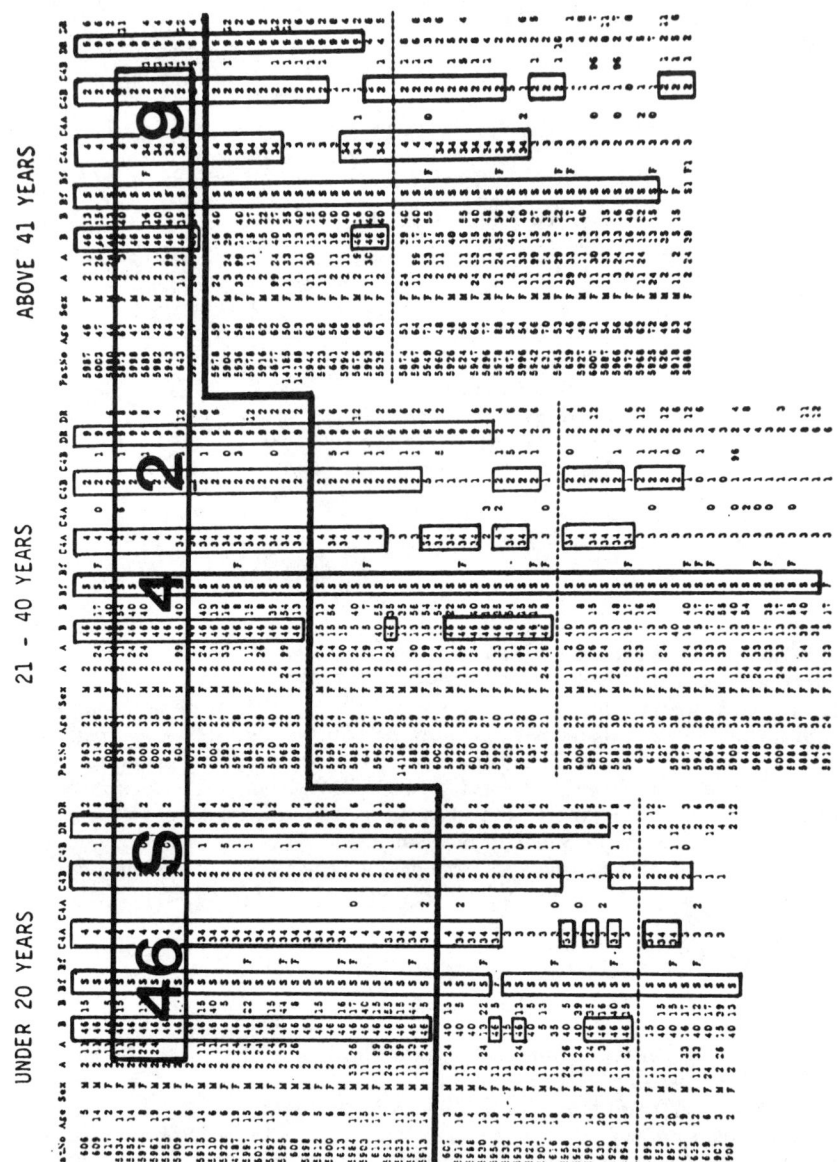

FIGURE 1. HLA Bw46,BfS,C4A4,C4B2,DRw9 supratype and age in myasthenia gravis in the Chinese.

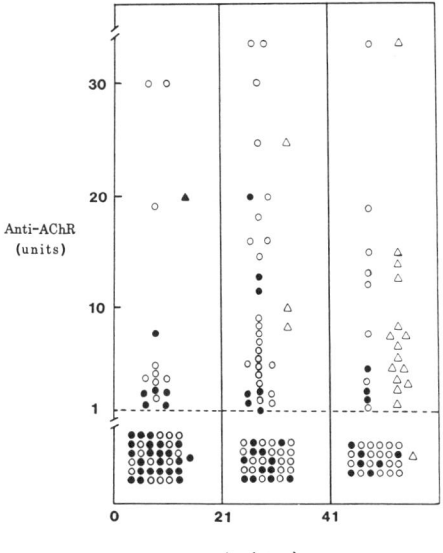

**FIGURE 2.** Anti-AChR is relatively more frequent in older patients without the 46,S,4,2,9 supratype (*open*) but with anti-Str (*triangles*). The 46,S,4,2,9 supratype (*closed*) is positively associated with younger age and lower anti-AChR.

it remains possible that the two supratypes share an allele that protects against the development of anti-Str and probably thymoma.

## REFERENCES

1. DAWKINS, R. L. 1980. Myasthenia Gravis Disease Report. *In* Histocompatibility Testing 1980. P. I. Terasaki (Ed): 662-667. UCLA Tissue Typing Laboratory, Los Angeles, CA.
2. HAWKINS, B. R., W. Y. CHAN-LUI, E. K. K. CHOI & A. Y. HO. 1986. Strong association of HLA Bw46 with juvenile onset myasthenia gravis in Hong Kong Chinese. J. Neurol. Neurosurg. Psychiatry **49**: 316-319.
3. THAJEB, P., C. Y. CHEE & C. C. HUANG. 1987. The distribution of HLA A,B,DR antigens in Chinese myasthenia gravis. Tissue Antigens **29**: 273-279.
4. ZHANG, W. J., P. H. KAY, T. J. COBAIN & R. L. DAWKINS. 1988. C4 allotyping on plasma or serum: Application to routine laboratories. Human Immunol. **21**: 156-171.
5. TOKUNAGA, K., G. SAUERACKER, P. H. KAY, F. T. CHRISTIANSIEN, R. ANAND & R. L. DAWKINS. Extensive deletions and insertions in different MHC supratypes detected by pulsed field gel electrophoresis. J. Exp. Med., in press.

# Synthetic Peptide of Human Acetylcholine Receptor α-Subunit Sequence 125-147 (Methionine 144), a More Potent Autoantigen Than Its Norleucine 144 Analog[a]

VANDA A. LENNON,[b] ZHONG-XIAN HUANG,[b]
DANIEL J. McCORMICK,[c] GUY E. GRIESMANN,[b]
NAOKI FUJII,[b] AND EDWARD H. LAMBERT [d]

[b]Departments of Immunology, Neurology,
[c]Biochemistry and Molecular Biology
Mayo Clinic
Rochester, Minnesota 55905
[d]Department of Neurology
University of Minnesota
Minneapolis, Minnesota 55455

A decrease in functional nicotinic acetylcholine receptors (AChR) at the motor endplate causes the defect in neuromuscular transmission that is characteristic of myasthenia gravis (MG). This loss of AChR is caused by anti-AChR autoantibodies.[1] The AChR α-subunit has been implicated as the major target for pathogenic autoantibodies in MG.[2]

We are using a synthetic peptide strategy to define antigenic sites on the AChR of human muscle that can activate helper T cells for the production of pathogenic autoantibodies. The region encompassing residues 125-147 of the α-subunit was the first defined myasthenogenic region of the AChR.[3,4] Myasthenogenicity does not depend on intramolecular cyclization through cysteines 128 and 142[4]; experimental autoimmune MG (EAMG) can be induced by the 17 amino acid peptide encompassing only residues 131-147.[5] Because methionine (Met) is potentially susceptible to oxidation, we substituted norleucine (Nle) at position 144 in our previous peptide syntheses.[3-5] We now report the antigenic properties of a synthetic peptide corresponding to the native sequence of the human AChR, that is, with Met at position 144. The sequence of human AChR α-subunit region 125-147 is as follows:

$^+$NH$_3$-Lys-Ser-Tyr-Cys-Glu-Ile-Ile-Val-Thr-His-Phe-Pro-Phe-Asp-
  125                    131

---

[a]This work was supported by grants from the National Institutes of Health (NS 15057, V.A.L.; NS 24694, D.J.M.; NS 23691, E.H.L.) and The William K. Warren Foundation.

Glu-Gln-Asn-Cys-Ser-Met-Lys-Leu-Gly-COO⁻
                    ---
                    144           147

Peptide analogs tested included some with Nle substituted for Met at position 144, and some with a tripeptide "cap" (Lys-Gly-Gly or Lys-Lys-Gly) added to the N terminus to enhance solubility.

Peptides were synthesized by standard solid phase procedures using t-BOC-L-amino acids.[4] Those containing Met were purified in reducing conditions. Female Lewis rats, aged about 10 weeks, were inoculated intradermally with unconjugated peptides emulsified in complete Freund's adjuvant, with *Bortedella pertussis* vaccine

TABLE 1. Microelectrophysiologic and Biochemical Evidence of EAMG in Tail Muscle of Rats Immunized with Peptide Hα125-147 or the Analog [¹⁴⁴Nle] Hα125-147 (*Nle → 144*)

| Immunogen | No. of Rats | Clinical Signs of EAMG[a] | MEPP[a] Amplitude (mV) | AChR Extracted[a] Total (fmol/g) | % Complexed with Ig |
|---|---|---|---|---|---|
| Adjuvants | 12 | 0/12 | 0.63 ± 0.031 | 438 ± 27 | 0 ± 0 |
| Denatured T AChR | 6 | 4/6 | <u>0.29 ± 0.057</u> | <u>180 ± 27</u> | <u>37 ± 11</u> |
| Hα125-147[c] | 5 | 1/5 | <u>0.37 ± 0.019</u>[e] | <u>152 ± 11</u>[e] | <u>17 ± 5</u> |
| [¹⁴⁴Nle] Hα125-147[d] | 7 | 0/7 | <u>0.46 ± 0.049</u> | <u>204 ± 26</u> | <u>21 ± 7</u> |

[a] Chronic progressive weakness, worsened by exercise and relieved by rest, accompanied by weight loss secondary to impaired chewing.

[b] Values are mean ± SE. Those underlined are significantly different from adjuvant control values ($p < 0.01$).

[c,d] Additional tripeptides at the N termini (Lys-Gly-Gly[c] and Lys-Lys-Gly[d]) did not influence the antigenicity of the peptide in terms of T-cell responses (TABLE 2) or antipeptide antibody responses (data not shown). Hα125-147 refers to peptide of native sequence (i.e., Met 144).

[e] Rats immunized with Hα125-147[c] had significantly greater loss of AChR from tail muscle (i.e., lower MEPP amplitudes and lower yields of extractable AChR) than did rats immunized with the Nle analog ($p < 0.05$). Values for Hα125-147[c]-immunized rats did not differ significantly from those of rats immunized with denatured *Torpedo* AChR.

injected subcutaneously.[6] Control rats received denatured *Torpedo* (T) AChR[3] or adjuvants only. Antigen-induced proliferation of T cells was assayed using lymph node cells.[5] Miniature endplate potential (MEPP) amplitudes in tail muscles were measured *in vitro*,[3] and AChR were quantitated by immunoprecipitation after detergent extraction and complexing with ¹²⁵I-α-bungarotoxin.

Despite Met's potential for oxidation, its incorporation at position 144 in synthesizing human AChR α-subunit peptide 125-147 did not compromise antigenicity. In fact, synthetic peptide 125-147 of native sequence was a more potent autoantigen than was the Nle 144 analog. Unlike the Nle analog, the Met peptide induced electrophysiologic and biochemical signs of EAMG equivalent to those induced by denatured T AChR (TABLE 1). Furthermore, T cells primed by denatured T AChR were stimulated by the Met peptide but not by the Nle analog (TABLE 2). The fact that denatured T AChR is myasthenogenic in rats contrasts with findings in rabbit studies.[7]

TABLE 2. T-Cell Proliferative Responses[a] of Rats Immunized with Synthetic Peptides Corresponding to Region 125-147 of Human (H) AChR α-Subunit with or without Nle Substituted for Met at Position 144

| Immunogen | No. of Rats | Lymphocyte Incorporation of $^3$H-Thymidine (Mean Stimulation Index ± SE) in the Presence of: | | | | | |
|---|---|---|---|---|---|---|---|
| | | Hα125-147 | Hα125-147[b] | [$^{144}$Nle] Hα125-147[c] | [$^{144}$Nle] Tα125-147[c] | T AChR | Tuberculin PPD |
| Adjuvants | 14 | 0.9 ± 0.1 | 1.2 ± 0.2 | 0.8 ± 0.1 | 1.0 ± 0.1 | 1.2 ± 0.1 | 7.6 ± 1.4 |
| d.T AChR | 6 | NT[d] | 3.1 ± 0.3 | 1.7 ± 0.7 | 1.4 ± 0.4 | 11 ± 2.7 | 8.3 ± 2.4 |
| Hα125-147 | 6 | 13 ± 4.8 | 13 ± 3.7 | 13 ± 4.2 | 7.1 ± 1.1 | 1.2 ± 0.2 | 9.3 ± 2.6 |
| Hα125-147[b] | 21 | 7.5 ± 1.4 | 12 ± 2.1 | 11 ± 1.8 | 7.3 ± 0.8 | 1.3 ± 0.1 | 6.6 ± 0.6 |
| [$^{144}$Nle] Hα125-147[c] (Nle → 144) | 13 | 10 ± 3.5 | 15 ± 3.2 | 14 ± 3.1 | 8.3 ± 1.3 | 1.1 ± 0.1 | 8.0 ± 1.4 |

[a] Lymph node cells were tested ($8 \times 10^5$ cells per microculture) 13 to 63 days after primary inoculation. Responses between days 10 and 63 did not differ significantly. Each antigen was tested in quadruplicate cultures.

$$\text{Stimulation Index} = \frac{\text{mean cpm with antigen}}{\text{mean cpm without antigen}}$$

Values underlined indicate significant stimulation by comparison with adjuvant control values ($p < 0.01$). Rats immunized with d.T AChR responded to Hα125-147[b] but not to the Nle analog peptides ($p < 0.05$).

[b,c] Hα125-147 indicates peptide of native sequence (i.e., Met 144). Additional tripeptides at the N termini (Lys-Gly-Gly[b] and Lys-Lys-Gly[c]) did not influence the specificities of T-cell responses ($p > 0.05$ for comparison of differences between responses to individual peptides, Student's $t$ test).

[d] NT = not tested.

## REFERENCES

1. LENNON, V. A. 1979. Immunological mechanisms in myasthenia gravis — a model of a receptor disease. *In* Clinical Immunology Update: Reviews for Physicians, E. Franklin, Ed.: 259-289. Elsevier North Holland, New York.
2. TZARTOS, S. J., M. E. SEYBOLD & J. M. LINDSTROM. 1982. Specificities of antibodies to acetylcholine receptors in sera from myasthenia gravis patients measured by monoclonal antibodies. Proc. Natl. Acad. Sci. USA **79:** 188-192.
3. LENNON, V. A., D. J. MCCORMICK, E. H. LAMBERT, G. E. GRIESMANN & M. Z. ATASSI. 1985. Region of peptide 125-147 of acetylcholine receptor $\alpha$ subunit is exposed at neuromuscular junction and induces experimental autoimmune myasthenia gravis, T-cell immunity and modulating autoantibodies. Proc. Natl. Acad. Sci. USA **82:** 8805-8809.
4. MCCORMICK, D. J., G. E. GRIESMANN, Z. HUANG, E. H. LAMBERT & V. A. LENNON. 1987. Myasthenogenicity of human acetylcholine receptor $\alpha$ subunit peptide 125-147 does not require intramolecular disulfide cyclisation. J. Immunol. **139:** 2615-2619.
5. LENNON, V. A., G. E. GRIESMANN, D. J. MCCORMICK, Z. HUANG, H. FENG & E. H. LAMBERT. 1987. Definition of myasthenogenic sites of the human acetylcholine receptor using synthetic peptides. Ann. N. Y. Acad. Sci. **505:** 439-449.
6. LENNON, V. A., J. LINDSTROM & M. E. SEYBOLD. 1976. Experimental autoimmune myasthenia gravis: Cellular and humoral immune responses. Ann. N. Y. Acad. Sci. **274:** 283-299.
7. BARTFELD, D. & S. FUCHS. 1977. Immunological characterization of an irreversibly denatured acetylcholine receptor. FEBS Lett **77:** 214-218.

# Probing for the Main Immunogenic Region of the Human Acetylcholine Receptor

H. ENG,[a] H. JÖRNVALL,[b] M. CARLQUIST,[c]
AND A. K. LEFVERT[a]

[a]*Department of Medicine*
*Karolinska Hospital*
*Stockholm, Sweden*
*Departments of* [b]*Medical Chemistry and*
[c]*Biochemistry*
*Karolinska Institute*
*Stockholm, Sweden*

In individuals with myasthenia gravis (MG) the nicotinic acetylcholine receptor (AChR) at the neuromuscular junction is the target for an autoimmune response. Although the antireceptor antibody (Ab) response is heterogeneous, one extracellular region of the alpha subunit, designated as the main immunogenic region (MIR), binds over 60% of the anti-AChR Ab in patients with MG and in rats with experimental autoimmune MG.[1,2] Although the exact location of the MIR is unknown, the mouse MIR was recently localized to residues 5-85 of the alpha subunit.[3] Two peptides corresponding to residues 66-79 (peptide 1) and 44-59 (peptide 2) of the human alpha subunit were synthesized as possible sites of the MIR.

Rat monoclonal Ab 35, specific for the MIR, reacted with both peptides, although it displayed a stronger reaction to peptide 2 both in titer and in direct binding (FIG. 1). As those peptides that react with a monospecific Ab may comprise the individual components of a conformational epitope, it is likely that the MIR is composed of at least two sites, localized within peptides 1 and 2, that are in close spatial proximity. Binding of mAb 35 to both peptides was inhibited by the addition of MG sera (data not shown), suggesting the antipeptide antibodies from both sources bound at or near the same peptide epitope.

The sera of 18 patients with MG, on examination, also bound peptides 1 and 2 but displayed individual variation as to which peptide was more antigenic (FIG. 2). Such variation in reactivity confirms the observation that the MIR elicits a heterogeneous immune response.[4] Peptide 2 was able to inhibit the binding of sera of two patients with MG to torpedo AChR coated ELISA plates by as much as 70%, whereas the addition of peptide 1 had much less of an inhibitory effect.

Thus, the human MIR, as defined by mAb 35, appears to be composed of at least two regions, comprising residues 44-59 and 66-79 which in the native receptor may be in close spatial orientation. Monoclonal Ab 35 binds more strongly to peptide 2 than peptide 1, whereas MG sera exhibit variation as to which peptide is more antigenic. Complete elucidation of the MIR using mAb and patient sera will further our understanding of the AChR antigenic sites and of the pathology involved in MG.

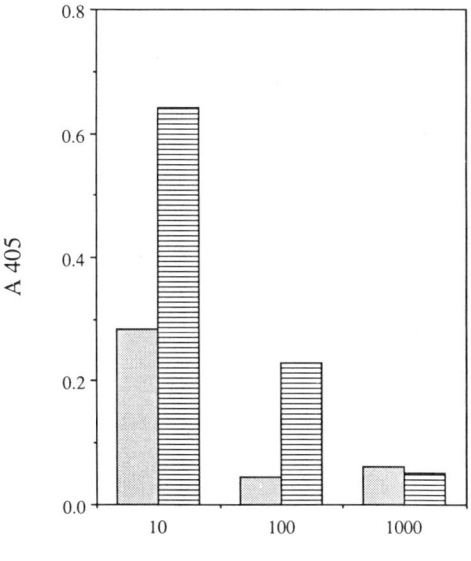

**FIGURE 1.** Binding of anti-MIR mAb 35 to peptides 1 (▒) and 2 (≡) as determined by ELISA and expressed as $A_{405}$.

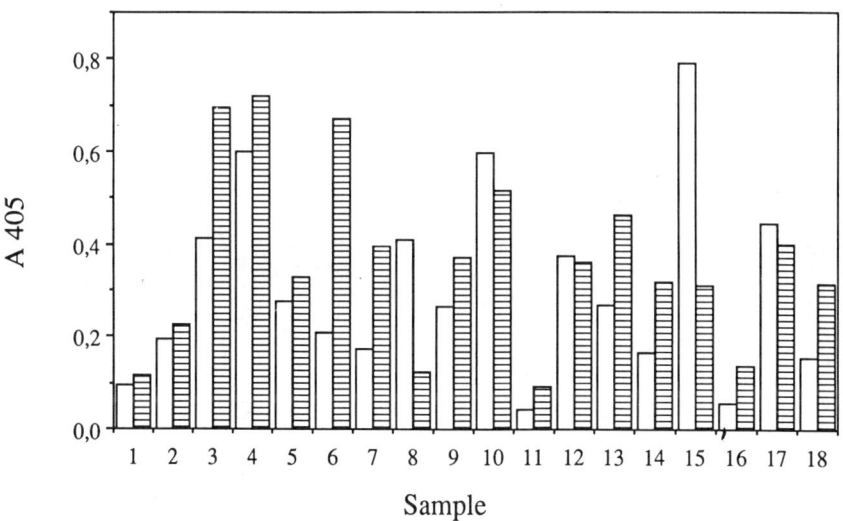

**FIGURE 2.** Reactivity of the sera of 18 patients with MG for peptides 1 (□) and 2 (≡). The presence of antipeptide Ab was determined by ELISA and expressed as $A_{405}$.

## REFERENCES

1. TZARTOS, S. J., D. E. RAND, B. E. EINARSON & J. M. LINDSTROM. 1981. Mapping of surface structures of electrophorus acetylcholine receptor using monoclonal antibodies. J. Biol. Chem. **256:** 8635-8645.
2. TZARTOS, S. J., M. E. SEYBOLD & J. M. LINDSTROM. 1982. Specificity of antibodies to acetylcholine receptors in sera from myasthenia gravis patients measured by monoclonal antibodies. Proc. Natl. Acad. Sci. **79:** 188-192.
3. BARKAS, T., A. MAURON, B. ROTH, C. ALLIOD, S. J. TZARTOS & M. BALLIVET. 1987. Mapping the main immunogenic region and toxin binding site of nicotinic acetylcholine receptor. Science **235:** 77-80.
4. KILLEN, J. A., S. M. HOCHSCHWENDER & J. M. LINDSTROM. 1985. The main immunogenic regions of acetylcholine receptors does not provoke the formation of antibodies of a predominant idiotype. J. Neuroimmunol. **9:** 229-241.

# *In Vitro* Blockade of Neuromuscular Transmission by Monoclonal Anti-Acetylcholine Receptor Antibodies

RICARDO A. MASELLI, BRIAN JOW,
DAVID P. RICHMAN, AND DEBORAH J. NELSON

*Departments of Neurology and Medicine
and
The Brain Research Institute
The University of Chicago
Chicago, Illinois 60637*

Autoantibody-induced loss of neuromuscular transmission in myasthenia gravis (MG) has been attributed to an increase in acetylcholine receptor (AChR) turnover as well as complement-mediated destruction of the receptor-enriched postsynaptic membrane, with little emphasis on the role of functional receptor blockade. Gomez and Richman[1] described a hyperacute animal model of experimental autoimmune myasthenia gravis (EAMG) in chicken hatchlings that is characterized by profound weakness leading to death within minutes after injection of monoclonal antibodies (mAb) that block alpha bungarotoxin ($\alpha$-BTX) binding. Unlike the classically described passive transfer EAMG, these animals develop paralysis in the absence of an accompanying inflammatory response or subsynaptic membrane destruction, suggesting the possible functional importance of antibodies capable of altering ion channel activation in the pathology of MG. We chose to study the *in vitro* effects of the mAb 370A, which induces the hyperacute form of EAMG and which was previously reported to be a competitive blocker of both agonist and $\alpha$-BTX binding,[2] as representative of a class of autoantibodies that are capable of pharmacologic (functional) receptor blockade.

The *in vitro* electrophysiologic effects on normal chicken endplates of mAb 370A and of control anti-AChR mAb 132A, which does not interfere with either agonist or $\alpha$-BTX binding,[1] were compared. Miniature endplate potentials (MEPPs) as well as endplate currents (EPCs) were recorded in the posterior latissimus dorsi muscle under high magnification ($\times$ 250) interference contrast optics before and after exposure of the preparation to antibody. Following incubation of the electrophysiologic preparation with mAb 370A (5-50 $\mu$g/ml), MEPPs and EPCs were reduced by 42 and 63%, respectively, without alteration in the rate constant describing EPC decay or in the reversal potential of the nerve-impulse evoked currents. The EPC time constant was 5.9 $\pm$ 0.6 ms (SEM) ($n = 10$) before incubation with mAb 370A and 6.0 $\pm$ 0.9 ms (SEM) ($n = 28$) afterwards. The change in membrane potential required to produce an e-fold change in EPC decay was 128 $\pm$ 2.3 mV (SEM) ($n = 6$) before incubation compared to 125 $\pm$ 6.6 mV (SEM) ($n = 24$) after incubation. Experiments with mAb 132A, which is capable of inducing the classically described passive transfer EAMG, produced no significant change in MEPP amplitude, EPC amplitude, time constant describing EPC decay, or EPC reversal potentials.

From the foregoing data, we conclude that the mAb 370A-induced weakness in the hyperacute animal model can be attributed to a block of acetylcholine-induced ion channel activity in the postsynaptic membrane. Furthermore, the single-channel properties of the receptors that remain activatable in the presence of antibody are unmodified. Therefore, the disordered neuromuscular transmission that is observed in MG as well as its experimental model EAMG is likely to be the result of a combination of antibody-mediated mechanisms, one of which is the direct block of ion channel activation.

## REFERENCES

1. GOMEZ, C. & D. P. RICHMAN. 1983. Proc. Natl. Acad. Sci. USA **80:** 4089-4093.
2. MIHOVILOVIC, M. & D. P. RICHMAN. 1987. J. Biol. Chem. **262:** 4979-4986.

# Antibodies Against the Acetylcholine Receptor also in Nonmyasthenic Autoimmune Disease

## ANN-CHARLOTT SUNDEWALL AND ANN KARI LEFVERT

*Department of Internal Medicine
Karolinska Hospital
Stockholm, Sweden*

Antibodies binding to the acetylcholine receptor of human skeletal muscle were found in patients with different kinds of mitochondrial antibodies. In patients with primary biliary cirrhosis (PBC), the prevalence of these antibodies is high.[1] The antibody activity was found in monomeric and pentameric IgM as well as in IgG, whereas patients with other kinds of mitochondrial antibodies had antireceptor antibodies of predominantly the IgG class.[2]

The PBC sera were tested for reactivity against receptor from other species. IgG class antibodies reacting with mouse receptor were found only in association with antibody activity against human receptor. Antibodies of IgM class were more commonly directed against mouse receptor. One patient had IgG class antibodies against the torpedo receptor but no antibody activity against human or mouse receptors. Two other sera contained IgM class antibodies against the torpedo receptor.

Passive transfer of purified immunoglobulins from patients with PBC resulted in a reduction of receptors in mouse muscle comparable to the reduction observed with immunoglobulins from patients with myasthenia gravis (MG) (FIG. 1).

The antibody affinity was in the same order of magnitude of PBC as in MG, but populations with different affinities were more common in PBC.

Primary biliary cirrhosis antibodies were also recognized by anti-idiotypic antibodies raised against antibodies from patients with MG, but the repertoire was markedly different from that found in MG (TABLE 1). For example, the anti-idiotypic antibody AI 21, raised against an antibody directed against the toxin binding site on the receptor, reacted with only 3 of the 19 PBC sera, but it is the most commonly found idiotype in MG, 60%. In addition, some of the PBC antibodies showed a multireactivity not found in MG.

Cell lines, produced by EBV transformation of peripheral blood lymphocytes from PBC patients, produced antimitochondrial antibodies, antibodies reacting with acetylcholine receptor, antibodies reacting with anti-idiotypic antibodies, and anti-idiotypic antibodies reacting with monoclonal receptor antibodies.

The antibody repertoire produced by the clones differed from that found in serum from the patient. Some idiotypes not present in sera were detectable in the clones; reversedly one idiotype present in sera was not shown in the clones. Anti-idiotypic antibodies of IgG class were more common.

The antibody activity against torpedo acetylcholine receptor would be inhibited

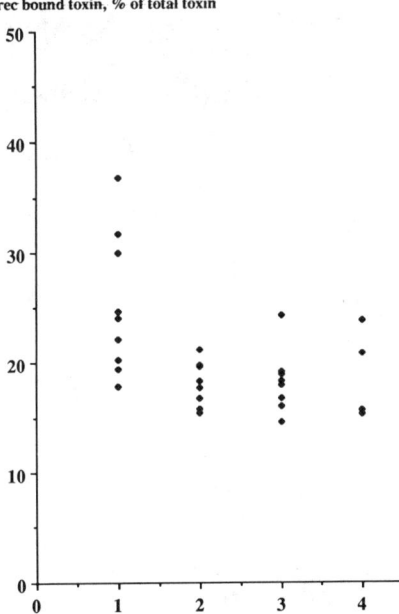

**FIGURE 1.** The amount of free receptor (rec) measured as toxin bound to receptor in the percentage of total toxin concentration in (1) mice transfused with normal Ig, (2) mice transfused with Ig from patients with myasthenia gravis (MG) in complete remission, (3) mice transfused with Ig from severely ill patients with MG, and (4) mice transfused with Ig from patients with primary biliary cirrhosis.

**TABLE 1.** Prevalence of Receptor-Related Idiotypes Binding to Monoclonal Antiidiotypic Antibodies in Primary Biliary Cirrhosis and Myasthenia Gravis (MG)

| Patient | IgG | | | | | | IgM | | | | | |
|---|---|---|---|---|---|---|---|---|---|---|---|---|
| | AI 21 | AI 3 | AI 8 | AI 24 | AI 41 | AI 45 | AI 21 | AI 3 | AI 8 | AI 24 | AI 41 | AI 45 |
| 1  | − | − | − | − | − | − | − | + | − | − | + | + |
| 2  | − | − | − | − | − | − | − | + | − | − | − | − |
| 3  | − | − | − | − | − | − | − | − | − | − | − | − |
| 4  | − | − | − | − | − | − | − | − | − | − | − | − |
| 6  | + | + | + | + | + | + | − | − | − | + | − | − |
| 7  | − | − | − | − | − | − | − | − | − | + | − | − |
| 8  | − | − | − | − | − | − | − | − | − | + | − | − |
| 9  | − | − | − | − | − | − | − | − | − | + | − | − |
| 10 | + | + | + | + | + | + | + | + | + | + | + | − |
| 11 | − | − | − | − | − | − | + | + | − | + | + | + |
| 12 | − | − | − | − | − | − | − | − | − | − | − | − |
| 13 | − | − | − | − | − | − | − | − | − | − | − | − |
| 14 | − | − | − | − | − | − | − | − | − | − | − | − |
| 15 | − | − | − | − | − | − | − | + | − | − | + | − |
| 16 | − | − | − | − | − | − | − | − | − | − | − | + |
| 17 | + | + | + | + | + | + | + | + | + | + | + | + |
| 18 | − | − | − | − | − | − | − | − | − | − | − | − |
| 19 | − | − | − | − | − | − | − | − | − | − | − | − |
| 20 | − | − | − | − | − | − | − | − | − | − | + | + |
| Total % | 16 | 16 | 16 | 16 | 16 | 16 | 16 | 32 | 11 | 37 | 32 | 26 |
| MG %    | 60 | 27 | 30 | 36 | 14 | 14 | −  | −  | −  | −  | −  | −  |

by preincubation of sera with potential cross-reacting substances. One serum with IgM class activity against the receptor was tested. The activity was inhibited by several substances: cardiolipin, ssDNA, Poly[I], and poly[A]-poly[U]. Another serum with IgG class activity showed inhibition only with cardiolipin; this was also the case with serum from a patient with MG with IgG class activity against the torpedo receptor. This activity was inhibited to some extent by cardiolipin.

Also, the ability of monoclonal anti-idiotypic antibodies to bind the idiotypes in sera, in an ELISA system, could be reduced.

## REFERENCES

1. SUNDEWALL, A.-C., A. K. LEFVERT & R. OLSSON. 1985. Acta Med. Scand. **217:** 519-525.
2. SUNDEWALL, A.-C., A. K. LEFVERT & R. NORBERG. J. Clin. Immunol. Immunpathol. In press.

# Standardization of Acetylcholine Receptor Antibody Measurement

E. BONIFACIO, R. L. DAWKINS, M. S. GRIFFITHS, AND T. J. COBAIN

*Departments of Clinical Immunology*
*Royal Perth Hospital*
*Queen Elizabeth II Medical Centre*
*and*
*University of Western Australia*
*Perth, Australia*

A variety of assays are used to detect the autoantibodies to the acetylcholine receptor (anti-AChR) that occur in patients with myasthenia gravis (MG). Both precision and accuracy are important when using the assay for diagnosis or to monitor sequential changes.

To evaluate intra- and inter-laboratory variation, 10 coded sera were distributed to each of the participating laboratories. These sera included four "standards" prepared

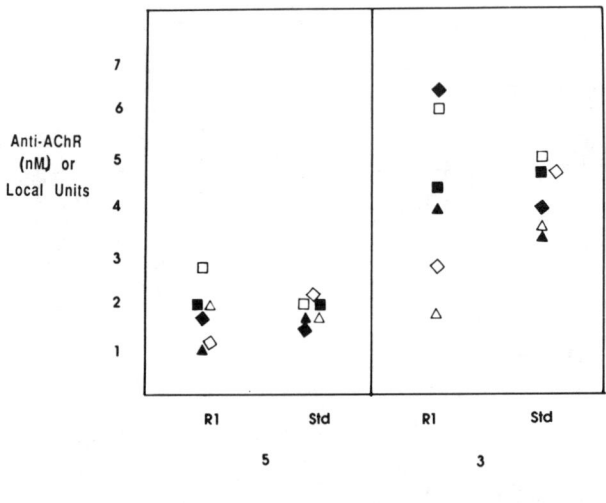

**FIGURE 1.** Effect of standardization. The results for anti-acetylcholine receptor (anti-AChR) reported by the six cooperating laboratories (represented by different symbols) are compared. The raw results as reported by each laboratory (R1) and the results after correction from the standard curve (STD) are given for two sera: 5 and 3.

by serially diluting a pool of MG sera in a negative serum, four samples from MG patients including one duplicate, one sample from a possible MG patient, and one sample from a blood donor. The assays used by the participating laboratories were similar,[1] in that all used human AChR as the antigen and iodine-125-labeled alpha bungaratoxin. However, different incubation conditions, precipitation techniques, and methods of interpreting the raw data were employed.

Analysis of the raw results received from the six cooperating laboratories showed considerable scatter in the results as well as differences in the method of expressing the amount of antibody. Despite this, all laboratories generally ranked the sera in the same order from low to high, and intra-laboratory precision as determined by the replicate was reasonably good. Results for the diluted standards showed good linearity for four laboratories and a tendency for the remaining two to plateau; however, there was considerable variation in slope.

Little improvement was achieved by the use of a standard precipitating antibody distributed with the test sera; however, when the individual standard curves were used to correct the results of the remaining samples, considerable reduction of the scatter was achieved (FIG. 1).

Preliminary results from a subsequent exchange indicate that some improvement was achieved at least in the area of the dilution curves, where improved concordance of slope and linearity was seen. However, each laboratory's interpretation of its own results from the current exchange indicate a need for further evaluation to determine suitable cut-offs for positivity. (8742)

## REFERENCES

1. PATRICK, J., J. LINDSTROM, B. CULP & J. MCMILLAN. 1973. Studies on purified eel acetylcholine receptor antibody. Proc. Natl. Acad. Sci. USA **70**: 3334-3338.

WORKSHOP 10. IMMUNOTHERAPY OF AUTOIMMUNE DISEASES

# Specific Suppression of the Antibody Response to Acetylcholine Receptor *in Vitro* and *in Vivo* by Daunomycin-Acetylcholine Receptor Conjugates

DIANE SHELTON, YOSHITAKA FUJII,
WOLFGANG KNOGGE, AND JON LINDSTROM

*The Salk Institute for Biological Studies
San Diego, California 92138*

Although currently accepted methods of therapy for myasthenia gravis (MG) frequently result in clinical improvement, they are not a cure, they lack specificity, and they are not without adverse side effects. One approach to the elimination of only the abnormal cells is the use of toxin conjugates containing an antigen that targets the response coupled to a toxin that results in specific cell killing. Experimental autoimmune MG (EAMG) is a good model for the initial development and testing of toxin conjugates, because the mechanisms of immune damage at the neuromuscular junction and the cellular immunology of the immune response are well described. Daunomycin (DM), an anthracycline antibiotic, is a DNA-intercalating agent that has been used in cancer chemotherapy. It has the advantage that it is a small molecule (MW 564) and can readily cross cell membranes to inhibit cell growth. DM-acetylcholine receptor (AChR) and DM-keyhole limpet hemocyanin (KLH) conjugates were prepared according to the method of Shen and Ryser.[1] DM, when conjugated with a targeting antigen by an acid-sensitive spacer, remains inactive at an intravascular pH of 7.4, but is activated following cleavage within the acidic lysosomal environment of the target cell. Using the EAMG model, we tested the ability of DM-AChR conjugates to specifically suppress the immune response to AChR in AChR-sensitized lymph node cell cultures and to prevent the onset of EAMG in intact rats.

DM-AChR conjugates containing 40-60 DM molecules per AChR specifically suppressed the production of antibodies to AChR by lymphocyte cultures. When compared with antibody production by AChR-sensitized lymphocyte cultures treated with AChR only, conjugate-treated sensitized lymphocytes produced 50-90% less AChR antibody without any nonspecific suppression. The conjugates did not suppress T-cell proliferation.

Rats were pretreated with either saline solution, DM-AChR, or DM-KLH and then immunized with either AChR or KLH (TABLE 1). In the DM-AChR pretreated group immunized with AChR, only one of nine rats showed the weakness characteristic of EAMG at 6 weeks postimmunization. All AChR-only rats that were not pretreated and three of four DM-KLH pretreated rats that were immunized with AChR developed severe clinical weakness. Serum antibody titers against *Torpedo* AChR at 2, 4, and 6

TABLE 1. Schedule of Conjugate Pretreatments and AChR Immunization

| Treatment Groups[a] | Treatments | | EAMG Expected? | EAMG Observed (at 6 weeks) | Severity of EAMG (average) |
| --- | --- | --- | --- | --- | --- |
| | Pretreatment Days 1 and 4 (20 μg DM) | Immunization Day 7 (100 μg AChR or KLH) | | | |
| 1 | None | AChR | Yes | 4/4 | +++ |
| 2 | DM-KLH | AChR | Yes | 3/4 | +++ |
| 3 | DM-AChR | AChR | No | 1/9 | 0 |
| 4 | DM-AChR | KLH | No | 0/4 | 0 |

ABBREVIATIONS: AChR = acetylcholine receptor; DM = daunomycin; EAMG = experimental autoimmune myasthenia gravis; KLH = keyhole limpet hemocyanin.

[a] Treatment groups: (1) untreated EAMG control; (2) control treatment with an irrelevant DM conjugate; (3) specific immune suppression with a DM-AChR conjugate; and (4) control treatment with a DM-AChR conjugate in the absence of specific immunization.

weeks postimmunization are shown in FIGURE 1. At all time points, the DM-AChR-treated rats had lower serum antibody titers than did controls pretreated with only AChR or DM-KLH. By 6 weeks, the difference between controls and treated rats was significant ($p < 0.005$). Using a crude preparation of denervated rat AChR, the cross-reacting antibody response was also significantly lower in DM-AChR conjugate-treated rats than in untreated AChR-immunized rats ($p < 0.005$). Those treated with the DM-AChR conjugate, however, had a high titer against KLH as measured by ELISA. Because these conjugates were effective in decreasing AChR antibody titers

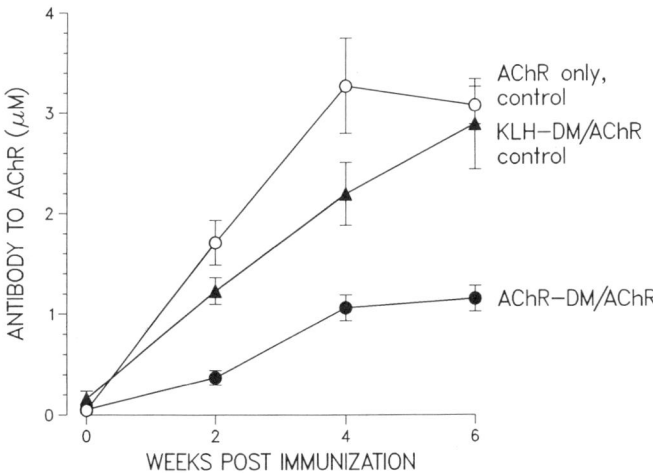

FIGURE 1. Pretreatment of rats with daunomycin-acetylcholine receptor (DM-AChR) specifically inhibits the production of antibodies in response to subsequent immunization with AChR. Antibody titers were measured in triplicate by standard immunoprecipitation methods using purified *Torpedo* AChR. Data are plotted as the mean titer for all animals in a group ± SE. KLH = keyhole limpet hemocyanin.

while allowing a normal immune response to KLH, they have the required specificity. By optimizing conditions in chronic EAMG, these conjugates should theoretically be effective.

**REFERENCE**

1. SHEN, W. & J. RYSER. 1981. Cis-aconityl spacer between daunomycin and macromolecular carriers: A model of pH-sensitive linkage releasing drug from a lysosomotrophic conjugate. Biochem. Biophys. Res. Commun. **102:** 1048.

# Effect of Lymphoid Irradiation on Clinical Course, Lymphocyte Count, and T-Cell Subsets in Chronic Progressive Multiple Sclerosis

S. D. COOK, C. DEVEREUX, R. TROIANO,
C. ROHOWSKY-KOCHAN, G. ZITO, AND
P. C. DOWLING

*University of Medicine and Dentistry of New Jersey*
*New Jersey Medical School*
*Newark, New Jersey*

*Veterans Administration Medical Center*
*East Orange, New Jersey*

*Clara Maass Medical Center*
*Belleville, New Jersey*

In a double-blinded study, 45 patients with chronic progressive multiple sclerosis (CPMS) were randomized into either a total lymphoid irradiation (TLI) treatment group (2,000 rads) or a control group treated with a sham TLI protocol. Patients were well matched for sex, age, and duration of disease. The code was broken in August 1986, and thereafter physicians and patients were not blinded, but were unaware of absolute lymphocyte count or T-cell subsets. In a subsequent, ongoing, open pilot study, other patients with CPMS were given total body irradiation (15 rads twice weekly for 5 weeks) plus prednisone ($\leq 30$ mg/day).

Immediately before treatment, patients were scored clinically on a practical functional scale. After treatment, the patients were clinically evaluated at monthly intervals for 6 months and then every 3 months. Immediately before treatment and periodically after treatment, blood was obtained to assess absolute lymphocyte count and T-cell subsets.

## RESULTS

### Total Lymphoid Irradiation

Patients with TLI showed significantly less rapid functional deterioration than did sham-irradiated controls ($p < 0.05$). When clinical results were reanalyzed by comparing the relation between mean absolute blood lymphocyte count and functional scale, even greater differences between groups were noted. Patients whose mean absolute lymphocyte count was less than 900 over the first 3 months after treatment (all TLI) predictably did significantly better at all time intervals up to 30 months after therapy than did those whose lymphocyte count was above this level (TLI plus sham).

During the first year after treatment, Th/Ts ratios were significantly higher in the group of sham control patients whose condition worsened clinically than in either the group of TLI-treated patients or sham controls whose condition was clinically stable ($p < 0.005$). The significantly higher post-treatment Th/Ts ratios in the control patients whose condition worsened was the net result of a decrease in the percentage of suppressor cells in these patients in contrast to a decrease in the percentage of helper cells in TLI-treated patients whose condition remained stable.

*Preliminary Data on TBI and Low Dose Prednisone*

Six patients with CPMS received TBI with prednisone ($\leq$ 30 mg/day). Although the follow-up period after therapy is short to date, these patients have remained in functionally stable condition and have generally shown a sustained lymphocytopenia, a decline in Th/Ts ratio, and a decrease in percentage of T-cell suppressor-inducer cells.

## CONCLUSIONS

In summary, TLI as well as TBI plus low doses of steroids produce alterations in the immune system in patients with CPMS. These changes are associated with transient stabilization in functional determination. Although these therapies are crude, invasive, and may be palliative rather than curative, if their beneficial effects in CPMS are confirmed, they may prove to be useful in the management of some patients with this disorder. In addition, these results provide indirect evidence that CPMS is an immune-mediated disorder and suggest that the absolute blood lymphocyte count may be a valuable barometer in monitoring immunosuppressive therapy in CPMS.

# Cumulative Experience with High-Dose Intravenous Cyclophosphamide and ACTH Therapy in Chronic Progressive Multiple Sclerosis

JONATHAN L. CARTER, DAVID M. DAWSON, DAVID A. HAFLER, ROBERT J. FALLIS, LYNN STAZZONE, JOHN ORAV, AND HOWARD L. WEINER

*Center for Neurological Diseases*
*Brigham and Women's Hospital*
*Boston, Massachusetts 02115*

*Department of Neurology*
*Mayo Clinic Scottsdale*
*Scottsdale, Arizona 85259*

Multiple sclerosis (MS) is postulated to be an immune-mediated disease, and clinical trials have focused on modulation of the immune system in an attempt to influence the history of the disease.[1] Cyclophosphamide was shown to be of benefit in MS in both controlled and uncontrolled clinical trials.[2-5] This report summarizes our experience at Brigham and Women's Hospital in treating 164 patients with rapidly progressive MS with a regimen of high-dose intravenous cyclophosphamide and ACTH therapy as previously published in earlier studies.[4,5] Patients were treated with 500 mg of cyclophosphamide daily until their total white blood cell count fell below 4,000 cells/mm$^3$, at which time the medication was stopped. A 21-day tapering course of intravenous ACTH was given concurrently. The mean total dose of cyclophosphamide was 6.3 g, and the mean white count nadir was 1,486 cells/mm$^3$.

Improvement or worsening after treatment was defined as a 1-point change in the modified Kurtzke Disability Status Scale or the Ambulation Index.[4] The results 1 year after the first treatment in the 100 patients in whom all clinical and laboratory data were available at the time of this review were as follows: 24% improved; 57% stable; and 19% worse. Fifty-eight patients were treated a second time, and the results in 27 patients in whom the 1-year follow-up point had occurred were as follows: 15% improved; 55% stable; and 30% worse. Sixty-nine percent of patients who responded to the initial treatment showed evidence of disease reprogression, with a mean time to reprogression of 17.6 months. Thirty-three percent of patients progressed between 6 and 12 months after treatment, 27% between 12 and 18 months after treatment, 17.5% between 18 and 24 months after treatment, 17.5% between 24 and 30 months after treatment, and 5% after 30 months of treatment. Seventy-four percent of all patients were improved or stable at 2 years after the initial treatment, and 55% of all patients were improved or stable at 3 years after initial treatment.

The complications of treatment and their frequencies in 164 patients were as follows: alopecia (100%), minor infections (26%), nausea (27%), nausea and vomiting (20%), complications of ACTH (5%), microscopic hematuria (6%), macroscopic hematuria (5%), mucositis (3%), major infections (1%), and fever alone (1%). Four patients were unable to complete the treatment, three because of persistent macroscopic hematuria and one because of nausea and vomiting. The incidence of complications with a second course of treatment was not significantly different from that with the first treatment. A single patient developed breast carcinoma 37 months after treatment, but no hematologic malignancies have been observed to date. No fatalities have occurred in association with therapy.

In summary, high-dose intravenous cyclophosphamide and ACTH therapy produced stabilization of the disease for a least 1 year after treatment in 81% of patients with rapid disease progression before treatment. The regimen was generally well tolerated, and only 2% of patients were unable to complete treatment. Research protocols currently under development include the use of monthly cyclophosphamide maintenance boosters titrated to the leukocyte count and treatment of patients with lower initial disability scores.

## REFERENCES

1. WEINER, H. L. & D. A. HAFLER. 1988. Immunotherapy of multiple sclerosis. Ann. Neurol. **23:** 211-222.
2. HOMMES, O. R., K. J. B. LAMERS & P. REEKERS. 1980. Effect of intensive immunosuppression on the course of chronic progressive multiple sclerosis. J. Neurol. **233:** 177-190.
3. GONSETTE, R. E., L. DEMONTY & P. DELMONTTE. 1980. Intensive immunosuppression with cyclophosphamide in remittent forms of multiple sclerosis. A followup of 134 patients for 2-10 years. *In* Progress in Multiple Sclerosis Research. Springer-Verlag, Berlin.
4. HAUSER, S. L., D. M. DAWSON, J. R. LEHRICH *et al.* 1983. Intensive immunosuppression in progressive multiple sclerosis. N. Engl. J. Med. **308:** 173-180.
5. WEINER, H. L., S. L. HAUSER, D. A. HAFLER *et al.* 1985. The use of cyclophosphamide in the treatment of multiple sclerosis. Ann. N. Y. Acad. Sci. **436:** 373-381.

# Suppressor Cell Regulation of Chronic Relapsing Experimental Allergic Encephalomyelitis

RUTH H. WHITHAM, DENNIS N. BOURDETTE,
HALINA OFFNER, CHARLES K. MESHUL, AND
ARTHUR A. VANDENBARK

*VA Medical Center
and
Oregon Health Sciences University
Portland, Oregon 97201*

Suppressor cells may be important in the regulation of chronic relapsing experimental allergic encephalomyelitis (CR-EAE) in SJL/J mice. *In vitro* culture of lymphocytes with cyclosporin A (CsA) and antigen has been shown in other systems to generate suppressor cells.[1-3] We investigated whether suppressor cells with *in vitro* and *in vivo* activity could be generated in the CR-EAE model system.

Antigen-specific T-cell lines were derived from lymph node cells of 6- to 12-week-old female SJL/J mice, using a modification of a previously published protocol.[4] Spleen cells were obtained from normal 6- to 12-week-old female SJL/J mice and from mice inoculated 11-14 days previously with guinea pig myelin basic protein

TABLE 1. *In Vitro* Suppression of Antigen-Specific T-Cell Lines by Spleen Cells

| Immunization of Spleen Cell Donors | *In Vitro* Treatment[a] of Spleen Cells | T-Cell Line | Proliferation[b] (cpm $\times 10^{-3}$) | Percentage of Suppression[c] |
|---|---|---|---|---|
| None | Medium | BP line + BP | 83 ± 5 | 29 |
| None | CsA + BP | BP line + BP | 52 ± 4 | 40 |
| BP-CFA[d] | Medium | BP line + BP | 64 ± 37 | 38 |
| BP-CFA | CsA + BP | BP line + BP | 3.3 ± 0.4 | 96[e] |
| BP-CFA | CsA + BP | PPD line + PPD | 0.8 ± 0.3 | 99 |
| OA-CFA[d] | CsA + OA | OA line + OA | 0.5 ± 0.1 | 98 |
| OA-CFA | CsA + OA | BP line + BP | 5.6 ± 1.1 | 95 |

[a] Splenocytes were cultured *in vitro* with medium or with cyclosporin A (CSA) 200 ng/ml and basic protein (BP) 50 μg/ml or ovalbumin (OA) 50 μg/ml for 7 days.

[b] $10^5$ spleen cells were added to wells containing $2 \times 10^4$ antigen-specific line cells and appropriate antigen (BP 50 μg/ml, OA 50 μg/ml, or PPD 25 μg/ml).

[c] Percentage of suppression was calculated as:
(1 - cpm [spleen cells + line cells + antigen]/cpm [line cells + antigen]) × 100.

[d] Mice were inoculated with 400 μg of guinea pig BP or 400 μg of OA in complete Freund's adjuvant (CFA).

[e] This population of spleen cells was used for *in vivo* experiments.

TABLE 2. Treatment of Chronic Relapsing EAE with Suppressor Cells

| Animals | Regimen | Onset of Disease | Clinical Score[a] First Attack | Percentage with Relapse | DTH to BP[b] | Histology[b] |
|---|---|---|---|---|---|---|
| Group 1 | 10^7 BP line day 0 | day 15 ± 4 | 3.7 ± 0.9 | 33 | + | 2.7 ± 1.2 |
| Group 2 | 10^8 suppressors[d] day −3<br>10^7 BP line day 0 | day 50 ± 5 | 1.3 ± 0.9 | 0 | + | 0.8 ± 0.6 |

[a] 0 = normal, 1 = flaccid tail, 2 = mild hindlimb weakness (HLW), 3 = moderate HLW, 4 = moderately severe HLW, 5 = severe HLW, and 6 = paraplegia.
[b] Ear testing for delayed-type hypersensitivity (DTH) to basic protein (BP) was performed on day 55.
[c] Spinal cord sections from animals sacrificed on day 55 or 63 were stained with toluidine blue and graded for the severity of demyelination on a scale of 0–4 by an evaluator unaware of the treatment group.
[d] Spleen cells from BP-CFA donors were treated for 7 days *in vitro* with cyclosporin A and basic protein, as outlined in TABLE 1.

(BP) or ovalbumin (OA). Splenocytes were then cultured *in vitro* for 7 days with medium or with CsA and antigen. To evaluate the effects of spleen cells on *in vitro* proliferation of T-cell lines to antigen, $10^4$ to $10^5$ washed spleen cells were added to microtiter wells containing appropriate antigen, $2 \times 10^4$ antigen-specific line cells, and $1 \times 10^6$ irradiated thymocytes as antigen-presenting cells and cultured for 3 days. Tritiated thymidine was added for the last 18 hours of culture, and counts per minute (cpm) were determined in triplicate wells. To evaluate the *in vivo* effects of processed spleen cells, 6- to 12-week-old naive female SJL/J mice were injected intraperitoneally (IP) with $10^8$ spleen cells, followed 3 days later by $10^7$ BP-specific line cells. Control mice received only $10^7$ BP-specific line cells, a dose that was shown previously to passively transfer CR-EAE.[5]

Results of *in vitro* proliferation assays for normal and immune donor spleens are shown in TABLE 1. Maximal suppression of BP-specific T-cell line proliferation to BP required immune spleens and *in vitro* culture of spleen cells with CsA and antigen. Suppression was not antigen specific for responder cells. A ratio of 2.5:1 or more of suppressor cells to line cells was necessary for suppression to occur (data not shown). Spleen cells with *in vitro* suppressive activity were plastic nonadherent and radiation resistant and also suppressed the proliferation of antigen-specific T-cell lines to concanavalin A (data not shown). Normal spleen cells incubated with CsA, 200 ng/ml for 2 or 24 hours, did not significantly alter the *in vitro* proliferation of BP-specific lines to BP, suggesting that CsA carry-over by spleen cells was not the explanation for the suppressive effects we observed. Results of the *in vivo* treatment with suppressor cells are shown in TABLE 2. Suppressor cells ameliorated the course of CR-EAE, with reduced incidence and severity of clinical disease, delayed onset of disease, and less severe histopathologic changes.

This is the first report of successful treatment of CR-EAE with suppressor cells. Using a modification of a previously published protocol,[3] we were able to generate suppressor cells that inhibited encephalitogenic helper T lymphocytes both *in vitro* and *in vivo*. These CsA-induced suppressor cells were radiation resistant and antigen nonspecific, findings that agree with those of some previous reports[6,7] but not others.[1-3,6,8] This approach may prove to be promising in the treatment of autoimmune diseases such as multiple sclerosis.

## REFERENCES

1. HESS, A. D., P. J. TUTSCHKA & G. W. SANTOS. 1981. J. Immunol. **126:** 961-968.
2. DOS REIS, G. A. & E. M. SHEVACH. 1982. J. Immunol. **129:** 2360-2367.
3. MCINTOSH, K. & D. DRACHMAN. 1986. Science **232:** 401-403.
4. VANDENBARK, A. A., T. GILL & H. OFFNER. 1985. J. Immunol. **135:** 223-228.
5. BOURDETTE, D., H. OFFNER, R. WHITHAM *et al.* 1987. Neurology 37 (Suppl. 1): 233.
6. BEN-NUN, A. & I. COHEN. 1982. J. Immunol. **128:** 1450-1457.
7. WANG, B. S., E. H. HEACOCK *et al.* 1982. J. Immunol. **128:** 1382-1385.
8. HUTCHINSON, I. F., C. A. SHADUR *et al.* 1981. Transplantation **32:** 210-216.

# Attenuated T-Lymphocyte Lines As Vaccinating Agents Against Experimental Autoimmune Encephalomyelitis[a]

HALINA OFFNER, RICHARD JONES, AND ARTHUR A. VANDENBARK

*Oregon Health Sciences University
Departments of Neurology and Microbiology and Immunology
and
Veterans Administration Medical Center
Portland, Oregon*

Experimental autoimmune encephalomyelitis (EAE) is a paralytic disease that is mediated by myelin basic protein specific T lymphocytes. With the development of BP-specific T-cell lines and clones,[1,2] naive recipient animals can reportedly be "vaccinated" against active and passive EAE, using attenuated encephalitogenic T cells.[3] In this study, we evaluated several vaccination protocols for protecting Lewis rats against EAE.

Guinea pig basic protein (GP-BP) specific T-cell lines were selected, as described previously,[2] and were administered by one of the following protocols: (1) two doses of $20 \times 10^6$ encephalitogenic T cells were lethally irradiated (2,500 R) and injected (intraperitoneally or intravenously) 7 days apart; (2) three doses of $20 \times 10^6$ T cells were pressure treated (1300A, 15 minutes), lethally irradiated, and administered weekly; (3) a single dose of $10^3$-$10^5$ activated T cells was injected intravenously; or (4) $2$-$5 \times 10^6$ encephalitogenic T cells were injected to induce passive EAE. After 7-14 days, control and experimental groups of rats (154 total) were challenged with GP-BP in complete Freund's adjuvant (active EAE) or $2$-$5 \times 10^6$ activated, encephalitogenic T cells (passive EAE).

Rats vaccinated with lethally irradiated T cells (protocol 1) were partially protected against active but not passive EAE (data not shown), but animals injected with low (nonencephalitogenic) doses of T cells (protocol 3) were not resistant to either active or passive disease (data not shown). Animals that had recovered from passive EAE (protocol 4) were resistant to actively induced EAE, the animals most severely affected during the first bout being the most resistant to the second challenge (data not shown).

By far the most effective protocol was to vaccinate with pressurized activated encephalitogenic cells (purportedly to cause aggregation of membrane antigens[3]) and then to lethally irradiate (protocol 2). The final irradiation step was found to be essential to the vaccination protocol, because pressure-treated, nonirradiated T cells

---

[a] This work was supported by National Institutes of Health Grants NS23444, NS23221, and the Veterans Administration.

remained viable, proliferated in the presence of interleukin-2 (IL-2), and transferred mild but definite signs of EAE (TABLE 1). After attenuation, however, these pressurized cells induced resistance to active EAE in dramatic fashion (TABLE 2). Vaccination with either the BP line or the D9 clone, both encephalitogenic before pressure treatment and irradiation, protected completely against challenge with BP-CFA.

Protection against passive EAE could also be induced in some cases after vaccination with pressurized, attenuated T cells. When the D9 clone was used to vaccinate, complete protection was induced against D9-induced EAE, although no protection was observed against BP-line-mediated EAE (TABLE 2). Conversely, vaccination with BP line cells produced significant but unimpressive resistance against BP-line-induced EAE (TABLE 2).

Vaccinated rats and controls were also tested for delayed-type hypersensitivity (DTH) reactions against the vaccinating T cells. Highly significant DTH reactions

TABLE 1. Pressure-Treated Cells Proliferate *in vitro* and Transfer EAE

| Treatment | Clinical Disease | Time (h) | Proliferation (cpm $\times 10^{-3}$) | Viability |
|---|---|---|---|---|
| None | $2.7 \pm 0.8^a$ | 24 | $167 \pm 4.0$ | 96 |
| | | 48 | $133 \pm 0.5$ | 94 |
| | | 72 | $37 \pm 0.8$ | 81 |
| | | 96 | $8.1 \pm 1.3$ | 75 |
| Pressure[b] | $1.5 \pm 0^c$ | 24 | $9.3 \pm 0.5$ | 57 |
| | | 48 | $47 \pm 0.8$ | 11 |
| | | 72 | $93 \pm 2.5$ | 45 |
| | | 96 | $42 \pm 5.8$ | 41 |
| Pressure[b] and Irradiation[d] | $0 \pm 0^c$ | 24 | $4.9 \pm 0.2$ | 33 |
| | | 48 | $1.9 \pm 0.1$ | 7 |
| | | 72 | $0.5 \pm 0.02$ | 0 |
| | | 96 | $0.2 \pm 0.02$ | 0 |

[a] Clinical disease transferred with $3 \times 10^6$ stimulated cells.
[b] 1,300 atmospheres for 15 minutes.
[c] Clinical disease transferred with $20 \times 10^6$ stimulated cells.
[d] 2,500 rads.

were observed in treated rats against both the vaccinating T cells as well as the cells of other antigen specificities. These results demonstrate clearly that the vaccinating T cells were autoimmunogenic, but they suggest that the most prominent autoantigens were shared among T cells of various specificities and were not restricted to idiotypes.

In conclusion, we confirm previous reports[3] that attenuated, encephalitogenic T cells can vaccinate against EAE. It is our experience, however, that pressure treatment alone cannot attenuate the vaccinating T cells, and that effective vaccination requires additional lethal irradiation. Before similar vaccination protocols are applied in human diseases such as multiple sclerosis, it will be important to define relevant T-cell specificities to determine if vaccination can affect ongoing disease, and to evaluate which molecules and epitopes on the T cells are relevant to the protection phenomenon.

TABLE 2. Vaccination Against EAE Using Pressure-Treated, Irradiated Encephalitogenic T Cells

| Vaccinating T Cells: Protocol 2 | Disease Induction[a] | Clinical Disease[b] |
|---|---|---|
| Experiment 1 | | |
| None | BP 20 Line | 2.5 ± 0.8 |
| | D9 Clone | 4.0 ± 0.0 |
| | Active | 3.5 ± 0.7 |
| D9 Clone[c] | BP-20 Line | 3.3 ± 0.3 |
| | D9 Clone | 0 ± 0 |
| | Active | 0 ± 0 |
| Experiment 2 | | |
| None | BP 20 Line | 4.0 ± 0 |
| | Active | 3.0 ± 0.5 |
| BP-20 Line[c] | BP-20 Line | 2.8 ± 1.0 |
| | Active | 0 ± 0 |

[a] Passive or active disease induced on day 28.
[b] Clinical signs scored as: 0 = no signs; 1 = flaccid tail; 2 = weakness; 3 = paralysis; 4 = death.
[c] Stimulated cells were exposed to 1,300 Atm for 15 minutes followed by irradiation with 2,500 rads. $20 \times 10^6$ cells were administered intraperitoneally on days 0, 7, and 14.

## REFERENCES

1. BEN-NUN, A., H. WEKERLE & I. R. COHEN. 1981. Eur. J. Immunol. **9:** 195-199.
2. VANDENBARK, A. A., T. GILL & H. OFFNER. 1985. J. Immunol. **135:** 223-229.
3. LIDER, O., M. SHINITZKY & I. R. COHEN. 1986. Proc. N.Y. Acad. Sci. **275:** 267-273.

# Inhibition of Passive Allergic Encephalomyelitis by Sulfated Polysaccharides

## DAVID O. WILLENBORG [a,b] AND CHRISTOPHER R. PARISH [c]

[a] *Neurosciences Research Unit*
*Royal Canberra Hospital*
*and*
[b] *Departments of Experimental Pathology and* [c] *Microbiology*
*John Curtin School of Medical Research*
*Australian National University*
*Canberra, Australia*

Experimental allergic encephalomyelitis (EAE), whether induced actively by injection of encephalitogen plus adjuvant or passively by transfer of T lymphocytes from such sensitized animals, results in the accumulation of inflammatory cells within the central nervous system (CNS). There are two crucial steps in the development of these inflammatory lesions: (1) the arrest of neural antigen-specific T lymphocytes in the CNS vasculature, and (2) their subsequent movement across the endothelium and through the subendothelial extracellular matrix into the parenchyma of the white matter. This process is analogous to the metastasis of tumor cells, which also requires binding to and migration through the endothelium. Because of recent studies showing the inhibition of experimental metastasis by sulfated polysaccharides, we examined the ability of some of these polysaccharides to inhibit the neuroinflammatory response of EAE (TABLE 1).

TABLE 1. Effect of Sulfated Polysaccharides on Adoptively Transferred EAE[a]

| Treatment[b] | No. with EAE/Total | Mean Day of Onset | Mean Clinical Score | Mean Duration of Disease |
|---|---|---|---|---|
| Control | 7/7 | 4.4 ± 0.2 | 4.1 ± 0.9 | 5.0 ± 0.4 |
| Chondroitin-4-sulfate (20 mg/ml) | 5/5 | 5 | 3.5 ± 0.2 | 5.0 ± 0.4 |
| Pentosan sulfate (20 mg/ml) | 5/5 | 6.2 ± 0.3 | 2.4 ± 0.2 | 3.0 ± 0.4 |
| Fucoidan (20 mg/ml) | 0/6 | — | — | — |
| Heparin (20 mg/ml) | 0/8 | — | — | — |
| Periodate oxidized heparin (20 mg/ml) | 5/5 | 6.4 ± 0.2 | 1.6 ± 0.2 | 2.4 ± 0.4 |

[a] $30 \times 10^6$ concanavalin-A-activated EAE spleen cells given intravenously.
[b] Osmotic pumps containing sulfated polysaccharides were implanted day 3 after cell transfer. Pumps hold 2 ml and deliver 10 µl/h for 7 days.

Heparin and fucoidan both completely inhibited passive EAE even when treatment was begun 3 days after transfer of cells. Pentosan sulfate was partially inhibitory, whereas chondroitin-4-sulfate had no effect. Not only was clinical disease inhibited, but also examination of some 80 sections through the lower thoracic/upper lumbar spinal cord from three heparin-treated rats revealed not a single lesion (FIG. 1b), whereas controls had numerous lesions in virtually every low power field (FIG. 1a).

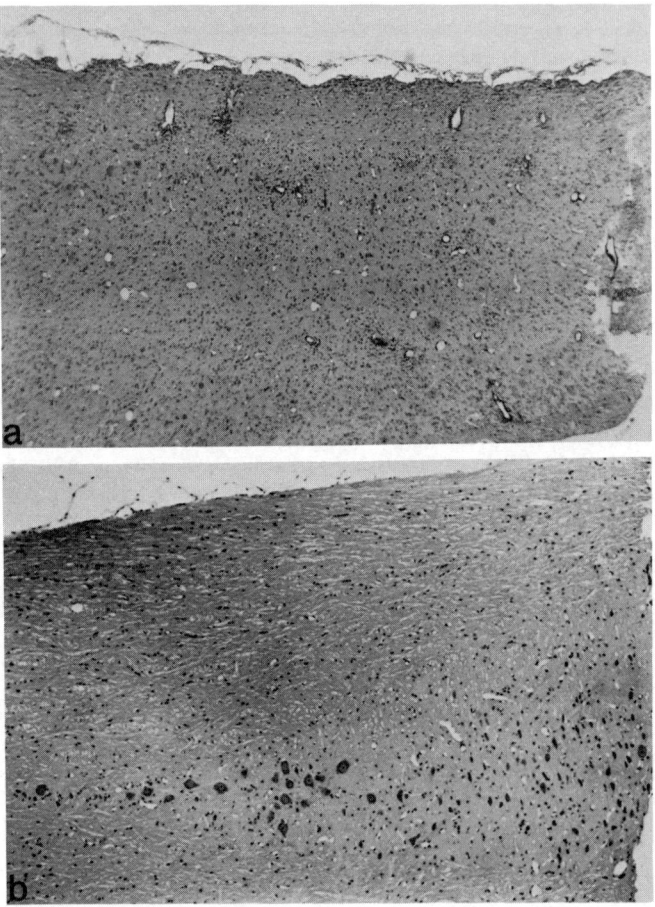

**FIGURE 1.** Lower thoracic/upper lumbar spinal cord from (**a**) untreated control rats with EAE or (**b**) heparin-treated rats that failed to develop clinical signs. Note the total absence of any inflammatory lesions in **b**.

Inhibition was not merely due to killing of effector cells by the sulfated polysaccharides, because active sensitization 14 days after cell transfer resulted in an early onset of disease, indicating the persistence of transferred cells as memory cells (data not shown).

Although all three inhibitory polysaccharides are anticoagulants, it appears that this function is not **solely** responsible for inhibition because a heparin preparation devoid of anticoagulant activity also partially inhibited EAE (periodate oxidized heparin; TABLE 1).

The ability of anticoagulant-free heparin to significantly inhibit passive EAE is of considerable interest. At least two mechanisms are possible. First, CNS venules may have receptors for sulfated polysaccharides, as do high endothelial venules of lymphoid tissue,[1] and exogenous polysaccharides may bind to these receptors and prevent lymphocyte binding through complementary structures on their surface. Secondly, inhibition may not be in binding to, but at the level of passage of lymphocytes through the endothelium.

Studies on tumor metastasis have demonstrated that the sulfated polysaccharides shown to inhibit EAE also inhibit metastasis. Furthermore, in the tumor system, the sulfated polysaccharides did not inhibit adhesion of tumor cells[2] to the vascular endothelium, but blocked tumor cell-derived heparanases involved in the penetration of the vascular basement membrane by tumor cells.[3] Similar to EAE, the anticoagulant activity of heparin played a minor role in its antimetastatic activity, anticoagulant-free heparin being a potent antimetastatic agent and heparanase inhibitor.[2]

With respect to lymphocyte emigration, it was shown[4] that activated T lymphocytes express an endoglycosidase, heparanase, which also degrades the heparan sulfate side chains of the proteoglycan scaffold of the ECM. This heparanase activity may indeed facilitate passage of activated T cells (e.g., EAE effector cells) across the blood-brain barrier into the parenchyma of the CNS. Heparin as well as other sulfated polysaccharides may inhibit EAE by being potent inhibitors of lymphocyte heparanases by occupying and blocking the active site of the enzyme.

## REFERENCES

1. BRENAN, M. & C. R. PARISH. 1986. Modification of lymphocyte migration by sulphated polysaccharides. Eur. J. Immunol. **16:** 423-430.
2. COOMBE, D. R., C. R. PARISH, I. A. RAMSHAW & J. M. SNOWDEN. 1987. Analysis of the inhibition of tumour metastasis by sulphated polysaccharides. Int. J. Cancer. **39:** 82-88.
3. PARISH, C. R., D. R. COOMBE, K. B. JAKOBSEN & P. A. UNDERWOOD. 1987. Evidence that sulphated polysaccharides inhibit tumour metastasis by blocking tumour cell-derived heparanases. Int. J. Cancer, in press.
4. NAPARSTEK, Y., I. R. COHEN, Z. FUKS & I. VLODAVSKY. 1984. Activated T-lymphocytes produce a matrix-degrading heparan sulfate endoglycosidase. Nature **310:** 241-244.

# Suppression of Experimental Allergic Neuritis by Cyclosporin A

### H. NAKAYASU, K. OTA, H. TANAKA, H. IRIE, AND K. TAKAHASHI

*Division of Neurology*
*Institute of Neurological Sciences*
*Tottori University School of Medicine*
*Yonago 683, Japan*

Cyclosporin A (CyA) is reported to prevent the development of experimental allergic neuritis (EAN) during the course of its administration.[1,2] After the cessation of CyA, however, EAN developed. In this study, we are reporting how the administration of CyA modulates the course of EAN and why relapse of EAN occurs after the cessation of CyA.

## MATERIALS AND METHODS

In actively induced EAN, inbred Lewis rats were sensitized with 2 mg of bovine peripheral nerve myelin. In passively transferred EAN, $1 \times 10^9$ lymphoid cells, obtained 10 days after sensitization, were injected into each recipient rat intraperitoneally. Rats were divided into three groups. Control groups were given olive oil only. Groups receiving CyA for prophylactic use were given 50 mg/kg of CyA orally every other day from the day of inoculation or transfer. Groups receiving CyA for therapeutic use were given CyA after manifestation of clinical signs.

## RESULTS

In actively induced EAN (FIG. 1), prophylactic use of CyA completely prevented the development of paresis, histologic lesions, and elevation of antimyelin antibody titers. When CyA was given for therapeutic use, the severity of EAN was reduced. However, after the cessation of CyA administration, paresis developed in the groups given CyA prophylactically and it exacerbated in the groups given CyA therapeutically.

In passively transferred EAN (FIG. 2), all control groups and groups receiving therapeutic CyA developed paresis and recovered monophasically. None of the groups receiving CyA prophylactically developed paresis during the course of CyA administration or after its cessation. However, there were slight histologic lesions, and antimyelin antibody titers were elevated.

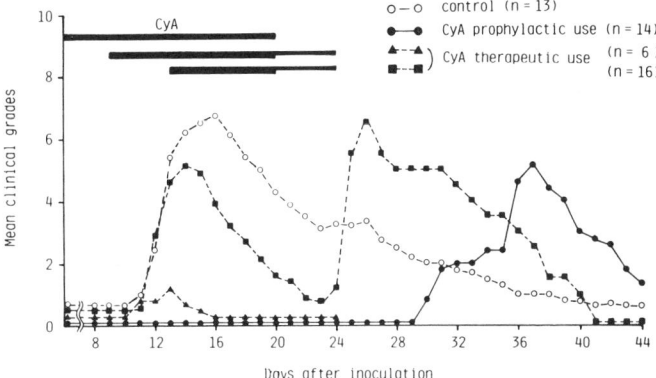

**FIGURE 1.** The mean clinical grades of actively induced EAN in the four groups of rats. *Open circles* = control groups; olive oil was given from the day of inoculation. *Closed circles* = groups receiving CyA prophylactically; CyA was given from the day of inoculation. *Closed triangles* = groups receiving CyA therapeutically; CyA was given from 9 days after inoculation. *Closed squares* = groups given CyA therapeutically; CyA was given from 13 days after inoculation.

## COMMENTS

1. EAN did not develop after cessation of CyA dosing when antigen stimulation was removed. The development of EAN after the cessation of CyA dosing is thought to be caused by remaining antigen in actively induced EAN.

2. CyA prevented the development of EAN and the production of antibodies when administered from the day of inoculation.

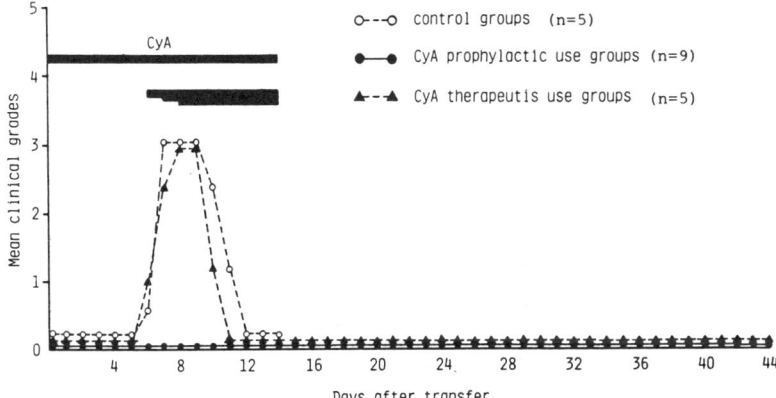

**FIGURE 2.** The mean clinical grades of passively transferred EAN for three groups of rats. *Open circles* = control groups; olive oil was given from the day of transfer. *Closed circles* = groups receiving CyA prophylactically; CyA was given from the day of transfer. *Closed triangles* = groups receiving CyA therapeutically; CyA was given from the day limp tail appeared.

3. CyA reduced the severity of EAN without suppressing antibody production when administered after the establishment of sensitization. These findings are consistent with the actions of CyA, which are considered to inhibit the production of interleukin-2 and gamma-interferon.

## REFERENCES

1. TOMPKINS, C., R. H. M. KING et al. 1980. Modification of experimental allergic neuritis by cyclosporin A. Neuropathol. Appl. Neurobiol. **6:** 240.
2. KING, R. H. M., R. I. CRAGGS et al. 1983. Suppression of experimental allergic neuritis by Cyclosporin-A. Acta Neuropathol. **59:** 262.

# Low-dose Cyclosporin A Induces Relapsing Experimental Allergic Encephalomyelitis in the Lewis Rat

CHRISTINE D. DIJKSTRA,[a] C. J. A. DE GROOT,[a]
J. C. KOETSIER,[b] I. MATTHAEI,[b] C. H. POLMAN,[b]
AND T. SMINIA[a]

[a]*Department of Histology and* [b]*Neurology*
*Free University*
*Amsterdam, The Netherlands*

Experimental allergic encephalomyelitis (EAE) in Lewis rats is an acute autoimmune disease of the CNS, which generally has a monophasic course.[1] It serves as a model for multiple sclerosis in humans. The administration of large doses of cyclosporin A (CsA) reduces the incidence and severity of symptoms of EAE in Lewis rats.[2] However, its usefulness in humans is limited because of the nephrotoxicity of such doses of CsA.[3] Therefore, we studied the effect of smaller doses of CsA on the clinical and pathologic findings in EAE.

## MATERIALS AND METHODS

Male Lewis rats were immunized by a single subcutaneous injection of guinea pig spinal cord homogenate with complete Freund's adjuvant.[4] CsA suitable for subcutaneous injection[5] was obtained from J.C.J.M. Stokvis, Sandoz, The Netherlands. Seven animals received low doses of CsA on alternate days from day 0 to day 22 after immunization; seven animals did not receive any medication.

Clinical signs were scored from 1 (loss of tail tonus, unsteady gait) to 4 (death resulting from EAE) during the course of the disease; scoring of both groups was continued until day 50 after immunization, when all the animals were sacrificed (if they had not died in the course of the disease or been killed for other reasons). Brains were frozen in liquid nitrogen. Infiltrates in the CNS were analyzed using monoclonal ED1, ED2, and ED3 against macrophages,[6] OX4 against Ia antigen, and W3/13, W3/25, and OX8 against T lymphocytes in a two-step immunoperoxidase method.[4]

## RESULTS

All animals in the control group showed a monophasic course of the disease with clinical signs from day 11 to day 16 after immunization; none of them (0/7) had relapses. In the CsA-treated group the clinical signs developed somewhat later (an average of 2 days), and all animals (7/7) showed at least one severe relapse about 1 week after recovery from the first attack and in most cases it was followed by a second or third relapse.

Immunohistochemical analysis of infiltrates in the CNS revealed that the brains of CsA-treated animals at day 50 showed (after one or more relapses) an enormous expression of Ia antigen when compared with those of untreated animals. Application of monoclonal antibodies against lymphocytes and macrophages on parallel sections revealed that these cells were responsible for only part of the Ia antigen expression. In contrast to the perivascular infiltrates, Ia antigen in the CNS parenchyma was expressed by neuroglial cells and not by infiltrated cells.

## CONCLUSION

Low-dose CsA treatment does not prevent the induction of EAE in Lewis rats; on the contrary, it induces an exceedingly high relapse rate.

This severe course of EAE after CsA treatment is acompanied by persistent expression of Ia antigen in the CNS by infiltrated lymphocytes and macrophages as well as by neuroglial cells within the brain tissue.

### REFERENCES

1. RAINE, C. S. 1985. Demyelinating disease. *In* Handbook of Clinical Neurology, Vol. 7. J. C. Koetsier, Ed.: 429-466. (Rev. Ser. 3.) Elsevier, Amsterdam.
2. BOLTON, C., J. F. BOREL, M. L. CUZNER, A. N. DAVISON & A. M. TURNER. 1982. J. Immunol. Sci. **56**: 147.
3. MYERS, B. D., J. ROSS, L. NEWTON, J. LUETSCHER & M. PERLROTH. 1984. N. Engl. J. Med. **311**: 699.
4. POLMAN, C. H., C. D. DIJKSTRA, T. SMINIA & J. C. KOETSIER. 1986. J. Neuroimmunol. **11**: 215.
5. WASSEF, R., Z. COHEN & B. LANGER. 1985. Transplantation **40**: 489.
6. DIJKSTRA, C. D., E. A. DÖPP, P. JOLING & G. KRAAL. 1985. Immunology **54**: 589.

# Treatment of Experimental Allergic Myasthenia Gravis with a New Immunosuppressant: 15-Deoxyspergualin[a]

YASUNORI ISHIGAKI,[b] TAKESHI SATO,[b] SONG TONG-LIN,[b] AND KYOZO HAYASHI[c]

[b] *Department of Neurology*
*Juntendo University School of Medicine*
*Tokyo, Japan*

[c] *Department of Biology*
*Gifu Pharmaceutical University*
*Gifu, Japan*

Myasthenia gravis (MG) is an autoimmune disease in which antibodies inhibit the acetylcholine receptor (AChR) of neuromuscular junctions. Currently, treatment of MG commonly involves the use of anticholine esterase, thymectomy, and immunosuppressive agents, such as adrenocorticosteroids and azathioprine. Combined therapy during the early stage is generally effective in controlling MG, but about 5% of patients with severe MG do not show improvement despite long-term high-dose therapy with such immunosuppressive drugs. In view of this limitation, an effective new immunosuppressive agent was needed in the treatment of MG.

15-Deoxyspergualin (15-DSP) is a new immunosuppressant developed as an antitumor antibiotic by Umezawa *et al.*[1] in 1981. It was discovered in culture filtrates of bacterial BMG 162-aF2, which is related to *Bacillus laterosporus*. It is known to have antitumor effects in treating mouse leukemia, rat hepatoma, and other tumors in animals and to have strikingly immunosuppressive effects on graft skin rejection and other acquired autoimmune disease models.[2] The toxicity of 15-DSP is low. The LD50 by intraperitoneal injection is about 150 mg/kg in mice. In our research, we produced experimental allergic myasthenia gravis (EAMG) rat models, immunized with AChR prepared from electric organ of *Torpedo californica,* and administered 15-DSP to them in order to find a practical application to human MG.

Four groups—15, 10, 5, and 5 rats in each—were treated, respectively, as follows: (1) MG immunized by AChR; (2) MG + 5.0 mg/kg per day of 15-DSP; (3) complete Freund's adjuvant (CFA) + 5.0 mg/kg per day of 15-DSP; and (4) CFA. Anti-AChR antibody assays and histologic observation of EDL muscle specimens were performed.

Anti-AChR antibody was detected neither in the controls nor in the 15-DSP-

---

[a] This work was supported in part by a grant in aid for New Drug Development Research from the Ministry of Health and Welfare, Japan.

treated MG group. In the MG group, the levels of anti-AChR antibodies began to increase 2 weeks after the initial immunization (FIG. 1). The levels of anti-AChR correlated with the clinical states.

The neuromuscular junctions of the controls and CFA + 15-DSP group were normal. Acetylcholine receptors were detected on the primary and secondary synaptic clefts stained with peroxidase-labeled α-bungarotoxin. In nerve terminals, synaptic

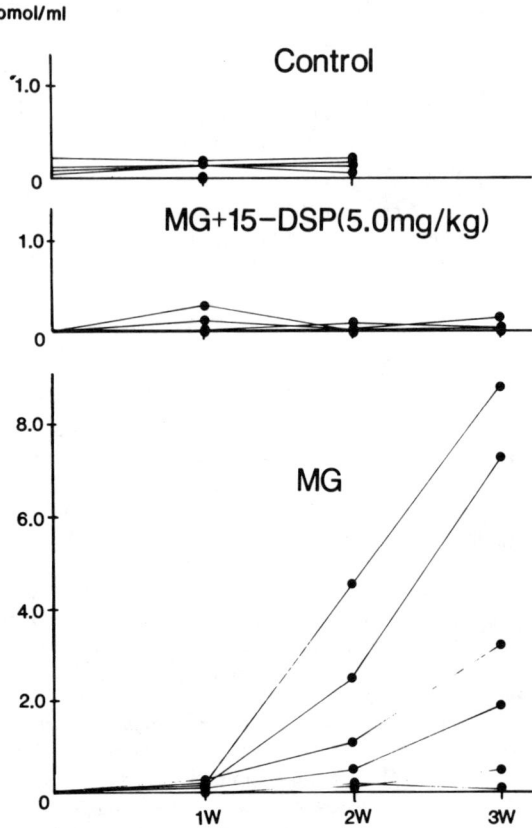

**FIGURE 1.** Levels of antiacetylcholine receptor antibody. *Upper* (control) and *middle* (EAMG-treated with 15-DSP) *panels* show no elevation of anti-AChR antibodies. *Lower panel* (EAMG) shows that anti-AChR antibodies begin to elevate 2 weeks after immunization.

vesicles and mitochondria could be observed. In the MG group, biopsied at the chronic phase, 4 weeks after the booster, the neuromuscular junctions were severely degenerated and remarkably decreased. On the postsynaptic clefts, few AChRs remained. Detached parts in the intersynaptic space were also observed. However, the nerve terminals, including synaptic vesicles and mitochondria, appeared not to be affected.

In conclusion, 15-DSP can prevent the elevation of anti-AChR antibodies and histologic changes in EAMG. Less than 5.0 mg/kg per day of 15-DSP may be useful in treating human MG.

## REFERENCES

1. UMEZAWA, H., K. MORIMOTO, N. SHIMADA, H. NAGANAWA & T. TAKITA. 1981. A new antitumor antibiotic, spergualin: Isolation and antitumor activity. J. Antibiotics **34**: 1619-1621.
2. UMEZAWA, H., M. ISHIZUKA, T. TAKEUCHI, F. ABE, K. NEMOTO, K. SHIBUYA & T. NAKAMURA. 1985. Suppression of tissue graft rejection by spergualin. J. Antibiotics **38**: 283-284.

# Therapeutic Immunoadsorption of Acetylcholine Receptor Antibodies in Myasthenia Gravis[a]

## TAKESHI SATO,[b] YASUNORI ISHIGAKI,[b] TADATOSHI KOMIYA,[b] AND HIROSHI TSUDA [c]

[b] Departments of Neurology and [c] Internal Medicine
Juntendo University
Tokyo, Japan

The first reports by Sato et al.[1,2] in 1983 indicated that acetylcholine receptor (AChR) antibodies are adsorbed selectively by a new immunoadsorbent (tryptophane-conjugated polyvinyl alcohol, IM-T). However, only a minimal amount of antibody is adsorbed with phenylalanine-conjugated polyvinyl alcohol resin.

Seven patients with severe generalized myasthenia gravis (MG) were treated with plasmapheresis (PF), using IM-T for selective removal of AChR antibodies. Although these patients were treated with both thymectomy and corticosteroids, they remained in serious condition and most of them required respiratory assistance. Six patients had thymoma and one had thymous hyperplasia. Five patients showed high levels of AChR antibodies. The conditions of all patients were maintained with an optimal dosage of anticholine esterase and corticosteroids before and after PF.

Two methods of PF were used: (1) double membrane filtration (DF) (plasma separator and plasma filter), and (2) IM-T (plasma separator and IM-T column). The separated plasma was perfused through the IM-T column and returned to the blood circuit. In each treatment, 3 liters of plasma were perfused in 3 hours. Each series of PF was carried out over 3 days. Furthermore, a subsequent series of PF was performed 4 weeks later.

Remarkable clinical improvements occurred in six of seven patients just after each series of PF. Treatment by IM-T and DF methods of PF resulted in almost the same grades of improvement. The reduction rate of AChR antibodies was almost the same with both methods, whereas the rates of IgG, IgA, and IgM were greater with DF, in which 10-20 g of albumin supplementation were required (FIG. 1).

Post-PF AChR antibody titers were reduced by a mean reduction of 68.1 ± 17.1% in DF and by 78.9 ± 7.2 in IM-T. The reduction in AChR antibodies was selective. The reduction rates of IgG, IgA, IgM, and C3, while remaining low in the IM-T, were higher in DF.

Long-term PF was feasible and effective in controlling one patient with chronic MG. This patient was treated monthly over 14 months with PF combined with steroids and azathioprine. The AChR antibody levels, after each series of PF, were remarkably decreased and followed by clinical improvements (FIG. 2). Complications associated with PF using IM-T include a decrease in the concentration of fibrinogen and an

[a] This work was supported in part by a grant from the Ministry of Health and Welfare, Japan.

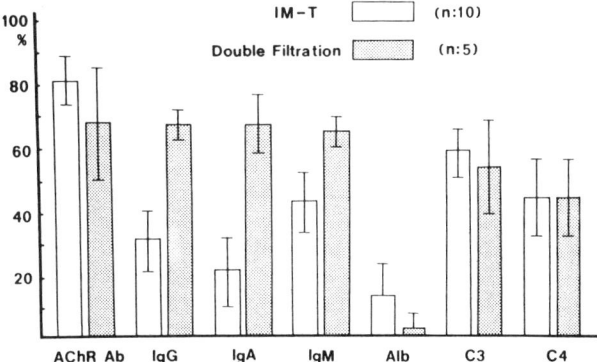

**FIGURE 1.** Reduction rate of acetylcholine receptor (AChR) antibodies, immunoglobulins, albumin, and complements before and after successive plasmapheresis by tryptophane-conjugated polyvinyl alcohol (IM-T) and double filtration method.

increase in the number of white blood cells which cleared within 24 hours without serious sequelae.

The present study demonstrated that IM-T adsorbs a high concentration of AChR antibodies, but the adsorption rate of IgG remains at a lower level. These data suggest that certain differences may exist between AChR antibodies and other immunoglobulins. Further study will be required to elucidate the mechanism of selective adsorption of AChR antibodies with IM-T column.

In conclusion, IM-T shows selective removal of AChR antibodies from sera in patients with MG. The use of IM-T may be very useful physiologically and serve as a more efficient alternative to other previous methods of PF.

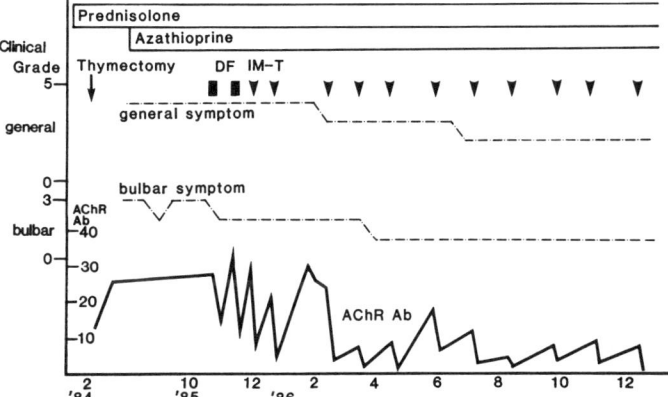

**FIGURE 2.** Level of acetylcholine receptor (AChR) antibodies and grades of clinical state in case 1 after long-term intermittent plasmapheresis combined with prednisolone and azathioprine.

## REFERENCES

1. SATO, T., M. ANNO, et al. 1983. Progress in Artificial Organs (Cleveland): 719-722.
2. SATO, T., J. NISHIMIYA, et al. 1983. In Therapeutic Plasmapheresis III. T. Oda, Ed.: 565-568. F. K. Schattauer, Verlag, Stuttgart.

# Anti-CD4 and Anti-CD2 Monoclonal Antibody Infusions in Subjects with Multiple Sclerosis

## Immunosuppressive Effects and Human Antimouse Responses

DAVID A. HAFLER AND HOWARD L. WEINER

*Center for Neurologic Diseases*
*Division of Neurology*
*Department of Medicine*
*Brigham and Women's Hospital*
*and*
*Harvard Medical School*
*Boston, Massachusetts*

Monoclonal antibodies (mAb) that recognize T-cell-specific surface determinants have been used in animals as immunosuppressive agents that can reverse experimental models of organ transplant rejection and autoimmune diseases.[1-4] The mechanisms responsible for immunologic suppression have not been well established. Infusions of murine antibodies in humans usually result in modulation of T-cell surface markers without significant T-cell destruction.[5,6] In contrast, in rat mAb infusions in mice, significant cell loss does occur.[4] Sensitization against murine monoclonal antibodies is another problem that can abrogate the therapeutic effectiveness of therapy.[5,8]

In these series of experiments, we examined the immunologic responses to infusions of anti-CD2 (T11) and anti-CD4 (T4) monoclonal antibodies to specifically address the following issues: (1) Is there evidence of immunosuppression using *in vitro* measure of immune function after infusion of anti-CD2 or anti-CD4 mAb? and (2) What is the host response to repeated infusion of murine mAb?

Eight subjects received five daily infusions (0.2 mg/kg per day) of either anti-T11 (CD2) or anti-T4 (CD4) murine monoclonal antibody. *In vitro* pokeweed mitogen (PWM) induced immunoglobulin synthesis was used to measure the immunosuppressive effects of the anti-T4 and anti-T11 mAb infusions. There was significant suppression in PWM-induced Ig synthesis up to 2 weeks after infusions of anti-T4 mAb (FIG. 1). There were no consistent changes in PWM Ig synthesis after anti-T11 infusions. The CD2 activation pathway was measured by stimulating whole mononuclear cells with a combination of anti-T11$_2$ and anti-T11$_3$ mAb. There was suppression of the CD2 pathway 4-7 days after anti-T11 mAb infusions (FIG. 2). In contrast, this suppression was not observed after anti-T4 mAb infusions.

The sera from each subject were measured for their specificity against different murine antibody isotypes. There was cross-reactivity between the different IgG iso-

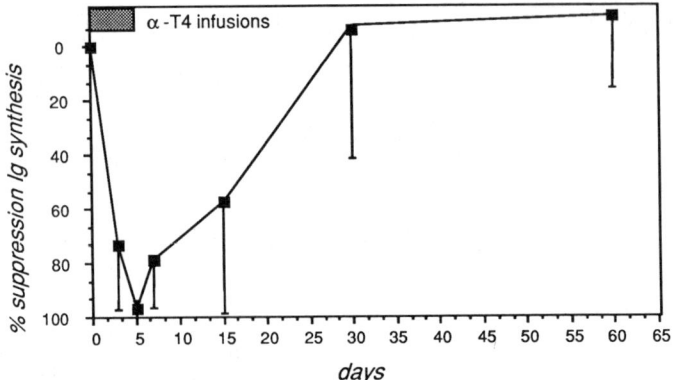

**FIGURE 1.** Four subjects were infused with αT4 monoclonal antibodies for 5 days. One hundred thousand MNC obtained from blood samples on the days indicated were cultured for 7 days with pokeweed mitogen; supernatants were harvested and Ig concentration determined by ELISA. The percentage of inhibition of Ig synthesis to preinfusion values is shown ( ± SEM). (Reprinted, with permission, from J. Immunol., reference 9.)

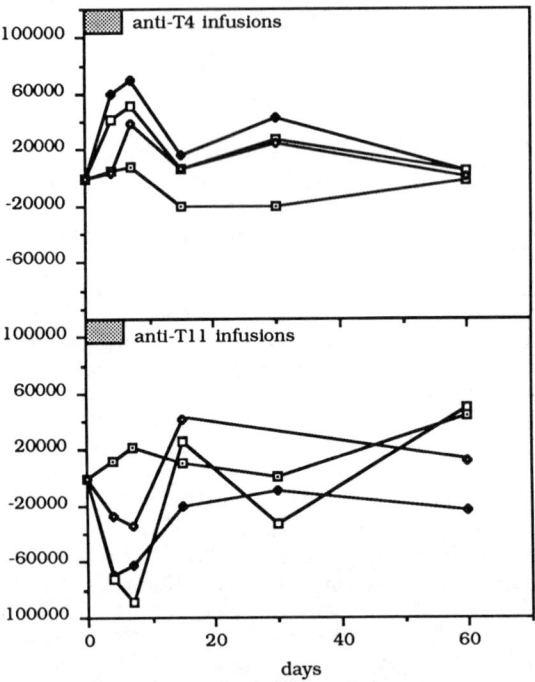

**FIGURE 2.** Four subjects were infused for 5 consecutive days with anti-T4 (*top*) or anti-T11 (*bottom*) monoclonal antibody. One-hundred thousand MNC were incubated with anti-T11$_2$ and anti-T11$_3$ mAbs for 4 days and tritiated thymidine was added during the last 18 hours of incubation. Each line represents a separate subject and each data point represents the counts per minute compared to pre-treatment values.

types, whereas there was less reactivity to the IgM class. The sera were then assayed for their ability to inhibit the binding of fluoresceinated anti-T11 to T cells. Low levels of blocking activity were observed after the first series of infusions in two subjects. There was nearly total inhibition of fluoresceinated anti-T11 binding to T cells in this *in vitro* assay by the sera of two subjects after the second series of mAb infusion, which was not observed in a third subject. The isotype of anti-mouse human antibodies was measured serially. The earliest human anti-T11 response was observed between 15 days and 2 months after the initial anti-T11 infusions. The majority of the human anti-mouse response was of the IgG isotype.

The antigenicity of anti-T11 and anti-T12 mAb after infusions in different subjects was compared. A significantly higher anti-mouse response was observed in subjects receiving anti-T12 (IgM) as opposed to anti-T11 (IgG2b mAbs). The anti -T12 human response was predominantly directed (IgM/($\alpha$T12)) against determinants. There were no significant differences between the anti-mouse response observed after anti-T4 and that after anti-T11 mAb infusions.

In summary, our studies demonstrated that murine mAbs can be differentially immunosuppressive in humans without eliminating the target T-cell population. Possible mechanisms include the induction of negative signals via T-cell surface structures as well as blocking or modulating T-cell receptors for ligands that are important in T-cell activation. However, human anti-mouse responses may in certain circumstances prevent continued administration of the mAb in chronic diseases. In the future, it will be important to develop strategies that effectively block the induction of anti-idiotype responses after infusion of anti-T-cell mAb in humans.

## REFERENCES

1. JONKER, M., P. NEUHAUS, C. ZURCHER, A. FUCELLO & G. GOLDSTEIN. 1985. OKT4 and OKT4A antibody treatment as immunosuppression for kidney transplantation in rhesus monkeys. Transplantation **39**: 247-253.
2. BROSTOFF, S. W. & D. W. MASON. 1984. Experimental allergic encephalomyelitis: Successful treatment in vivo with a monoclonal antibody that recognized T helper cells. J. Immunol. **133**: 1938-1942.
3. WALDOR, M. D., S. SRIRAM, R. HARDY *et al.* 1985. Reversal of experimental allergic encephalomyelitis with monoclonal antibody to a T-cell subset market. Science **227**: 415-417.
4. SRIRAM, S. & C. A. ROBERTS. 1986. Treatment of established chronic relapsing experimental allergic encephalomyelitis with anti-L3T4 antibodies. J. Immunol. **136**: 4464-4469.
5. HAFLER, D. A., R. J. FALLIS, D. M. DAWSON, S. F. SCHLOSSMAN, E. L. REINHERZ & H. L. WEINER. 1986. Immunologic responses of progressive multiple sclerosis patients treated with an anti-T-cell monoclonal antibody, anti-T12. Neurology **36**: 777-784.
6. CHATENOUD, L., M. F. BAUDRIHAYE, N. CHKOFF, H. KREIS & J. F. BACH. 1983. Immunologic follow-up of renal allograft recipients treated prophylactically by OKT3 alone. Transplant. Proc. **15**: 643-645.
7. CHATENOUD, L., M. F. BAUDRIHAYE, N. CHKOFF, H. KREIS, G. GOLDSTEIN & J. F. BACH. 1986. Restriction of the human in vivo immune response against the mouse monoclonal antibody OKT3. J. Immunol. **137**: 830-838.
8. CHATENOUD, L., M. JONKER, F. VILLEMAIN, G. GOLDSTEIN & J. F. BACH. 1986. The human immune response to the OKT3 monoclonal antibody is oligoclonal. Science **232**: 1406-1408.
9. HAFLER, D. A., J. RITZ, S. F. SCHLOSSMAN & H. L. WEINER. Anti-CD4 and anti-CO$^2$ monoclonal antibody infusions in subjects with multiple sclerosis. J. Immunol., in press.

# Effects on Experimental Allergic Neuritis in Rats by *in Vivo* Treatment with Monoclonal Anti-T-Cell Antibodies

T. OLSSON,[a] K. STRIGÅRD,[a] P. LARSSON,[b]
R. HOLMDAHL,[a] AND L. KLARESKOG[a]

[a]*Department of Neurology*
*Huddinge University Hospital*
*Karolinska Institutet*
*Stockholm, Sweden*

[b]*Department of Med. Phys. Chem.*
*University of Uppsala*
*Uppsala, Sweden*

T lymphocytes play a crucial role in disease induction in experimental allergic neuritis (EAN).[1] T cells and their subsets occur in close proximity to cells in endoneuria that express class II (Ia) transplantation antigens, giving morphologic requisites for local T-cell activation within nerves.[2,3] The number of endoneurial T lymphocytes correlates with functional nerve deficits.[4] One way to study T-cell function *in vivo* is to selectively manipulate these cells by *in vivo* treatment with monoclonal antibodies (mAb) directed against T-cell surface antigens.[5] We here describe such immune manipulations using single injections of anti-rat CD4 (W3/25)-T helper cells, anti-Ia (0 × 6), W3/13-pan T cells, anti-rat CD5 (0 × 19)-pan T cells, and anti-rat CD8 (0 × 8)-T suppressor/cytotoxic cells, during various phases of EAN[6] and after $P_2$-induced protection against EAN.

Lewis rats were immunized with bovine peripheral myelin and complete Freund's adjuvant for induction of EAN. One milligram of mAb was injected into each animal at days 0, 9 (before the expected onset of disease), or 15 (at the height of the disease) after immunization. Other Lewis rats were pretreated with $P_2$ in incomplete Freund's adjuvant, 4 weeks later rechallenged with neuritogenic doses of myelin in adjuvant, and simultaneously injected with 1 mg of 0 × 19 or 0 × 8. Rats were examined daily for clinical signs of EAN. Selected spleens were sampled for immunohistochemical staining of lymphocyte phenotypes.

Several mAbs, W3/13, W3/25, 0 × 8 as well as 0 × 6 partly prevented clinical signs of EAN when given shortly before the expected onset of disease, whereas W3/13 and 0 × 8 given at the height of disease did not further affect disease development. Both 0 × 19 treatment day 9 and day 15 after immunization dramatically exaggerated the duration and severity of the disease. When given on day 0 after immunization, a slight decrease in disease symptoms occurred. $P_2$-induced protection against neuritogenic immunization was broken by 0 × 19 injection (FIG. 1). Immunohistochemistry showed abolished staining for CD5 lymphocyte surface receptors in spleens 4 days or more after the 0 × 19 treatment, in spite of preserved staining with another pan T-cell marker, arguing for surface receptor modulation and not physical elimination on the T cell as the consequence of 0 × 19 treatment. Treatment with 0 × 8, however, did not terminate $P_2$-induced protection against EAN. Immunohistochemistry showed physical elimination of CD8-positive cells after this treatment.

This study demonstrates that *in vivo* mAb treatment may produce profound effects in an autoimmune demyelinating disease. This finding should encourage further studies with mAb to modulate both experimental and human disease. However, the sometimes unexpected results that depend on which type of mAbs are used and in what phase of disease they are injected emphasize the need for further detailed experimental data

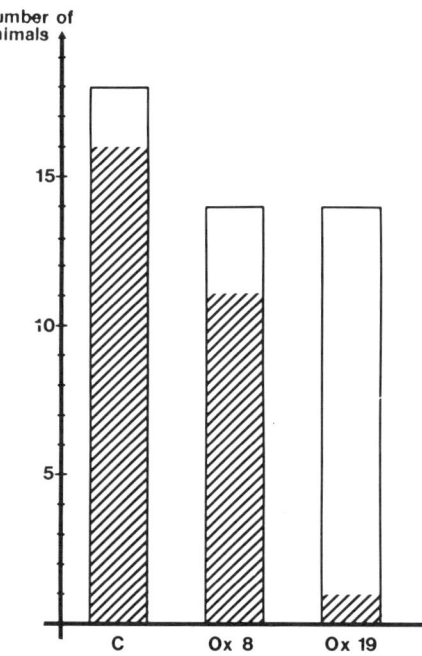

FIGURE 1. Lewis rats were immunized with $P_2$ in incomplete Freund's adjuvant. Four weeks later they obtained neuritogenic immunization with bovine peripheral myelin in complete Freund's adjuvant. Thereby, 16 of 18 control animals (C) were protected from clinical signs of experimental allergic neuritis (EAN) (*shadowed area*). After anti-CD8 (0 × 8) injection simultaneously with reimmunization, 11 of 14 rats were protected. In contrast, anti-CD5 (0 × 19) injection terminated $P_2$-induced protection against EAN in 13 of 14 animals.

in this area. The results may also indicate a direct role of the CD5 lymphocyte surface receptor in down-regulation of the neuritogenic response. T cells in target tissue, sciatic nerves, do not express the CD5 receptor during the onset of EAN; reexpression occurs later.[4] Artificial down-regulation of this receptor, as now performed, may have exaggerated the neuritogenic response. In contrast, CD8-positive T cells apparently do not suppress this response *in vivo*.

## REFERENCES

1. LININGTON, C., S. IZUMO, M. SUZUKI, K. UYEMURA, R. MEYERMANN & H. WEKERLE. 1984. A permanent rat T cell line that mediates experimental allergic neuritis in the Lewis rat in vivo. J. Immunol. **133:** 1946.

2. OLSSON, T., R. HOLMDAHL, L. KLARESKOG & U. FORSUM. 1983. Ia-expressing cells and T lymphocytes of different subsets in peripheral nerve tissue during experimental allergic neuritis in Lewis rats. Scand. J. Immunol. **18:** 339.
3. OLSSON, T., R. HOLMDAHL, L. KLARESKOG, U. FORSUM & K. KRISTENSSON. 1984. Dynamics of Ia-expressing cells and T lymphocytes of different subsets during experimental allergic neuritis in Lewis rats. N. Neurol. Sci. **66:** 141.
4. STRIGÅRD, K., T. BRISMAR, T. OLSSON, K. KRISTENSSON & L. KLARESKOG. 1987. T lymphocyte subsets, function deficits and morphology in sciatic nerves during experimental allergic neuritis. Muscle & Nerve **10:** 329.
5. HOLMDAHL, R., T. OLSSON, T. MORAN & L. KLARESKOG. 1985. In vivo treatment of rats with monoclonal anti T cell antibodies. Immunohistochemical and functional analysis in normal rats and in experimental allergic neuritis (EAN). Scand. J. Immunol. **22:** 157.
6. STRIGÅRD, K., T. OLSSON, P. LARSSON, R. HOLMDAHL & L. KLARESKOG. 1988. Effects on experimental allergic neuritis in rats by in vivo treatment with monoclonal anti-T-cell antibodies. J. Neurol. Sci., **83:** 283.

# Suppression of P2-T-Cell Line Mediated Experimental Autoimmune Neuritis by Interleukin-2 Receptor Blockade

H. P. HARTUNG,[a] B. SCHÄFER,[a] T. DIAMANTSTEIN,[b]
W. FIERZ,[c] K. HEININGER,[a] AND K. V. TOYKA[a]

[a]*Department of Neurology*
*University of Düsseldorf*
*Düsseldorf, West Germany*

[b]*Institute of Immunology*
*FU Berlin*
*Berlin, West Germany*

[c]*Division of Clinical Immunology*
*University Hospital*
*Zurich, Switzerland*

Experimental autoimmune neuritis can be produced by adoptive transfer of P2-reactive T-lymphocyte line cells.[1] As an animal model of the acute Guillain-Barré syndrome, it can serve to evaluate novel therapeutic strategies for more specific immunosuppression in autoimmune disease of the peripheral nervous system. We examined whether interference with T-cell activation achieved through administration of the monoclonal antibody ART 18 directed to the $\beta$-chain of the interleukin-2 receptor would prevent or mitigate adoptive transfer EAN.[2]

## METHODS

Eight-week-old Lewis rats were injected with $5 \times 10^6$ cells from a freshly activated P2-T-cell line.[1] Each treatment group comprised six animals. ART 18 (IgG$_1$ from mouse, 1 mg/kg) was injected intraperitoneally shortly before cell transfer (group 1) as well as on day 1 (group 2) through day 3 after transfer. Animals were inspected for clinical signs of the disease and were serially monitored electrophysiologically for evolving changes in the functional properties of the sciatic nerve.[3] Rats were perfused on day 9 after transfer. Epon sections of roots and sciatic nerves were assessed semiquantitatively for morphologic alterations (cellular infiltration, demyelination, edema, and axonal damage).[4]

## RESULTS AND DISCUSSION

Sham-treated rats developed full-blown disease, with paraparesis and neurographical conduction slowing and failure, temporal dispersion and delay of H reflex, F T wave, and S response of lumbar somatosensory evoked potentials. By contrast, *in vivo* administration of ART 18, even one single injection, markedly suppressed or completely prevented the development of the disease as evidenced by clinical, electrophysiologic, and histopathologic examination (FIGS. 1 and 2). No changes were noted in the distribution of lymphocyte subsets.

The role of T cells in the pathogenesis of EAN is well established. Previous attempts to modulate the course of this disease have utilized monoclonal antibodies directed to specific T-cell subsets. The advantage of interleukin-2 receptor-targeted monoclonal antibody therapy lies in its exclusive blockade of recently activated T cells expressing this antigen. Administration of this antibody thus allows specific immunosuppression of experimental autoimmune disease of the peripheral nervous system. Our findings may have implications for future immunomodulatory therapy in the Guillain-Barré syndrome in humans.

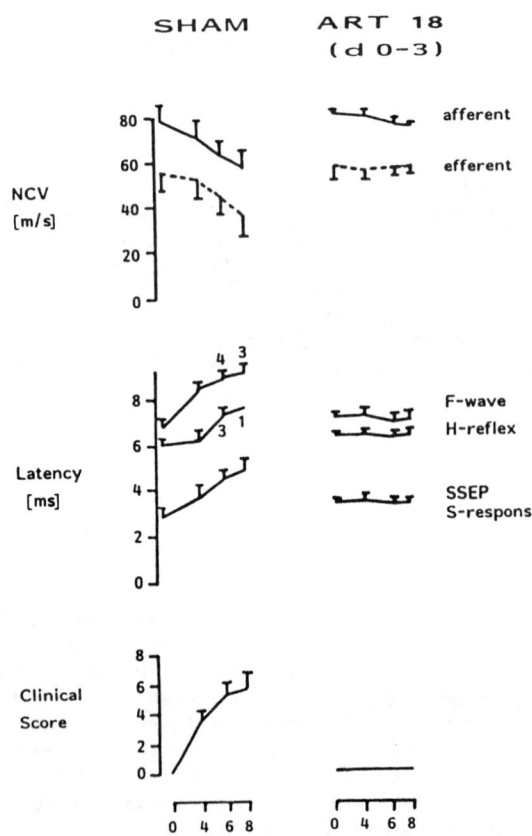

**FIGURE 1.** Serial nerve conduction studies in sham- and ART-18-treated rats. *Top to bottom:* NCV-motor nerve conduction velocities of the sciatic nerve on stimulation at the sciatic notch (efferent NCV) and mixed afferent nerve conduction velocities of the sciatic nerve after stimulation at the malleolus. Latencies of F waves, H reflex, and S response of lumbar somatosensory evoked potentials recorded at the D12/L1 spinal level. Comparison of results obtained in sham-treated rats and those that received ART 18 from day 0 through 3 after cell transfer. Note that on day 6 it was possible only in four (three) rats to obtain an F response/H reflex, whereas on day 8 F responses could be elicited in three and an H reflex in only one of six sham-treated rats. Clinical score according to King et al.[5]: 0 = normal; 10 = death. Sham-treated rats developed severe paraparesis.

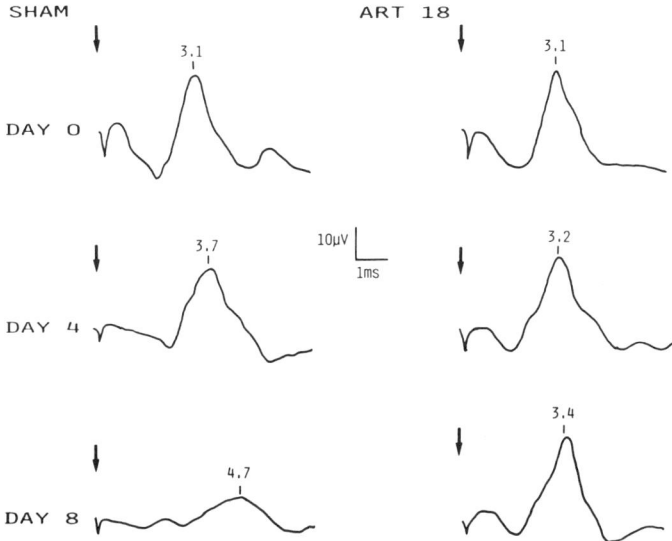

**FIGURE 2.** Serial studies on S response of lumbar somatosensory evoked potentials in sham- and ART-18-treated rats. The S response was recorded after stimulation at the malleolus at D12/L1 and was averaged. Sham-treated rats exhibited increasing delay and temporal dispersion as well as loss of amplitude of the S response. In contrast, rats that received injection of ART 18 from day 0-3 after cell transfer showed marginal changes only. Numbers indicate latencies in milliseconds.

## REFERENCES

1. LININGTON, C., S. IZUMO, M. SUZUKI et al. 1984. A permanent rat T cell line that mediates experimental allergic neuritis in the rat in vivo. J. Immunol. **133:** 1946.
2. DIAMANTSTEIN, T. & H. OSAWA. 1986. The interleukin-2 receptor, its physiology and a new approach to a selective immunosuppressive therapy by interleukin-2 receptor monoclonal antibodies. Immunol. Rev. **92:** 5.
3. HEININGER, K., G. STOLL, C. LININGTON, et al. 1986. Conduction failure and nerve conduction slowing in experimental allergic neuritis induced by P2-specific T-cell lines. Ann. Neurol. **19:** 44.
4. HEININGER, K., B. SCHÄFER, H. P. HARTUNG et al. 1988. The role of macrophages in experimental autoimmune neuritis induced by a P2 specific T cell line. Ann. Neurol. **23:** 326.
5. KING, R. H. M., R. I. CRAGGS, L. P. GROSS et al. 1983. Suppression of experimental allergic neuritis by cyclosporin A. Acta Neuropathol. (Berl.) **59:** 262.

# Sindbis Virus Neutralization

## M. E. WESTARP, J. STANLEY, AND D. E. GRIFFIN

*Department of Neurology*
*Johns Hopkins School of Medicine*
*Baltimore, Maryland 21205*

The single-stranded RNA alphavirus, sindbis virus, is transmitted by arthropods and causes acute encephalitis in mice, and fever, rash, and arthritis in man. The sindbis virus envelop consists of 240 heterodimers of two glycoproteins, E1 (439 aa) and E2 (423 aa), which undergo conformational changes during the virus life cycle.[1-3]

The mechanism of recovery from alphavirus infection is the production of antibodies to the surface glycoproteins. Using monoclonal antibodies (mAbs) it was shown that both neutralizing and non-neutralizing anti-E1 and anti-E2 mAbs are protective.[4]

## MATERIAL AND METHODS

Our current studies use three strains of virus that differ in virulence for mice: SBRL (avirulent[5]), SV (moderately virulent[6]), and NSV (highly virulent[7]). Single amino acid differences in their surface glycoproteins determine these virulence characteristics.[8]

Our purpose was to define the regions on the surface of the E1 and E2 glycoproteins that elicit neutralizing and protective antibodies. For these studies we used mouse mAbs and rabbit polyclonal antisera to synthetic peptides of 12-16 amino acids each. With more than a dozen mAbs to E1 and E2 and eight partially overlapping peptides to regions E2 (175-202) and E2 (45-60), we asked the following questions:

1. Do mAbs recognize any synthetic peptide?
2. Can we correlate the neutralizing activity of mAbs with conformational changes in E1-E2 introduced through SDS denaturation, Triton-X treatment, or cell surface expression of viral antigens?
3. How do neutralizing and non-neutralizing mAbs act on the different steps of the infectious cycle? Do they interfere with virus attachment to the cell surface, or do they alter later steps in replication?
4. Can our peptide antisera identify antigenic and/or functionally important sites on the viral surface?
5. Do strain-specific peptides elicit strain-specific antibodies?

## RESULTS

The answers so far are:

1. None of our mAbs recognizes any of our eight peptides, whether glutaraldehyde cross-linked, Triton-X treated, or KLH coupled.
2. Binding of anti-E2 mAbs is more sensitive to conformational changes than is binding of anti-E1 mAbs; antigen treatment with anionic or nonionic detergents, or cell surface expression of antigens, often abrogates anti-E2, but not anti-E1 mAb binding.
3. Neutralization is very rapid, taking place within minutes, but neutralizing and non-neutralizing mAbs both inhibit viral adsorption to cells.
4. Two antigenic sites have been identified on E2 with antipeptide sera. One (45-60) is a functional neutralizing site, but this antibody does not provide *in vivo* protection.
5. A single amino acid change at the E2 (45-60) binding site can seriously alter the predicted conformation of the protein; neutralizing antisera raised against strain-specific peptides were cross-neutralizing.

## REFERENCES

1. STRAUSS, E. G., C. M. RICE & J. H. STRAUSS. 1984. J. Virol. **133:** 92-110.
2. SCHMALJOHN, A. J., K. M. KOKUBUN & G. A. COLE. 1983. Virology **130:** 144-154.
3. FULLER, S. D. 1987. Cell **48:** 923-34.
4. STANLEY, J., S. J. COOPER & D. E. GRIFFIN. 1986. J. Virol. **58:** 107-115.
5. OLMSTEDT, R. A., W. J. MEYER & R. E. JOHNSON. 1986. Virology **148:** 245-254.
6. TAYLOR, R. M., H. S. HURLBUT, T. H. WORK *et al.* 1955. Am. J. Trop. Med. Hyg. **4:** 844-862.
7. GRIFFIN, D. E. & R. T. JOHNSON. 1977. Immunology **118:** 1070-1075.
8. DAVIS, N. L., F. J. FULLER, W. G. DOUGHERTY *et al.* 1986. Proc. Natl. Acad. Sci. USA **83:** 6771-6775.

# Tumor Necrosis Factor Mediates Myelin Damage in Organotypic Cultures of Nervous Tissue[a]

KRZYSZTOF SELMAJ [b,c] AND CEDRIC S. RAINE [b]

[b] Department of Pathology (Neuropathology)
Albert Einstein College of Medicine
New York, New York

[c] Department of Neurology
Medical Academy of Lodz
Lodz, Poland

In view of the active role played by infiltrating cells in the pathogenesis of the multiple sclerosis (MS) lesion and its experimental analogs, immune system products have been suspected as participants in the observed myelin damage in these diseases. Tumor necrosis factor (TNF) is one member of a growing family of cytokines currently implicated in several disease processes in which immune cytolytic mechanisms are operative. This study examines the effect of a number of cytokines upon myelin *in vitro*. Recombinant human TNF, gamma-interferon (IFN-$\gamma$), and interleukin-2 (IL-2), as well as T-cell supernatants, were all compared for myelinolytic effect in myelinated cultures of mouse spinal cord. In addition, the patterns were compared with antiserum-induced (antigalactocerebroside) demyelination.[1] Although cultures exposed to normal nutrient medium displayed regularly myelinated fibers (FIG. 1), those exposed to TNF ($1 \times 10^3$ to $1 \times 10^4$ U/ml) displayed a type of myelin dilatation unique to this system (FIG. 2) which appeared to result from the influx of water into the internodal periaxonal space (FIG. 3). The effect of TNF upon myelin had a delayed onset (18-24 hours after exposure) and was accompanied by the selective necrosis of oligodendrocytes. Neurons were not affected, but astrocytes became hypertrophic and participated in the phagocytosis of oligodendroglial debris. Some myelinated fibers progressed to demyelination by 72 hours of exposure. The myelin lesion was not reversed by returning the cultures to normal feeding medium for 3 days.

In contrast to TNF, IFN-$\gamma$ and IL-2 had little or no effect on myelinated CNS cultures. T-cell supernatants induced some myelin fragmentation over 72 hours but no dilatation of the type produced by TNF. The pattern of myelin disintegration induced by antigalactocerebroside antiserum differed markedly from the TNF picture in that by 4 hours of exposure, total lysis of myelin with little or no bubbling was achieved with the lytic process beginning in the outer layers of the sheath.

We suggest that the myelin changes resulting from exposure to TNF are related to a selective activity upon ion channels on the surface of the axon or the oligodendrocyte, and this leads to water influx into the periaxonal space. Thus, TNF produces a physiologic demyelination (not structural, as is the case with antiserum) initially

[a] This work was supported by NMSS RG 1001-F-6, and HHS NS 08952 and NS 11920.

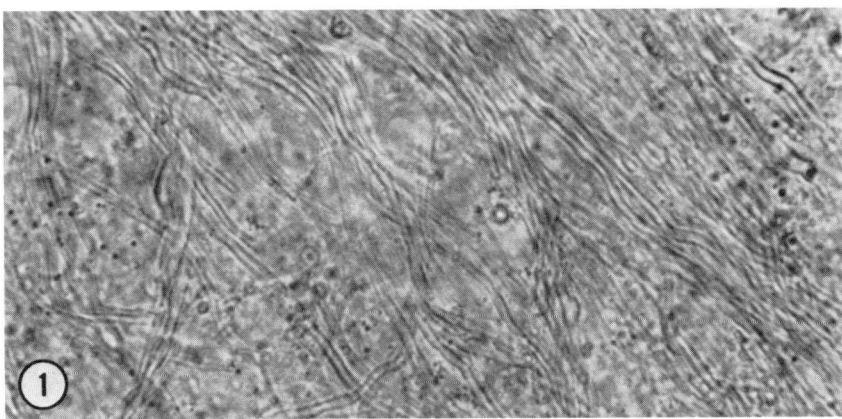

**FIGURE 1.** An area from a mouse spinal cord culture exposed to normal nutrient medium displays abundant long stretches of normally myelinated nerve fibers (18 days *in vitro;* living culture; magnification × 450).

without overt damage to the myelin membrane. Similar effects of TNF on water and electrolytes have been demonstrated,[2] and its effects upon transmembrane potentials are documented.[3] The present morphologic picture is also similar to that produced by batrachotoxin, a sodium channel neurotoxin.[4] Such an ionic channel dysfunction in MS might help explain the eventual depletion of oligodendrocytes and some axons in the long-standing lesion.

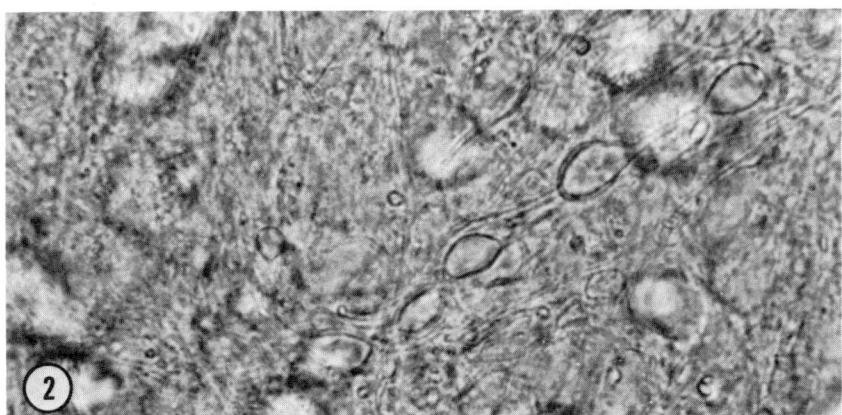

**FIGURE 2.** After 24 hours of exposure to $2 \times 10^3$ U/ml recombinant human tumor necrosis factor, this sister culture shows many regions of myelin sheaths to be dilated and to appear as regularly spaced bubbles. The blurred profiles are macrophages at a different level of focus (living culture; magnification × 450).

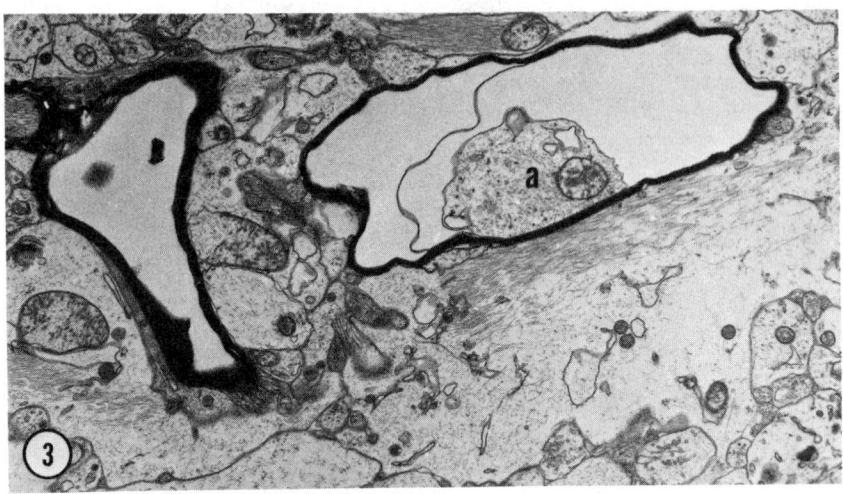

**FIGURE 3.** An electron micrograph from a culture exposed for 20 hours to $1 \times 10^3$ U/ml of tumor necrosis factor reveals the myelin dilatation to involve swelling between the periaxonal space and the inner layer of myelin. The axon (**a**) is unaffected. Processes from hypertrophic astrocytes are also present (magnification $\times$ 10,000).

## REFERENCES

1. RAINE, C. S., A. B. JOHNSON, D. M. MARCUS, A. SUZUKI & M. B. BORNSTEIN. 1981. J. Neurol. Sci. **52:** 117-131.
2. BEUTLER, B. & A. CERAMI. 1987. N. Engl. J. Med. **316:** 379-385.
3. TRACEY, K. J., S. F. LOWRY, B. BEUTLER, et al. 1986. J. Exp. Med. **164:** 1368-1373.
4. MOORE, G. R. W., R. J. BOEGMAN, D. M. ROBERTSON & C. S. RAINE. 1986. J. Neurocytol. **15:** 573-583.

# Recombinant Human Lymphokines Induce Changes in Visual Evoked Potentials in the Rabbit[a]

C. F. BROSNAN,[b,c] K. SELMAJ,[b,d] C. E. SCHROEDER,[c]
M. LITWAK,[c] C. S. RAINE,[b,c] AND J. C. AREZZO [c]

[b] *Department of Pathology*
*and*
[c] *Department of Neuroscience*
*Albert Einstein College of Medicine*
*Bronx, New York*

[d] *Department of Neurology*
*Medical Academy of Lodz*
*Lodz, Poland*

In response to antigenic stimulation, lymphocytes and macrophages secrete an array of inflammatory mediators that serve to activate and effect an immune response. The success achieved in cloning the genes for many of these mediators has led to the availability of relatively pure products and an increased understanding of the role that they play in the inflammatory process. Much of this information has been obtained from experimentation *in vitro* or from subcutaneous or systemic injection *in vivo* However, less is known about the effect of these cytokines on central nervous system (CNS) function.

To establish a system that would permit longitudinal assessment of the role of cytokines in inducing electrophysiologic and structural changes associated with inflammation in the CNS, we explored the use of epidural visual evoked potentials (VEPs) in the rabbit. The rabbit visual system offers several advantages for these studies: the visual pathways are almost entirely crossed, which permits the response of one eye to be distinguished from the response in the other, allowing one eye to function as an internal control; the visual cortex is on the dorsolateral surface of the brain, which results in large amplitude cortical VEPs and a clearly defined topographic distribution of monocular and binocular responses; and factors to be tested can be injected into the vitreous, circumventing the blood-brain barrier with minimal trauma. In addition, axons of the retina are myelinated, which permits a study of the effect of inflammatory mediators on myelinated portions of the primary sensory axons.

Injection of 1,000 U of recombinant human gamma-interferon (rhIFN-γ) increased the peak latency of the cortical response by 2 ms within 10 minutes of injection. No change in the morphology of the waveform was evident. Cortical responses were still delayed 3 hours postchallenge but had returned to baseline values by 24 hours postchallenge. The response could be reinduced by reinjection of rhIFN-γ and again reversed within 24 hours. Injection of 1,000 U of tumor necrosis factor (rhTNF)

---

[a] This work was supported by USPHS grants NS11920 and NS23247.

produced a similar delay and recovery in VEPs except that the response was not evident until 3 hours postchallenge. No long-term changes were observed in animals for up to 2 months postchallenge. Injection of 1,000 U of interleukin-2 (rhIL-2) produced a subtle alteration only after 48-72 hours. The effects induced by rhIL-2 showed partial recovery by 96 hours.

Pathologic examination of the tissue suggests that the primary effect of these lymphokines is on the vasculature. Animals challenged with rhIFN-$\gamma$ or rhTNF showed proliferation of vascular adventitia but little or no inflammation. In the electron microscope there was evidence of capillary damage, duplication of basal lamina, collagen deposition, increased pinocytotic activity of large veins, and opening of endothelial cell junctions. Increased granularity of the Muller cells was observed in animals that had received multiple injections. Pathologic examination of rabbits injected with rhIL-2 revealed the presence of increased adhesion of mononuclear cells to the endothelium and perivascular inflammation. There was no evidence that the results were due to the presence of endotoxin in the preparations. These findings illustrate the sensitivity of the system and demonstrate that rhIFN and rhTNF induce acute and characteristic alterations that can be differentiated from the inflammatory effects of IL-2.

# Intracerebral Beta-Interferon in Brain Tumor Therapy

## Monitoring Cerebral Function with Compressed Spectral Analysis[a]

ROBERT L. KNOBLER,[b] FRED D. LUBLIN,[b]
LEOPOLD J. STRELETZ,[b] MICHAEL ZIMMER,[b]
JEYMOHAN JOSEPH,[b] CONCETTA D'IMPERIO,[b]
BRUCE NORTHRUP,[c] GIANCARLO BAROLAT,[c] AND
STEPHEN G. MARCUS[d]

[b]*Department of Neurology*
*Jefferson Medical College*
*Philadelphia, Pennsylvania*

[c]*Department of Neurosurgery*
*Jefferson Medical College*
*Philadelphia, Pennsylvania*

[d]*Triton Biosciences, Inc.*
*Alameda, California*

Human recombinant beta-interferon (Betaseron, Triton Biosciences, Inc.) was administered intracerebrally to four patients with biopsy-proven glioblastoma multiforme to test the safety and efficacy of this form of interferon. Prior encouraging results in preliminary clinical trials,[1] the demonstration of cytotoxic antitumor effects *in vitro*,[2] and known immunomodulatory effects[3] of natural beta-interferon provided a strong stimulus for undertaking this study. In contrast, there were several reports that systemic administration of natural alpha- or beta-interferons could lead to neurologic symptoms and electroencephalographic changes.[4-6] Therefore, we sought to learn about the biology of the intracerebral response to Betaseron to gain clinical experience and to determine the relative safety of this route of administration for potential use in this and other intracerebral clinical applications.

Each of the four patients had tumor debulking and placement of a Rickham reservoir and catheter before the onset of therapy. Primary cultures of the tumors were established to test the effectiveness of Betaseron *in vitro*. Escalating doses *in vitro* demonstrated a direct cytotoxic effect with $10^5$ U/ml (~0.01 mg/ml) (TABLE 1).

---

[a]This work was supported by Teacher Investigator Development Award K07 NS 00961 from the NINCDS, The Mary L. Smith Charitable Lead Trust, the Arthur L. Swim Foundation, and Triton Biosciences, Inc.

TABLE 1. Betaseron Treatment *in Vitro* Limits Cell Survival and Proliferation in a Dose-Dependent Fashion

| No. of Cells Treated | Betaseron Treatment | Duration of Treatment (days) | No. of Cells Recovered |
|---|---|---|---|
| $5 \times 10^4$ | Medium alone | 4 | $2 \times 10^4$ |
| $5 \times 10^4$ | $10^3$ U/ml | 4 | $1.2 \times 10^4$ |
| $5 \times 10^4$ | $10^4$ U/ml | 4 | $1 \times 10^3$ |
| $5 \times 10^4$ | $10^5$ U/ml | 4 | 0 |

Betaseron doses into the tumor bed were escalated over a 4-week schedule, with dosing twice weekly. Doses increased from $0.5 \times 10^6$ to $50 \times 10^6$ units, and then were maintained at a dose of $50 \times 10^6$ units twice weekly until side effects or tumor recurrence required stopping this treatment protocol. Electroencephalography with compressed spectral analysis (CSA),[7] a power spectrum from 0-100%, was a measure of EEG activity. It was evaluated each week during the escalation period, at 0.5, 2, 10, and $50 \times 10^6$ units, and 4-6-week intervals thereafter, assessing possible complications of intratumor interferon therapy.

Although the EEG with CSA was abnormal in all four patients from the onset of the study (low percentage of EEG power), reflecting the underlying tumor, there was no evidence of either immediate or cumulative toxic effects ("interferon encephalopathy")[4-6] due to beta-interferon administered intracerebrally. There was no reduction in the percentage of EEG power immediately after dosing, comparing the responses at 2 and 5 months (FIG. 1). However, the EEG with CSA proved a sensitive and valuable tool for assessing tumor recurrence, because it revealed a decreased

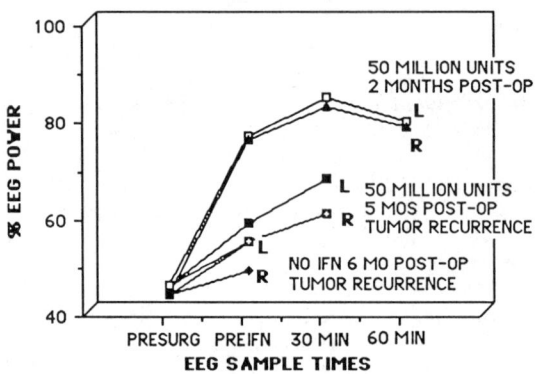

FIGURE 1. Tumor recurrence versus interferon encephalopathy. L = left cerebral hemisphere, nontumor-bearing in this patient. R = right cerebral hemisphere, tumor-bearing in this patient. Power spectra are shown at the following times, presurgically, when first presenting clinically, before dosing with Betaseron at 2, 5 and 6 months postoperatively, and both 30 and 60 minutes after interferon administration at 2 and 5 months postoperatively. At 2 months this patient had received a cumulative dose of just under $500 \times 10^6$ units ($\sim 50$ mg of protein). At 5 months this patient had received a cumulative dose of just over $1500 \times 10^6$ units ($\sim 150$ mg of protein). He was beginning to show signs of tumor recurrence, a reduced percentage of EEG power, which necessitated drop out from the study because of treatment failure at 6 months.

percentage of EEG power as the initial indicator of further tumor growth, apparent at 5 months (FIG. 1). These changes were observed even before tumor recurrence was apparent on computerized tomographic scans or magnetic resonance imaging.

Beta-interferon intracerebrally in the dose range used in the present study was not therapeutic in any of the four patients treated. This may reflect greater drug delivery to the necrotic tumor bed rather than to the more proliferative tumor periphery. Nevertheless, these findings demonstrate the relative safety of beta-interferon administered intracerebrally and point to the effectiveness of the EEG with CSA as an early indicator of tumor recurrence.

## REFERENCES

1. MAHALEY, M. S., M. B. URSO, R. A. WHALEY, M. BLUE, T. E. WILLIAMS, A. GUASPARI & R. G. SELKER. 1985. Immunobiology of primary intracranial tumors. Part 10. Therapeutic efficacy of interferon in the treatment of recurrent gliomas. J. Neurosurg. **63:** 719-725.
2. COOK, A. W., W. A. CARTER, F. NIDZGORSKI & L. AKHTAR. 1983. Human brain tumor-derived cell lines: Growth rate reduced by human fibroblast interferon. Science **219:** 881-883.
3. STIEHM, E. R. 1982. Interferon: Immunobiology and clinical significance. Ann. Int. Med. **96:** 80-93.
4. SMEDLEY, H., M. KATRAK, K. SIKORA & T. WHEELER. 1983. Neurological effects of recombinant human interferon. Br. Med. J. **286:** 262-264.
5. ROHATINER, A. Z. S., P. F. PRIOR, A. C. BURTON, A. T. SMITH, F. R. BALKWILL & T. A. LISTER. 1983. Central nervous system toxicity of interferon. Br. J. Cancer **47:** 419-422.
6. SUTER, C. C., B. F. WESTMORELAND, F. W. SHARBROUGH & R. C. HERMAN. 1984. Electroencephalographic abnormalities in interferon encephalopathy: A preliminary report. Mayo Clin. Proc. **59:** 847-850.
7. STEBEN, J. D., L. J. STRELETZ & R. G. FARIELLO. 1985. Multiprocessing computer system for sensory evoked potentials and EEG spectral analysis for clinical neurophysiology laboratory. J. Med. Systems **9:** 347-363.

# Clonal Modulation of Experimental Allergic Encephalomyelitis by a Monoclonal Antibody Directed to the T-Cell Receptor

E. HEBER-KATZ, M. OWHASHI, M. P. HAPP,
F. BURNS, N. SHEN, AND X. LI

*The Wistar Institute*
*Philadelphia, Pennsylvania 19104*

The discovery by Cohen and his colleagues[1] that experimental allergic encephalomyelitis (EAE) can be modulated by immunizing the host with antigen-specific T-cell lines suggests a role for idiotypic regulation in this disease model. A natural explanation is that this regulatory response is directed against the T-cell receptor (TcR) and consequently that the T-cell repertoire to the encephalitogenic determinant is of limited clonality. We have pursued these issues and examined T cells from Lewis rats reactive to the 68-88 encephalitogenic determinant of guinea pig myelin basic protein (GP MBP). First, we looked at the fine specificity patterns of the clonal T-cell response to interspecies MBPs and nested peptides and examined TcR gene usage by these clones. Secondly, we made an antireceptor antibody to one of these T-cell clones and examined the ability of this antibody to modulate disease. This paper briefly describes these findings and discusses the implications for therapy of an autoimmune disease in man.

## T-CELL REPERTOIRE OF THE LEWIS RAT TO THE ENCEPHALITOGENIC DETERMINANT OF GP MBP

Lewis rats were immunized with GP MBP, and proliferating lymph node T cells were hybridized through fusion with the mouse AKR thymoma, BW5147. About 75% of MBP-reactive T hybridomas were directed to the 68-88 encephalitogenic determinant.[2] Southern blot analysis (for beta-chain gene DNA rearrangements) and fine specificity antigen-reactivity patterns revealed a polyclonal response. There were two clusters of bands which we have interpreted as meaning usage of at least two different V regions with multiple J regions.[3] These findings were difficult to reconcile with the Cohen study until a surprising result was obtained with a monoclonal anti-TcR antibody.

## A MONOCLONAL ANTIBODY AGAINST THE T-CELL RECEPTOR OF ONE CLONE CAN PROTECT ANIMALS FROM EAE

Although our T-cell data did not support the idea that an antibody against a V beta TcR gene segment would bind to all 68-88 reactive T cells, it was still possible that the disease-causing cells could share an idiotype or that all of the disease-relevant clones could use the same V alpha TcR gene. Thus, we made a monoclonal antibody directed at one T-cell hybridoma (5.10) specific for the 68-88 determinant.[4] This antibody immunoprecipitated a disulfide-linked heterodimer with molecular weights of 45 and 40 kd. Furthermore, the antibody could block antigen-specific stimulation of 5.10 but not an OVA-specific T-cell hybridoma and could also stimulate 5.10 but not the OVA clone in the absence of antigen or antigen-presenting cells when coupled to sepharose beads. This antibody binds to only a very small percentage of normal lymph node cells ($<1\%$), indicating that the binding was to a restricted population of T cells but could bind to almost all of the 68-88 clones tested. By all criteria, this antibody appeared to be directed to a common idiotope, the TcR of 68-88 reactive T-cell clones.

This antibody was then tested for its *in vivo* effects on active EAE. Initial experiments using ascites (estimated at 100 µg of antibody per rat) resulted in almost complete elimination of clinical disease. This occurred with only a single injection of antibody intraperitoneally, either at the time of MBP administration or 5 days after MBP was given. Purified antibody did not seem to be as potent, but multiple injections of only 0.03µg of purified antibody per rat every other day for 12 days completely eliminated all symptoms. The ability to block disease with such a low concentration of anti-idiotypic antibody may indicate a network response as opposed to directly eliminating cells. One finding that we feel is very important considering the possibility of disease treatment using anti-idiotypes is that in cases in which we had induced a submaximal disease state with MBP, the antibody was able to *enhance* the symptoms dramatically. Thus, animals with floppy tails were driven to full paralysis in the presence of antibody. At present, we do not know what the antibody is binding to or how it is functioning. We have cloned and sequenced rat alpha and beta TcR messenger RNA from the 5.10 T-cell hybridoma and are attempting to map the binding specificity of the antibody by *in situ* hybridization and immunohistochemistry of MBP-specific T-cell hybridomas and normal T-cell populations.

### REFERENCES

1. COHEN, I. R., A. BEN-NUN, J. HOLOSHITZ, R. MARON & R. ZERUBAVEL. 1983. Vaccination against autoimmune disease using lines of autoimmune T lymphocytes. Immunol. Today **4:** 227-230.
2. HAPP, M. P. & E. HEBER-KATZ. 1988. Differences in the repertoire of the Lewis rat T cell response to self and non-self myelin basic proteins. J. Exp. Med. **167:** 502.
3. HAPP, M. P., A. KIRALY, H. OFFNER, A. VANDENBARK & E. HEBER-KATZ. 1988. The autoreactive T cell population in experimental allergic encephalomyelitis: T cell receptor B chain rearrangements. J. Neuroimmunol., in press.

# Inhibition of Experimental Allergic Encephalomyelitis by a New Anti-Inflammatory Compound—SK&F 86002

M. J. DiMARTINO, C. E. WOLFF,
G. K. CAMPBELL, JR., AND N. HANNA

*Department of Immunology & Anti-infectives Therapy
Smith Kline and French Laboratories
King of Prussia, Pennsylvania 19406-2799*

Experimental allergic encephalomyelitis (EAE) is characterized by cell-mediated immune responses to central nervous system tissue antigens, resulting in hindleg paralysis. In Lewis rats EAE can be prevented by immunosuppressive agents (e.g., methotrexate) or corticosteroids, but not by nonsteroidal anti-inflammatory cyclooxygenase inhibitors such as indomethacin.[1] Previous studies demonstrated that SK&F 86002, [6-(4-fluoropheny)2,3-Dihydro-5(4-Pyridinyl)imidazo(2, 1-b) thiazole], a dual lipoxygenase and cyclooxygenase inhibitor,[2] is effective in inhibiting mast cell mediator release (unpublished observations) and immune and nonimmune-mediated inflammatory responses that are insensitive to selective cyclooxygenase inhibitors.[3] Therefore, the present studies were performed to evaluate SK&F 86002 for its ability to inhibit the induction and progression of EAE in female Lewis rats. Methotrexate, prednisolone, and indomethacin were also evaluated for comparative purposes.

Experimental allergic encephalomyelitis was induced in female (Charles River) Lewis rats by a single intradermal injection of 0.1 ml of an emulsion consisting of equal parts of a 50% w/v homogenate of guinea pig spinal cord and midbrain in 0.5% aqueous phenol and complete Freund's adjuvant (4 mg/ml killed, dried *Mycobacterium butyricum*) into a hindpaw (left) footpad. The level of significant difference in hindleg paralysis between the treatment and control groups was determined by a chi square test. Compounds, homogenized in 0.5% aqueous gum tragacanth, or control vehicle were administered orally in a total volume of 10 ml/kg of body weight by intubation. Drug doses are expressed as milligrams per kilogram of body weight.

As shown in TABLE 1, prophylactic administration of SK&F 86002 (60 mg/kg per day) or methotrexate (0.3 mg/kg per day) markedly suppressed the development of hindleg paralysis, whereas indomethacin, even at a high anti-inflammatory dose level (2 mg/kg per day), was ineffective. In a dose response study, SK&F 86002 administered at dose levels of 60, 30, 15, or 7.5 mg/kg per day from day 0-17 inhibited the incidence of hindleg paralysis in 12/12, 9/12, 5/12, and 3/12 rats, respectively.

The therapeutic efficacy of SK&F 86002 was assessed further by administering the compound to female Lewis rats with established clinical symptoms of EAE, which is characterized by fluctuating periods of remissions and relapses of hindleg paralysis. As shown in TABLE 2, SK&F 86002 (60 mg/kg per day) administered after the initial

TABLE 1. Effect of SK&F 86002 on Hindleg Paralysis in Experimental Allergic Encephalomyelitis Induced in Female Lewis Rats

| Compound (Dose)[a] | Hindleg Paralysis—Cumulative Incidence[b] | |
| --- | --- | --- |
| | Days 14-18 | Days 20-22 |
| SK&F 86002 (60) | 0/11[c] | 8/11 |
| Indomethacin (2) | 10/11 | 9/11 |
| Methotrexate (0.3) | 0/11[c] | 0/11[c] |
| Control | 14/16 | 12/16 |

[a] mg/kg per day; days 0-4, 7-11, and 14-18.
[b] The number of animals with paralysis out of the total number treated.
[c] Significantly different from control ($p < 0.01$).

occurrence of hindleg paralysis on day 12 markedly suppressed the relapsing hindleg paralysis occurring 17-26 days after sensitization. Similar effects were produced by methotrexate (0.3 mg/kg per day) and prednisolone (20 mg/kg per day). In contrast, indomethacin (2 mg/kg per day) either had no effect or enhanced the incidence of relapsing hindleg paralysis.

Although the exact mechanism by which SK&F 86002 inhibits EAE has not been fully elucidated, its therapeutic effect in this model is probably related to its corticosteroid-like anti-inflammatory properties[3] which may be due, at least in part, to inhibition of lipoxygenase-generated products or mast cell mediator release, or both. Thus, novel nonsteroidal anti-inflammatory compounds, such as SK&F 86002, may provide effective therapy for autoimmune-mediated inflammatory diseases, including those involving the CNS.

TABLE 2. Effect of SK&F 86002 on Relapsing Hindleg Paralysis of Experimental Allergic Encephalomyelitis Induced in Female Lewis Rats[a]

| Compound (Dose)[b] | Hindleg Paralysis—Cumulative Incidence[c] | |
| --- | --- | --- |
| | Days 17-20 | Days 20-26 |
| SK&F 86002 (60) | 0/10 | 0/10[d] |
| Indomethacin (2) | 12/14[d] | 12/14 |
| Methotrexate (0.3) | 0/14[e] | 1/14[d] |
| Prednisolone (20) | 0/14[e] | 0/14[d] |
| Control | 6/18 | 12/18 |

[a] On day 12 (pre-drug), the incidence of paralysis in each group was 100% but decreased to <7% by day 16. Relapsing hindleg paralysis in the control group started to occur by day 19.
[b] mg/kg per day from day 12-26.
[c] The number of animals with paralysis out of the total number treated.
[d] Significantly different from control ($p < 0.01$).
[e] Significantly different from control ($p < 0.05$).

## REFERENCES

1. ROSENTHALE, M. E. et al. 1969. Arch. Int. Pharmacodyn. **179:** 251-275.
2. GRISWOLD, D. E. et al. 1987. Biochem. Pharmacol. **36:** 3463-3470.
3. DiMARTINO, M. J. et al. 1987. Agents Action **20:** 113-123.

# Anti-CD4 Monoclonal Antibody Therapy of Experimental Allergic Encephalomyelitis in Longtailed Macaques[a]

LYNN M. ROSE,[b,c] ELLSWORTH C. ALVORD, JR.,[c]
SARKA HRUBY,[c] SUSANNE L. JACKEVICIUS,[b]
ROSEMARIE PETERSEN,[c] NOEL WARNER,[d] AND
EDWARD A. CLARK [b,e]

*University of Washington
School of Medicine
Departments of Microbiology [b] and Pathology[c]
Becton Dickinson Monoclonal Center,[d] and the University of
Washington Regional Primate Research Center [e]
Seattle, Washington*

Experimental allergic encephalomyelitis (EAE), an autoimmune inflammatory and demyelinating disease of the central nervous system (CNS), is a model for the human demyelinating disease multiple sclerosis (MS). Experimental allergic encephalomyelitis can be induced in a variety of species by sensitization with myelin basic protein in complete Freund's adjuvant (CFA). The form of EAE induced in monkeys appears to have many immunologic features in common with MS,[1] especially an association between disease activity and depletions of circulating T cells. In addition, because monkeys are outbred, they react differently to sensitization with myelin basic protein than do inbred species of rodents. This difference provides a unique opportunity to assess the effectiveness of therapies on a wide range of clinical signs, with visual, cerebellar, spinal, and brain stem syndromes such as those encountered in humans with MS. In this study, we tested the effectiveness of two anti-CD4 monoclonal antibodies (mAbs), OKT4a (Ortho Pharmaceuticals) and Leu3a (Becton Dickinson Monoclonal Center), in the treatment of EAE in nonhuman primates. Anti-CD4 mAbs were selected because $CD4^+$ cells appear to be involved in the pathogenesis of EAE and because anti-CD4 mAbs have been successful in reversing EAE in inbred mice and rats.[2,3] The fact that leukocyte differentiation antigens are highly conserved in primate evolution[4] makes it possible to use the same monoclonal antibodies to treat humans and nonhuman primates.

---

[a] This work was supported by National Institutes of Health Grant CA 39935, National Multiple Sclerosis Society Grants RG-1708-A-21 and RG-1829-A-1, Regional Primate Center NIH Core Grant RRD0166, and Becton Dickinson Monoclonal Center, Inc.

## METHOD

Experimental allergic encephalomyelitis was induced by intradermal injection of 0.15 ml of a water-in-oil emulsion of CFA containing 7.5 mg of monkey myelin basic protein (BP) and 0.75 mg of heat-killed *Mycobacterium tuberculosis* (H37Ra, Difco) divided among three sites in the ankle. The animals were bled weekly to analyze lymphocyte subsets (using FITC-conjugated antibodies and a flow cytometer) and to measure serum anti-BP antibody titers. When the animals developed clinical signs of EAE, treatment was administered.[5] Each animal received a loading dose of mAb of 2.0 mg/kg intravenously for 4 hours. Immediately afterwards, a continuous intravenous infusion was started at 2.0 mg/kg per day for 7 days. Blood samples were taken 1, 2, 4, 7, 10, and 14 days after the start of treatment for serum assays and subset analysis. Blood samples continued to be taken at weekly intervals thereafter until a maximum of 5 weeks had elapsed since the onset of EAE. The sera were assayed for circulating murine mAb and for host antibody to murine mAb and myelin BP.

## RESULTS

All of the animals treated with mAb or saline solution developed clinical signs of EAE ranging in severity from ± to + before treatment was started. TABLE 1 sum-

TABLE 1. Course of Experimental Allergic Encephalomyelitis in Monkeys Treated with Continuous Intravenous Infusion of Monoclonal Antibody

| | | Onset of EAE | | Response to Treatment | |
|---|---|---|---|---|---|
| Animal No. | mAb | Days after Sensitization | Severity at Onset | Severity at End of Treatment | Days of Survival after Onset |
| *Group I:* | | | | | |
| 84254 | Leu3a | 21 | ± | ± | 26 |
| 84283 | 2.0 mg/kg | 23 | + | + | 13 |
| 84269 | | 18 | ± | ? | 29 |
| 84285 | | 18 | + | D | 8 |
| 85169 | Leu3a | 25 | + | ± | >30 |
| 86144 | low dose | 18 | + | D | 2 |
| 86148 | 0.5 mg/kg | 32 | + | D | 2 |
| 86156 | | 28 | + | ± | 30 |
| 84299 | OKT4a | 15 | ± | D | 5 |
| 84270 | 2.0 mg/kg | 14 | + | ? | 17 |
| 84213 | | 12 | + | D | 4 |
| *Group II:* | | | | | |
| 84253 | Leu2a | 16 | + | D | 1 |
| 84273 | 2.0 mg/kg | 16 | + | D | 5 |
| 84228 | Saline | 13 | + | D | 5 |
| 84291 | | 25 | + | D | 2 |
| 84218 | | 19 | + | D | 5 |
| 86140 | | 26 | ± | D | 3 |

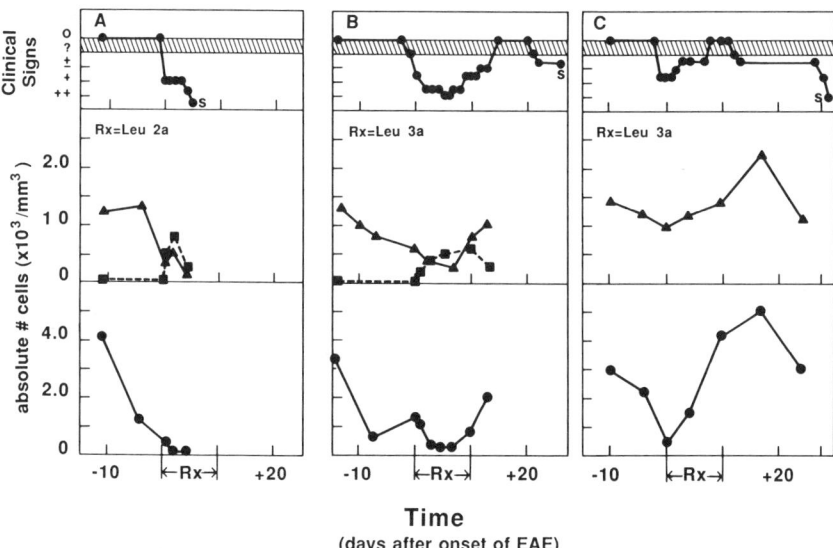

**FIGURE 1.** Comparison of T-cell subsets in macaques with experimental allergic encephalomyelitis (EAE) treated with either Leu2a anti-CD8 mAb (A-84273) or Leu3a anti-CD4 mAb (B-84254, C-84269). The total leukocytes and cell differentials were obtained for each animal. The absolute numbers of $CD4^+$ (▲), and $CD8^+$ (●) and mouse IgG (■)-coated cells were calculated by multiplying the percentage of each subset by the absolute lymphocyte number per cubic millimeter of whole blood. The daily clinical evaluations for each animal are given in the *upper panels.* The onset of EAE is indicated by the day treatment (Rx) was started. An "s" indicates that the animal was sacrificed.

marizes the major features of the clinical course and survival times of two groups of animals: group I, treated with anti-CD4 mAb, and group II, the control group, treated with saline solution or anti-CD8 mAb. The mean survival time of the control animals (group II) was 3.5 days, whereas the mean survival time of animals treated with anti-CD4 mAb was 15 days.

The dose of mAb given to the animals in all cases was sufficient to maintain significant levels of free murine antibody in the circulation. The amount of circulating antibody varied and seemed to depend on the frequency of $CD4^+$ cells in the peripheral blood. Seven to 10 days after the start of infusion, the injected mAb was no longer detectable in the circulation. The disappearance of the murine mAb coincided with the appearance of monkey antimouse IgG antibodies in the circulation. In some animals the monkey antimouse IgG response appeared to be directed against both isotypic and idiotypic determinants.

In untreated animals with EAE there is a depletion of both $CD4^+$ and $CD8^+$ T lymphocytes before the onset of EAE.[1] Longitudinal analysis of CD4 and CD8 T cells in treated animals revealed a return to presensitization levels 10-15 days after treatment was started (FIG. 1). There was no sustained depletion of $CD4^+$ cells following treatment with either the OKT4a or Leu3a mAbs. This was determined by measuring the frequency of mAb-coated cells with FITC-goat anti-mouse IgG and by measuring the frequency of $CD4^+$ cells with mAb to a different epitope from that recognized by the treatment antibody. Leu3a and OKT4a recognize different epitopes on the CD4 molecule and do not block each others' binding to $CD4^+$ cells.

## CONCLUSIONS

These studies were initiated to provide a basis for the development of immunologic strategies in the treatment of human demyelinating disease such as MS. We have used mAb to the human CD4 surface antigen associated with helper T cells to treat acute EAE in nonhuman primates. Treatment with anti-CD4 mAbs had a significant effect on the survival of animals with EAE when compared with untreated animals and animals treated with anti-CD8 mAb. In addition to increasing survival times, anti-CD4 mAb therapy appeared to reverse the depletion of $CD4^+$ and $CD8^+$ T cells caused by the development of EAE.[5] These treatments did not induce immunologic tolerance to mouse IgG because all of the anti-CD4-treated animals produced high titers of anti-mouse IgG antibodies. These results suggest that $CD4^+$ cells are important in the pathogenesis of EAE in macaques and that manipulation of this subset with mAbs may provide effective treatment of human demyelinating disease.

### REFERENCES

1. ROSE, L. M., E. A. CLARK, S. HRUBY & E. C. ALVORD, JR. 1987. Clin. Immunol. Immunopathol. **44:** 93.
2. WALDOR, M. K., S. SRIRAM, R. HARDY, L. A. HERZENBERG, L. A. HERZENBERG, L. LANIER, M. LIM & L. STEINMAN. 1985. Science **227:** 415.
3. BROSTOFF, S. W. & D. W. MASON. 1984. Immunology **133:** 1938.
4. HAYNES, B. F. 1981. Immunol. Rev. **57:** 126.
5. ROSE, L. M., E. C. ALVORD, JR., S. HRUBY, S. L. JACKEVICIUS, R. PETERSEN, N. WARNER & E. A. CLARK. 1987. Clin. Immunol. Immunopathol. **45:** 405.

WORKSHOP 12. CLINICAL IMMUNOGENETICS

# Blood Lymphocyte β-Adrenergic Receptors in Multiple Sclerosis

### BARRY G. W. ARNASON, MARGARET BROWN, RICARDO MASELLI, JOE KARASZEWSKI, AND ANTHONY REDER

*Department of Neurology
University of Chicago
and
The Brain Research Institute
Chicago, Illinois*

We hypothesize that immune abnormalities in multiple sclerosis (MS), such as the reduction in suppressor cell function observed when disease is active, are linked to central nervous system (CNS) lesions that arise during the disease. The immune system is innervated by the sympathetic nervous system (SNS). Could strategically situated lesions, acting via the SNS, impair suppressor cell function and thereby favor progression? Many patients with MS have an exacerbating-remitting course at the outset and a progressive one later. We postulate that SNS-mediated signals may be involved. Abrogation of this SNS innervation in mice by chemical axotomy with 6-hydroxydopamine alters immune function and causes splenic T and B cells to increase their β-adrenergic receptors severalfold, that is, they develop denervation hypersensitivity.

β-adrenergic receptor density in healthy humans is threefold greater on suppressor T cells ($CD8^+$, $9.3^-$) than on cytotoxic T cells ($CD8^+$, $9.3^+$). It seems reasonable to postulate that SNS influence on suppressor cells would predominate over its influence on other T-cell types. Could CNS damage in MS decrease SNS "tone" and in this way compromise suppressor function, thus setting the stage for a progressive course? Sympathetic nervous system ablation augments antibody production and up-regulates β-adrenergic receptor density on lymphocytes. Moreover, SNS ablation increases the severity of experimental allergic encephalomyelitis (EAE). (See paper by Schorr *et al.* in these proceedings.) We therefore thought it of interest to determine β-adrenergic receptor density on lymphocytes from patients with progressive MS.

## METHODS

Peripheral blood lymphocytes were collected from patients with MS, diabetes mellitus with peripheral neuropathy, and healthy controls. Mononuclear cells as well as T-cell subsets were studied. T-cell subsets are obtained from sheep red cell-rosetted cells followed by a panning technique to isolate $CD4^+$ and $CD8^+$ subsets. Following fractionation, cell populations were resuspended in incubation buffer (150 mM of saline solution, 20 mM of Tris, and 1 mM of ascorbic acid). For each population, 5 × 10⁵ cells were incubated with different concentrations of [$^{125}$I]cyanopindolol (CYP) (6-200 pM) in a total volume of 300 µl of incubation buffer at pH 7.4, 30°C for 90 minutes.

Nonspecific binding is determined in duplicate samples of cells in the presence of dl-propranolol (Sigma) at a final concentration of $6 \times 10^6$ M. Following incubation the reaction is terminated by diluting samples with 4.5 ml of cold incubation buffer. The samples are then harvested by vacuum filtration through GF/C Whatman glass fiber filters. Each sample tube is rinsed with an additional 4.5 ml of cold buffer, and the filters are washed with 30 ml of cold buffer. Radioactive standards are also run through the filters to determine the amount of nonspecific binding of the ligand to the glass fiber filter. The filters are counted in a Beckman Gamma 4000 counter.

The sympathetic skin response (SSR) was determined in patients as previously described (Muscle and Nerve, October 1987).

## RESULTS AND DISCUSSION

Patients with MS have abnormal cardiovascular responses to the Valsalva maneuver, presumably because of a defect in autonomic regulation. We have found the SSR to electrical stimulation is absent in 50% of patients with progressive MS. The data are given in FIGURE 1. The SSR is a complex reflex that depends on somato-

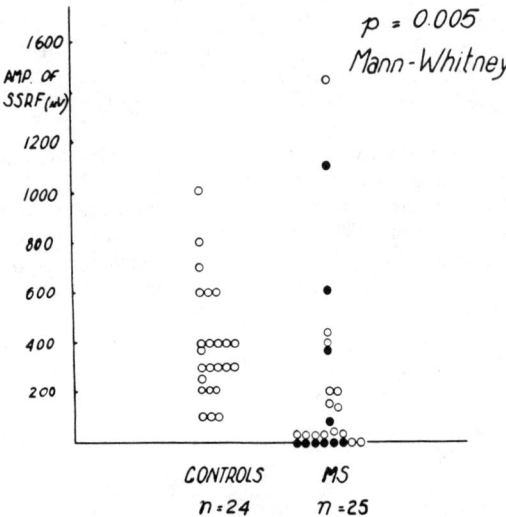

**FIGURE 1.** Sympathetic skin response of the foot (SSRF) following electrical stimulation in healthy controls and in patients with MS. ○ = rapidly progressive MS (a decline of >1 point on the Kurtzke scale in the prior year); ● = slowly progressive MS (<1 point decline). Nonparametric statistics were used because of the severe skew in the MS values. (NOTE: Patients with Shy Drager syndrome, characterized by degeneration of the preganglionic sympathetic neurons in the spinal cord, had completely absent responses. Data not shown.

TABLE 1. Beta Receptor Concentration versus Concanavalin A (Con A) Suppression in Patients with Progressive Multiple Sclerosis and in Healthy Controls

| Multiple Sclerosis | | | Controls | | |
|---|---|---|---|---|---|
| β-Adrenergic Receptor[a] | Kd | % Con A Suppression | β-Adrenergic Receptor | Kd | % Con A Suppression |
| 24.4 | 55 | 37 | 10.9 | 35 | ND |
| 22.4 | 58 | 20 | 9.1 | 35 | 83 |
| 8.6 | 57 | 20 | 7.5 | 40 | 59 |
| 8.6 | 48 | ND | 6.9 | 32 | 79 |
| 22.5 | 105 | 13 | 7.4 | 41 | ND |
| 10.0 | 39 | ND | 10.6 | 54 | 92 |
| 17.8 | 47 | 39 | 6.5 | 17 | 55 |
| 47.4 | 361 | 32 | 15.0 | 38 | ND |
| 20.2 ± 4.5[b] | 96 ± 38[c] | 27 ± 4[b] | 9.2 ± 1.0 | 37 ± 40 | 74 ± 7 |

[a] pM/6 × 10⁵ mononuclear cells.
[b] Mean ± SEM; $p < 0.03$, unpaired $t$ test.
[c] No difference between MS and controls.
[d] $p < 0.001$.

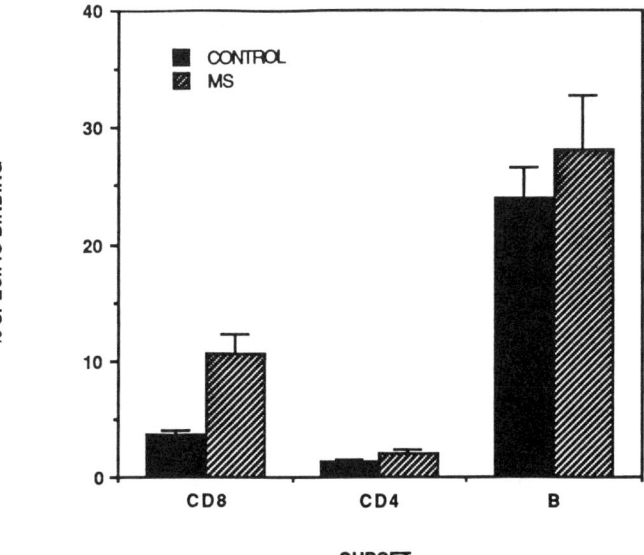

**FIGURE 2.** Specific iodo[$^{125}$I]cyanopindolol ([$^{125}$I]CYP) binding to subsets of lymphocytes in patients with MS and controls. Cells (5 × 10⁵) were incubated in the presence of increasing concentrations of [$^{125}$I]CYP at 30°C for 90 minutes. Specific binding was determined as the difference in [$^{125}$I]CYP binding in the absence and presence of 6 μm DL-propranolol. For CD8 cells, $B_{max}$ = 3.6 ± 0.4 fmol/10⁶ cells in controls and 10.6 ± 1.9 fmol/10⁶ in patients with MS ($p < 0.01$, $n = 10$); for CD4, $B_{max}$ = 1.3 ± 0.1 fmol/10⁶ in controls and 2 ± 0.3 fmol/10⁶ in patients with MS ($p < 0.05$, $n = 10$); and for B cells, $B_{max}$ = 23.9 ± 3.9 fmol/10⁶ in controls and 28.1 ± 4.5 fmol/10⁶ in patients with MS (ns, $n = 6$).

sympathetic pathways with spinal, medullary, and suprabulbar components. Therefore, we interpret our finding as evidence of abnormal sympathetic function.

Because of these abnormalities, we reasoned that decreased SNS function in MS could produce (1) denervation hypersensitivity of lymphocytes, and (2) up-regulation of immune responses through loss of $CD8^+$, $9.3^-$ suppressor influence.

We studied the first hypothesis by measuring $\beta$-adrenergic receptors on mononuclear cells from eight patients with progressive MS and from eight normal controls. Mononuclear cells from patients with MS had higher numbers of $\beta$ receptors than did the control cells ($p < 0.03$) (TABLE 1). There was no obvious correlation of $\beta$ receptor level with the level of concanavalin A suppression (done at a separate time) in individual patients with MS or with the tempo of worsening of MS over the preceding 2 years. All eight patients had lower limb spasticity. Patients receiving amitriptyline or baclofen and patients on no medication showed no significant differences in $\beta$-adrenergic density on their lymphocytes.

We next turned our attention to lymphocyte subsets. Cells from 10 patients with MS, 10 age-matched controls, and 7 patients with varying degrees of diabetic neuropathy and SNS involvement were examined. The data are given in FIGURE 2. It was known from our earlier work in mice that B cells have more $\beta$-adrenergic receptors than T cells, and this was found in man as well. The greatest difference between MS and control values in the present study was found for $CD8^+$ cells, with $\beta$-adrenergic receptors increased threefold in progressive MS compared with controls. $CD4^+$ cells had few receptors in all groups. Subfractionation of $CD8^+$ cells into $9.3^+$ (cytotoxic) and $9.3^-$ (suppressor) groups is planned.

Thus, we have evidence that the SNS is abnormal in MS and that $\beta$-adrenergic receptors are up-regulated on cells within the $CD8^+$ T-cell subset. In earlier work we showed that this subset is responsible for abnormal suppressor cell function in MS. These $CD8^+$ cells may be under strong regulatory control by the SNS and its neurotransmitters.

# ACTH Production by Human Mononuclear Cells

ANTHONY T. REDER, SUSMITHA PINAMANENI,
WILLIAM SMYKA, AND DANIEL NUTTER[a]

*The University of Chicago and the Brain Research Foundation*
*Chicago, Illinois 60637*

The mononuclear cells of mice and men can produce adrenocorticotrophic hormone (ACTH). Newcastle disease virus (NCDV) infection causes mouse spleen cells to exhibit ACTH-like immunoreactivity and induces physiologic levels of corticosterone.[1] *In vitro* stimulation of human mononuclear cells (MNC) with NCDV, corticotrophin-releasing factor (CRF), or lipopolysaccharide (LPS) has similar effects.

We investigated ACTH immunoreactivity in MNCs from normal, virally infected, and multiple sclerosis (MS) subjects using indirect immunofluorescence and Western blots obtained with rabbit anti-ACTH serum. Virus-infected patients and those with MS were used because their lymphocytes are activated *in vivo*.

ACTH-like immunofluorescence was present but not clearly different in intensity in freshly isolated lymphocytes from all three subject groups. All MNC subsets (OKT3$^+$, OKT4$^+$, and OKT8$^+$ cells) exhibited perinuclear staining.

PMA stimulation for 18 hours intensified staining. Synthetic ACTH 1-24 added to E+ cells for 2 hours resulted in a thin rim of fluorescence without intracellular staining.

The most intense bands on Western blots occurred at molecular weights of ~16 to 17 kd. Moderate bands were at 32-36 kd and weak bands at ~4.5 kd especially in cells that had been lysed without protease inhibitors. Unstimulated MNCs from patients with MS tended to have more intense bands than did those from normal controls. PMA further increased the intensity of both the 16-17 and 32-36 kd bands in patients with MS and one virus-infected control. RNA dot blots and Northern analysis showed mRNA production by lymphocytes; MS and PMA-induced cells again produced more.

The immune and neuroendocrine systems interact and form a complex feedback network. The ACTH-like immunoreactivity seen in fixed MNCs has ACTH bioactivity.[1] PMA, which induces ACTH secretion by mouse pituitary tumor cells, increased the immunofluorescence of cells from all three groups of subjects. PMA, through the protein kinase C pathway, might be expected to cause ACTH production by activating MNCs *in vivo*.[2]

All MNC stained for ACTH. ACTH has been detected in NCDV-stimulated mouse spleen cells, in LPS-stimulated human (B) cells, and in unstimulated mouse monocytes.[1] Background ACTH production may have been due to *in vivo* stimuli (e.g., viral infections). The addition of ACTH-unstimulated MNCs for several hours resulted

[a] This work was supported by the Multiple Sclerosis Society Harry Weaver Award (JF 2027-A1) and NIH-CIDA 1 KO8 NS 01068-01.

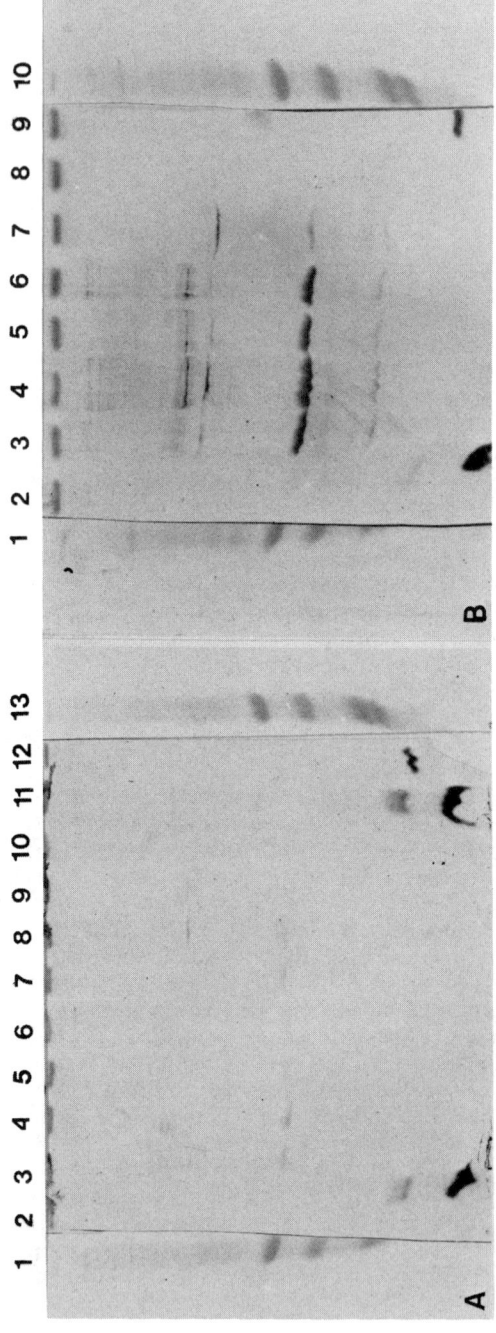

**FIGURE 1.** Western blot of mononuclear cell lysates stained for ACTH. Western blots were performed on 10 μl of lysate from $5 \times 10^7$ cells/ml. Gels run through 20% SDS-polyacrylamide gels were transblotted onto nitrocellulose filters and stained with rabbit anti-ACTH followed by goat antirabbit-Ig-peroxidase.

(A) *Lane 1:* low molecular weight SDS standard (16.95, 14.4, 8.16, 6.21, and 2.51 kd); *2:* ACTH 1-24; *3:* stable MS (7 days before exacerbation); *4:* stable MS (before exacerbation) after 25 ng/ml of PMA for 18 hours; *5:* remitting MS (during prednisone therapy); *6:* remitting MS (on 30 mg of prednisone orally every day) plus PMA; *7:* progressive MS; *8:* progressive MS plus PMA; *9:* normal control; *10:* NL plus PMA; *11:* NL lysate mixed with ACTH 1:24; *12:* ACTH 1-39; *13:* SDS molecular weight standard. Note bands at ~16 and ~35 kd.

(B) *Lane 1:* SDS molecular weight standard; *2:* ACTH 1-24; *3:* MS during early remission; *4:* MS during early remission plus PMA; *5:* stable MS (see note for A, lane 3); *6:* stable MS (see A, lane 4) plus PMA; *7:* NL; *8:* NL plus PMA; *9:* ACTH 1-39; *10:* SDS molecular weight standards.

NOTE: (1) Glycosylated peptides may show high apparent molecular weights, and (2) small peptides may migrate erratically.

in staining of the cell membrane only, without the perinuclear staining seen after PMA stimulation. This rim of fluorescence is likely to be due to ACTH receptor-ACTH-anti-ACTH complexes.

Processing of human proopiomelanocortin (POMC) may differ in lymphocytes. Western blotting revealed discrete bands at 16-17 kd and, less strongly, at 32-36 kd which correspond to ACTH precursors in man. Weak bands at ~4.5 kd (ACTH 1-39) correspond to secreted forms of ACTH. PMA induced more intense staining at 16-17 kd and at 32-36 kd (*de novo* at times). The highest molecular weight bands presumably represented newly synthesized POMC that had not yet been processed. Note that the cell lysates and fixed cells contained ACTH that had not been secreted and could therefore tend to be weighted toward higher molecular weight precursors present in the golgi and endoplasmic reticulum.

PMA stimulation seemed to preferentially affect MS lymphocytes in this limited number of subjects. If MS cells were preactivated or more easily activated by stimuli that cause ACTH secretion, chronic excessive cortisol secretion could result in DST abnormalities and also subsensitivity of lymphocytes to cortisol regulation.[3]

## ACKNOWLEDGMENTS

We thank Tom Roszman for helpful suggestions and Mary Witt for typing the manuscript.

### REFERENCES

1. BLALOCK, J. E. *et al.* 1985. J. Neurol. **10:** 31-40.
2. HARBOUR-MCMENAMIN, D. *et al.* 1985. Infect. & Immunol. **10:** 813-817.
3. REDER, A. T. *et al.* 1987. Neurology **37:** 849-853.

# Identification of Myelin Basic Protein-Specific Oligoclonal Bands in Multiple Sclerosis

KEISUKE MORIMOTO,[a] SHIN-ICHIRO IKEBE,[a] AND TAKESHI SATO [b]

[a] Department of Neurology
National Fuji Hospital
Fujinomiya City, Shizuoka, Japan

[b] Department of Neurology
Juntendo University School of Medicine
Tokyo, Japan

The antigen causing the synthesis of oligoclonal bands (OB) in multiple sclerosis (MS) has not been identified. To detect whether myelin basic protein (MBP)-specific IgG OB exists in patients with MS we developed a sensitive method of isoelectric focusing combined with affinity-mediated immunoblotting. Briefly, nitrocellulose paper strips were coated with human MBP and then blocked with 0.1 M phosphate buffer containing 1% of bovine serum albumin, 0.1% of histone, and 0.5% Tween 80. Immediately after agarose isoelectric focusing, MBP-coated nitrocellulose paper was placed on the agarose gel for 30 minutes. After washing the nitrocellulose paper with

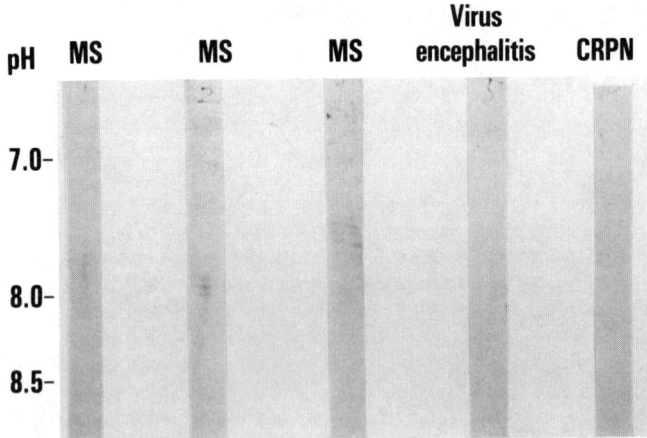

**FIGURE 1.** Myelin basic protein-specific IgG bands are seen in the sera of three patients with MS (columns 1-3), whereas sera from both viral encephalitis and chronic relapsing polyneuropathy (CRPN) are negative (columns 4 and 5).

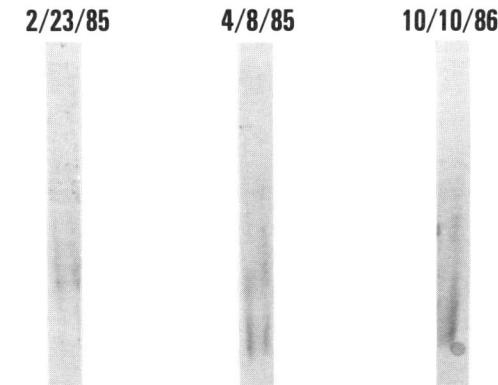

**FIGURE 2.** Sera obtained serially from one 44-year-old male patient with MS show a different distribution of MBP-specific IgG bands.

1.2% NaCl solution and 0.05% Tween 80, IgG reacting with MBP on the nitrocellulose paper was stained with rabbit antihuman IgG and the avidin-biotin system. This method clearly demonstrates MBP-specific IgG OB when rabbit antihuman MBP serum is applied. Either absorption with human MBP before applying the sample or the layering of other basic protein (lysozyme or histone) made the bands invisible. In the sera in 8 of 13 patients with MS (62%), MBP-specific IgG OB was detected. Five patients (38%) had both MBP-specific bands in sera and IgG OB in cerebrospinal fluid. In two patients (15%), however, both were negative. Three patients (23%), none of whom had IgG OB in cerebrospinal fluid, demonstrated MBP-specific bands in sera, whereas three patients (23%) with IgG OB in the cerebrospinal fluid showed no MBP-specific bands in sera. Serial observation in one patient for 1.5 years showed a different IgG spectrum. No positive findings were noted in the control group except in two cases: one case of viral encephalitis and one case of myelopathy with autoantibody (anti-extractable nuclear antigens). In both cases, nonetheless, MBP-specific bands were transient. These findings suggest that MBP-specific IgG bands are fairly specific to MS. This conclusion, however, needs to be confirmed by further detailed investigation because the number of our cases was restricted. Analysis of antigen-specific humoral immunity may lead to a clearer understanding of the pathogenesis of MS.

## REFERENCES

1. ROSTROEM, B. 1981. Acta Neurol. Scand. **63** (suppl. 86): 1-84.
2. VARTDAL, F. & B. VANDVIK. 1982. J. Neurol. Sci. **54:** 99-107.
3. NEWCOMBE, J. et al. 1982. J. Neurochem. **39:** 1192-1194.
4. DOERRIES, R. & V. TER MEULEN. 1984. J. Neuroimmunol. **7:** 77-89.
5. MOYLE, S. et al. 1984. Biosci. Rep. **4:** 505-510.
6. GROOME, N. P. 1980. J. Neurochem. **35:** 1409-1417.

# Human T-Cell Response to Human and Heterologous Myelin Basic Proteins

### E. TOURNIER-LASSERVE,[a] G. HASHIM,[b] AND M. A. BACH [a]

[a]*Unité de Pathologie de l'Immunité*
*Institut Pasteur*
*Paris, France*
[b]*St. Luke's Roosevelt Hospital Center*
*New York, New York*

Multiple sclerosis (MS) is a human demyelinating disease sharing some pathologic features with experimental allergic encephalomyelitis (EAE). Thus, an autoimmune response directed against the myelin basic protein (BP) might be involved in the demyelinating process as it is in EAE.[1,2] We are presenting some data suggesting that the T-cell response to BP is quantitatively and qualitatively different in patients with MS from that in healthy subjects.

## MATERIAL AND METHODS

*Subjects.* The patients included in this study had definite MS (Schumacher's criteria). Healthy subjects were blood bank donors or staff members.

*Basic Protein-Triggered T-Cell Lines.* These lines were established as described elsewhere by culturing peripheral blood mononuclear cells (PBMC) with human BP in the presence of interleukin-2 (IL-2).[3] Their proliferative response was measured by $^3$H-thymidine incorporation in a 48-hour assay in the presence of human or heterologous BP and of autologous irradiated PBMC used as antigen-presenting cells.

## RESULTS AND DISCUSSION

*T-Cell Response to Human Basic Protein* (TABLE 1). Although BP-triggered T-cell lines in patients with MS grew faster than those in healthy subjects, once the lines were established, the proliferative response of both groups to human BP was not significantly different.

These observations confirm previous work[3,4] and indicate that T-cell autoreacting to BP is a physiologic phenomenon.

TABLE 1. Proliferative Response to Human Basic Protein (BP) of Human BP-Triggered T-Cell Lines from Healthy Subjects and Patients with MS

|  | Antigen Added | | |
|---|---|---|---|
| Subjects | None | Human BP | Stimulation Index |
| Healthy subjects ($n = 5$) | $1,075 \pm 600^a$ | $12,656 \pm 1,635$ | $25.3 \pm 26.1$ |
| Patients with MS ($n = 8$) | $3,395 \pm 4,575$ | $17,553 \pm 11,407^b$ | $12.6 \pm 11.4^b$ |

[a] Mean ± SD. Stimulation index = cpm with antigen/cpm without antigen.
[b] $p > 0.1$ (compared to healthy subjects).

*T-Cell Response to Heterologous Basic Protein* (TABLE 2). The proliferative response of human BP-triggered T-cell lines to several heterologous BPs was compared with that triggered by human BP in the same experiment. Healthy subject lines did respond to all BPs tested equally well, in all but one case, or even better than to human BP. Conversely, lines in 6 of 7 patients with MS showed a weak response or no response at all to either rat or monkey BP or both. This occurred in patients with active disease as well as in patients in remission. A low response to bovine BP was also observed, but only in patients with relapse or progressive aggravation.

These data suggest that the T cells of healthy subjects compared with patients with MS preferentially recognize conserved peptide sequences of BP. Strain variations in the T-cell repertoire to BP have been described in rat and mouse.[5,6] The relevance of these peculiarities in the T-cell response of patients with MS to the pathophysiology of the disease remains unknown. The release of BP products, as a consequence of demyelination, could have expanded a pool of T-cell clones reacting to BP epitopes normally not exposed. Alternatively, some patients with MS perhaps display a T-cell repertoire to human BP that includes the recognition of potentially encephalitogenic peptides and that favors the development of the disease.

TABLE 2. Proliferative Response of T-Cell Lines to Heterologous Basic Protein (BP) as Compared to Human BP in Patients with MS and Healthy Subjects

|  | BP Source | | |
|---|---|---|---|
|  | Monkey | Rat | Beef |
| Healthy subjects | $-20 \pm 31^a$ ($n = 5$) | $-18 \pm 86$ ($n = 5$) | $+29 \pm 64$ ($n = 5$) |
| Patients with MS (all cases) | $-67 \pm 34$ ($n = 8$) | $-67 \pm 37$ ($n = 7$) | $-2 \pm 69$ ($n = 8$) |
| Patients with active disease only | $-57 \pm 25$ ($n = 5$) | $-49 \pm 36$ ($n = 5$) | $-46 \pm 35$ ($n = 5$) |

[a] Percentage of variation of the response as compared with that obtained with human BP within the same experiment (mean ± SD). Significant values ($p < 0.05$) are underlined.

## REFERENCES

1. PATERSON, P. Y. 1966. Adv. Immunol. **5:** 131.
2. LISAK, R. P., B. ZWEIMAN, J. B. BURNS, A. ROSTAMI & D. H. SILBERBERG. 1985. Ann. N.Y. Acad. Sci. **436:** 221.
3. TOURNIER-LASSERVE, E., C. JACQUE, D. FRADELIZI & M. A. BACH. 1986. Ann. N.Y. Acad. Sci. **475:** 404.
4. BURNS, J. B., A. ROSENZWEIG, B. ZWEIMAN & R. P. LISAK. 1983. Cell. Immunol. **81:** 435.
5. BERAUD, E., T. RESHEF, A. A. VANDENBARK, H. OFFNER, R. FRITZ, C. H. JEN CHOU, D. BERNARD & I. R. COHEN. 1986. J. Immunol. **136:** 511.
6. ZAMVIL, S., P. A. NELSON, D. J. MITCHELL, R. L. KNOBLER, R. B. FRITZ & L. STEINMAN. 1985. J. Exp. Med. **162:** 2107.

# Changes in Immune Function in Relapsing Multiple Sclerosis Correlate with Disease Activity As Assessed by Magnetic Resonance Imaging

J. OGER,[a] M. O'GORMAN,[a] E. WILLOUGHBY,[a,b]
D. LI,[c] AND D. W. PATY[a]

[a]*Department of Medicine and*
[c]*Department of Radiology*
*University of British Columbia*
*Vancouver, BC, Canada*

The extent to which the immune system is affected in multiple sclerosis (MS) has been a controversial subject for the last 15 years.[1] *In vitro* tools used to study the immune system have been applied to the study of MS at variable stages of their development. Studies involving patients with MS have long been hampered by the lack of correlation between the clinical presentation and the pathologic process. Magnetic resonance imaging (MRI) has recently made the MS lesions recognizable *in vivo* and thus permitted closer monitoring of the disease process. Since this technique has been used, not only has the accuracy of the clinical diagnosis been greatly improved,[2] but also some insight has been gained in the changes occurring in lesions over time.[3] We have noted that in some patients with relapsing remitting MS large rounded lesions can appear and disappear over a few weeks' time without any clinical correlate.[3,4] We report here that when *in vitro* immune function in these patients was studied, fluctuations that were time related to the changes recognized on MRI occurred. Changes in immune function do not precede the development of these large lesions, but they do seem to appear once the maximum extent of the lesion has been reached.

## TECHNIQUES

We prospectively followed 15 patients with relapsing remitting MS monthly or twice monthly by clinical examination, MRI examination of the head, and *in vitro* measurement of their suppressor cell activity as well as their immunoglobulin G secretion capability. Each patient was studied for 4-6 months. The MRI was performed

[b]Kroc Visiting Professor; permanent address: Auckland, New Zealand.

TABLE 1. Con A Suppression and IgG Secretion in 11 Patients Separated into Two Groups According to the Longitudinal Results of the MRI

|  | Group 1:<br>MRI Stable ($n = 5$) | Group 2:<br>MRI Large Lesion ($n = 6$) |
|---|---|---|
| Con A suppression (%) | 37.8 ± 5.3 | 23 ± 6.0 |
| IgG secretion (ng/ml) | 1,893 ± 458 | 662 ± 78[a] |

[a] Different from group 1 ($p < 0.05$).

NOTE: Con A suppression appeared lower in patients who had MRI changes, but this did not reach significance. IgG secretion was lower when the group with new active lesions was compared with the MRI-stable group.

on a Picker 200 cryogenics with a field strength of 0.15 Tesla. Careful repositioning was done. Concanavalin A suppressor cell assay and IgG secretion assay were performed on peripheral mononuclear cells (MNC) as described by Oger et al.[5] except that IgG secretion in in vitro cultures was also set up for 10 days with both pokeweed mitogen (PWM) and *Staphylococcus aureus* Cowan I (SAC) stimulation.

## RESULTS

The patients were divided into two groups according to the results of their MRI scanning: group 1, stable ($n = 5$); group 2, waxing and waning of a single isolated lesion ($n = 6$). Results of Con A and IgG secretion are presented in TABLE 1.

We have suggested that changes in immune function could be temporary.[6,7] To see if these changes coincided with MRI lesions, we selected three times according to MRI findings. These corresponded to the initial appearance of the new lesion, the maximum extent of the lesion, and the first scan showing a decrease in size. At these time points we averaged the individual results in the six patients studied and compared these values with those obtained in patients whose MRI remained stable. Values were matched retrospectively by date; the value generated by assays set up at the closest date was used for comparison (TABLE 2).

TABLE 2. Con A Suppression (%) at Three Time Points in the Appearance and Disappearance of Large MRI Lesions

|  | Initial Appearance of Lesion | Maximum Extent of Lesion | Decrease in Size of Lesion |
|---|---|---|---|
| Patients with large MRI lesions | 31.2 ± 6 (5)[a] | −49 ± 22[b] (4) | 26.2 ± 6.6 (5) |
| Patients with stable MRI | 45.4 ± 13 (5) | 24.3 ± 12.1 (5) | 49 ± 10.1 (5) |

[a] Number of data points available for calculation.
[b] $p < 0.05$ from stable MS.

TABLE 3. IgG Secretion in Culture (ng/ml) Induced by Pokeweed Mitogen (PWM) at 7 and 10 Days and by *Staphylococcus aureus* Cowan I (SAC)

| | Initial Appearance of Lesion | Maximum Extent of Lesion | %[a] | Decrease in Size of Lesion | %[b] |
|---|---|---|---|---|---|
| MS with large MRI lesions | | | | | |
| PWM 7 | 978 ± 288 (5) | 373 ± 99 (5) | 62 | 429 ± 120 (5) | 56 |
| PWM 10 | 2,476 ± 828 (4) | 1,146 ± 719 (4) | 54 | 929 ± 483 (4) | 63 |
| SAC 10 | 5,835 ± 2,301 (4) | 3,290 ± 1,390 (4) | 44 | 2,096 ± 1,644 (4) | 64 |
| MS with stable MRI | | | | | |
| PWM 7 | 1,455 ± 645 (5) | 2,379 ± 1,380 (5) | NR[c](3) | 897 ± 291 (5) | 38 |
| PWM 10 | 6,333 ± 3,175 (4) | 7,109 ± 3,204 (4) | NR | 3,796 ± 818 (4) | 40 |
| SAC 10 | 6,368 ± 2,151 (4) | 7,036 ± 2,404 (4) | NR | 7,567 ± 2,236 (4) | NR |

[a] Percentage of reduction when compared with levels of IgG secretion found at the time of appearance of the lesion.
[b] Number of data points available for calculation.
[c] NR = no reduction.

It is apparent from these results that a drastic change in Con A inducible suppression function occurred as a function of time and that a maximum reduction in Con A suppression occurred at the time of maximal extent of the lesion. B-cell stimulation was also performed using the polyclonal activator PWM for 7 or 10 days of culture as well as using SAC. Results are shown in TABLE 3.

IgG secretion *in vitro* varied in both groups, but there was a great reduction in the amount of IgG secreted in patients exhibiting a lesion that appeared and disappeared at the time when a large MRI lesion developed. This was not observed in time-matched patients who had no changes on their MRI. We[8] have defined the limits of high response following PWM stimulation and 7 days of incubation as being 1,000 ng. A high responder (HR) secretes more than 1,000 ng; a low responder (LR) secretes less than 1,000 ng. Controls are relatively stable over time and generally remain HR or LR. It is noteworthy that among the MRI-stable patients two of five were HRs and they did not change to LRs. On the contrary, four of five patients showing large MRI lesions were HRs at some point in the 6-month study, but none of five were HRs when their MRI lesion was active.

## DISCUSSION

We have shown in this group of patients with relapsing remitting MS followed serially by MRI that changes in Con A suppression and IgG secretion accompany the development of MRI lesions. Con A suppressor cell function as well as IgG secretion *in vitro* were both depressed when the lesion showed its maximum extent on MRI. As these changes were not present at the time the lesions were initially recognizable (even though small), we think these acute changes are secondary to the MRI-recognized lesion and not the cause of it. We currently have no indication of the nature of these waxing and waning lesions even though their evolution suggests an inflammatory process. The concurrent reduction of both functions could come from the trapping in these large lesions of effector (B) and regulatory cells (T suppressor) necessary for these *in vitro* immune functions. From parallel computerized tomography and MRI results as well as from MRI using a maker of the blood-brain barrier, others have shown that similar lesions do exhibit blood-brain barrier leakage. An alternative explanation would be the leakage of a biologic product from the site of the lesion.

### REFERENCES

1. O'GORMAN, M. & J. OGER. 1987. Cell-mediated immune functions in multiple sclerosis. Pathol. Immunopathol. Res. **6:** 241-272.
2. PATY, D. W., J. OGER, L. F. KASTRUKOFF *et al.* 1988. MRI in the diagnosis of MS: A prospective comparison of clinic evaluation, evoked potentials, oligoclonal banding and computerized tomography. Neurology **38:** 180-185.
3. PATY, D. W., C. D. ISAAC, E. GROCHOWSKI *et al.* 1986. A serial study of relapsing remitting patients with quantitative measurement of lesion size. Neurology **36**(suppl.1): 177.
4. WILLOUGHBY, E., E. GROCHOWSKI, D. LI, J. OGER, L. KASTRUKOFF & D. PATY. 1987. A prospective study of MRI scanning in multiple sclerosis. Neurology **37**(suppl.1): 231.
5. OGER, J., L. KASTRUKOFF, M. O'GORMAN & D. W. PATY. 1986. Progressive multiple

sclerosis: Abnormal immune function in vitro and aberrant correlation with enumeration of lymphocyte subpopulations. J. Neuroimmunol. **12:** 37-48.
6. OGER, J., L. KASTRUKOFF & D. W. PATY. 1986. Multiple sclerosis: relationship between suppressor cell function, Ig secretion in vitro and the attacks of multiple sclerosis (MS) as studied by serial clinical and MRI examinations. Ann. Neurol. **20:** 162.
7. OGER, J., L. KASTRUKOFF & D. W. PATY. 1986. Multiple sclerosis: Relationship between suppressor cell function, Ig secretion in vitro and the attacks of multiple sclerosis as studied by serial clinical and MRI examinations. Can. J. Neurol. Sci. **4:** 371.
8. OGER, J., J. ANTEL & B. G. W. ARNASON. 1982. Effect of imuran therapy on in vitro immune function of MS patients. Ann. Neurol. **11:** 177-181.

# Immunodiagnosis and Immunotherapy in Autistic Children[a]

V. K. SINGH,[b,c] H. H. FUDENBERG,[b] D. EMERSON,[b]
AND M. COLEMAN[d]

[b]*Medical University of South Carolina*
*Charleston, South Carolina 29425*

[d]*Georgetown University School of Medicine*
*Washington, DC 20010*

The etiology and pathogenesis of the autistic syndrome are not known. On the basis of our current work with other neuropsychiatric disorders,[1,2] we hypothesized that autism is a syndrome, and at least one subset thereof may be immunologic in origin. This hypothesis is supported by our immunologic studies reported herein.

Our studies included 20 patients with well-diagnosed autistic syndrome; the onset of symptoms was 16-18 months. Detailed immunologic testing included: (a) enumeration of total T (SRBC rosettes), interactive T (Raji rosettes), and surface membrane orosomucoid positive (Om+) T cells; (b) DNA synthesis in response to stimulation by mitogens (phytohemagglutinin [PHA], pokeweed mitogen [PWM], and concanavalin A [Con A]) or B cells and monocytes in autologous mixed lymphocyte reaction (AMLR); and (c) detection of antoantibodies to neuron-axon filament proteins (NAFP). The methods of the various test procedures are described elsewhere.[3,4]

The numerical data on various types of T cells are given in FIGURE 1. The values in autistic patients were normal for total T cells; lower than siblings' in 9 of 20 patients for interactive T cells; and lower in 10 of 20 or higher in 5 of 20 patients for Om+ T cells. We showed that Om is an immunoregulatory protein.[5] The data on DNA synthesis stimulated by PHA, PWM, or Con A mitogen were abnormally distributed in many patients. Compared with siblings, many patients displayed an abnormally high or low AMLR response (FIG. 1) presumably because of abnormal function of suppressor T cells.

Approximately 67% of the autistic sera contained antibodies to NAFP as detected by the immunoblot technique (TABLE 1 and FIG. 2). The reactivity was directed against a neurofilament protein (200 kd) or additional proteins (40-60 kd and 21 kd) whose nature is not known. Antibodies to NAFP were found in almost all patients with abnormal cell-mediated immunity (CMI). In many cases (FIG. 2), the sera from household contacts were also positive for anti-NAFP (46% of the siblings or 55% of the parents). Antibodies to NAFP were found in neurotropic slow virus diseases (kuru and Creutzfeld-Jacob disease) of man.[6] As reported herein, anti-NAFP was highly prevalent among the household contacts of autistic patients and, like the

---

[a]This work was supported in part by the Immunohematology Research Foundation.

[c]New address: D.C.H.P. and Department of Biology, Utah State University, Logan, UT 84322.

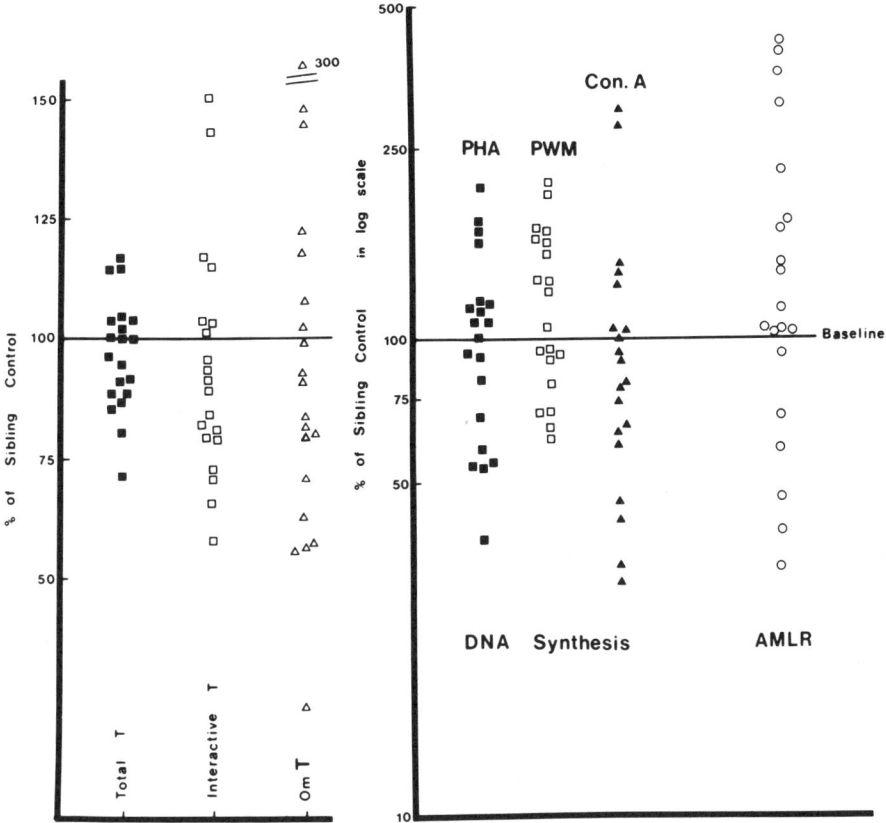

**FIGURE 1.** Distribution of various T cells and cell-mediated immunity responses in autistic patients.

household contacts of most patients with degenerative disorders of the brain,[4,6] suggests the association of an infectious agent (slow virus) in the etiology of the disease.

Based on this premise, eight patients (six with abnormal CMI and two without this defect) were placed on immunomodulant therapy. In six patients, the defect in AMLR and other parameters of T-cell function was partially corrected. Notably, these

**TABLE 1.** Distribution of Antibodies to Neuron-Axon Filament Proteins in Autistic Patients and Family Controls

| Patient Group | No. of Sera Tested | No. of Sera Positive | Positive Sera (%) |
|---|---|---|---|
| Autistic syndrome | 15 | 10 | 67 |
| Family controls | 33 | 17 | 52 |
| Parents | 20 | 11 | 55 |
| Siblings | 13 | 6 | 46 |

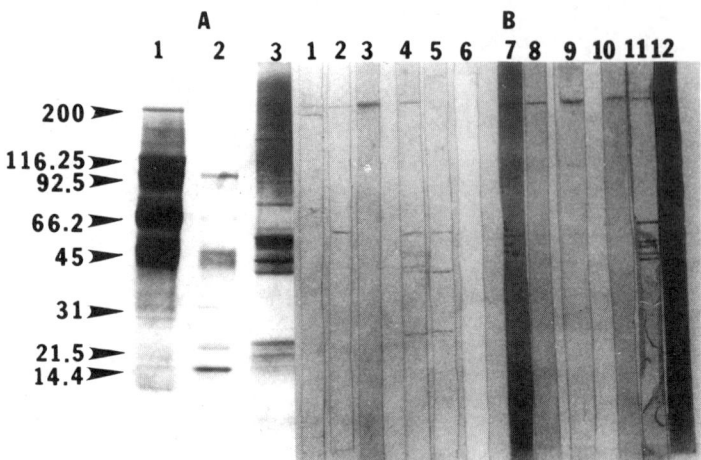

**FIGURE 2.** Serum autoantibodies to neuron-axon filament proteins (NAFP) in autistic patients. (A) Molecular weight reference markers. (B) Immunoblots of sera from patients and family controls: (1) Autistic, (2) Sibling, (3) Father, (4) Autistic, (5) Sibling, (6) Father, (7) Autistic, (8) Sibling, (9) Mother, (10) Autistic, (11) Sibling, and (12) Mother.

six patients also had improvement in their clinical status in terms of speech, sleep, or attention (eg, after 8 weeks they could speak more than one command, after 16 weeks they were able to write complete sentences, and all had increased span of sleep or attention). The other two patients without abnormal CMI were nonresponders. These observations suggest that AMLR and anti-NAFP may be important predictors of autistic patient's responsiveness to this new form of immunomodulant therapy.

### REFERENCES

1. SINGH, V. K. & H. H. FUDENBERG. 1986. J. Clin. Psychiatr. **47:** 592.
2. SINGH, V. K. & H. H. FUDENBERG. 1986. Prog. Drug Res. **30:** 345.
3. SINGH, V. K. et al. 1987. Mech. Age. Develop. **37:** 257.
4. GALBRAITH, G. M. P. et al. 1986. J. Clin. Invest. **78:** 865.
5. SINGH, V. K. & H. H. FUDENBERG. 1987. Clin. Immunol. Newslett. **8:** 164.
6. TOH, G. H. et al. 1985. Proc. Natl. Acad. Sci. USA **82:** 3485.

# Long-Term Follow-up Study of Relapse in Symptoms and Reelevation of Acetylcholine Receptor Antibody Titers in Patients with Myasthenia Gravis[a]

## TADATOSHI KOMIYA AND TAKESHI SATO

*Department of Neurology*
*Juntendo University School of Medicine*
*Tokyo, Japan*

This study presents the results of a long-term follow-up study of clinical states and antiacetylcholine receptor (AChR) antibody titers in patients with myasthenia gravis (MG) who underwent thymectomy and steroid therapy alone or combined with plasma exchange (PE).

Fifty-one patients, aged 11 to 57 years, with generalized MG (39 with nonthymoma and 12 with thymoma, including 4 with invasive thymoma) were analyzed (TABLE 1). Thirty-six patients (seven with thymoma) were treated with thymectomy and steroids (Group A); 15 patients (5 with thymoma including 4 with invasive thymoma) were treated with PE in addition to thymectomy and steroids (Group B). Plasma exchange by a bag system was performed in patients with severe disease, and 1.5-2 liters of plasma were exchanged daily for a period of 7-14 days. The AChR antibodies were measured using the Lindstrom *et al.* assay system.

[a] This work was supported in part by a grant from the Ministry of Health and Welfare, Japan.

TABLE 1. Classification of Patients with Myasthenia Gravis[a,b]

|  | Age (yr) at Onset | Sex | Duration; Onset to Thymectomy (yr) | Duration; Onset to PE (yr) | Thymic Histology | |
|---|---|---|---|---|---|---|
| Group A (n = 36) | 12-56 (32) | M 9 F 27 | 0.3-12 (3.4) |  | Nonthymoma Thymoma | 29 7 |
| Group B (n = 15) | 11-57 (26) | M 5 F 10 | 0.2-11 (3.3) | 0.3-11 (3.6) | Nonthymoma Thymoma | 10 5[4] |

[a] Group A = 36 patients treated with thymectomy and steroids; Group B = 15 patients treated with plasma exchange (PE) in addition to thymectomy and steroids. The mean duration from thymectomy to PE was about 4 months.

[b] Figures in parentheses are the mean; figures in brackets indicate number with invasive thymoma.

FIGURE 1 indicates changes in AChR antibody levels and clinical states of patients in both groups.

All Group A patients showed a maximum decrease in mean titers of AChR antibodies at the end of the first year after thymectomy (reduction rate 46 ± 15%). All Group B patients except one showed markedly decreased titers with clinical improvement just after PE (reduction rate 70 ± 20%).

Two patterns were noted in the AChR antibody levels of both groups during the 5-year period after thymectomy.[1] One pattern is consistently decreased titers in patients (60%) and the other is a reelevation of titers (40%).

Of both groups, 30% of the patients with titer reelevation had relapse in proportion to the tapering off of steroids after long-term remission, and all of them, except one,

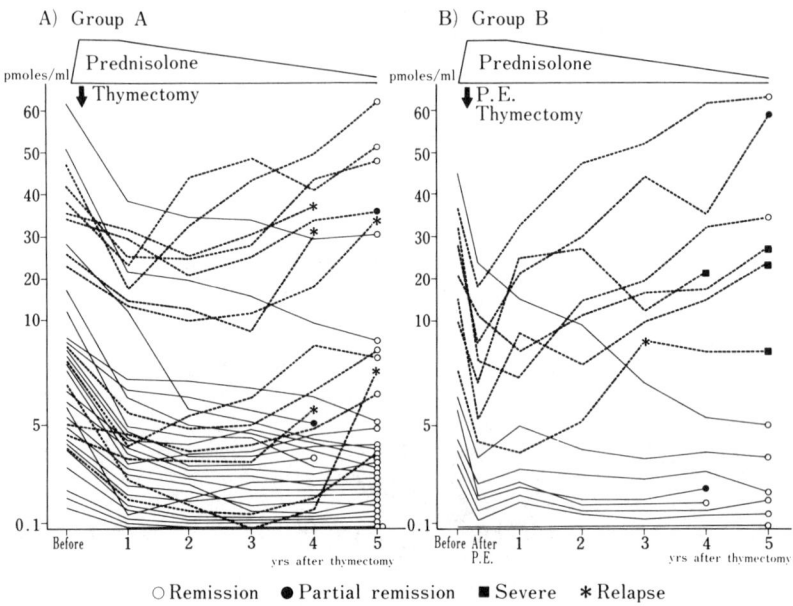

○ Remission ● Partial remission ■ Severe ∗ Relapse

**FIGURE 1.** Long-term changes in acetylcholine receptor antibody levels and clinical states 4 to 5 years after thymectomy. *Solid lines* = patients who showed decreased titers. *Dotted lines* = patients who showed reelevation of titers.

had thymoma (four noninvasive and one invasive). All patients with invasive thymoma were incurable and required high-dose steroid therapy. Sixty-five percent of patients with titer reelevation had high levels of AChR antibodies before treatment.

Ninety percent of both groups of patients with titer reduction showed remission at 5 years after thymectomy, so that steroids could be tapered off quickly. The remission rate of patients without thymoma was 95% at 5 years after treatment, but that of patients with thymoma was only 50%.

We have made it clear that the factors involved in titer reelevation and relapse in myasthenic symptoms are as follows: (1) the tapering off of steroids; (2) high titers before treatment; and (3) thymoma. Our results indicate that (1) we should be careful to note a relapse in myasthenic symptoms in patients who have thymoma and show a reelevation of titers, even after thymectomy and steroid therapy; and (2) PE is a very useful method for decreasing AChR antibodies and controlling patients with severe disease.

## REFERENCE

1. KOMIYA, T., T. SATO et al. 1986. In Therapeutic Plasmapheresis. T. Oda, Ed.:471-475. F. K. Schattauer Verlag, Stuttgart.

# Lymphocyte Subsets after Stroke

A. CZŁONKOWSKA, J. KORLAK,
AND A. KUCZYŃSKA

*Institute of Psychiatry and Neurology*
*Sobieskiego 1/9*
*02 957 Warsaw, Poland*

In this study we investigated the influence of cerebral stroke on the distribution of lymphocytes in peripheral blood, paying particular attention to the hemispheric localization of the brain lesion.

## MATERIALS AND METHOD

Sixty-three patients with stroke (mean age 67.80 ± 14.88) were studied. In 54, stroke was caused by cerebral infarction and in 9 by cerebral hemorrhage. In 54 cases a primary cerebral lesion was localized in the cerebral hemispheres (21 right and 33 left) and in 9 cases in the cerebral stem.

The control group consisted of 23 subjects over 45 years of age (mean age 71.47 ± 11.68), all of whom were in good physical condition.

The following monoclonal antibodies produced by Becton Dickinson were used as lymphocyte markers: Leu 4a (T cells), Leu 2a (cytotoxic/suppressor cells), Leu 3a (T helper/inducer cells), HLA-DQ (B cells, macrophages), HLA-DR (B cells, macrophages, and activated T cells).

To identify the cells that bound the monoclonal antibodies, immunoperoxidase slide assay was used.

## RESULTS

The distribution of lymphocyte populations in patients based on the hemispheric localization of the vascular event is given in TABLE 1.

One week after the vascular event patients with a right hemispheric lesion were found to have a significant decrease in T cells $T_h$, $T_s$, $T_h/T_s$ ratio compared with patients with a left hemispheric lesion and the control group. A decrease in the percentage of B cells with HLA-DQ markers was found during the entire observation period in patients with a left hemispheric lesion.

TABLE 1. Influence of the Location of the Lesion in the Left or Right Hemisphere on the Lymphocyte Subsets in Blood (Mean ± SD)

| Group<br>Type<br>of<br>Lymphocytes | Right Hemisphere Lesion | | | Left Hemisphere Lesion | | | Oder<br>Control<br>($n = 23$) |
|---|---|---|---|---|---|---|---|
| | 48 Hours<br>($n = 21$) | 1 Week<br>($n = 21$) | 3 Weeks<br>($n = 15$) | 48 Hours<br>($n = 33$) | 1 Week<br>($n = 33$) | 3 Weeks<br>($n = 22$) | |
| Leu 4<br>(%) | 64.76<br>± 8.78 | 51.10[a,b,c]<br>±26.21 | 64.40<br>± 8.51 | 63.30[a]<br>± 9.28 | 63.97[a]<br>± 8.77 | 68.18<br>±10.35 | 69.48<br>± 6.86 |
| Leu 2a<br>(%) | 22.86[c]<br>± 4.12 | 17.43[a,b,c]<br>± 9.34 | 23.93<br>± 4.73 | 27.03[a]<br>± 7.33 | 24.67<br>± 6.73 | 24.09<br>± 5.28 | 24.00<br>± 3.02 |
| Leu 3a<br>(%) | 35.33<br>± 6.61 | 27.19[a,b,c]<br>±15.02 | 35.47<br>± 6.62 | 37.79<br>± 7.51 | 35.76[b]<br>± 5.96 | 37.05<br>± 6.06 | 38.78<br>± 6.83 |
| Leu 3a/Leu 2a | 1.58<br>± 0.36 | 1.27[a,b]<br>± 0.65 | 1.54<br>± 0.45 | 1.48<br>± 0.39 | 1.52<br>± 0.38 | 1.62<br>± 0.46 | 1.63<br>± 0.33 |
| HLA-DQ<br>(%) | 17.00[c]<br>± 4.39 | 14.67<br>± 8.27 | 15.40<br>± 4.62 | 14.42[a]<br>± 4.55 | 13.36[a]<br>±10.02 | 13.45[a]<br>± 3.79 | 18.52<br>± 5.94 |
| HLA-DR<br>(%) | 11.39<br>± 5.47 | 10.61<br>± 7.90 | 13.00[b]<br>± 5.12 | 11.87<br>± 4.08 | 13.60[b]<br>± 5.26 | 12.57<br>± 4.37 | 12.09<br>± 3.76 |

[a] $p < 0.05$ vs. control.
[b] $p < 0.05$ vs. first investigation.
[c] $p < 0.05$ vs. left side.

## DISCUSSION

Differences in cell population were found in stroke patients, depending on whether the cerebrovascular event occurred in the right or left hemisphere. In both groups of patients with lesion of the left and right hemisphere, there was a similar proportion of patients with good and bad outcomes and concomitant infections. Therefore, the effect of disease severity in these groups can be excluded, making it more likely that the differences observed were due to the actual location of the lesion.

In animal experiments it was shown that ablation of the neocortex results in changes in immunologic response, and that these changes depend on the site of the lesion.[1]

In humans there are few investigations in the effect of lateralization on immunologic response. Left-handed persons and their families have a greater proportion of learning disabilities and immunologic diseases.[2]

The influence of the cerebral cortex on the function of the immune system is unclear. Injuries to different hemispheres may lead to different changes in neurotransmitters as well as a disturbance in the function of the hypothalamic-pituitary axis and subsequent release of peptides.

### REFERENCES

1. NEUEV, P. J. et al. 1986. Modulation of mitogen induced lymphoproliferation by cerebral neocortex. Life Sci. **38:** 1907.
2. GESCHWIND, N. 1984. Immunological associations of cerebral dominance. In Neuroimmunology. P. Behan & F. Spreafico, Eds. Raven Press, New York.

WORKSHOP 13. NEUROIMMUNOLOGY OF AIDS AND SLOW VIRUS INFECTION

# Human Immunodeficiency Virus gp120 and p24 Oligoclonal Antibody in Acquired Immunodeficiency Syndrome Cerebrospinal Fluid and Sera[a]

LUIGI M. E. GRIMALDI,[b] RAYMOND P. ROOS,[b]
ADRIANO LAZZARIN,[c] MARIO MORONI,[c] JAMES M.
CASEY,[d] AND SUSHILKUMAR G. DEVARE[d]

[b]University of Chicago
Department of Neurology
Chicago, Illinois

[c]Universitá di Milano
Clinica Malattie Infettive
Milano, Italy

[d]Abbott Laboratories
North Chicago, Illinois

Over 90% of patients with acquired immunodeficiency syndrome (AIDS) have evidence of central or peripheral nervous system disease.[1] The neurologic diseases complicating AIDS can be divided into those related to opportunistic infections and neoplasms and those related to the AIDS dementia complex (ADC), a syndrome presumed secondary to direct infection of the central nervous system (CNS) by HIV. The neurologic diseases are reflected in a variety of immunologic abnormalities in the cerebrospinal fluid (CSF), including intrathecal immunoglobulin synthesis, elevated levels of anti-HIV antibody, and the presence of oligoclonal IgG bands.[2]

The aims of this study were to further characterize the humoral immune response of patients with AIDS and to determine whether the oligoclonal IgG bands detected in CSF and in serum were directed against major HIV proteins.

## MATERIALS AND METHODS

Paired CSF and sera were collected from 24 patients with AIDS, 9 with and 15 without ADC. HIV antibody was detected in the serum of all AIDS patients by the ELISA test and confirmed by Western blot.

[a]This work was supported in part by the Brain Research Foundation, an affiliate of the University of Chicago.

The presence of oligoclonal bands was detected by isoelectric focusing (IEF) on polyacrylamide (PAG) plates (L.K.B., Bromma, Sweden) followed by silver staining, as previously described.[3] The antibody response to viral proteins was evaluated by an IEF-antigen overlay technique[4] with the following modifications. After PAG-IEF and transfer to nitrocellulose paper, 5% nonfat dry milk was used to block free sites on nitrocellulose paper. From 50,000-250,000 cpm per lane of $^{125}$I-labeled purified HIV gp120 or p24 were incubated in 5% nonfat dry milk for 3-6 hours. All HIV proteins were purified as previously described[5,6] and $^{125}$I labeled by the chloramine T method. After extensive washes with 5% nonfat dry milk, the nitrocellulose paper was processed for autoradiography.

## RESULTS

Serum oligoclonal bands were detected in 3 of 9 ADC-positive and 7 of 13 ADC-negative patients (FIG. 1a). Cerebrospinal fluid oligoclonal bands were present in 4 of 9 ADC-positive and 7 of 15 ADC-negative AIDS patients, for a total of 11 of 24 patients (FIG. 1c); 5 patients had bands in both CSF and serum.

Anti-gp120 antibody activity was found in 19 of 22 sera (FIG. 1b) and in 14 of 24 CSF (FIG. 1d). Anti-p24 antibody activity was detected in only 2 of 24 CSF and 3 of 22 sera from AIDS patients, at a different pI than that of anti-gp120 antibody activity (FIG. 1e-g). Anti-HIV gp120 and p24 antibody activities appeared very restricted in pI distribution.

When CSF and serum anti-gp120 antibody IEF patterns were compared, they were often dissimilar, suggesting an intrathecal synthesis of HIV antibody. Silver-stained oligoclonal bands were compared to IEF-antigen overlay autoradiograms to determine whether they coincided with detectable anti-HIV protein activity. None of the AIDS' CSF and serum oligoclonal bands had antibody reactivity to radiolabeled HIV gp120 or p24 (FIG. 1a-b and c-d). The bands were presumably not directed against other HIV components, because they failed to react with a $^{125}$I-labeled disrupted purified HIV (data not shown).

The presence of ADC among AIDS patients did not correlate with any of the immunologic parameters evaluated in our study.

## DISCUSSION

Our findings indicate that the CSF antibody response to two major HIV proteins (gp120 and p24) in AIDS patients is locally produced in the CNS and is of restricted heterogeneity. This restricted response contrasts with the broadly distributed herpes simplex virus (HSV) glycoprotein (g)B response in patients with HSV encephalitis (FIG. 1h). This restricted response may explain the relatively low titers of neutralizing antibody found in AIDS sera.[7] The response to p24 was less frequently detected and even more restricted than that to gp120, indicating the presence of a limited number of anti-p24 antibody-producing clones. The limited number of p24 clones may render them more vulnerable to progressive immunosuppression and explain the disappearance of anti-p24 antibody activity seen in frank AIDS.[8]

We demonstrated that silver-stained oligoclonal bands are not directed against HIV proteins. This observation contrasts with our findings with HTLV-1-associated myelopathy, a CNS disease caused by another retrovirus and in which the CSF oligoclonal bands possess anti-HTLV-I p24 antibody activity (data not shown). It is possible that the AIDS CSF oligoclonal bands are directed against agents responsible for opportunistic infections; this is presently under study. Another possibility is that the oligoclonal bands represent "nonsense" antibody, unrelated to any etiologic antigen or autoimmunogen, and result from immunodysregulation. "Nonsense" bands are present in CSF from patients with multiple sclerosis,[9] a disease in which retroviral involvement has recently been proposed.[10]

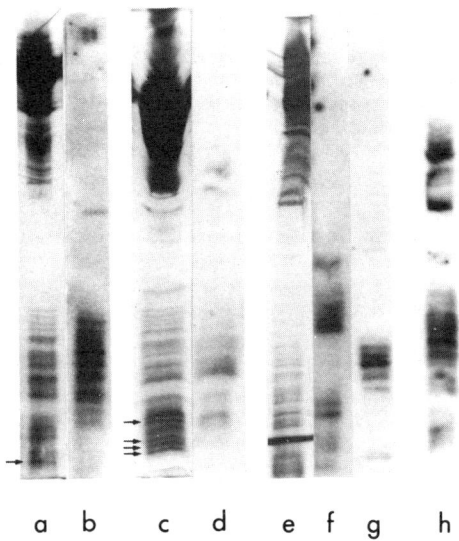

**FIGURE 1.** Representative silver-stained isoelectric focusing (IEF) gels and autoradiograms after IEF-antigen overlay. AIDS patient serum following IEF (*lane a*) and autoradiography showing anti-gp120 antibody activity (*lane b*); AIDS patient CSF following IEF (*lane c*) and autoradiography showing anti-gp120 antibody activity (*lane d*). Arrows indicate silver-stained oligoclonal bands not reacting to gp120. AIDS patient serum following IEF (*lane e*) and autoradiography showing anti-gp120 (*lane f*) and anti-p24 (*lane g*) antibody activities. Note the different pI distribution of the two anti-HIV protein antibody patterns. Autoradiography demonstrating anti-HSV gB antibody activity of CSF from an HSV encephalitis patient (*lane h*). Note that the broad pI distribution contrasts with the more restricted response of the anti-HIV gp120 and p24 antibody activity. The very darkly stained lane in *lane e* is an artifact.

## REFERENCES

1. NAVIA, B. A., E-S. CHO, C. K. PETITO & R. W. PRICE. 1986. Ann. Neurol. **19:** 525.
2. RESNICK, L., F. DIMARZO-VERONESE, J. SCHUPBACH, W. W. TOURTELLOTTE, D. D. HO, F. MULLER, P. SHAPSHAK, M. VOGT, J. E. GROOPMAN, P. D. MARKHAM & R. C. GALLO. 1985. N. Engl. J. Med. **313:** 1498.
3. ROOS, R. P. & M. LICHTER. 1983. J. Neurosci. Method **8:** 375.

4. Roos, R. P., E. A. Nalefski, S. Nitayaphan, R. Variakojis & K. K. Singh. 1987. J. Neuroimmunol. **13**: 305.
5. Robey, W. G., L. O. Arthur, T. J. Matthews, A. Langlois, T. D. Copeland, N. W. Lerche, S. Oroszlan, D. P. Bolognesi, R. V. Gilden & P. J. Fishinger. 1986. Proc. Natl. Acad. Sci. USA **83**: 7023.
6. Casey, J. M., Y. Kim, P. R. Anderson, K. F. Watson, L. Fox & S. G. Devare. 1985. J. Virol. **55**: 417.
7. Wahren, B., L. Morfeldt-Masson, G. Biberfeld, L. Moberg, A. Sonnerborg, P. Ljungman, A. Werner, R. Kurth, R. C. Gallo & D. Bolognesi. 1987. J. Virol. **61**: 2017.
8. Weber, J. N., R. A. Weiss, C. Roberts, I. Weller, R. S. Tedder, P. R. Clapham, D. Parker, J. Duncan, C. Carne, A. Pinching & R. Cheingsong-Popov. 1987. Lancet **i**: 119.
9. Roos, R. P. 1985. Arch. Neurol. **42**: 73.
10. Koprowski, H., E. C. DeFreitas, M. E. Harper, M. Sandberg-Wollheim, W. A. Sheremata, M. Robert-Guroff, C. W. Saxinger, M. B. Feinberg, F. Wong-Staal & R. C. Gallo. 1985. Nature **318**: 154.

# Intrathecal Synthesis of Anti-HIV Oligoclonal IgG in HIV-Seropositive Patients Having No Signs of HIV-Induced Neurologic Diseases

P. GALLO,[a] A. DE ROSSI,[b] P. CADROBBI,[c]
E. FRANCAVILLA,[c] L. CHIECO-BIANCHI,[b] AND
B. TAVOLATO[a]

*Department of Neurology,[a]
Department of Oncology,[b] and
Infectious Diseases Unit,[c]
University Hospital of Padova
Padova, Italy*

The peculiar neurotropism of human immunodeficiency virus (HIV) has been proved by (a) the isolation of HIV from the brain, spinal cord, and cerebrospinal fluid (CSF) of patients with acquired immunodeficiency syndrome (AIDS) and encephalopathy,[1] and (b) the evidence that the AIDS dementia complex can be the presenting or sole manifestation of HIV infection, suggesting that a direct brain infection may occur early in the course of systemic virus spread.[2] Few data have so far been produced on CSF antibodies of HIV-seropositive patients having no signs of HIV-induced neurologic diseases (i.e., AIDS dementia complex, vacuolar myelopathy, and inflammatory demyelinating peripheral neuropathy). Therefore, a study was undertaken to identify an early CSF marker that could reflect a latent infection of the nervous system in such patients.

## MATERIAL AND METHODS

Twenty-two subjects were included in this study (TABLE 1) and were classified according to the Walter-Reed criteria for HIV infection[3]: 2 WR1 (asymptomatic), 4 WR2, 1 WR3, 1 WR4, 2 WR5, and 12 WR6. None had clinical signs and symptoms of neurologic disorders due to HIV infection at the time of CSF sampling. The following tests were performed: detection of HIV antibodies (HIV-ab) by Western blot and ELISA in serum and CSF; demonstration of intrathecal IgG synthesis by quantitative formulas (IgG index and intra-blood-brain barrier [BBB] IgG synthesis rate) and by agarose isoelectric focusing (i.e., IgG oligoclonal bands); and detection of HIV-specific oligoclonal IgG by affinity-driven transfer of focused IgG to HIV-antigen precoated nitrocellulose membranes.

TABLE 1. Cerebrospinal Fluid Data of the 22 Seropositive Patients Included in the Study[a]

| Patients | | Neurologic Complications | Increased CSF/Serum Albumin Ratio ($n \leq 5.5$) | Increased IgG Index ($n \leq 0.7$) | IgG Oligoclonal Bands Positive | CSF HIV ab Positive |
|---|---|---|---|---|---|---|
| WR 1: | 2  | 0/2   | 0/2   | 0/2  | 0/2  | 1/2   |
| WR 2: | 4  | 1/4   | 1/4   | 2/4  | 2/4  | 4/4   |
| WR 3: | 1  | 0/1   | 0/1   | 0/1  | 0/1  | 1/1   |
| WR 4: | 1  | 0/1   | 0/1   | 0/1  | 0/1  | 1/1   |
| WR 5: | 2  | 1/2   | 1/2   | 0/2  | 0/2  | 2/2   |
| WR 6: | 12 | 8/12  | 8/12  | 5/12 | 5/12 | 9/12  |
|       | 22 | 10/22 | 10/22 | 7/22 | 7/22 | 18/22 |

[a] Patients were grouped according to the Walter-Reed (WR) criteria for HIV infection.

## RESULTS

Eighteen patients (82%) had detectable levels of HIV-ab in their CSF, whereas 4 (1 WR1 and 3 WR6) had negative results in repeated controls. The presence of a blood-brain barrier damage did not influence the positivity as well as the pattern of HIV-ab detected by Western blot. In fact, the CSF of two patients was HIV-ab negative despite the presence of BBB damage, which was severe in one case. Intrathecal IgG synthesis was demonstrated in 8 of 12 WR6 patients (3 with increased formulas, 3 with IgG oligoclonal bands, and 2 with both), in 2 WR2 patients (both with increased formulas and oligoclonal IgG), and in one WR3 patient (increased formulas) (FIG.

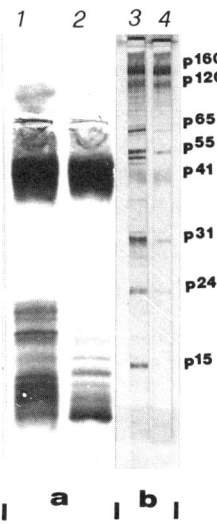

**FIGURE 1.** (a) Serum (1) and CSF (2) IgG patterns of a WR6 patient studied by agarose isoelectric focusing and anti-IgG (Fc) immunofixation. Additional IgG oligoclonal bands are clearly visible in CSF, suggesting an intrathecal synthesis of IgG. (b) Patterns of HIV antibodies detected in serum (3) and CSF (4) of the same patient.

1). One asymptomatic, one WR2, and two WR6 patients had superimposable IgG patterns in CSF and serum, likely due to expression of a systemic polyclonal B-cell activation. The seven HIV-ab positive CSF (5 WR6, 2 WR2) that showed IgG oligoclonal bands on isoelectric focusing were also studied by means of affinity-driven transfer. It was noted that most IgG bands were antibodies against HIV antigens (HIV-ag). However, not all bands were absorbed by HIV-ag, suggesting a CNS segregation of B cells having specificities other than HIV and likely activated by a polyclonal mechanism.

Summarizing, our data extend and confirm previous reports[4] on the intrathecal HIV-ab production by HIV-seropositive patients. The high number of HIV-positive CSF, the increased IgG indexes, the detection of IgG oligoclonal bands as well as the demonstration of HIV-specific oligoclonal IgG in patients with low WR staging provided evidence for an early infection of the CNS by HIV. Moreover, the finding of intrathecal HIV-ab synthesis can be of prognostic importance and may help to understand the contribution of HIV in the genesis of the neurologic syndrome related to this virus. Therefore, a complete CSF examination, as reported herein, may be useful in predicting the outcome in HIV-seropositive patients.

## REFERENCES

1. Ho, D. D., T. R. Rota, R. T. Schooley, et al. 1985. Isolation of HTLV-III from cerebrospinal fluids and neural tissues of patients with neurologic syndromes related to the acquired immunodeficiency syndrome. N. Engl. J. Med. **313:** 1493-1497.
2. Navia, B. A. & R. W. Price. 1987. The acquired immunodeficiency syndrome dementia complex as the presenting or sole manifestation of human immunodeficiency virus infection. Arch. Neurol. **44:** 65-69.
3. Redfield, R. R., D. C. Wright & E. C. Tramont. 1986. The Walter-Reed staging classification for HTLV-III/LAV infection. N. Engl. J. Med. **314:** 131-132.
4. Resnick, L., F. di Marzio-Veronese, J. Schüpbach et al. 1985. Intra-blood-brain barrier synthesis of HTLV-III specific IgG in patients with neurologic symptoms associated with AIDS or AIDS-related complex. N. Engl. J. Med. **313:** 1498-1504.

# Intrathecal Immunity in 37 Patients Seropositive for Anti-HIV-1 Antibody[a]

J. REBOUL,[b] E. SCHULLER,[b] G. PIALOUX,[c] M. A. REY,[c] P. LEBON,[d] AND F. BRUN-VEZINET[c]

[b]*Laboratory of Neuro-Immunology*
*Hôpital de la Salpêtrière*
*75651 Paris Cedex 13, France*

[c]*Laboratory of Virology*
*Hôpital Claude Bernard*
*75019 Paris, France*

[d]*Laboratory of Virology*
*Hôpital Saint-Vincent-de-Paul*
*75674 Paris, Cedex 14, France*

## MATERIALS AND METHODS

### Population

Thirty-eight paired samples of sera and cerebrospinal fluid from 37 men aged 18 to 65 years (mean 38.6 ± 11.5) were used in the study. Clinically 11 had subacute encephalitis (9 AIDS, 2 ARC), 10 peripheral neuropathies (3 AIDS, 6 ARC, 1 seropositive), 1 myelopathy (AIDS), 3 cerebral tumors, and 3 neuromeningeal infections (all with AIDS) and 9 without neurologic or psychiatric symptoms (7 AIDS, 1 ARC, and 1 seropositive).

### Assessment of Intrathecal Immunity

1. *Intrathecal synthesis of immunoglobulins and complement components:* These were calculated by applying the mathematical formulas established previously[1] giving the percentages of intrathecal IgG synthesis and, by deduction, the percentage of plasmatic IgG in the CSF.

2. *Antibody-specific activity:* The antibody-specific activity (ASA) expresses the

---

[a] This research was supported by the Institut National de la Santé et de la Recherche Médicale (INSERM) and the Association pour la Recherche sur la Sclérose en Plaques (ARSEP).

antibody power of an immunoglobulin for a concentration of 1 mg/1. It is calculated, in units, as:

$$\frac{\text{reciprocal of serologic titer}}{\text{Ig (mg/1)}}$$

This activity, calculated in the serum and CSF, is, by convenience, expressed in $10^{-3}$ units.

Thus, intrathecal ASA equals:

$$\frac{\text{CSF ASA} - (\text{Serum ASA} \times \text{percentage of plasmatic Ig})}{(\text{percentage of intrathecal Ig})}$$

## RESULTS

The results are summarized in TABLE 1.

### Serum

1. IgA concentrations higher than 6 g/1 are observed in three patients, reaching 13 g/1 in one of them.
2. C4 increase is very frequently noted and statistically correlated ($p < 0.05$) with a C3 decrease. Such complement changes to our knowledge have never been described in any neuroimmunologic disease.
3. Anti-HIV ASA was high ($>200$) in 8 patients: no correlation ($r = -0.09$) was found with serum IgG levels, suggesting a specific immune answer not related to a more or less important IgG synthesis. Anti-herpes ASA was high ($>200$) in 10 patients: a significant ($p < 0.001$) *negative* correlation ($r = -0.56$) with serum IgG was evidenced.

### Intrathecal Immunity

The classification[1] of the 38 CSF patterns was: normal (3), transudate (1), inflammatory (13), and meningitis (21). Intrathecal IgA synthesis (mean 1.9 ± 0.7 mg/1) was high and frequent (42%) and correlated ($p < 0.05$) with the serum IgA increase. Intrathecal changes of complement components are very similar to those observed in serum: C3 decrease and intrathecal C4 synthesis were very frequent but not statistically correlated. Intrathecal anti-HIV ASA was higher than serum anti-HIV ASA in all but 3 patients: in 8 patients it was 100 times higher, in 10 patients between 20 and 100 times higher, and in 14 patients 2 to 20 times higher. A significant ($p < 0.01$) negative correlation ($r = -0.31$) was calculated with local IgG synthesis. Finally, this intrathecal ASA was not correlated ($r = 0.12$) with serum anti-HIV ASA. Intrathecal anti-herpes ASA (calculated in 19 patients only) was higher than serum anti-herpes ASA in 6 patients only and not established in 9 others: no correlation ($r = -0.18$) was found with local IgG synthesis.

### Interferon

Alpha-interferon was detected in 14 of 20 sera investigated (range 5-52 IU) and in 13 CSF samples (range 3-150). No significant correlations were found with intrathecal synthesis of immunoglobulins or with anti-HIV ASA.

TABLE 1. Protein Abnormalities in 38 HIV-Seropositive Patients

|  | Normal Limits | Abnormalities Observed | No. of Patients | Percentage |
|---|---|---|---|---|
| Serum (g/l) |  |  |  |  |
| Prealbumin[a] | 0.25-0.35 | <0.25 | 18 | 60 |
| Albumin | 30-50 | <30 | 10 | 26 |
| IgA | 1-4 | >4 | 7 | 18 |
| IgG | 10-15 | >15 | 27 | 71 |
| IgM | 0.5-1 | >1 | 15 | 39 |
| C3 | 0.7-1.2 | <0.7 | 18 | 47 |
| C4 | 0.15-0.40 | >0.4 | 26 | 68 |
| CSF (mg/l) |  |  |  |  |
| Albumin | 126-294 | >294 | 22 | 58 |
| IgA | 2-5 | Intrathecal synthesis | 16 | 42 |
| IgG | 15-30 | Intrathecal synthesis | 34 | 89 |
| IgM | 0.2-0.5 | Intrathecal synthesis | 14 | 37 |
| C3 | 2-4 | Intrathecal decrease | 21 | 55 |
| C4 | 1-3 | Intrathecal synthesis | 29 | 76 |

[a] Thirty patients only

### Calculation of Intrathecal IgG Synthesis: Comparison of Three Formulas

Using our formula, intrathecal IgG synthesis was detected in 34 CSF samples (89%), Link's index[2] was abnormal (>0.65) in 25 (66%), and Tourtellotte's formula[3] (>3.3 mg/day) gives pathologic results in 27 (71%).

*Clinical Correlations*

No clinical correlations were established between any of the immunologic or virologic data and the clinical data.

## DISCUSSION

*Specific Activity of HIV:* The most remarkable fact is the presence of an intrathecal HIV ASA in 33 patients presenting an intrathecal synthesis of IgG. This local anti-HIV ASA was higher than the serum ASA in 29 of 33, which suggests that this ASA was linked to a local antigenic stimulation and not to a nonspecific immune response.

These results are in agreement with the results of two previous studies suggesting intrathecal synthesis of such antibodies in both AIDS patients[4] or HIV healthy carriers.[5] There is therefore little doubt that this fact constitutes an early testimony of HIV disease in the CNS.

*Intrathecal synthesis of immunoglobulins* is very particular: compared to IgG intrathecal synthesis, that of IgM appears relatively modest and rare. However, IgA intrathecal synthesis, correlated with serum IgA increases, is a very particular characteristic of AIDS disease and seems more important than that observed during infections with viruses such as herpes virus, Epstein-Barr virus, varicella-zona, cytomegalovirus, or rubella.

*Intrathecal variations of C3 and C4:* It is very probable that intrathecal synthesis of C4 is a witness of the activation of macrophages. C3 decrease suggests formation of a possible immune complex.

*Specific intrathecal anti-herpes activity,* when higher than that noted in the serum of the same patients, suggests the possibility of HSV replication.

## CONCLUSION

This first study confirms the practically constant and therefore probably early invasion of the CNS by HIV, but the prognostic value of intrathecal HIV ASA remains unclear. The IgA and C4 complement components' increases are important, but their significance remains unknown. The possibility of other intrathecal associated infections (as HSV) should be discussed.

### REFERENCES

1. SCHULLER, E., S. BENEBDALLAH, H. J. SAGAR, J. REBOUL & L. TÖMPE. 1987. IgG synthesis within the central nervous system. Arch. Neurol. **44:** 600-604.
2. TIBBLING, G., H. LINK & S. OHMAN. 1977. Principles of albumin and IgG analyses in neurological disorders. I. Establishment of reference values. Scand. J. Clin. Lab. Invest. **37:** 385-390.

3. TOURTELLOTTE, W. 1970. On cerebrospinal fluid immunoglobulin G (IgG) quotients in multiple sclerosis and other diseases: A review and a new formula to estimate the amount of IgG synthesized per day by the central nervous system. J. Neurol. Sci. **10:** 279-304.
4. ACKERMANN, R., M. NEKIC & R. JÜRGENS. 1986. Locally synthesized antibodies in cerebrospinal fluid of patients with AIDS J. Neurol. **233:** 140-141.
5. GOUDSMIT, J., E. C. WOLTERS, M. BAKKER, L. SMIT, J. VAN DER NOORDAA, E. A. H. HISCHE, J. A. TUTUARIMA & H. J. VAN DER HELM. 1986. Intrathecal synthesis of antibodies to HTLV-III in patients without AIDS or AIDS related complex. Br. Med. J. **292:** 1231-1234.

# Cerebrospinal Fluid Changes in HIV-1 Infection

MATS ANDERSSON,[a] TOMAS BERGSTRÖM,[b]
CHRISTIAN BLOMSTRAND,[a] SVANTE
HERMODSSON,[b] CHARLES HÅKANSSON,[c] AND
GUN-BRITT LÖWHAGEN[c]

*[a]Department of Neurology*
*[b]Department of Clinical Virology, and*
*[c]Department of Dermatology*
*University of Gothenburg*
*Sahlgren's Hospital*
*Gothenburg, Sweden*

Thirty-four consecutive HIV-1-seropositive patients were studied by neurologic examination and lumbar puncture. Fifteen patients fulfilled the criteria for the lymphadenopathy syndrome. Only four of the patients had neurologic symptoms that could possibly be related to HIV infection. Nine patients had previously been treated for syphilis. All but four were seronegative for syphilis. Two patients had herpes zoster 5 and 6 months before the lumbar puncture. Twenty-two patients had antibodies to hepatitis B, and 2 were HBs ag positive. In 23 cases the duration of HIV infection could be estimated. The population was divided into four groups with a duration of < 1, 1-3, > 3 years, and unknown.

## METHODS

Lymphocyte subpopulations CD4 and CD8 were determined in blood using monoclonal antibodies. Cytologic examination of cerebrospinal fluid (CSF) cells was performed. CSF and serum proteins were analyzed with isoelectric focusing (IEF) in polyacrylamide gels, quantification of albumin and IgG (electroimmunodiffusion), and beta$_2$-microglobulin (ELISA). Intrathecal IgG production was calculated as IgG index according to Link and according to Tourtellotte's formula for IgG production. IgG antibodies to HIV-1 were detected with ELISA and Western blot. Antibody screening in serum and CSF was made against CMV, HSV 1 and 2, VZV, Morbilli, Epstein-Barr virus, *Toxoplasma gondii*, Borrelia, syphilis, and hepatitis B. Virus isolation was attempted from CSF and blood leukocytes. Pitmans nonparametric permutation test was used in the statistical analysis.

## RESULTS

All patients but one had CSF antibodies to HIV-1 detectable with ELISA. All patients had CSF HIV antibodies detectable with Western blot (two patients only against one protein band). Ten patients had a stronger reaction in CSF than in serum against one or more bands, when the strips were incubated with equal amounts of

TABLE 1. Laboratory Findings in 34 HIV-1-Infected Individuals[a]

| Findings | Group | | | |
|---|---|---|---|---|
| | I ($n = 3$) | II ($n = 8$) | III ($n = 12$) | IV ($n = 11$) |
| CSF mononuclear cells ($<5/\mu l$) | 0/3<br>3 | 3/8<br>4 ± 3.4 | 9/12<br>12.4 ± 9 | 9/11<br>15.3 ± 14 |
| Pathologic CSF cytology | 1/3 | 5/8 | 11/12 | 10/11 |
| IEF with CSF enriched gamma bands | 1/3 | 5/8 | 10/12 | 6/11 |
| N:o bands | 0.7 | 2.9 ± 3 | 6.6 ± 5.3 | 5 ± 5.9 |
| IgG index (Link <0.7) | 0/3<br>0.61 ± 0.09 | 5/8<br>0.78 ± 0.13 | 9/12<br>0.97 ± 0.28 | 6/11<br>0.88 ± 0.18 |
| IgG production (Tourtellotte <3 mg/day) | 0/3<br>0 ± 3.5 | 4/8<br>4.9 ± 7.4 | 10/12<br>33 ± 47 | 6/11<br>12 ± 22 |
| CSF beta$_2$-microglobulin (<2.22 mg/l) | 0/3<br>1.43 ± 0.33 | 2/8<br>1.95 ± 0.61 | 8/12<br>2.83 ± 1.31 | 6/11<br>2.66 ± 1.08 |
| Serum beta$_2$-microglobulin (<2.36 mg/l) | 0/3<br>1.74 ± 0.30 | 3/8<br>2.85 ± 1.42 | 6/12<br>2.93 ± 1.22 | 4/11<br>2.26 ± 0.70 |
| Blood CD4/CD8 ratio (<1.0) | 0/3<br>1.31 ± 0.28 | 6/8<br>0.75 ± 0.37 | 10/12<br>0.49 ± 0.30 | 10/11<br>0.58 ± 0.28 |

[a]Values represent the number of pathologic tests/total number of tests, and mean ± SD.

IgG, indicating intrathecal synthesis. No signs of opportunistic infections were found at serologic screening of CSF or in attempts to isolate virus. Only six patients had an increased CSF to serum albumin ratio. CSF lymphocytosis was found in 21 of 34 patients and increased IgG index in 20 of 34 patients. A significant positive correlation was found between the duration of HIV infection and an increase in CSF mononuclear cells ($p < 0.01$), increased intrathecal IgG production expressed as IgG index ($p < 0.05$) or according to Tourtellotte's formula ($p < 0.05$), number of CSF-enriched gamma bands at IEF ($p < 0.05$), and CSF beta$_2$-microglobulin ($p < 0.05$). A significant negative correlation was found between the duration of HIV infection and the blood lymphocyte CD4/CD8 ratio ($p < 0.01$). See TABLE 1 and FIGURE 1.

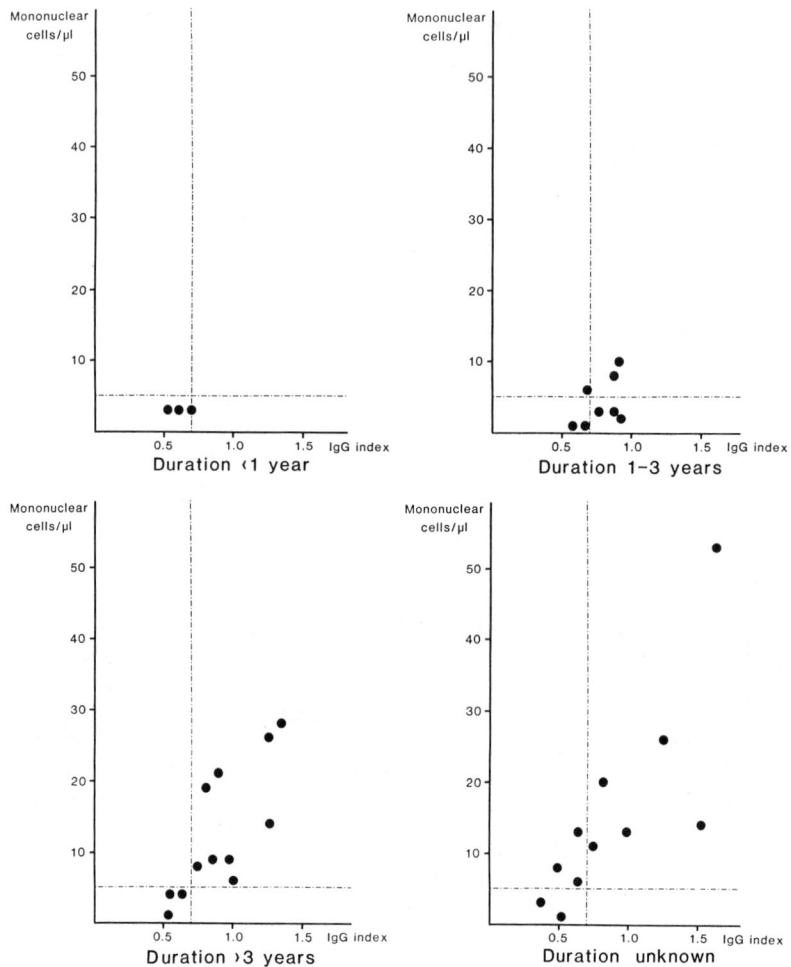

**FIGURE 1.** Correlation between cerebrospinal fluid mononuclear cells per microliter and immunoglobulin G production expressed as IgG index (CSF IgG/serum IgG)/(CSF albumin/serum albumin) in the four groups with different durations of HIV infection.

## CONCLUSIONS

A majority of the investigated HIV-1-seropositive but neurologically asymptomatic individuals had CSF lymphocytosis and increased IgG production as signs of intrathecal B-lymphocyte activation. These CSF abnormalities significantly correlated with the duration of HIV infection and could not be explained by other infections.

## HYPOTHESIS

Intrathecal B-cell activation as a consequence of persistent HIV infection of the nervous system is part of the natural history of the infection preceding stages of progressive neurologic symptoms.

# An AIDS Virus-Associated Antigen Localized in Human Fetal Brain[a]

W. D. LYMAN, Y. KRESS, W. K. RASHBAUM,
T. A. CALVELLI, E. STEINHAUER, J. M. KASHKIN,
C. E. HENDERSON, AND A. RUBINSTEIN

*Albert Einstein College of Medicine
The Bronx, New York 10461*

Because most children with acquired immunodeficiency syndrome (AIDS) exhibit signs of neurologic dysfunction, experiments were conducted to test the hypothesis that the causative agent of AIDS, human immunodeficiency virus (HIV), can be transmitted from mother to fetus and that HIV has a tropism for the central nervous system (CNS). Although many children with congenital HIV infections develop chronic and progressive subacute encephalopathy, it is unclear if the neuropathology is the result of HIV infection of neural cells or the consequence of "bystander" pathogenic mechanisms. The findings that over 80% of patients at autopsy have neuropathologic abnormalities including perivascular inflammation, multinucleated giant cells, and microglial nodules tend to support a pathogenic role for HIV-infected hematogenous cells invading the CNS and causing "bystander" pathology. In contrast, CNS tissue from AIDS patients can also show hypertrophy of oligodendrocyte nuclei, demyelination, gliosis, and disseminated necrotic foci, which suggests that neural cells can also be infected by HIV.

## MATERIALS AND METHODS

Central nervous system tissue from elective pregnancy terminations of HIV-seropositive and control females of unknown serostatus was studied. Sections of frontal cortex were fixed in glutaraldehyde for light and electron microscopy (LM and EM). Two monoclonal antibodies (mAbs) that recognize the p24 core protein of HIV were used as immunocytochemical probes. These mAbs were chosen because a convenient specificity control exists in an analogous mAb that recognizes the p24 core protein of human T-cell lymphotrophic virus-1 (HTLV-1). As positive and negative controls, two cell lines, H-9 cells infected with HIV and C10/MJ cells infected with HTLV-1, were used.

[a] This work was supported in part by grants DA 04583; NS 11920; CP-31041-03; and HL07060-10.

## RESULTS

Light microscopic examination of frontal cortex derived from a 23-week-old abortus of an HIV-seropositive female revealed a significant decrease in CNS parenchymal cell number when compared with that of equivalent sections from control abortuses. The decrease seemed to be selective for germinal plate cells, although astrocyte-like cells were also fewer. There was also an increase in extracellular space consistent with edema. No evidence of overt inflammation was found; however, a multinucleated cell was seen in one section. Electron microscopy revealed prominent pathologic changes consistent with cytolysis in the sections from the HIV abortus but not in equivalent abortus tissues from control patients. HIV-like particles were observed and contained an electron-dense nucleoid. The cerebral vasculature remained morphologically intact in the HIV abortus in that endothelial cells had normal appearing cytoplasm, mitochondria, and junctional complexes. Immunocytochemical results showed that fetal CNS tissue obtained from the HIV-seropositive female was positive for HIV p24 but negative for the equivalent HTLV-1 protein. The anti-HIV p24 mAb revealed positive staining in both the nucleus and the cytoplasm of CNS cells of the HIV abortus. Nuclear staining was localized to the nucleolus and heterochromatin, whereas in the cytoplasm mainly to ribosomes. Control abortus tissue, possibly normal but of unknown HIV status, also had some staining. Anti-HTLV-1 p24 did not stain abortus tissue. Control experiments showed that mAbs used to identify HIV and HTLV-1 specific antigens do not cross-react.

## CONCLUSIONS

Human immunodeficiency virus can infect fetal CNS tissue during gestation, and the consequences of this infection may be significant neuropathology. The staining of control abortus tissue by the mAbs for HIV p24 suggests three possibilities. The first is that the mAbs may not be specific for HIV. The second is that the control abortus tissue was not normal but infected with HIV. Thirdly, an HIV cross-reacting epitope is expressed in normal tissue during gestation. These points are currently under investigation.

# Pathogenesis of Human Immunodeficiency Virus (HIV)-Associated Brain Lesions

## A Neuropathologic Evaluation

HERBERT BUDKA

*Division of Special Neuropathology*
*Neurological Institute*
*University of Vienna*
*A-1090 Vienna, Austria*

Neuropathologic examination of autopsy brain tissue of 100 subjects with human immunodeficiency virus (HIV) infection revealed in 38 brains lesions attributable to HIV, in 17 brains without other pathologies.[1] These lesions were characterized as multifocal giant cell encephalitis[2] (MGCE) and/or progressive diffuse leukoencephalopathy[3] (PDL), both featuring multinucleated giant cells as evidence of the local presence and cytopathic action of HIV[2] on monohistiocytes (as confirmed by electron microscopic detection of retroviral particles in four MGCE cases and immunocytochemical detection of HIV proteins in two MGCE brains[1]). Gray matter changes were found as diffuse glial/glioneuronal poliodystrophy in 51 brains.[1]

HIV-associated brain tissue lesions represent a novel syndrome in which opportunistic agents can be excluded and which can be differentiated from hitherto established brain lesions found in the immunocompromised host, such as progressive multifocal leukoencephalopathy (PML) and nodular (subacute) encephalitis (in most cases cytomegalovirus [CMV] or toxoplasma detectable).

Features that are important in the evaluation of the pathogenesis of HIV-associated lesions (MGCE and PDL) comprise:

1. Monohistiocytes/macrophages, including multinucleated giant cells and "rod cells," all of which were labeled by an antimacrophage antibody, are the predominant cells in the lesions (FIGS. 1A, 1B, and 2B).

2. Parenchymal damage is usually seen as demyelination (FIG. 2A); close attachment of macrophages to damaged myelin is suggestive of myelin stripping. However, neurons, axons, and oligodendroglia remain intact even in the proximity of macrophages (FIG. 1B).

3. Focal lesions of MGCE have a perivascular site (FIGS. 1A and 1B); occasionally, fibrinous streaks are seen extending from the vessel wall, somewhat similar to vasculitis.

These morphologic characteristics do not seem to support a hypothesis of primary neurocytopathy by HIV. Rather, they suggest secondary events related to the predominant cell in the lesion, the monohistiocyte/macrophage, which appears to be attracted to areas of focal vascular damage, possibly by endothelial HIV infection.

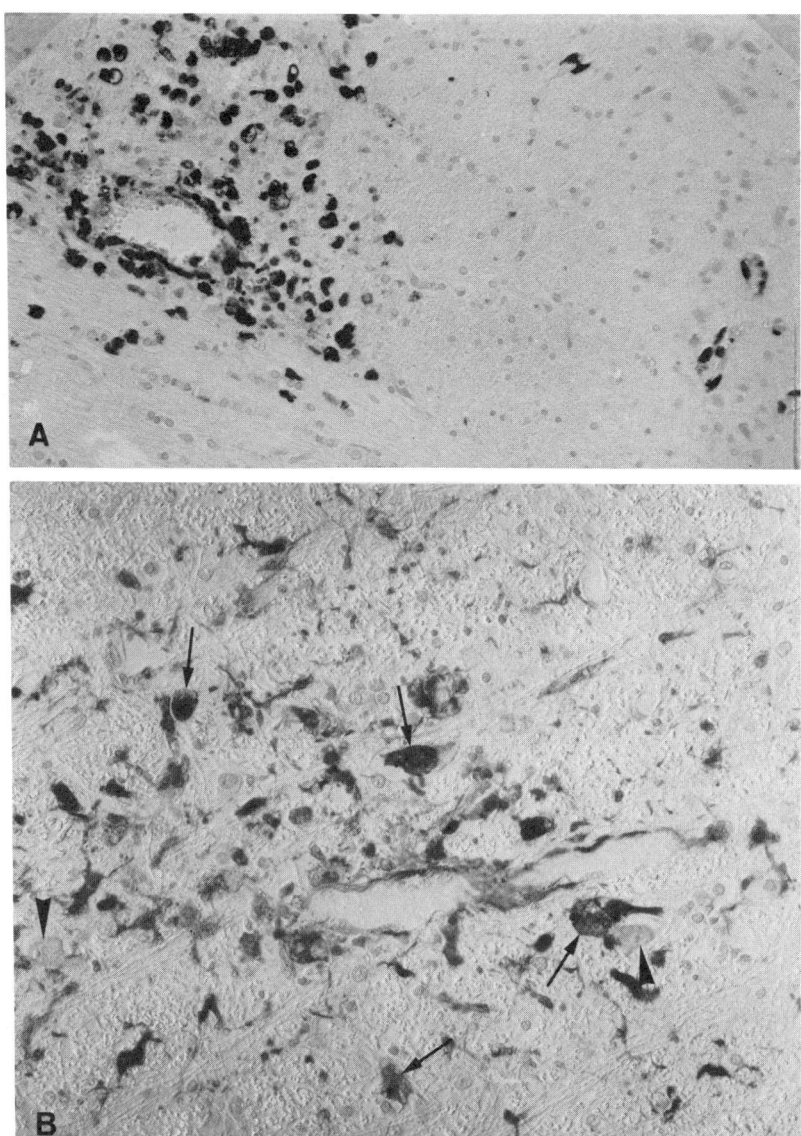

FIGURE 1. Multifocal giant cell encephalitis (MGCE), pons, two different cases. (A) Encephalitic focus around a vessel is predominantly composed of monohistiocytes/macrophages labeled with an antimacrophage antibody (a-mph). Immunocytochemical-labeled biotin-avidin technique, slight hemalum counterstain, original magnification × 160, reduced by 68%. (B) Numerous cells labeled by a-mph exhibit prominent formation of cellular processes. Labeled mono- and multinucleated giant cells (*arrows*) are adjacent to intact neurons (*arrowheads*). Same stain as in A, Nomarski optics, original magnification × 250.

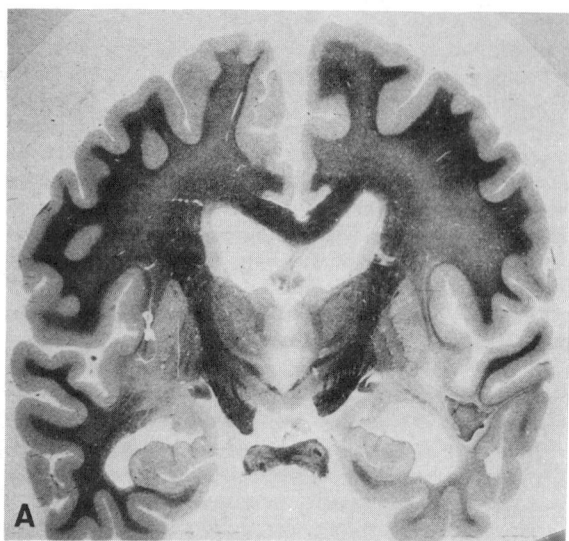
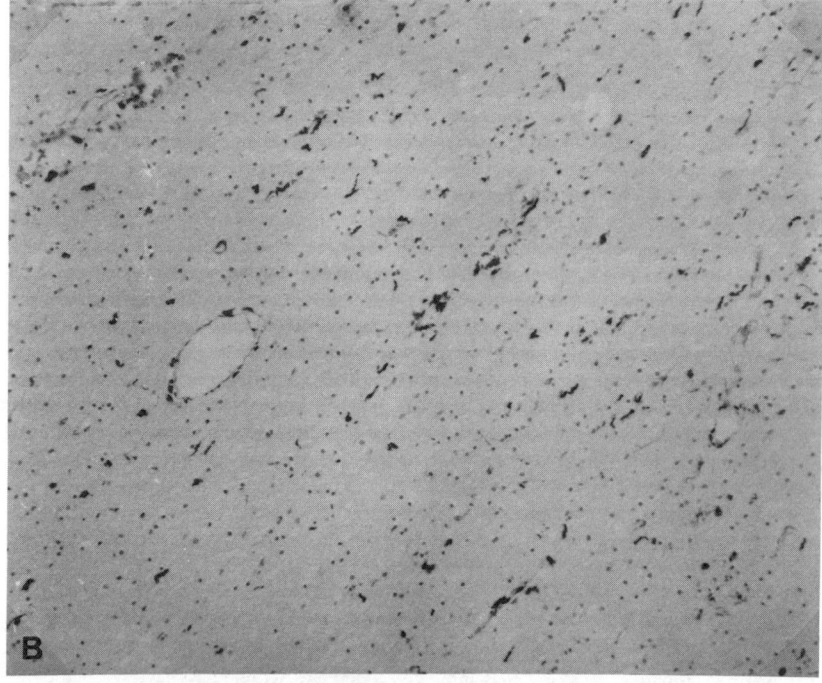

**FIGURE 2.** Progressive diffuse leukoencephalopathy (PDL). (**A**) Bihemispheric coronal section through the cerebrum stained for myelin. Diffuse symmetrical demyelination of deep cerebral white matter; subcortical fibers, basal ganglia, and brain stem are less affected. Heidenhain stain, original magnification × 0.6, reduced by 65%. (**B**) Perivascular and diffuse infiltration of the damaged white matter by monohistiocytic cells labeled with a-mph. Same stain as in FIGURE 1, original magnification × 100.

Focal edema and release of enzymes or mediator substances (e.g., interleukin-1) by macrophages could contribute to dysfunction and tissue damage. In addition, the present macrophages could attack adjacent myelin in the way of the "innocent bystander demyelination."

Diffuse changes in the gray matter including the cerebral cortex (glial/glioneuronal poliodystrophy) have been largely neglected; their pathogenesis is obscure. Occasional minor nerve cell loss might be interpreted as a sign of direct HIV neuronopathy; however, the disproportionate astroglial reaction and the occasional infiltration of mono- and multinucleated macrophages[1] could suggest that similar pathomechanisms, as just suggested for MGCE and PDL, might also operate diffusely in the gray matter.

In sum, this neuropathologic study suggests major HIV-induced brain pathology (MGCE and PDL) as a secondary macrophage-mediated disease triggered by the local presence of HIV.

## REFERENCES

1. BUDKA, H., G. COSTANZI, S. CRISTINA, A. LECHI, C. PARRAVICINI, R. TRABATTONI & L. VAGO. 1987. Brain pathology induced by infection with the human immunodeficiency virus (HIV). A histological, immunocytochemical, and electron microscopical study of 100 autopsy cases. Acta Neuropathol. **75:** 185-198.
2. BUDKA, H. 1986. Multinucleated giant cells in brain: A hallmark of the acquired immune deficiency syndrome (AIDS). Acta Neuropathol. **69:** 253-258.
3. KLEIHUES, P., W. LANG, P. C. BURGER, H. BUDKA, M. VOGT, R. MAURER, R. LÜTHY & W. SIEGENTHALER. 1985. Progressive diffuse leukoencephalopathy in patients with acquired immune deficiency syndrome (AIDS). Acta Neuropathol. **68:** 333-339.

# Host-Virus Interaction in Caprine Arthritis-Encephalitis

## M. C. ZINK AND O. NARAYAN

*Division of Comparative Medicine*
*Johns Hopkins Medical Institutions*
*Baltimore, Maryland 21205*

Caprine arthritis-encephalitis (CAE) virus is a lentivirus that causes chronic, progressive encephalomyelitis, interstitial pneumonia, and synovitis/arthritis in goats.[1] The virus infects cells of the monocyte-macrophage system *in vivo*. CAE virus is unable to replicate in monocytes, where it exists as proviral DNA. As monocytes mature to macrophages in tissues, the cells become more susceptible to viral replication, producing viral RNA. If these macrophages are then cultured *in vitro*, the cells begin to generate infectious virions.[2] This *in vivo* restriction of replication appears to be associated with the production of an interferon (LV-IFN) which is produced when fresh lymphocytes are added to a culture of CAEV-infected goat macrophages.[3] LV-IFN has physical and functional attributes of both alpha- and gamma-interferon in addition to some unique characteristics.

Preliminary studies showed that peripheral blood monocytes cultured *in vitro* in the presence of LV-IFN for several days did not develop the morphologic characteristics of macrophages. LV-IFN also induced the expression of Ia antigen on transformed sheep alveolar macrophages.[4] The purpose of this study was to characterize the actions of LV-IFN on monocyte maturation and CAEV replication to clarify its possible role in the pathogenesis of caprine arthritis-encephalitis.

Adherent goat mononuclear cells cultured in medium with or without 10% LV-IFN were sampled after 1, 2, 4, and 6 days of incubation, and the degree of cell maturation was assessed by measuring cell size and testing for the presence of Fc receptors and production of $PGE_2$. The effect of LV-IFN on CAEV replication was assessed by performing infectious center assays and *in situ* hybridization on infected, LV-IFN-treated monocyte-macrophages and by measuring the infectivity of their culture supernatant.

Monocytes cultured in the presence of LV-IFN were smaller, and fewer of these cells expressed Fc receptors, indicating that LV-IFN inhibited the maturation of monocytes to macrophages. Treated macrophages secreted $PGE_2$, whereas control macrophages did not. LV-IFN blocked the replication of CAEV in mature macrophages at the level of transcription and also inhibited viral replication indirectly by inhibiting monocyte maturation.

The results of this study suggest that LV-IFN may play an important role in the induction and maintenance of inflammation within infected target organs. By restricting macrophage maturation and viral replication, it may slow the tempo of disease and at the same time contribute to the persistence of virus within the host. LV-IFN may also suppress disease manifestations by the induction and/or maintenance of $PGE_2$ production by macrophages. Conversely, by virtue of its ability to induce Ia antigen expression on macrophages, LV-IFN may facilitate the presentation of viral antigen to helper T cells. These cells may then initiate the cascade of events that leads to the influx of lymphocytes and macrophages into the target tissue, resulting in the characteristic pathologic changes seen in affected tissues.

## REFERENCES

1. NARAYAN, O. & L. C. CORK. 1985. Lentiviral diseases of sheep and goats. Chronic pneumonia, leukoencephalomyelitis and arthritis. Rev. Infect. Dis. **7:** 89-98.
2. NARAYAN, O., J. S. WOLINSKY, J. E. CLEMENTS, J. D. STRANDBERG, D. E. GRIFFIN & L. C. CORK. 1982. Slow virus replication: The role of macrophages in the persistence and expression of visna viruses in sheep and goats. J. Gen. Virol. **59:** 345-356.
3. NARAYAN, O., D. SHEFFER, J. E. CLEMENTS & G. TENNEKOON. 1985. Restricted replication of lentiviruses, Visna viruses induce a unique interferon during interaction between lymphocytes and infected macrophages. J. Exp. Med. **162:** 1954-1969.
4. KENNEDY, P. G. E., O. NARAYAN, Z. GHOTBI, J. HOPKINS, H. E. GENDELMAN & J. E. CLEMENTS. 1985. Persistent expression of Ia antigen and viral genome in visna-maedi virus-induced inflammatory cells. Possible role of lentivirus-induced interferon. J. Exp. Med. **162:** 1970-1982.

# HTLV-I Myelitis: Isolation of Virus, Genomic Analysis, and Infection in Neural Cell Cultures

T. SAIDA, K. SAIDA, M. FUNAUCHI,
E. NISHIGUCHI, M. NAKAJIMA, S. MATSUDA,
M. OHTA, K. OHTA, H. NISHITANI, AND
M. HATANAKA

*Utano National Hospital and Institute for Virus Research
Kyoto University
Kyoto, Japan*

Human T-lymphotropic virus type I (HTLV-I) is an exogenous retrovirus originally associated with an endemic malignancy termed adult T-cell leukemia (ATL). More recently recognized HTLV-I myelitis (HTLV-I M)[1,2] is characterized by perivascular infiltration of lymphocytes and foamy cells and predominant involvement of white matter usually without association with ATL. Western blotting analysis of sera from patients with ATL and of sera and cerebrospinal fluid (CSF) of patients with HTLV-I M revealed similar antibody binding patterns to HTLV-I antigens.

To elucidate the pathogenic mechanism of HTLV-I M, we established virus-producing T-cell lines from the peripheral blood and CSF mononuclear cells of 25 patients with HTLV-I M. All cell lines were positively stained with HTLV-I M sera, ATL sera, and monoclonal antibodies to HTLV-I gag proteins p15, p19, and p24, and revealed type C viral particles by electron microscopic studies. Cytofluorographic analysis showed most of the line cells have T3$^+$, T4$^+$, 2H4$^-$, T8$^-$, T11$^+$, Tac$^+$ (IL-2R$^+$), and Ia$^+$ helper inducer surface markers.

By restriction map analysis, we found two major subgroups of HTLV-I: MT-2[3] type and ATK-1 type.[4] They were almost equally distributed among the patients with HTLV-I M. We also found two types of the provirus in DNA derived from fresh peripheral blood lymphocytes of patients with ATL. It was concluded that two subgroups of HTLV-I exist in Japan, and both have the ability to cause both ATL and HTLV-I M (FIGS. 1 and 2).

Cultured human endothelial cells and glial line cells (GFAP-positive and GFAP-negative) were infected by HTLV-I and showed syncithium formation, degenerative changes, and cell lysis when co-cultured with HTLV-I-producing T-cell lines derived either from HTLV-I M or ATL. GFAP-positive astrocytes in dissociated newborn rat brain cell cultures were also infected with HTLV-I derived from either of the two diseases. Galactocerebroside-positive oligodendrocytes rapidly disappeared in these cultures within a few days after application of irradiated virus-producing T cells, although HTLV-I-antigen-positive oligodendrocytes were only rarely recognized by a double-staining indirect immunofluorescence technique. Application of the conditioned medium of HTLV-I-infected T-cell line cultures did not suppress oligodendrocyte

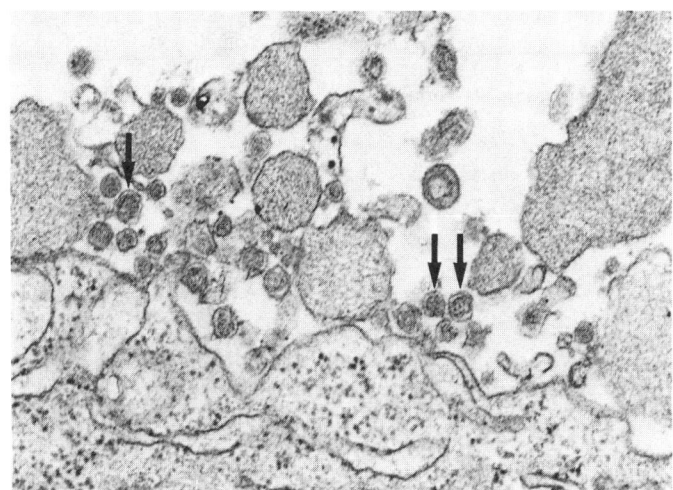

**FIGURE 1.** Thin-section election micrograph of HTLV-I-infected line cells established by co-cultivating cerebrospinal fluid cells from a patient with HTLV-I myelitis and peripheral lymphocytes from a healthy male. Mature extracellular type C virus particles (*arrows*) 100 to 110 nm in diameter have condensed; a centrally located nucleoid is surrounded by an outer membrane separated by an electron-lucent area (original magnification × 45,000)

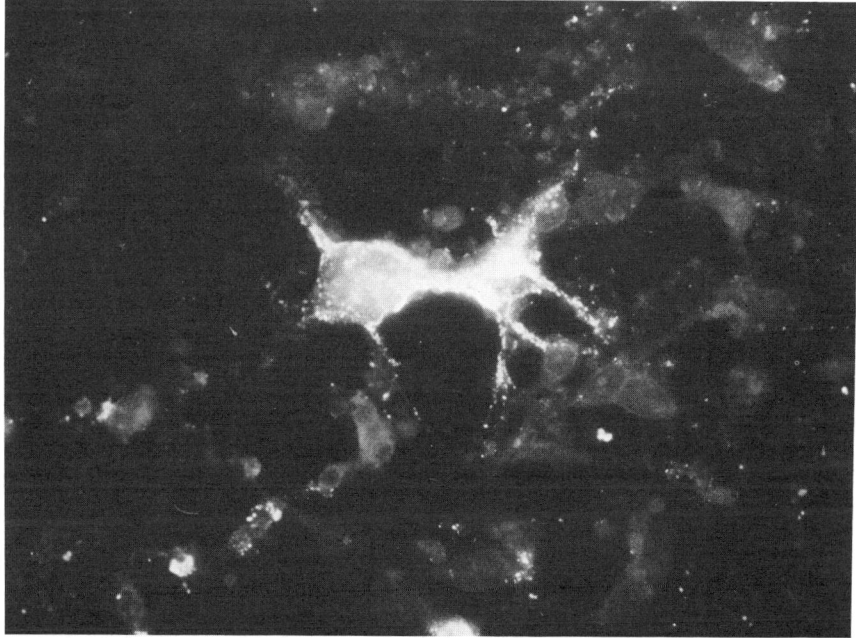

**FIGURE 2.** An HTLV-I infected glioma cell line (U251MG, GFAP-positive). An HTLV-I core protein is immunostained with anti-p19 monoclonal antibodies by an indirect immunofluorescence technique 3 days after the application of an irradiated HTLV-I-producing T-cell line.

proliferation, but enhanced the formation of cell processes in number as well as in length, as was reported previously. The reason oligodendrocytes in HTLV-I-infected cultures are destroyed without apparent infection of the oligodendrocyte itself remains to be elucidated. Infection was inhibited by the application of antisera to HTLV-I into the culture medium.

## REFERENCES

1. OSAME, M., K. USUKU, S. IZUMO et al. 1986. HTLV-I associated myelopathy: A new clinical entity. Lancet **1:** 1031-1032.
2. AKIZUKI, S., O. NAKAZATO, Y. HIGUCHI et al. 1987. Necropsy findings in HTLV-I associated myelopathy. Lancet **1:** 156-157.
3. SEIKI, M., S. HATTORI, Y. HIRAYAMA et al. 1983. Proc. Natl. Acad. Sci. USA **80:** 3618-3622.
4. RATNER, L., S. F. JOSEPHS, B. STARCICHI et al. 1985. J. Virol. **54:** 781-790.

# Sera from Patients with Multiple Sclerosis React with Human T-Cell Lymphotropic Virus-I GAG Proteins: Western Blotting and Solid-Phase Radioimmunoassay Analyses

M. OHTA,[a] T. SAIDA,[a] K. OHTA,[a] F. MORI,[a]
H. NISHITANI,[a] R. FUJINO,[b] AND M. IKEDA[b]

[a]*Clinical Research Center and Department of Neurology*
*Utano National Hospital*
*Kyoto, Japan*

[b]*Central Research Laboratories of Fujirebio Inc.*
*Tokyo, Japan*

We examined the presence of IgG and IgM antibodies reactive with HTLV-I viral antigens in sera from Japanese patients with multiple sclerosis (MS) in the Kyoto district, a nonendemic area for adult T-cell leukemia (ATL), using Western blotting analysis and a sensitive radioimmunoassay (RIA). Our data revealed that 11 (24%) of 46 patients with clinically definite MS had IgG and/or IgM antibodies reactive with antigens corresponding to the group-specific antigen (gag) proteins (p15, p19, and p24) by Western blotting analysis using disrupted virions from the virus-producing TCL Kan cells as antigens[1] (FIG. 1). Those seropositive MS patients consisted of four with IgG antibodies reactive mainly to the gag p24 and/or p15 protein, four with IgM antibodies reactive mainly to the gag p24 and/or p19 protein, and three with both IgG and IgM antibodies (TABLE 1). These immunostaining patterns of MS sera were clearly distinguishable from those of patients with ATL who had antibodies to the envelop (env) proteins and their precursors in addition to the gag proteins. The antibody in MS sera was generally of low titer and reactive at a high serum concentration (1/10 dilution). None of the sera from 9 patients with other neurologic diseases (OND) and from 11 healthy controls had the viral antibodies.

We also developed a simple and highly sensitive RIA for the detection of antibody to HTLV-I or p24 and surveyed 55 patients with clinically definite MS, 27 patients with OND, and 36 normal controls. The average age of patients with MS was 42.0 (range 14 to 69 years). Of all MS sera tested by RIA, 45% (25/55) had IgG and/or IgM antibodies against HTLV-I-disrupted virions, and 44% (24/55) had IgG and/or IgM antibodies against HTLV-I p24. This result is similar to that of Koprowski *et al.*[2] who used a sensitive EIA method. The levels of antibodies and the frequency were low in comparison with those in ATL, HTLV-I myelitis, or HTLV-I carriers. There was no apparent relation between the occurrence of the antibodies in MS and their clinical states. Immunologic specificity of antibodies to HTLV-I or p24 in MS sera was confirmed by a competitive inhibition RIA. Most of the sera from patients with OND and healthy controls reacted with neither of the viral antigens. We failed to detect HTLV-I antibodies in MS sera by our EIA using an MT-2 cell lysate, by a Japanese commercial EIA kit for HTLV-I antibodies (Eisai, Tokyo), and by a cell-based indirect immunofluorescence method. These failures are similar to those of other investigators[3,4] and are apparently the result of the low sensitivity of those assay systems.

These studies show that about half the Japanese patients with MS have IgG and/or IgM antibody reactive to a hitherto undefined agent related to, but distinct from, HTLV-I. The significance of the appearance of weak cross-reactivity to HTLV-I in MS sera is unclear. Further investigations of many other immunologic and neurologic diseases are in progress.

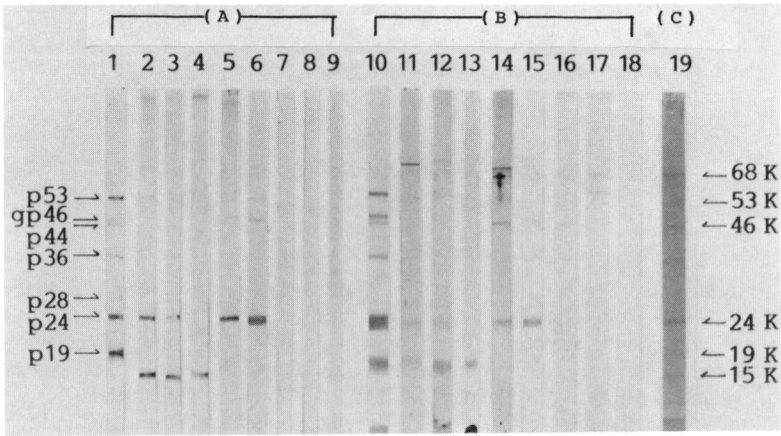

**FIGURE 1.** Western blotting patterns in serum samples from patients with multiple sclerosis (MS) using a peroxidase antiperoxidase (PAP) procedure. (**A**) IgG staining patterns. (**B**) IgM staining patterns. *Lanes 1 and 10,* serum from patients with ATL as positive control (1/500 dilution); *lanes 2 to 6* and *11 to 15,* sera from patients with MS (1/10 dilution); *lanes 7 to 9* and *16 to 18,* sera from healthy controls (1/10 dilution). (**C**) Coomassie Brilliant Blue staining of transblotted HTLV-I viral proteins obtained from TCL Kan cells. The PAP procedure was carried out as follows. The nitrocellulose sheet electrophoretically transferred viral proteins, was cut into small strips and incubated for 3 hours with 1 ml of a 1/10 dilution of test serum. In patients with ATL, serum was diluted at 1/500 for IgG staining and 1/100 for IgM staining. Strips were washed three times and incubated for 1 hour with a 1/500 dilution of rabbit antihuman IgG antibody and a 1/200 dilution of rabbit antihuman IgM, respectively. After washing as before, the strips were incubated with a 1/1,000 dilution of goat antirabbit IgG for 1 hour. After another wash, the strips were finally incubated with a 1/1,000 dilution of rabbit PAP complex for 1 hour. After a final washing step, the strips were allowed to react with 4-chloro-1-naphthol as a peroxidase color development reagent for about 10 minutes and were rinsed with distilled water. All reaction steps were performed at 37°C, and PBS containing 1% BSA and 0.05% Tween 20 was used as dilution and washing buffers during the experiment. (Reprinted, with permission, from Ohta *et al.*[1])

TABLE 1. Identification of Antibody Bands and Their Densities by Western Blotting Analysis in Sera from Patients with Multiple Sclerosis[a]

| Case No. | IgG Antibody | | | IgM Antibody | | |
|---|---|---|---|---|---|---|
| | p24 | p19 | p15 | p24 | p19 | p15 |
| 1 | ++[b] | − | ++ | + | + | − |
| 2 | + | − | + | − | − | − |
| 3 | − | − | + | − | − | − |
| 4 | ++ | − | − | + | − | − |
| 5 | +++ | − | − | − | − | − |
| 6 | − | − | − | + | ++ | − |
| 7 | − | − | − | + | ++ | − |
| 8 | − | − | − | − | + | − |
| 9 | − | − | − | +++ | − | − |
| 10 | + | + | + | + | + | + |
| 11 | − | − | + | − | − | − |

[a] Reprinted, with permission, from Ohta et al.[1]
[b] Densities of the staining of immunoblotting bands were estimated by visual observations and were expressed in three grades (+ to +++).

## REFERENCES

1. OHTA, M., K. OHTA, F. MORI et al. 1986. J. Immunol. **137:** 3440.
2. KOPROWSKI, H., E. C. DEFRETASA, M. E. HARPER et al. 1985. Nature **318:** 154.
3. HAUSER, S. L., C. AUBERT, J. S. BURKS et al. 1986. Nature **322:** 176.
4. KARPAS, A., U. KANPT, A. SIDEN, M. KOCH & S. POSER. 1986. Nature **322:** 177.

# Immune Effects of Intracerebral Infection with Mouse Hepatitis Virus[a]

### ROBERT L. KNOBLER, GEORGE C. BRAINARD, MARIELLE PERREAULT, CONCETTA D'IMPERIO, PAULA PHENIX, AND FRED D. LUBLIN

*Department of Neurology*
*Jefferson Medical College*
*Philadelphia, Pennsylvania*

Previous studies with mouse hepatitis virus type 4 (MHV-4), a neurotropic strain of murine coronavirus, demonstrated that there is involution of the thymus within 3-5 days after intracerebral inoculation of susceptible strains of mice. This involution is in part due to the direct infection of lymphocytes, epithelial cells, and macrophages of the thymus by the virus.[1] The degree of involution following intracerebral inoculation is better appreciated when compared with the limited changes observed after even 1,000-fold more virus delivered into the peritoneal cavity. The present series of experiments was undertaken to investigate potential mechanisms by which this difference could be explained.

Mice of the susceptible CXJ-8 strain,[2] in groups of four, were inoculated intracerebrally, under Avertin anesthesia, with 100 plaque-forming units (PFU) of MHV-4 in a volume of 0.05 ml. Control CXJ-8 mice received an equal volume of medium without virus. Another group of CXJ-8 mice were inoculated intraperitoneally with 0.1 ml of either 10,000 PFU of the virus or control medium. A group of unmanipulated CXJ-8 mice of the same 6-8-week age group were also studied. Only males were used for these studies. Plasma was collected from all mice at the time of sacrifice, 5 days after infection, for determination of corticosterone levels by radioimmunoassay.

Data on the thymic and splenic weights in the different groups at 5 days after treatment are presented graphically in FIGURE 1. Following virus intracerebrally (V-IC), there is involution of the thymus and spleen. Mean thymic weight in the V-IC group was 0.007 g compared with 0.036 g for the unmanipulated mice (NT = not treated). Mean splenic weight was 0.059 g compared with 0.190 g when untreated. The mean thymic weight following intraperitoneal inoculation of virus (V-IP) was 0.029 g. After intracerebral inoculation of medium (M-IC), mean thymic weight was 0.021 g, and after intraperitoneal inoculation of medium (M-IP) it was 0.041 g. The mean splenic weight following intraperitoneal injection of virus (V-IP) was 0.218 g, whereas following intracerebral injection of medium (M-IC) it was 0.132 g. After the intraperitoneal injection of medium (M-IP), the mean splenic weight was 0.161 g.

---

[a] This work was supported by research grant RG 1722-A-3 from the National Multiple Sclerosis Society, TIDA K07-NS00961 from the NINCDS, and a research award from The Arthur L. Swim Foundation.

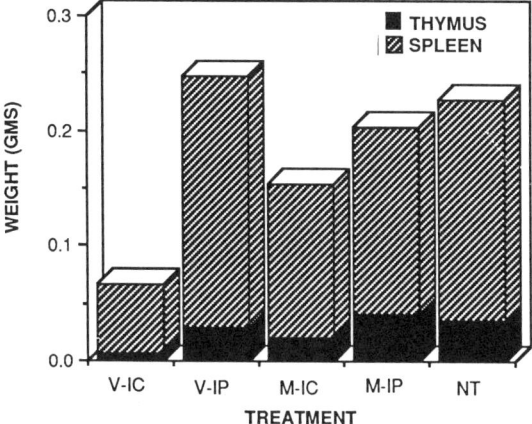

**FIGURE 1.** The mean weight of thymus (*solid*) and spleen (*hatched*) from groups of four mice each that were injected with virus intracerebrally (V-IC) or intraperitoneally (V-IP), injected with medium intracerebrally (M-IC) or intraperitoneally (M-IP), or not treated (NT).

Although the thymus did show some involutional changes at 5 days after intraperitoneal inoculation with MHV-4, the spleen does not involute. In fact, it appeared enlarged compared with spleens from unmanipulated or medium-inoculated mice. The thymus and spleen did show some effect from the intracerebral injection of medium, and therefore a response to stress by measuring corticosterone levels in the plasma of these mice was performed.

The corticosterone levels in three different groups of the mice are presented in FIGURE 2. These results demonstrate that the plasma corticosterone level is substantially higher in mice that had received virus intracerebrally (V-IC). There is also elevation after injection of the brain with medium alone, although it is not statistically

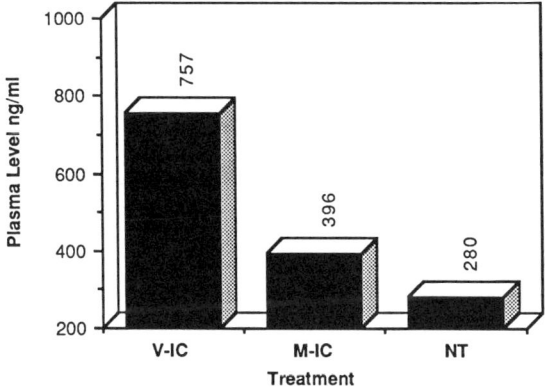

**FIGURE 2.** The mean plasma levels of groups of four mice each that were injected with virus intracerebrally (V-IC), medium intracerebrally (M-IC), or not treated (NT). The V-IC corticosterone level is significantly elevated over M-IC or NT at $p < 0.01$.

significant compared with the increase in unmanipulated mice. Therefore, intracerebral infection with MHV-4 appears to lead to involution of the lymphoid compartment both by direct infection, as previously demonstrated, and by a component due to a dramatic increase in corticosterone levels. The mechanism of this increase is currently under analysis.

This study demonstrates that there is involution of the central components of the immune system (thymus and spleen) following intracerebral, but not intraperitoneal (systemic), infection with MHV-4. Although this virus does infect the immune cells of the thymus and spleen directly, the infection alone does not account for the degree of involution observed. In mice that were intracerebrally infected with MHV-4, but not in controls receiving an intracerebral injection of medium alone, there was a significant elevation in plasma corticosterone levels. The combination of MHV-4 infection of immune cells with the hormonal milieu induced by intracerebral but not systemic virus infection suggests that virus replication in the brain can have a dramatic impact on the integrity of the immune system. This model will therefore be useful to investigate potential mechanisms by which virus replication in the brain can influence the development of acquired immunodeficiency syndrome.

## REFERENCES

1. KNOBLER, R. L. & M. B. A. OLDSTONE. 1987. Infection and involution of mouse thymus by MHV-4, *In* Coronaviruses. M. C. Lai & S. A. Stohlman, Eds.: 451-452. Plenum Pub Corp, New York.
2. KNOBLER, R. L., D. S. LINTHICUM & M. COHN. 1985. Host genetic regulation of acute MHV-4 encephalomyelitis and acute experimental autoimmune encephalomyelitis in CXJ (BALB/cKe × SJL/J) recombinant-inbred mice. J. Neuroimmunol. **8:** 15-28.

# Impaired Measles-Specific Cytotoxic T-Cell Response in Subacute Sclerosing Panencephalitis

### SUHAYL DHIB-JALBUT, STEVEN JACOBSON, DALE E. McFARLIN, AND HENRY F. McFARLAND

*Neuroimmunology Branch*
*NINCDS, National Institutes of Health*
*Bethesda, Maryland 20892*

Subacute sclerosing panencephalitis (SSPE) is a persistent measles virus (MV) infection of the nervous system. The role of the immune response, in particular the cellular immune response, to MV in the pathogenesis of SSPE is uncertain.[1] Recently, MV-specific HLA class II restricted cytotoxic T lymphocytes (CTL) were shown to represent the major component of the cellular immune response to MV in humans.[2] A defect in this response could contribute to MV persistence in SSPE. MV-CTL are generated *in vitro* by culturing peripheral blood lymphocytes (PBLs) with MV for 7 days. The CTL response is then demonstrated by the ability of sensitized PBLs to lyse MV-infected autologous or HLA class II matched Epstein-Barr virus transformed B-cell targets (which express HLA class II molecules) in a $^{51}$Cr-release assay as described.[2]

In this study the capacity of PBLs obtained from four patients with SSPE (RC, YB, BH, and RF) to proliferate to MV and to generate MV-specific CTLs was examined. The lymphoproliferative response to MV measured by $^3$H-thymidine uptake in the four patients was within the response range of the five healthy controls (stimulation indexes were 4.1, 21.5, 13.1, and 21.8 for RC, YB, BH, and RF, respectively, compared to a mean of 13.0 ± 4.9 in 5 controls).

The MV-CTL responses for the 4 patients with SSPE and 10 controls are shown in FIGURE 1. These responses were reduced in two of the four patients with SSPE (RC and YB). Patient BH showed significant lysis of uninfected targets, suggesting non-MV-specific lysis; in the fourth patient (RF), the MV-CTL response was similar to that of controls. The mean lysis of the patients with SSPE was lower than that in the controls (16.2 ± 9.5% compared to 27.6 ± 10.5%, respectively, at an effector to target ratio of 40:1). MV-infected SSPE targets were lysed by HLA class II matched MV-stimulated effectors from controls. The lysis was HLA class II restricted (FIG. 2A). These findings indicate that the reduced lysis found in patients with SSPE was not due to a defect in autologous MV-infected targets but in the generation of effector cells. Subsequent experiments have shown that lysis of control MV-infected targets by SSPE MV-stimulated effectors was not HLA restricted (FIG. 2B) and possibly mediated by cells other than CTL. To examine this possibility, FcR-positive cells were depleted from MV-stimulated effectors by adsorption to immune complexes. This reduced lysis of MV-infected targets in two patients with SSPE (73% reduction in YB and 61% in BH compared to 9% and 32% in two healthy donors). This was

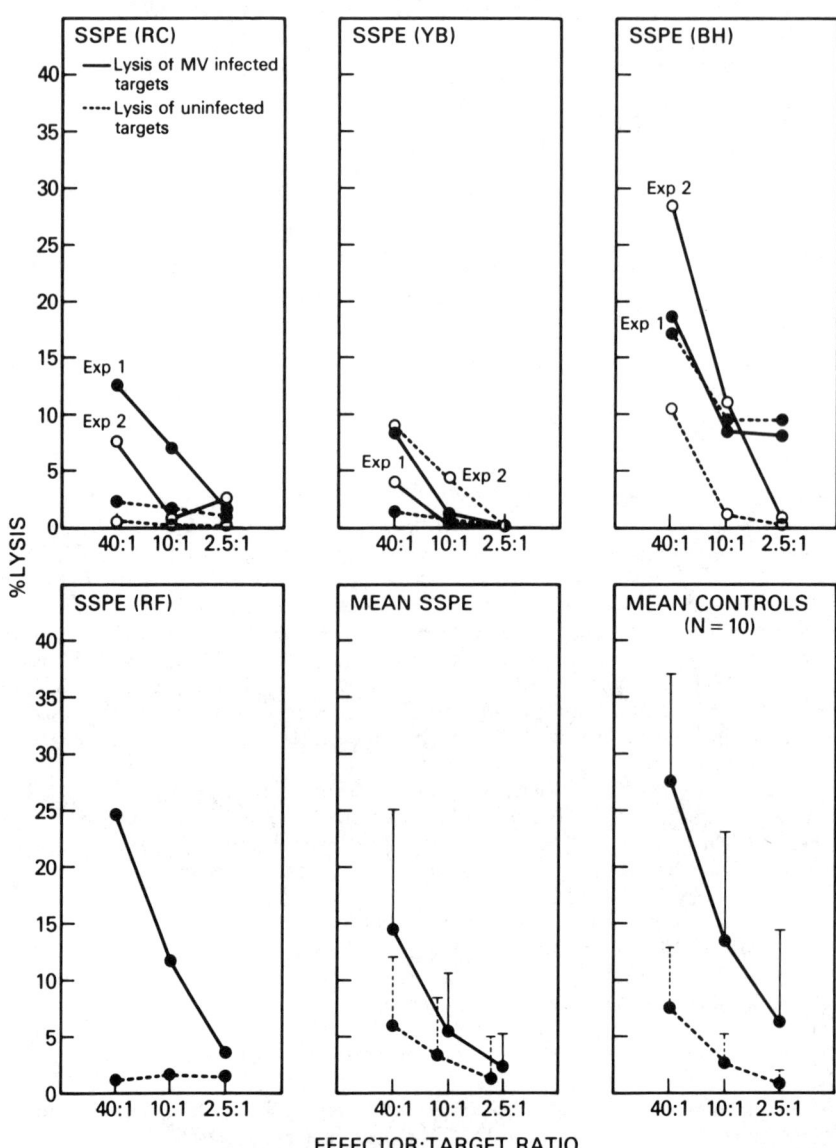

**FIGURE 1.** Measles virus-specific lysis of measles virus (MV) infected targets in four patients with subacute sclerosing panencephalitis (SSPE) and controls. Specific lysis is calculated as lysis of MV-infected targets by MV-stimulated effectors minus lysis by unstimulated effectors. Duplicate experiments were performed in patients RC, YB, and BH. Lysis of uninfected targets by MV-stimulated effectors is shown as interrupted lines.

consistent with the possibility that cytotoxicity in SSPE is mediated by natural killer (NK) cells.[3] NK activity tested on K562 targets in two patients (YB and BH) was comparable to that in controls, but the MV-CTL response was inhibited by unlabeled K562 cells which suggested that lysis of MV-infected targets by these two patients was mediated by NK cells. Generation of influenza virus and mumps-virus-specific

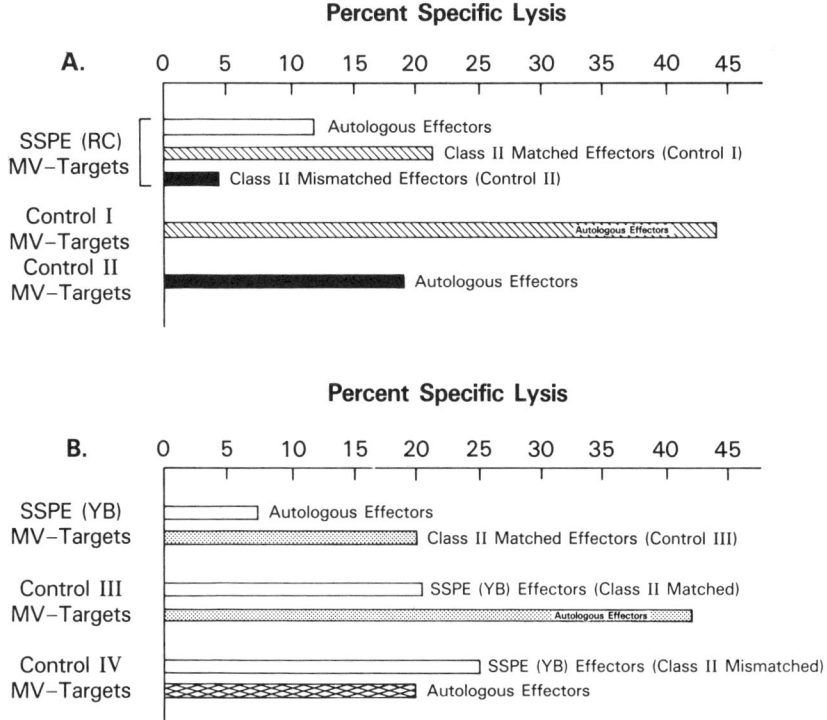

FIGURE 2. Percentage of measles-specific lysis of measles virus infected targets by autologous, matched, or mismatched effectors from two patients with subacute sclerosing panencephalitis (SSPE) and controls. The effector to target ratio was 40:1. (A) Inability of SSPE (RC) effectors to lyse autologous targets, whereas this patient's targets could be lysed by class II matched effectors from a healthy donor (control I) but not by class II mismatched effectors (control II). (B) SSPE (YB) effectors unable to lyse targets compared to effectors from a class II matched healthy donor (control III). Equal lysis of class II matched targets (control III) and class II mismatched targets (control IV) by SSPE (YB) effectors is shown.

CTL responses was normal in YB and BH, and generation of allogeneic specific CTL response was normal in RC. These results indicate that the defect in generation of CTLs in SSPE is MV specific.

This defect in the generation of HLA class II restricted MV-CTLs in some patients with SSPE may relate to MV persistence in SSPE. Possible mechanisms include: (1) sequestration of MV-CTLs in the CNS, (2) deletion of a subset of $T4^+$ cells that mediates MV-CTL, and (3) suppression of MV-CTL.

## REFERENCES

1. TER MEULEN, V., J. R. STEPHENSON & H. W. KRETH. 1983. Subacute sclerosing panencephalitis. Comp. Virol. **17:** 105.
2. JACOBSON S., J. R. RICHERT, W. E. BIDDISON, A. SATINSKY, R. J. HARTZMAN & H. F. MCFARLAND. 1984. Measles virus-specific T4$^+$ human cytotoxic T-cell clones are restricted by class II HLA antigens J. Immunol. **133:** 754.
3. KRETH, H. W. & G. WIEGAND. 1977. Cell-mediated cytotoxicity against measles virus in SSPE II. Analysis of cytotoxic effector cells. J. Immunol. **118:** 296.

WORKSHOP 14. MOLECULAR MIMICRY AND VIRUS-INDUCED DEMYELINATION

# Caprine Retroviral Encephalitis in Previously Infected and in Specific Pathogen-Free Goats

## G. C. JOHNSON,[a] D. S. ADAMS, AND T. C. McGUIRE

*Department of Veterinary Microbiology and Pathology*
*Washington State University*
*Pullman, Washington*

Caprine arthritis-encephalitis virus (CAEV), a lentivirus, produces natural disease characterized by demyelinating encephalomyelitis in young goats and progressive synovitis in adult animals. However, many seropositive adult goats have subclinical microscopic CNS lesions.[1] Morphologic characteristics of nonsuppurative inflammation and demyelination have been reproduced by intracerebral viral inoculation, but lesions have a more smoldering progressive course than does spontaneous disease.[2] Factors explaining the rapid evolution and severity of natural disease remain unknown, but immunization of goats before intrasynovial viral challenge causes accelerated tissue damage.[3]

Five cesarean-derived CAEV-free goats 4 days of age and four adult seropositive goats were inoculated in the right lateral ventricle of the brain with $10^{5.6}$ tissue culture infectious doses$_{50}$ CAEV; five other CAEV-free goats, inoculated with medium from uninfected goat synoviocyte cultures, served as controls. Cerebrospinal fluid (CSF) was drawn from the cisterna magna before infection and at weekly intervals thereafter. CSF leukocyte concentrations and differential cell counts were done using standard methods. Young goats were euthanized at 42 days postinoculation (PI), whereas adults were killed 7-28 days PI. Tissues were fixed in formalin for histopathologic evaluation.

As judged by CSF leukocyte counts (FIG. 1), meningoencephalitis developed more rapidly in seropositive adult goats than in those initially infected. Although lymphocytes were prevalent in CSF cytospins from both virus-inoculated groups, lymphoblasts and occasional plasma cells were evident in seropositive goats, with peak inflammation at 7 days PI. In contrast, initially infected goats developed transient mild leukocytosis, consisting of small lymphocytes and monocytoid cells, which was maximal at 14 days PI, and controls maintained low CSF leukocyte concentrations. CNS lesions in both infected groups compared with the controls were characterized by demyelination and nonsuppurative inflammation, but they were more severe and extensive in seropositive goats. Not only did lymphoplasmacytic cuffing, parenchymal inflammation, and loss of myelin staining occur adjacent to the site of inoculation, but also widespread foci occurred adjacent to the inoculated lateral and third ventricles well away from the

---

[a] Present address: Department of Veterinary Pathobiology, Ohio State University, Columbus, Ohio.

FIGURE 1. Leukocyte concentrations in CSF of caprine arthritis encephalitis virus-negative and seropositive goats following intraventricular inoculation and of controls inoculated with uninfected medium.

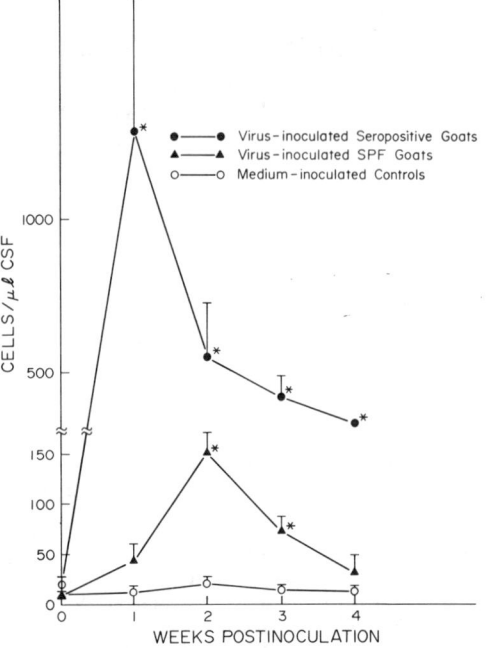

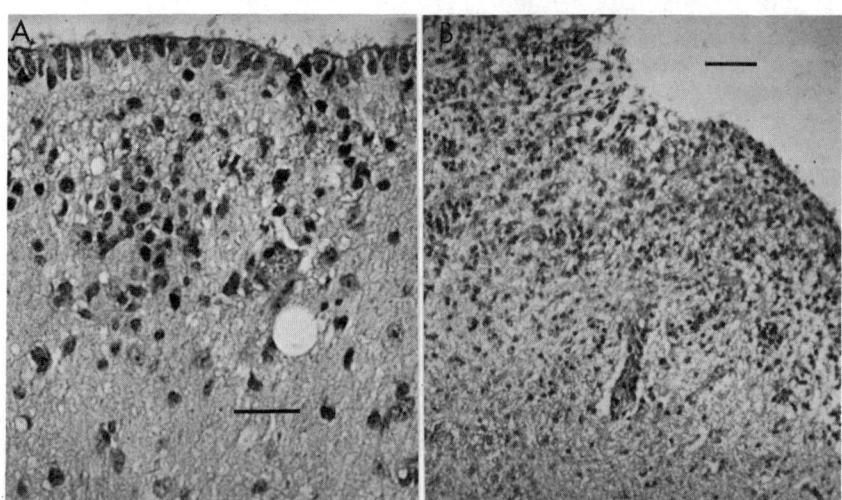

FIGURE 2. Periventricular demyelination and inflammation in a seronegative goat killed 42 days postinoculation (**A**) and a seropositive goat killed 28 days postinoculation (**B**). Bar = 50 μm in **A** and 100 μm in **B**.

injection site. The lesions were more severe than the occasional perivascular lymphocytic cuffs seen in brains of CAEV-seropositive goats (FIG. 2).

These findings indicate that lentiviral inoculation into the CNS of seropositive animals can intensify tissue damage compared with that seen in previously uninfected goats, much as in the arthritic form of disease, and suggests that periodic viral recrudescence may be capable of perpetuating retroviral encephalitis.

## REFERENCES

1. NARAYAN, O. & L. C. CORK. 1985. Rev. Infect. Dis. **7:** 89.
2. CORK, L. C. & O. NARAYAN. 1980. Lab. Invest. **42:** 596.
3. MCGUIRE, T. C., D. S. ADAMS et al. 1986. Am. J. Vet. Res. **47:** 537.

# Sequence Comparison of a Highly Virulent and a Less Virulent Strain of Theiler's Virus

## Amino Acid Differences on a Three-Dimensional Model Identifies the Location of Possible Immunogenic Sites

DANIEL C. PEVEAR,[a] JOSEPH BORKOWSKI,[a]
MING LUO,[b] AND HOWARD LIPTON[a]

[a]*Medical Neurology*
*Northwestern University Medical School*
*Chicago, Illinois*

[b]*Biological Sciences*
*Purdue University*
*W. Lafayette, Indiana*

Theiler's murine encephalomyelitis viruses (TMEV) are naturally occurring enteric pathogens of mice that can be divided into two subgroups based on their neurovirulence after intracerebral inoculation. Included in the first subgroup are the two most virulent viruses (FA and GDVII); they cause rapidly fatal encephalitis in mice. All other isolates, which constitute the second subgroup, are much less virulent but still cause CNS damage in the form of acute poliomyelitis (early onset) followed by chronic, inflammatory, demyelinating disease (late onset). The demyelinating disease is due to persistent infection wherein low levels of infectious virus can be recovered from the CNS for many months. TMEV-induced demyelinating disease is considered one of the best experimental animal models of human multiple sclerosis.

Determination of the complete nucleotide sequence of a demyelinating strain of TMEV (BeAn 8386)[1] showed that the TMEV are more closely related to cardioviruses (e.g., Mengovirus) than to any of the other picornaviruses. Computer-generated alignment of the capsid protein amino acids of BeAn and Mengoviruses revealed marked conservation of the structural backbone of the two viruses. Because the atomic structure of Mengovirus was recently determined,[2] these alignments were used in this study to construct a three-dimensional model of the BeAn virion on the atomic coordinates of Mengovirus.

We also determined the complete nucleotide and predicted amino acid sequence of the highly virulent GDVII virus. Differences in the amino acid residues of the three surface capsid proteins between BeAn and GDVII viruses were found to cluster in distinct regions on the three-dimensional model, indicating that sites on the surface of the virion mutate more rapidly than do nonsurface residues. These clusters are likely to represent neutralizing immunogenic sites (nIMs) on the virion, which have come under selective pressure from neutralizing antibodies to mutate. Four distinct clusters were identified in this study: the VP1 third corner, the VP2 "puff," and the VP3 first corner and "knob." All of these sites have been mapped as nIMs on human rhinovirus-14 or poliovirus by the use of monoclonal antibody escape mutants. Furthermore, the putative viral receptor binding site of the two TMEV stains was well conserved, suggesting that the markedly different pathogenicities of the two TMEV subgroups will map outside of this region.

## REFERENCES

1. PEVEAR, D. C., M. CALENOFF, E. ROZHON & H. L. LIPTON. 1987. J. Virol. **61:** 1507-1516.
2. LUO, M., G. VRIEND, G. KAMER, I. MINOR, E. ARNOLD, M. G. ROSSMANN, U. BOEGE, G. SCRABA, G. M. DUKE & A. C. PALMENBERG. 1987. Science **235:** 182-191.

# Herpes Simplex Virus Type 1 Induced Multifocal Demyelination of the Central Nervous System in Mice

L. F. KASTRUKOFF, A. S. LAU, AND S. U. KIM

*Department of Medicine*
*Faculty of Medicine*
*University of British Columbia*
*Vancouver, British Columbia*

Peripheral inoculation of herpes simplex virus type 1 (HSV 1) in the orofacial area of mice causes an ascending infection of the trigeminal nerve, ganglion, and descending tract of the brainstem.[1] Five to 8 days after infection, discrete demyelinative lesions associated with a mononuclear cell infiltrate are identified on the CNS side of the trigeminal root entry zone (TREZ).[2,3]

To determine if the pathologic appearance of the CNS following lip inoculation is genetically determined, inbred and congenic strains of mice were categorized on the basis of natural resistance to mortality.[4] The histologic appearance of representative strains from each group varied from focal collections of mononuclear cells in C57BL/6 (resistant) and unifocal demyelinating lesions at the TREZ in BALB/c (moderately resistant) to multifocal demyelinating lesions throughout the brain in A/J mice (susceptible).[5]

Serial viral titration studies in the three strains of mice implicate roles for both virus and the immune system in the development of lesions at TREZ, but the sequential appearance of the multifocal lesions at a time when infectious virus could not be isolated from the CNS suggests that the latter may be the result of immune mechanisms alone, possibly triggered by the acute infection.[5] Electron microscopic studies confirm the presence of virus in lesions at TREZ and the absence of virus in the multifocal lesions.

To determine if oligodendrocytes may also contribute to differences in resistance to HSV 1, primary murine oligodendrocyte cultures were derived from 20 strains of mice. $TCID_{50}$, immunofluorescence, and electron microscopic studies were performed on HSV-1-infected cultures. The results of the $TCID_{50}$ studies (FIGURE 1) and the immunofluorescence studies (TABLE 1) suggest that differences in resistance to HSV 1 do exist at the level of the CNS structural cells and may play a role in the pathogenesis of demyelinating lesions. A high degree of correlation was also observed between results *in vitro* and mortality results *in vivo*.[4]

## ACKNOWLEDGMENT

We would like to thank the MS Society of Canada for their contribution to this work.

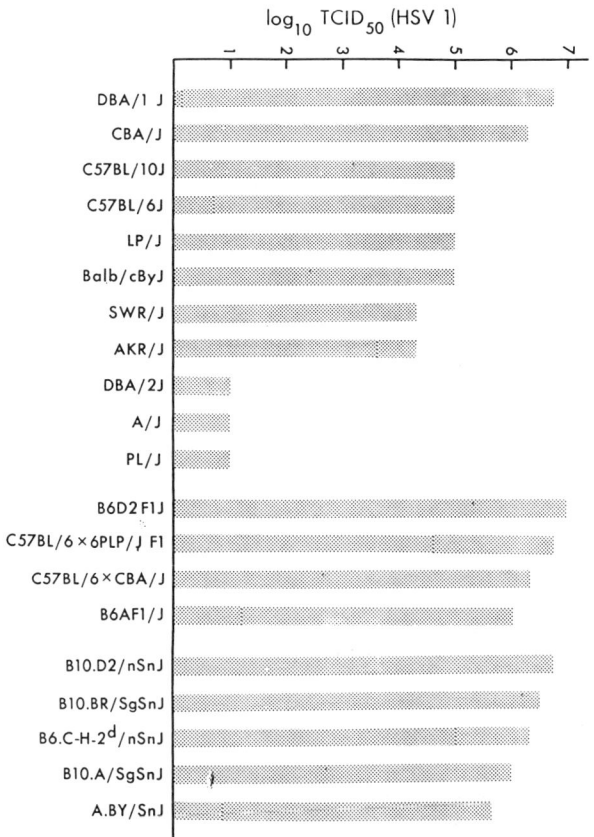

**FIGURE 1.** $TCID_{50}$ for primary oligodendrocyte cultures derived from different strains of mice and infected with HSV 1. Titers were determined using the method of Spearman-Karber (Dougherty, 1964).

TABLE 1. Immunofluorescence Studies of HSV-1-Infected Primary Murine Oligodendrocytes

| Murine Strain | Appearance of HSV 1 + Immunofluorescence (50% of cells) (hours after inoculation) |
|---|---|
| Inbred strains | |
| C57BL/10J | 42 |
| DBA/1J | 39 |
| CBA/J | 36 |
| LP/J | 33 |
| C57BL/6J | 30 |
| SWR/J | 27 |
| DBA/2J | 27 |
| AKR/J | 21 |
| Balb/cByJ | 21 |
| PL/J | 15 |
| A/J | 15 |
| F1 Hybrids | |
| (C57BL/6 × CBA/J)F1 | 42 |
| (C57BL/6 × LP/J)F1 | 39 |
| B6D2F1/J | 33 |
| B6AF1/J | 33 |
| Congenic strains | |
| B6.C-H-2$^d$/ByJ | 42 |
| B10.A/SgSnJ | 39 |
| B10.BR/SgSnJ | 39 |
| A.BY/SnJ | 36 |
| B10.D2/nSnJ | 30 |

## REFERENCES

1. COOK, M. L. & J. G. STEVENS. 1973. Infect. Immunol. **7:** 272-288.
2. KRISTENSSON, K. & A. VAHLNE. 1978. J. Neurol. Sci. **35:** 331-340.
3. TOWNSEND, J. J. 1981. J. Neurol. Sci. **50:** 435-441.
4. KASTRUKOFF, L. F., A. S. LAU & M. L. PUTERMAN. 1986. J. Gen. Virol. **67:** 613-621.
5. KASTRUKOFF, L. F., A. S. LAU & S. U. KIM. 1987. Ann. Neurol. **22:** 52-59.

# Enumeration and Distribution of T-Cell Subsets, Macrophages, and IgG Positive Cells in the CNS of SJL/J Mice Infected with Theiler's Virus[a]

### MARK D. LINDSLEY, ROGER L. THIEMANN, AND MOSES RODRIGUEZ

*Departments of Immunology and Neurology*
*Mayo Clinic and Mayo Foundation*
*Rochester, Minnesota 55905*

Infection with Theiler's murine encephalomyelitis virus (TMEV), a picornavirus, results in chronic demyelination in association with an intense inflammatory response.[1] The mechanism of demyelination is not clear, but it may involve either direct viral lysis of oligodendrocytes[2,3] or an immune response to virus or self-antigen. To further study the role of the cellular immune response, we enumerated mononuclear leukocytes (MNL) from the central nervous system (CNS) of TMEV-infected mice and examined their distribution.

## MATERIALS AND METHODS

SJL/J mice 4-6 weeks of age inoculated intracerebrally with $2 \times 10^5$ pfu TMEV (DA strain) were perfused with tissue culture medium prior to removal of CNS. After mechanical disruption of CNS tissue, a Percoll separation method[4] resulted in three fractions: a top myelin fraction, a middle glial fraction, and a bottom lymphocyte fraction. Cell fractions were placed on glass slides by cytocentrifugation and stained by immunoperoxidase for leukocyte antigens with monoclonal antibodies using the ABC technique (Vector Laboratories, Burlingame, California). For localization of MNL, brain and spinal cord from infected mice were quick frozen in isopentane chilled in liquid nitrogen.

## RESULTS AND DISCUSSION

Examination of cells recovered from the lymphocyte layer demonstrated a biphasic response (TABLE 1) as observed in the pathologic process by TMEV.[5] An increase

[a]This work was supported by grants CA 09127 and NS 00849 from the National Institutes of Health, RG 1878 from the National Multiple Sclerosis Society, and the Searle Foundation.

in Thy 1.2$^+$, L3T4$^+$, and Mac-1$^+$ cells was noted on days 7 and 27. Lyt 2$^+$ cells were not detected until day 13, but they continued to increase as the disease progressed. Because the glial fraction revealed many large leukocytes, we combined the number of cells isolated from glial and lymphocyte fractions to examine the total effect of the immune response (TABLE 1). The results were similar to those seen in the lymphocyte fraction except that a greater number of Mac-1$^+$ cells were detected.

To correlate these findings with the distribution of cells in pathologic lesions, immunoperoxidase studies were undertaken on frozen tissue sections. MNL infiltration was predominant in the brain by day 5 but declined to a low level by day 28 (TABLE 2). MNL were not observed in the spinal cord until day 13 and continued to increase through day 41. L3T4$^+$ cells were present in the brain during early infection and were common in the spinal cord throughout the course of disease. Lyt 2$^+$ cells, rare in the brain early, gradually increased in number in the demyelinating lesions. Both L3T4$^+$ and Lyt 2$^+$ cells were found in a perivascular distribution, whereas Lyt 2$^+$ cells more commonly infiltrated the white matter.

The importance of T-cell subsets during different phases of disease is being addressed by ongoing experiments from our laboratory.[6] Depletion of L3T4$^+$ cells during acute infection significantly worsens the disease and may result in death. Treatment of the chronic infection with anti-L3T4 antibody (clone GK1.5) slightly improves the demyelination. However, removal of Lyt 2$^+$ cells significantly diminishes inflammation and demyelination. Therefore, L3T4$^+$ and Mac-1$^+$ cells appear to be important in

TABLE 1. Number of Cells Recovered from the CNS of Mice Infected with TMEV by Percoll Gradient Technique

| Days after Infection | Number of Cells/Animal Positive for: | | | |
|---|---|---|---|---|
| | THY 1.2[a] | LYT 2[b] | L3T4[c] | MAC-1[d] |
| Lymph ($\times 10^4$)[e] | | | | |
| Uninfected | 0.8 | 0.01 | 0.03 | 1.0 |
| 7 | 50.0 | 0.0 | 40.0 | 8.0 |
| 13 | 40.0 | 4.0 | 22.0 | 0.6 |
| 20 | 11.0 | 1.0 | 5.0 | 2.0 |
| 27 | 46.0 | 12.0 | 36.0 | 6.0 |
| 35 | 20.0 | 6.0 | 27.0 | 5.0 |
| 41 | 29.0 | 21.0 | 18.0 | 4.0 |
| Total ($\times 10^5$)[f] | | | | |
| Uninfected | 0.4 | 0.04 | 0.08 | 0.46 |
| 7 | 35.0 | 0.0 | 25.0 | 15.8 |
| 13 | 10.7 | 3.4 | 6.2 | 2.0 |
| 20 | 9.1 | 2.0 | 3.5 | 1.4 |
| 27 | 9.0 | 2.6 | 6.6 | 3.2 |
| 35 | 8.0 | 1.5 | 11.7 | 3.9 |
| 41 | 6.9 | 3.0 | 2.2 | 2.2 |

[a] Pan T cells.
[b] Class I-restricted T cells.
[c] Class II-restricted T cells.
[d] Macrophages.
[e] Number of cells recovered from the lymphocyte fraction.
[f] Total number of cells recovered.

TABLE 2. Distribution of Inflammatory Cells in Brain and Spinal Cord from SJL/J Mice (Frozen Sections)

| Days after Infection | H&E | THY 1.2[a] | LYT 2 | L3T4 | MAC-1 | IgG |
|---|---|---|---|---|---|---|
| Brain | | | | | | |
| 1 | −[b] | −[c] | 1+ | − | 1+ | − |
| 3 | 2+ | 1+ | − | 1+ | 2+ | 1+ |
| 5 | 4+ | 1+ | 1+ | 2+ | 2+ | 2+ |
| 13 | 2+ | 1+ | 1+ | 1+ | 2+ | 2+ |
| 20 | 2+ | − | 1+ | − | 2+ | 1+ |
| 28 | 2+ | − | 1+ | 2+ | 2+ | − |
| 35 | 2+ | − | − | − | 3+ | 1+ |
| 42 | 1+ | 1+ | − | 1+ | 2+ | 1+ |
| Spinal cord | | | | | | |
| 1 | − | − | − | − | − | − |
| 3 | − | − | − | − | − | − |
| 5 | − | − | − | − | − | 1+ |
| 13 | 2+ | 1+ | 1+ | − | 2+ | 2+ |
| 20 | 1+ | 1+ | 1+ | 1+ | 2+ | 2+ |
| 28 | 2+ | 2+ | 2+ | 2+ | 3+ | 2+ |
| 35 | 3+ | 2+ | 1+ | 1+ | 2+ | 2+ |
| 42 | 3+ | 2+ | 2+ | 2+ | 3+ | 2+ |

[a] See Table 1.
[b] H&E: − = no inflammatory cells detected; 1+ = few inflammatory cells limited to meninges; 2+ = 1-10 lesions/40× field (LPF); 3+ = 10-20 lesions/LPF; 4+ = >20 lesions/LPF.
[c] Lymphocyte staining: − = no positive cells detected; 1+ = <5 positive cells/lesion; 2+ = <50% positive cells/lesion; 3+ = >50% positive cells/lesion.

the immune response during the early stages of infection, whereas Lyt $2^+$ cells may function as effectors in demyelination.

The importance of Lyt $2^+$ cells during TMEV infection is suggested by the differences in time-course appearance of these cells between susceptible and resistant strains of mice. Preliminary experiments indicate that Lyt $2^+$ cells can be isolated from resistant C57BL/10 mice during early infection (day 7) but not from susceptible SJL/J mice. Possible functions of Lyt $2^+$ cells during TMEV infection are: (1) cytotoxicity of viral infected targets which may limit viral infection during acute disease (C57BL/10) or cause demyelination during chronic infection (SJL/J), and/or (2) suppression of the immune response during chronic infection of SJL/J mice, thus allowing for viral persistence. Functional studies are in progress to answer these questions.

## REFERENCES

1. RODRIGUEZ, M., L. R. PEASE & C. S. DAVID. 1986. Immune-mediated injury of virus-infected oligodendrocytes. A model of multiple sclerosis. *Immunol. Today* **7**: 359-363.

2. Roos, R. P. & R. WOLLMAN. 1984. DA strain of Theiler's murine encephalomyelitis virus induces demyelination in nude mice. Ann. Neurol. **15:** 494-499.
3. ROSENTHAL, A., R. S. FUJINAMI & P. W. LAMPERT. 1986. Mechanism of Theiler's virus-induced demyelination in nude mice. Lab. Invest. **54:** 515-522.
4. SMYRNIS, E., S. U. KIM, M. W. KIM, J. OGER, S. SYLVESTER & D. W. PATY. 1986. Fluorescence-activated cell sorter analysis of bulk-isolated porcine oligodendrocytes. J. Neuroimmunol. **13:** 47-60.
5. LIPTON, H. L. 1975. Theiler's virus infection in mice: an unusual biphasic disease process leading to demyelination. Infect. Immunol. **11:** 1147-1155.
6. RODRIGUEZ, M. & S. SRIRAM. 1987. Treatment of TMEV-induced demyelination with monoclonal antibodies to T cell subsets. Neurology **37**(Suppl 1): 272.

# Borna Disease

## An Immunopathologic Response to Viral Infection in the CNS

### K. M. CARBONE, C. S. DUCHALA, AND O. NARAYAN

*The Johns Hopkins University Medical Institutions
Baltimore, Maryland 21228*

Borna disease is a sporadic infection of horses and sheep in Eastern Europe, characterized by a fatal meningoencephalomyelitis. The Borna disease agent has not been identified but it has the general properties of an enveloped virus.[1] In an experimental rat model, the Borna disease virus (BDV) produced a persistent infection exclusively of neurologic tissues. BDV induced a biphasic disease characterized by a period of agitation and aggression followed by chronic listlessness and ataxia.[1,2] We confirmed the unique neural tropism of the virus and examined the immunologic response of the host to BDV.

Antibodies directed against BDV antigens did not protect against infection with BDV *in vivo* and did not neutralize the ability of the virus to infect cell lines *in vitro*. Rats inoculated with ultraviolet-inactivated BDV in Freund's adjuvant produced anti-BDV antibody titers of 1:320 to 1:640 (measured in an indirect immunofluorescence assay on a persistently BDV-infected cell line). Despite prior immunization, over 90% of rats inoculated intranasally with BDV became infected and showed clinical signs of disease. Incubation of the agent with postinfection serum before inoculation into normal rats intracranially, normal rats intranasally, or cultures of fetal rabbit brain did not prevent infection with the virus. In addition, postinfection production of antibody does not eliminate the infecting agent, because BDV-infected rats developed persistent infection despite postinfection antibody titers of up to 1:2560.

We examined the immunopathologic basis for the behavior abnormalities and the disease syndrome. Injection of BDV into adult rats immunosuppressed by cyclophosphamide[2] or normal neonatal rats produced persistent infection of neurologic tissues without clinical signs of disease or the massive mononuclear cell inflammation seen after inoculation of normal adult rats.

In summary, BDV is an uncharacterized, exclusively neural pathogen that produces disease via immunopathologic responses to viral infection in the nervous system. There is no apparent role of antibody in this infection.

## REFERENCES

1. CARBONE, K. M., C. S. DUCHALA, J. W. GRIFFIN, A. L. KINCAID & O. NARAYAN. 1987. Pathogenesis of Borna disease in rats: Evidence that intra-axonal spread is the major route for virus dissemination and determinant for disease incubation. J. Virol. **61:** 3431-3440.
2. NARAYAN, O., S. HERTZOG, K. FRESE, H. SCHEEFERS & R. ROTT. 1983. Behavioral disease in rats caused by immunopathological responses to persistent Borna virus in the brain. Science **220:** 1401-1403.

# Coronavirus-JHM-Induced Demyelinating Encephalomyelitis in Rats

## Analysis of the Intrathecal Immune Response

R. DÖRRIES, S. SCHWENDER, H. WEGE, H. HARMS,
R. WATANABE, AND V. TER MEULEN

*Institut für Virologie und Immunbiologie der Universität
D-8700 Würzburg, FRG*

A clinically relevant, subacute, demyelinating encephalomyelitis can be induced in Lewis rats by intracerebral infection with the murine coronavirus JHM. The disease is characterized by hindleg paresis, ataxic gait, and decreased weight gain. Histopathologically, areas of primary demyelination are detectable in brain and spinal cord, infiltrated by mononuclear cells, and in close association with perivascular cuffs of lymphoid cells.[1] Several observations in recent years support the idea that besides the genetic background of the host and virus, the immune system seems to play a crucial role in the course of the disease. As we showed,[2] the transfer of basic myelin protein (BMP)-specific T-cell lines, generated from SDE-diseased Lewis rats, causes perivascular cuffing in healthy recipients, indicating autosensitization to brain antigens. Presentation of autoantigens may be associated with the induction of class II antigens on rat astrocytes by JHM virus, as shown in *in vitro* studies.[3] Because SDE-diseased animals reveal a clonally very restricted JHM-specific antibody response with a low titer in the central nervous system,[4] induction of Ia antigens on astrocytes by virus particles that have escaped neutralization is likely to happen *in vivo* as well. From these data, we wanted to determine the distribution of lymphocyte subsets in the brain of SDE-diseased Lewis rats in relation to virus-infected cells and for the brain cell type infected in or around a demyelinated area revealing intense lymphocyte infiltration.

By a combination of computer-aided cytophotometry and immunocytochemistry a multicolored topographic map of a representative demyelinated area in the cerebellum of an SDE animal was developed, revealing the following picture: Adjacent to a perivascular cuff, cytotoxic T cells distribute from the center of the focal demyelination, almost free of virus-infected cells versus the abundantly infected marginal zone. The rim of the plaque is the site where infiltrating T-helper cells are detected in close association with B lymphocytes and macrophages. However, the majority of macrophages show a strong affinity for the center of the plaque, indicating their function as a scavenger cell to eliminate cell debris. Because by double immunofluorescence oligodendrocytes were shown to be a major target for JHM virus in this area, we assume that immune-mediated killing of these cells takes place. This interpretation is further supported by preliminary observations that indicate that virus-infected cells in plaque areas express class I antigens in high density.

These data suggest that immune-mediated killing of JHM-infected oligodendrocytes may lead to the release of myelin components acting as autoantigens by presentation on astrocytes in the context of class II antigens.

## REFERENCES

1. WEGE, H., S. G. SIDELL & V. TER MEULEN. 1982. The biology and pathogenesis of coronaviruses. Curr. Top. Microbiol. Immunol., **99:** 165-200.
2. WATANABE, R., H. WEGE & V. TER MEULEN. 1983. Adoptive transfer of EAE-like lesions from rats with coronavirus-induced demyelinating encephalomyelitis. Nature **305:** 150-153.
3. MASSA, P. T., R. DÖRRIES & V. TER MEULEN. 1986. Viral particles induce Ia antigen expression on astrocytes. Nature **320:** 543-546.
4. DÖRRIES, R., R. WATANABE, H. WEGE & V. TER MEULEN. 1986. Murine coronavirus induced encephalomyelitides in rats: Analysis of immunoglobulins and virus-specific antibodies in serum and cerebrospinal fluid. J. Neuroimmunol. **12:** 131-142.

# Early Viral Proteins As Autoantigens

## Evidence from JC Virus Large T Antigen

G. L. STONER,[a] C. F. RYSCHKEWITSCH,[a]
D. L. WALKER,[b] D. SOFFER,[a,c] D. G. BRAUN,[d]
H. K. HOCHKEPPEL,[d] AND H. deF. WEBSTER[a]

[a]*Laboratory of Experimental Neuropathology, NINCDS,*
*National Institutes of Health*
*Bethesda, Maryland 20892*

[b]*Department of Medical Microbiology*
*University of Wisconsin Medical School*
*Madison, Wisconsin 53706*

[c]*Department of Pathology*
*Hadassah Medical Center*
*Jerusalem, Israel*

[d]*Pharmaceuticals Division*
*CIBA-GEIGY Limited*
*CH-4002 Basel, Switzerland*

In multiple sclerosis (MS) the target antigen in the CNS could be a normal component of glia or myelin. Alternatively, partial reactivation of a latent viral infection might allow the immune response to target an early viral antigen without virus replication. If an early viral protein induces immunopathology in the absence of virus particle production, it would mimic an autoantigen. Although the human polyomavirus JC virus (JCV) is not known to latently infect the brain, it occasionally reactivates in the kidney, and in progressive multifocal leukoencephalopathy (PML) it infects oligodendrocytes and astrocytes of immunocompromised adults.

Polyomavirus T antigens are early DNA-binding nuclear proteins that can also become targets of cytotoxic T lymphocytes at the cell surface. To study the relation of early and late viral gene expression, we developed a double-label method for simultaneous detection of JCV T antigen and capsid proteins in cryostat sections of PML brain.

PML was diagnosed in a 46-year-old man by computerized tomography and magnetic resonance imaging and confirmed pathologically at autopsy. For immunocytochemical methods see figure legends.

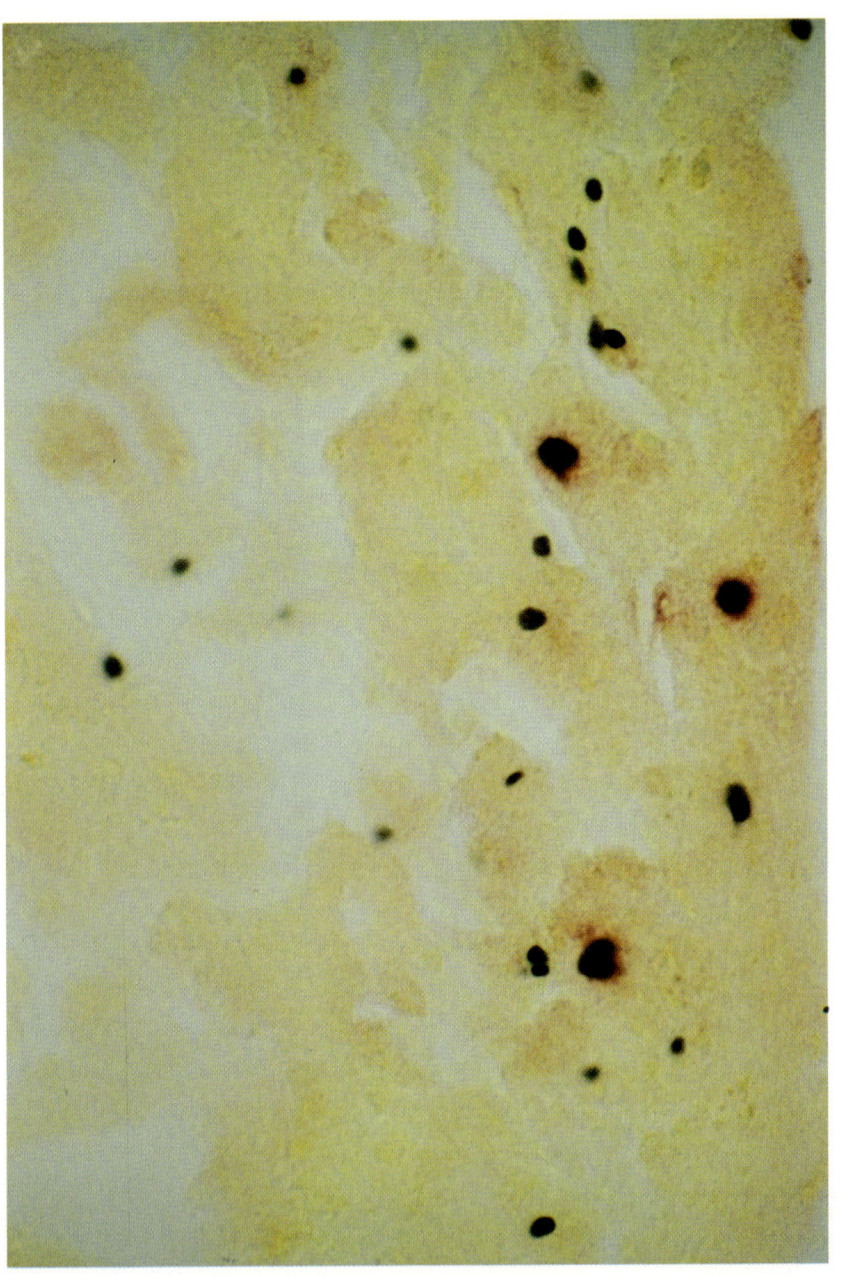

FIGURE 1. Cryostat section of PML brain incubated with monoclonal antibody to SV40 T antigen (PAb 1614),[2] followed by rabbit antibody to JCV capsid antigens.[1] Secondary antibodies applied mixed were goat antimouse IgG and biotinylated goat antirabbit IgG. Detection systems were mouse peroxidase-antiperoxidase (Clono-PAP, Sternberger-Meyer) and streptavidin-conjugated alkaline phosphatase (Zymed). The alkaline phosphatase substrate was Vector Red-I. The DAB reaction was enhanced with NiCl$_2$, giving a blue-black reaction product. Note three doubly labeled large cells. (T antigen: *blue-black*; capsid antigens: *red*.)

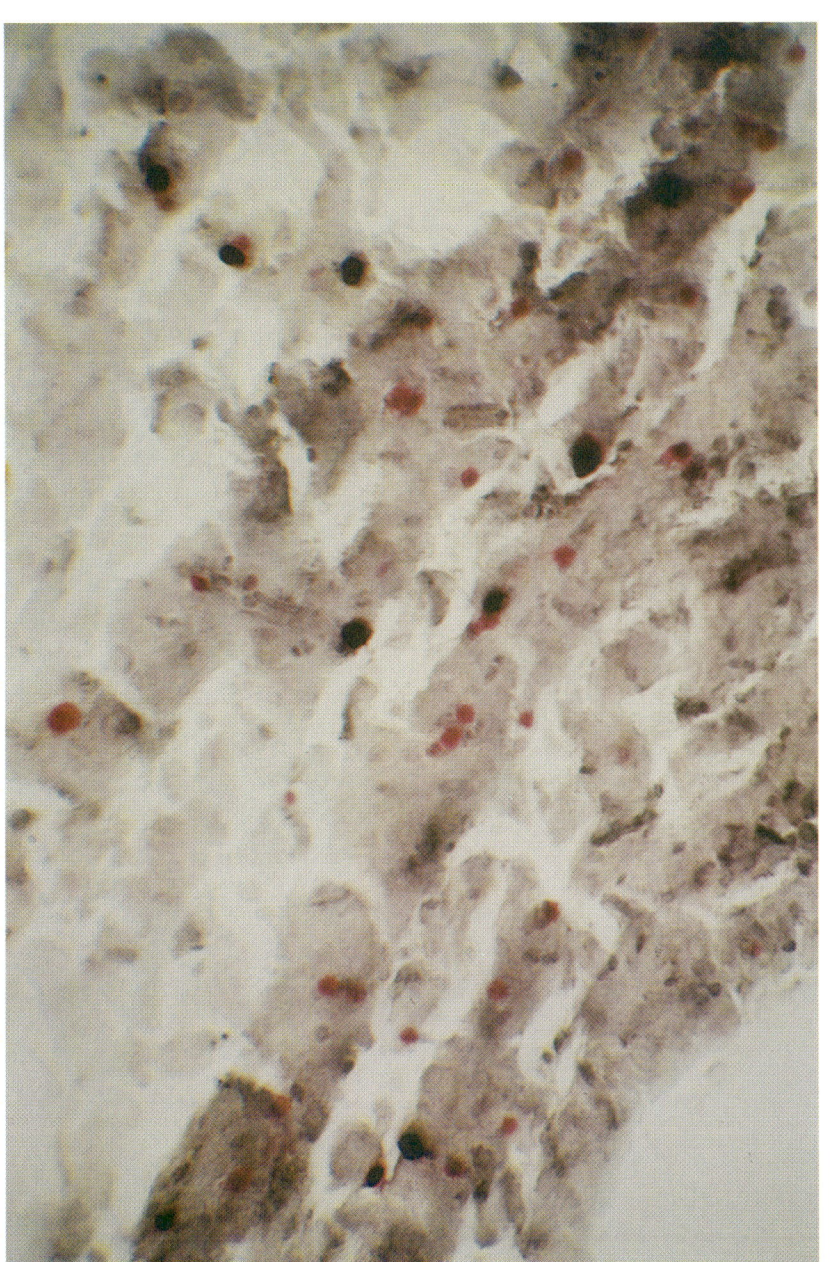

**FIGURE 2.** Cryostat section of the same tissue block shown in FIGURE 1 labeled with the same primary antibodies, but with the detection systems reversed. The monoclonal antibody to T antigen was detected by a biotinylated goat antimouse IgG followed by streptavidin-alkaline phosphatase. The rabbit antibody to capsid antigens was detected by goat antirabbit IgG followed by rabbit PAP. With the labels reversed, more large cells are doubly labeled, but the small cells expressing only T antigen persist. (T antigen: *red*; capsid antigens: *blue-black*.)

## RESULTS

Many smaller glial cells expressed T antigen in the nucleus without detectable capsid antigens (FIG. 1). A few larger cells were stained for both antigens. With the labels reversed (FIG. 2), more of the larger cells stained for both early and late (capsid) antigens, but many of the smaller cells still expressed T antigen alone. Our studies of CNS tissues from other PML cases indicate that extensive diffuse lesions such as this are not unique. In the more typical focal lesions, cells expressing capsid antigens occur around the necrotic center, with the cells expressing only T antigen located primarily in the periphery of the lesion.

## DISCUSSION

This double-label method demonstrates that JCV infection can be arrested for a time in the early antigen stage, and it confirms our earlier evidence that some cells in PML lesions express T antigen alone.[1]

In MS the role of viruses could be indirect, for example, by modulating the immune response, or direct, that is, through infection of glial cells. Failure to find virus particles in MS tissue is thought to support an indirect role for viruses. However, we find that in PML brain, JCV T antigen is detectable in many infected glial cells in the absence of late (capsid) proteins. This indicates a delay in progression through the infectious cycle and suggests an arrest in the early stage of infection. This delay slows the progress of a JCV infection in the CNS in the immunocompromised host. In a more competent host the delay might allow the immune response to target some infected cells before virion production. This may occur in the rare cases of "atypical" PML with cellular infiltration and prolonged survival.

A dissociation of early and late protein expression during CNS infection is unlikely to be unique to JC virus. For other viruses early proteins will also appear before DNA synthesis and without accompanying virus particle production. If this early antigen is targeted by the immune response, progression through the infectious cycle would be interrupted, and the link to a reactivating virus may be obscured. Thus, a search for early proteins and early mRNA of DNA viruses may provide clues to a viral etiology of immune-mediated diseases in which viral particles and even viral DNA are undetectable. If autoimmunity to a normal myelin or glial component cannot be shown in patients with MS, the targeting by the immune system of an early viral antigen selectively expressed in glial cells provides a useful alternate hypothesis.

## REFERENCES

1. STONER, G. L. *et al.* 1986. Proc. Natl. Acad. Sci. USA **83:** 2271-2275.
2. BALL, R. K. *et al.* 1984. EMBO J. **3:** 1485-1491.

# Increases in the Immune Responses to Theiler's Murine Encephalomyelitis Virus after Neonatal Treatment with Anti-T-Cell Receptor Antibody

### MARY CRANE,[a] STEPHEN MILLER,[b] HOWARD LIPTON,[c] AND BYUNG KIM [a,b]

*Departments of Pathology,[a] Microbiology-Immunology,[b] and Neurology[c]*
*Northwestern University Medical School*
*Chicago, Illinois 60611*

Intracerebral injection of susceptible mice with Theiler's murine encephalomyelitis virus (TMEV) is considered to be the most promising virally induced animal model system available for studying the pathogenesis of multiple sclerosis. The SJL mouse strain is the representative susceptible strain for this demyelinating disorder. Interestingly, the SJL mice have only one half the $V_\beta$ gene subfamilies, reflecting a huge deletion in the genome, including $V_\beta 5$ and $V_\beta 8$. In our preliminary studies using the CXJ (resistant BALB/c × susceptible SJL) recombinant inbred (RI) strains, we identified a strong linkage between the lack of $V_\beta 8$ subfamily genes and the susceptibility to TMEV-induced demyelinating disease (ref. 1 and data to be published). Previously, a linkage was demonstrated between susceptibility to disease and increased delayed type hypersensitivity (DTH) as well as antibody response to TMEV antigens.[2] BALB/c mice, which are resistant to the disease, exhibit a minimal virus-specific DTH response compared to that of sensitive mouse strains such as SJL. To study the role of $V_\beta 8$-bearing T-cell receptors in the resistance and susceptibility to this demyelinating disease, we treated resistant BALB/c adults as well as neonates with F23.1 monoclonal anti-$V_\beta 8$ antibody[3] to eliminate functional $V_\beta 8$-bearing T lymphocytes. Various treatment protocols were attempted in an effort to achieve maximum reduction of $V_\beta 8$ expression on peripheral T-cell populations. The most successful treatment scheme involving multiple administrations of anti-$V_\beta 8$ antibody results in a 100% reduction in $V_\beta 8$ expression on splenic T cells (TABLE 1). To study the functional effect of the elimination of $V_\beta 8^+$ T cells, virus-specific DTH as well as serum antibody titer was measured in BALB/c mice neonatally treated with anti-$V_\beta$ antibody. Preliminary experiments suggest that the level of virus-specific DTH as well as the serum antibody titer in the anti-$V_\beta 8$-treated animals is increased over that of control BALB/c mice (TABLE 2). Anti-$V_\beta 8$-treated neonates had an eightfold increase in serum antibody titer at 4 weeks after intracerebral injection compared to that in control treated animals. Interestingly, 5 weeks later the antibody titer of these same animals was equal. The fact that both the DTH and antibody responses have increased

TABLE 1. Analysis of Percentage of $V_\beta 8^+$ Cells after in vivo Treatment with Anti-$V_\beta 8$ Antibody[a]

|  | Experiment 1 | | Experiment 2 | |
| --- | --- | --- | --- | --- |
| Treatment | % $V_\beta 8^+$ | % Reduction | % $V_\beta 8^+$ | % Reduction |
| Control BALB/c | 25.85 | ... | 19.03 | ... |
| Anti-$V_\beta 8$-Treated BALB/c | | | | |
| Neonatal | 10.46 | 60 | 0 | 100 |
| Adult | 22.73 | 12 | 0 | 100 |
| Utero | 16.20 | 37 | ... | ... |
| Control SJL | 0 | ... | 0 | ... |

[a] Mice were treated with anti-$V_\beta 8$ and were ic injected with TMEV at 6 weeks of age. They were assayed for expression of $V_\beta 8$ at approximately 8–10 weeks. In Experiment 1 the neonatal treatment consisted of 3 intraperitoneal (ip) injections (5–10 µg each) of anti-$V_\beta 8$ antibody administered within the first week of life. The adult treatment consisted of 1 ip injection (20 µg) given at 5 weeks of age, and the in utero treatment involved an ip injection (20 µg) of a pregnant female (maximum day 15 of gestation).

In Experiment 2 the neonatal treatment consisted of 3 ip injections (15–30 µg each) as well as two additional injections (60–65 µg each) administered when mice were 6 and 9 weeks old. Adult mice were ip injected 3 times (60–65 µg each) at 6, 8, and 10 weeks of age.

in BALB/c animals after treatment with anti-$V_\beta 8$ suggests that $V_\beta 8^+$ T cells may confer resistancy to TMEV-induced demyelinating disease in BALB/c mice. Perhaps this T-cell population may be involved in the regulation of immune response to TMEV. Thus, the susceptibility of SJL mice to TMEV-induced demyelination may be partially attributable to the lack of T-cell populations bearing certain T-cell receptor variable region gene(s) (including $V_\beta 8$).

TABLE 2. Effect of Anti-$V_\beta 8$ Treatment on Anti-TMEV Immune Responses[a]

|  | DTH Response | | Antibody Response | |
| --- | --- | --- | --- | --- |
| Treatment | No. of Mice | Mean Ear Swelling[b] | No. of Mice | ELISA Titer[c] |
| Anti-$V_\beta 8$ plus TMEV (ic) | 6 | 19.5 ± 3.7 | 3 | 14.7 ± 0.3 |
| Control antibody plus TMEV (ic) | 6 | 7.4 ± 2.0 | 2 | 11.5 ± 0.5 |
| Anti-$V_\beta 8$ | 8 | 9.9 ± 2.3 | 2 | 8.3 ± 0.3 |

ABBREVIATION: ic = intracerebral.
[a] Mice were treated with anti-$V_\beta 8$ neonatally, then injected ic with TMEV at 5 weeks of age, and tested for antibody titer and DTH response at 4 weeks after ic injection.
[b] Mean ear swelling is measured in $\times 10^{-4}$ in. ± standard error of the mean.
[c] ELISA titer represents mean $\log_2$ ± standard error of the mean.

## REFERENCES

1. MELVOLD, R. W., D. M. JOKINEN, R. C. KNOBLER & H. L. LIPTON. 1987. J. Immunol. **138:** 1429.
2. CLATCH, R. J., R. W. MELVOLD, S. D. MILLER & H. L. LIPTON. 1985. J. Immunol. **135:** 1408.
3. STAERZ, U., H.-G. RAMENSEE, J. BENDETTO & M. BEVAN. 1985. J. Immunol. **134:** 3994.

# Semliki Forest Virus (A7[74]) Infection of Adult Mice Induces an Immune-Mediated Demyelinating Encephalomyelitis

J. K. FAZAKERLEY,[a,b] A. KHALILI-SHIRAZI,[b] AND
H. E. WEBB [b]

[a]*Department of Microbiology*
*University of Pennsylvania Medical School*
*Philadelphia, Pennsylvania 19104*

[b]*Neurovirology Unit*
*St. Thomas' Hospital*
*London, England*

The A7(74) strain of Semliki Forest virus (SFV) is avirulent in adult mice.[1] Infection results in a demyelinating encephalitis with occasional limb paralysis and is seen in several mouse strains.[2] Following intraperitoneal infection the virus replicates in peripheral tissues,[3] producing a plasma viremia, and infects the central nervous system (CNS) via the cerebral endothelial cells.[4] Virus is detectable in the CNS by infectivity assay for up to 12 days. The neuropathology is predominantly a mononuclear cell inflammatory response,[5] with foci of primary demyelination,[5,6] found throughout the brain, spinal cord, and optic nerves,[1,6-8] but not in the peripheral nerves (personal communication, Dr. S. Illavia). Demyelination is maximal at 14 days after infection, when virus is no longer detectable by infectivity. There is occasional, but limited destruction of CNS cells in the areas of inflammation.[5] Infected mice demonstrate a disturbance of the blood-brain barrier,[9] transient pleocytosis,[10] intrathecal antibody production,[11] and abnormal neurophysiology of the optic nerves.[12] Immunosuppression by total body irradiation results in very high brain titers without demyelination,[13] suggesting that the demyelination is immune mediated.

There is no CNS inflammatory reaction and no demyelination in SFV-infected $nu/nu$ mice up to 28 days after infection.[14] The present study extends this finding: Virus was detectable in the brains of SFV-infected $nu/nu$ mice throughout the life of the mouse and was as high as 6 logs at 6 months after infection. The brains of some of these aged "nude" mice showed some inflammatory changes and associated demyelination. Demyelination was not found in the absence of an immune response, despite persistent virus titers. Immunocompetent $nu/+$ mice have an infection essentially identical to that of other immunocompetent mice. Transfer of spleen cells ($8 \times 10^7$ nucleated splenocytes/mouse intraperitoneally) from $nu/+$ mice to $nu/nu$ mice 24 hours before infection reconstituted the CNS inflammatory reaction with maximal demyelination by day 15.[15] Transfer of spleen cells from $nu/+$ mice inoculated with SFV 7 days previously resulted in enhanced and earlier (maximal at day 7 post infection) demyelination. Depletion of T cells prior to transfer removed the ability to restore the demyelination; depletion of B cells had no effect. Repeated intraperitoneal inoculation of anti-SFV serum rapidly cleared the brain virus but produced no demyelination.[16] Depletion, with cobra venom, of complement in the first 4 days of infection prolonged the viremia. Decomplementation just before the time of maximal demyelination (days 10-14) did not affect the severity of demyelination. The outcome of infection in natural-killer-cell deficient beige mice was no different from that in normal immunocompetent mice.

The results demonstrate that the predominant mechanism of demyelination in these mice is one mediated probably directly by sensitized T lymphocytes. The antigen to which these cells react could be viral or autoantigen. Viral antigens have been demonstrated on the surface of myelin,[17] and SFV has been shown to cross-react with myelin glycolipids.[18,19]

## REFERENCES

1. BRADISH, C. J., K. ALLNER & H. M. MABER. 1971. J. Gen. Virol. **12:** 141-160.
2. SUCKLING, A. J., S. JAGELMAN, S. ILLAVIA & H. E. WEBB. 1980. Br. J. Exp. Pathol. **61:** 281-284.
3. PUSZTAI, R., E. A. GOULD & H. SMITH. 1971. Br. J. Exp. Pathol. **52:** 669-677.
4. PATHAK, S. & H. E. WEBB. 1980. Electron microscopy **2:** 492-493.
5. MACKENZIE, A., A. J. SUCKLING, S. JAGELMAN & A. M. WILSON. 1978. J. Comp. Pathol. **88:** 335-344.
6. KELLY, W. R., W. F. BLAKEMORE, S. JAGELMAN & H. E. WEBB. 1982. Neuropathol. Appl. Neurobiol. **2:** 43-53.
7. PATHAK, S., S. ILLAVIA & H. E. WEBB. 1983. *In* Immunology of Nervous System Infections. P. O. Behan, V. ter Meulen & F. C. Rose, Eds. Elsevier, Amsterdam, pp 237-254.
8. ILLAVIA, S., H. E. WEBB & S. PATHAK. 1982. *Neuropathol.* Appl. Neurobiol. **8:** 35-42.
9. PARSONS, L. M. & H. E. WEBB. 1982. J. Neurol. Sci. **57:** 307-318.
10. PARSONS, L. M. & H. E. WEBB. 1982. Neuropathol. Appl. Neurobiol. **8:** 395-401.
11. PARSONS, L. M. & H. E. WEBB. 1984. Microbiol. Letts. **25:** 135-140.
12. PESSOA, V. F. & H. IKEDA. 1984. Brain **107:** 433-446.
13. FAZAKERLEY, J. K. & H. E. WEBB. 1987. Br. J. Exp. Pathol. **68:** 101-113.
14. JAGELMAN, S., A. J. SUCKLING, H. E. WEBB & E. T. W. BOWEN. 1978. J. Gen. Virol. **41:** 599-607.
15. FAZAKERLEY, J. K., S. AMOR & H. E. WEBB. 1983. Clin. Exp. Immunol. **52:** 115-120.
16. FAZAKERLEY, J. K. & H. E. WEBB. 1987. J. Gen. Virol. **68:** 377-385.
17. BERGER, M. L. 1980. Infect. Immunol. **30:** 244-253.
18. KHALILI-SHIRAZI, A., N. GREGSON & H. E. WEBB. 1986. J. Neurol. Sci. **76:** 91-103.
19. WEBB, H. E. & J. K. FAZAKERLEY. 1984. Neuropathol. Appl. Neurobiol. **10:** 1-10.

# Fine Specificity of T-Cell-Mediated Immune Responses of Susceptible and Resistant Strains in Theiler's Murine Encephalomyelitis Virus-Induced Demyelinating Disease

STEPHEN D. MILLER, RICHARD J. CLATCH, AND
HOWARD L. LIPTON

*Departments of Microbiology-Immunology and Neurology*
*Northwestern University Medical School*
*Chicago, Illinois 60611*

Previous studies have shown a close correlation between susceptibility to Theiler's murine encephalomyelitis virus (TMEV)-induced demyelinating disease and the temporal development of chronically high levels of TMEV-specific, MHC class II-restricted delayed type hypersensitivity (DTH).[1,2] In this study, we examined the specificity of T-cell mediated immune (CMI) responses (DTH and splenic T-cell proliferative [Tprlf]) in TMEV-infected susceptible SJL mice to other picornaviruses and to the neuroantigens' myelin basic protein, proteolipid protein, and spinal cord homogenate. Neuroantigen-specific CMI responses were not detected in TMEV-infected mice before, during, or after the onset of clinical signs of demyelination. However, cross-reactive responses to closely related picornaviruses were seen. In contrast, SJL mice with chronic relapsing EAE exhibited significant CMI responses to all neuroantigens tested, but failed to show picornavirus-specific responses. The functionally defined CMI cross-reactivity pattern correlated with amino acid sequence homology between TMEV capsid proteins (VP1, VP2, and VP3) and other picornaviruses, but not with CNS myelin proteins.[3,4] These results are consistent with a TMEV-specific, DTH-mediated CNS pathology, but do not support a major role for CNS-specific autoimmune responses in the demyelinating process.

HPLC-purified virion proteins were used to *elicit* CMI responses in both susceptible SJL/J and resistant C57BL/6 mice in order to determine the fine antigenic specificity

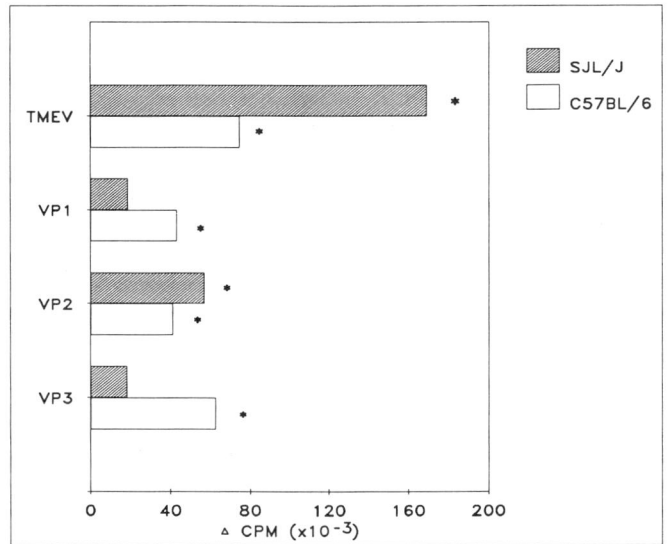

FIGURE 1. Virus protein (VP)-specificity of T-cell proliferative responses in susceptible SJL and resistant C57BL/6 mice peripherally immunized with UV-inactivated TMEV. Groups of 3-4 SJL/J and C57BL/6 mice were immunized with 25 μg of UV-inactivated TMEV emulsified in complete Freund's adjuvant (TMEV/CFA) subcutaneously at the base of the tail on day 0. On day +7, $4 \times 10^5$ draining (inguinal and periaortic) lymph node cells were cultured in modified Click's medium (0.2 ml per culture well) containing 0.5% fresh syngeneic mouse serum for 96 hours with 5 μg/well of intact TMEV, or the HPLC-purified virion proteins VP1, VP2, and VP3. Values shown are the delta counts per minute (Δ cpm) (i.e., no antigen backgrounds subtracted) following a 24-hour pulse with $^3$H-thymidine. *Responses significantly above background, $p < 0.001$.

of the T-cell repertoire. VP2 appeared to contain the major immunodominant T-cell determinant(s) in susceptible SJL/J mice either inoculated intracerebrally with viable TMEV or immunized peripherally with ultraviolet-inactivated TMEV as it elicited significantly higher DTH and Tprlf responses (FIG. 1) than did VP1 or VP3. VP2 was also significantly more efficient than VP1 or VP3 at *priming* susceptible SJL/J mice for DTH and Tprlf responses to the intact virion (FIG. 2). A major VP2 T-cell determinant has been preliminarily mapped to amino acids 189-208 of VP2 using synthetic peptides. In contrast, CMI responses in resistant C57BL/6 mice primed with intact TMEV were equally demonstrable to all three VPs (FIG. 1). These results

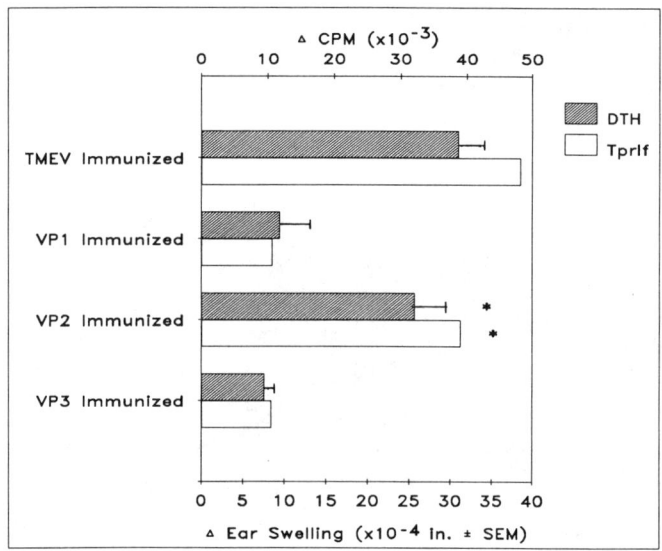

**FIGURE 2.** TMEV-specific cell-mediated immune responses in SJL/J mice peripherally immunized with intact TMEV and TMEV capsid proteins. Groups of 3-4 SJL/J mice were immunized with 25 μg of intact UV-inactivated TMEV or HPLC-purified virion proteins VP1, VP2, and VP3 emulsified in incomplete Freund's adjuvant (TMEV/CFA) subcutaneously at the base of the tail on day 0. On day +7, the mice were ear challenged with 5 μg of UV-inactivated TMEV, and the magnitude of the DTH response was determined 24 hours thereafter, using an ear swelling assay and expressed in units of $10^{-4}$ inches ± standard error of the mean (SEM).[1] Following ear measurement, $4 \times 10^5$ draining lymph node cells from each group were cultured in modified Click's medium (0.2 ml per culture well) containing 0.5% fresh syngeneic mouse serum for 96 hours with 5 μg per well of intact TMEV. Values shown are the delta counts per minute (Δ cpm) (i.e., no antigen backgrounds subtracted) following a 24-hour pulse with $^3$H-thymidine. *Responses significantly above background, $p < 0.01$.

suggest that susceptibility and resistance to TMEV-induced demyelinating disease may be influenced by the T-cell repertoire.

## REFERENCES

1. CLATCH, R. J., R. W. MELVOLD, S. D. MILLER & H. L. LIPTON. 1985. Theiler's murine encephalomyelitis virus (TMEV)-induced demyelinating disease in mice is influenced by the H-2D region: Correlation with TMEV-specific delayed-type hypersensitivity. J. Immunol. **135:** 1408.
2. CLATCH, R. J., H. L. LIPTON & S. D. MILLER. 1986. Characterization of Theiler's murine encephalomyelitis virus (TMEV)-specific delayed-type hypersensitivity responses in TMEV-induced demyelinating disease: Correlation with clinical signs. J. Immunol. **136:** 920.
3. MILLER, S. D., R. J. CLATCH, D. C. PEVEAR & H. L. LIPTON. 1987. Class II-restricted T cell responses in Theiler's murine encephalomyelitis virus (TMEV)-induced demyelinating

disease. I. Cross-specificity among TMEV substrains and related picornaviruses, but not myelin proteins. J. Immunol. **138:** 3776.
4. KENNEDY, M. K., R. J. CLATCH, M. C. DAL CANTO, J. L. TROTTER & S. D. MILLER. 1987. Monoclonal antibody-induced inhibition of relapsing EAE in SJL/J mice correlates with inhibition of neuroantigen-specific cell-mediated immune responses. J. Neuroimmunol. **16:** 345.

# A Study of Persistent Viral Infections Using Nude Mice and a Temperature-Sensitive Mutant of Vesicular Stomatitis Virus[a]

SHARON C. DOLL AND TERRY C. JOHNSON

*Division of Biology*
*Section of Virology and Oncology*
*Kansas State University*
*Manhattan, Kansas 66506*

Although the relation between the nervous and immune systems has yet to be defined in detail, it is evident that neuropeptides interact with immune components to enhance or suppress immune actions.[1] Hughes *et al.*[2] used bombesin to promote hypothermia to rescue temperature-sensitive (ts) viruses from the central nervous system (CNS) of persistently infected mice. Doll and Johnson[3] demonstrated that a single injection of 1 ng of neurotensin altered the course of CNS disease produced by ts vesicular stomatitis virus (VSV) in mice.

Similar to neurotensin with Swiss outbred mice,[3] a single intracerebroventricular injection of 100 ng of $\beta$-endorphin in BALB/c (+/+) mice 24 hours before an inoculation with $10^4$ PFU of tsG31-KS5 VSV dramatically altered the course of clinical disease. The introduction of $\beta$-endorphin caused an aggressive CNS disease, leading to the death of 70% of the animals within 15 days, whereas only 3% of the mice infected with only the ts VSV died (FIG. 1).

A role for the immune system in the progress of the CNS disease was illustrated by the use of BALB/c athymic nude mice (nu/nu). Unlike the immunocompetent (+/+) mice, almost all of the tsG31-KS5 VSV infected nude mice died within 25 days (FIG. 1). The animals had a slowly progressive and degenerative disease before dying with symptoms of paralysis, severe curvature of the spine, and wasting. Furthermore, an introduction of $\beta$-endorphin 24 hours before an intracerebral infection with the ts VSV did not alter the progression of CNS disease (FIG. 1). The inability of the neuropeptide to alter the course of CNS disease in nude mice may have reflected a lack of target cells for $\beta$-endorphin in the athymic animals.

Nude mice reconstituted with syngeneic T-lymphocyte-enriched splenocytes,[4] however, were relatively refractory to the CNS disease and over 90% survived 20 days and 70% lived beyond 25 days (FIG. 1). Animals that survived remained healthy at least 60 days after infection, and nude mice that were reconstituted with either 5 ×

---

[a] Supported by grant #441f722 from the Office of Naval Research and the Kansas Agricultural Experiment Station. This is contribution no. 86-384-J from the Kansas Agricultural Experiment Station, Kansas State University.

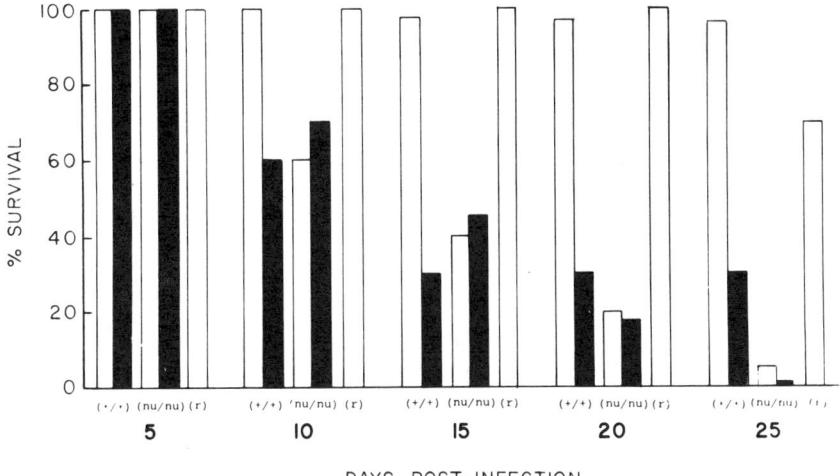

**FIGURE 1.** Mice received a single intracerebroventricular injection of 100 ng of β-endorphin in 10 μl of sterile distilled water (*shaded bars*) or with 10 μl of sterile distilled water alone (*open bars*). Twenty-four hours later all mice were infected with $10^4$ PFU of tsG31-KS5 VSV. r = nude (nu/nu) mice reconstituted with $5 \times 10^6$ syngeneic T lymphocytes 1 day before injection with vesicular stomatitis virus.

TABLE 1. Antibody and Vesicular Stomatitis Virus (VSV) in Persistently Infected Mice

| Mice | No. of T Cells | Days after Infection | Neutralizing Antibody | VSV in Brain |
|---|---|---|---|---|
| BALB/c (nu/nu) | 0 | 5 | 4/10[a] | 10/10[a] |
|  |  | 10 | 0/4 | 7/7 |
|  |  | 20 | 0/4 | 4/4 |
|  | $5 \times 10^6$ | 5 | 8/10 | 10/10 |
|  |  | 10 | 2/4 | 9/10 |
|  |  | 20 | 1/5 | 4/4 |
|  | $5 \times 10^7$ | 5 | 8/10 | 10/10 |
|  |  | 10 | 4/4 | 2/10 |
|  |  | 30 | 6/6 | 0/6 |
| BALB/c (+/+) | — | 5 | — | 0/6 |
|  | — | 10 | — | 0/5 |
|  | — | 20 | — | 0/10 |

[a] Number positive/total.

NOTE: Mice (nu/nu) were reconstituted with the indicated number of syngeneic T lymphocytes and 24 hours later inoculated with $10^4$ tsG31-KS5 VSV. After 5, 10, or 20 days of infection the animals were sacrificed, and their sera were measured for neutralizing antibody by a plaque reduction assay. Animals were scored positive if any neutralizing antibody was detected. Vesicular stomatitis virus in brain was determined by plaque assays of brain tissue homogenates on BHK cell monolayers incubated at 31°C, a permissive temperature for tsG31-KS5 VSV, and identification of the virus as VSV by antibody neutralization tests.

$10^6$ or $5 \times 10^7$ syngeneic T lymphocytes were provided with a similar degree of protection.

In nude mice not reconstituted with syngeneic lymphocytes, less than 50% of the animals had detectable levels of neutralizing antibody 5 days after infection, and by 10 days all animals were scored as negative (TABLE 1). Like outbred and BALB/c mice, most of the reconstituted nude mice had a brisk antibody response, but the presence of antibody was transient in those animals reconstituted with $5 \times 10^6$ lymphocytes (TABLE 1). Although virus could not be recovered from the brains of BALB/c (+/+) mice 5 through 20 days after infection, 90-100% of the nude mice reconstituted with $5 \times 10^6$ lymphocytes had a persistent CNS infection that endured. The latter animals appeared clinically healthy, and neutralizing antibody clearly played a minor, if any, role in maintaining the host-parasite relationship. More likely, a T-lymphocyte-mediated action must protect the animals from an aggressive form of the CNS disease, and this model system will allow the identification of subsets of immune components that are responsible for the protection and the effects of neuropeptides on the immune response.

## REFERENCES

1. VAN EPPS, D. E. & L. SALAND. 1984. J. Immunol. **130:** 3046-3053.
2. HUGHES, J., S. C. DOLL & T. C. JOHNSON. 1985. J. Virol. **53:** 781-785.
3. DOLL, S. C. & T. C. JOHNSON. 1985. J. Virol. **53:** 583-587.
4. JULIUS, H., E. SIMPSON & L. A. HERZENBERG. 1973. Eur. J. Immunol. **3:** 645-649.

WORKSHOP 15. NEUROIMMUNOMODULATION

# Potentiation of IL-1-Induced BALB/3T3 Fibroblast Proliferation by Substance P

### EDWARD S. KIMBALL AND M. C. FISHER

*Janssen Research Foundation
Spring House, Pennsylvania 19477*

Interleukin-1 (IL-1) is a peptide hormone whose wide spectrum of activities include activation of fibroblasts to proliferate and to secrete prostaglandins, collagenase, and plasminogen activator.[1] IL-1 is elevated in the synovial fluid of arthritic joints,[2] and it is possible that the fibroblast-activating properties of IL-1 might contribute to the synovial cell activation there, causing the development of pannus and further secretion of inflammatory mediators into the joint space. Substance P (SP) was also shown to have direct effects on fibroblasts,[3] macrophages,[4] and synovial cells,[5] and was indirectly shown to play a role in exacerbating experimental arthritis.[6] It was reasonable then to examine whether SP was able to amplify the fibroblast response to IL-1. In this report, we show that SP at nanomolar concentrations is able to enhance the proliferative response of BALB/3T3 fibroblasts to IL-1.

IL-1-induced fibroblast proliferation was followed by plating growth-arrested BALB/3T3 fibroblasts (clone A31) into 96-well plates at a density of 50,000 cells per well 24 hours before initiation of the assay. IL-1, in the presence or absence of SP, was added at various dilutions to the wells in triplicate and allowed to incubate for 66 hours in serum-free medium supplemented with Insulin-Transferrin-Selenium and 50 μM of indomethacin. At the end of this period, cells were pulsed with $^3$H-thymidine for an additional 6 hours.

FIGURE 1 shows the proliferative response of BALB/3T3 cells treated with increasing doses of SP in the presence or absence of a single dose of IL-1$_{beta}$. Substance P alone was only weakly effective in promoting incorporation of radioactive thymidine. However, the proliferative response to IL-1 was amplified approximately twofold by SP. The apparent bell-shaped dose responses observed at $>30$ ng/ml are typical of SP activity in other systems. FIGURE 2 shows the effect of 3 ng/ml of SP on the 3T3 proliferative response to increasing concentrations of recombinant IL-1$_{alpha}$. As with IL-1$_{beta}$, SP was able to potentiate the proliferative response to IL-1$_{alpha}$.

Both IL-1$_{alpha}$ and IL-1$_{beta}$ exhibited amplified proliferative responses in the presence of low concentrations of SP (i.e., $\leq 30$ ng/ml). Substance P alone showed only weak activity as a fibroblast mitogen at the concentrations tested. This result demonstrates that SP may contribute to the synovial hyperplasia associated with chronic rheumatoid arthritis as a result of its ability to amplify IL-1-induced fibroblast proliferation. Substance P is also able to elicit IL-1 production from the P388D1 macrophage cell line.[7] It is possible then that this neurokinin may be strongly involved in sustaining the chronic inflammatory state by promoting IL-1 release from infiltrating macrophages as well as by amplifying the biologic activity of any IL-1 thus secreted on

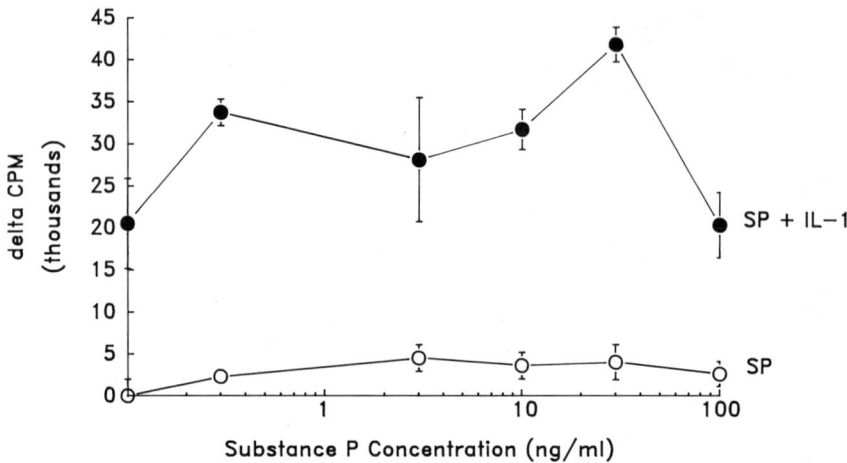

**FIGURE 1.** Amplification of IL-1$_{beta}$ by substance P (SP). Response of BALB/3T3 fibroblasts to increasing doses of substance P in the presence or absence of 1 unit/ml of IL-1$_{beta}$. Results shown are counts per minute (cpm) ± SE of $^3$H-thymidine incorporation for triplicate cultures.

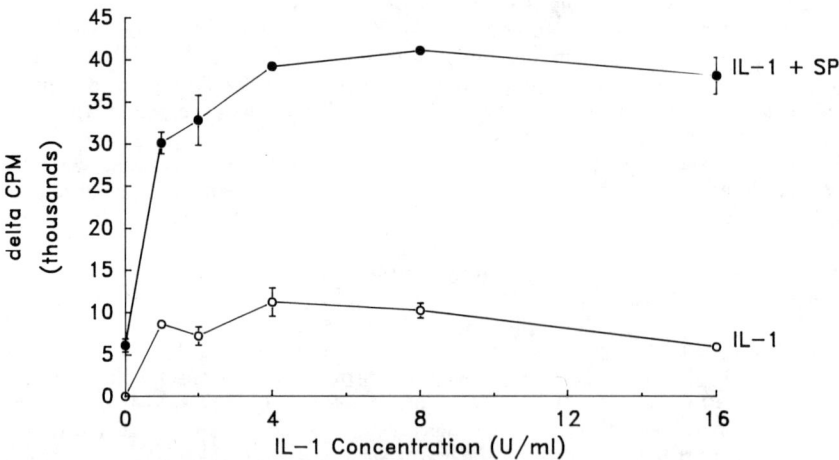

**FIGURE 2.** Amplification of IL-1$_{alpha}$ by substance P (SP). Response of BALB/3T3 fibroblasts to increasing doses of IL-1$_{alpha}$ in the presence or absence of SP (3 ng/ml). Results shown are counts per minute (cpm) ± SE of triplicate cultures.

synovial cells. Therefore, the combined actions of IL-1 and SP in the joint may directly contribute to, maintain, and sustain the pathology that occurs in the joint during chronic arthritic disease.

## REFERENCES

1. OPPENHEIM, J. J. & I. GERY. 1982. Immunol. Today **3:** 113.
2. WOOD, D. D., E. J. IHRIE, C. A. DINARELLO & P. L. COHEN. 1983. Arthritis Rheum. **26:** 975.
3. NILSSON, J., A. M. VON EULER & C. J. DALSGAARD. 1985. Nature **315:** 61.
4. HARTUNG, H.-P., K. WOLTERS & K. V. TOYKA. 1986. J. Immunol. **136:** 3856.
5. LOTZ, M., D. A. CARSON & J. VAUGHN. 1987. Science **235:** 893.
6. LEVINE, J. D., et al. 1984. Science **226:** 547.
7. KIMBALL, E. S., F. J. PERSICO & J. VAUGHT. 1988. Ann. N.Y. Acad. Sci., this issue.

# Suppression of Anaphylactic Shock by Enkephalins[a]

## DRAGAN MARIĆ AND BRANISLAV D. JANKOVIĆ [b]

*Immunology Research Center*
*Vojvode Stepe 458*
*11221 Belgrade, Yugoslavia*

Recent evidence has implicated opioid pentapeptides in the *in vivo* development of immune reactions,[1] including anaphylactic shock.[2,3] We are summarizing our results showing the antianaphylactic shock activity of methionine-enkephalin (Met-Enk) and leucine-enkephalin (Leu-Enk).

Male Wistar rats (200-250 g) were sensitized for systemic anaphylaxis with three subcutaneous injections of 10 μg of crystalline ovalbumin (OA) in aluminum hydroxide adjuvant with an interval of 14 days between injections. Nine days after the last sensitizing dose of OA, rats were injected intraperitoneally with 4 mg/kg of body weight of Met-Enk or Leu-Enk. Immunized controls were injected with saline solution. Enkephalin or saline solution was given every 12 hours for 5 consecutive days (a total of 10 injections per rat). Thirty minutes after the last injection of enkephalin or saline solution, each animal was challenged for anaphylactic shock with 0.6 mg of OA in 1 ml of saline solution injected into the tail vein. A separate group of rats received only one intraperitoneal injection of Met-Enk, Leu-Enk, or saline solution 30 minutes before injection of shocking dose of antigen. The development and severity of clinical signs,[3] and the mortality rate were recorded. Serum samples taken 12 hours before induction of shock were assayed for passive cutaneous anaphylaxis (PCA), ELISA, and precipitin anti-OA antibody titers. At autopsy, the omentum of each rat was dissected immediately after sacrifice and processed for mast cell degranulation examination.[3] The percentage of degranulated mast cells was determined microscopically.

Clinical, immunologic, and histomorphologic signs of anaphylactic shock were significantly suppressed by Met-Enk and Leu-Enk (FIGS. 1 and 2). However, antianaphylactic effect of Met-Enk was much more pronounced than that of Leu-Enk. Chronic treatment (10 injections) with Met-Enk completely protected the animals from fatal shock (FIG. 1), whereas acute treatment (one injection) with this peptide produced lower but still significant antishock activity. In contrast, one injection of Leu-Enk failed to prevent the incidence and severity of anaphylactic reaction. The level of circulating IgE (determined by PCA and ELISA assays) and precipitating anti-OA antibodies and the degree of mast cell degranulation (FIG. 2) decreased in rats given 10 injections of Met-Enk and Leu-Enk. This result implies that enkephalins exert their antianaphylactic action by suppressing antibody production[1,2] and sensitization of mast cells with specific IgE. It is also possible that enkephalins, and Met-

---

[a] This work was supported by the Republic of Serbia Research Fund, Belgrade, Yugoslavia, and Thymoorgan Pharmazie, Vienenburg, FRG.

[b] To whom correspondence should be addressed.

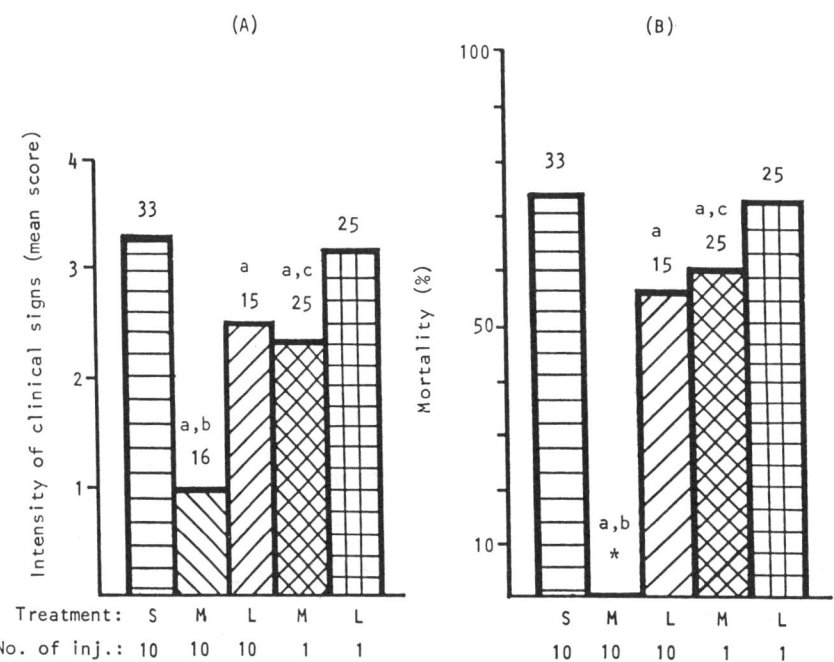

**FIGURE 1.** Intensity of clinical signs (**A**) and mortality rate (**B**) in sensitized rats treated with 4 mg/kg of body weight of Met-Enk (M) and Leu-Enk (L), and saline solution (S) and challenged with shocking dose of ovalbumin. *Numbers above the bars* indicate the number of animals in each group. *Asterisk* indicates that all animals treated with 10 injections of Met-Enk survived the shock. Statistically significant differences: $^{a}p < 0.001$, 1 injection of Met-Enk, or 10 injections of Met-Enk or Leu-Enk *vs* saline; $^{b}p < 0.001$, 10 injections of Met-Enk *vs* 10 injections of Leu-Enk; $^{c}p < 0.01$, 1 injection of Met-Enk *vs* 1 injection of Leu-Enk.

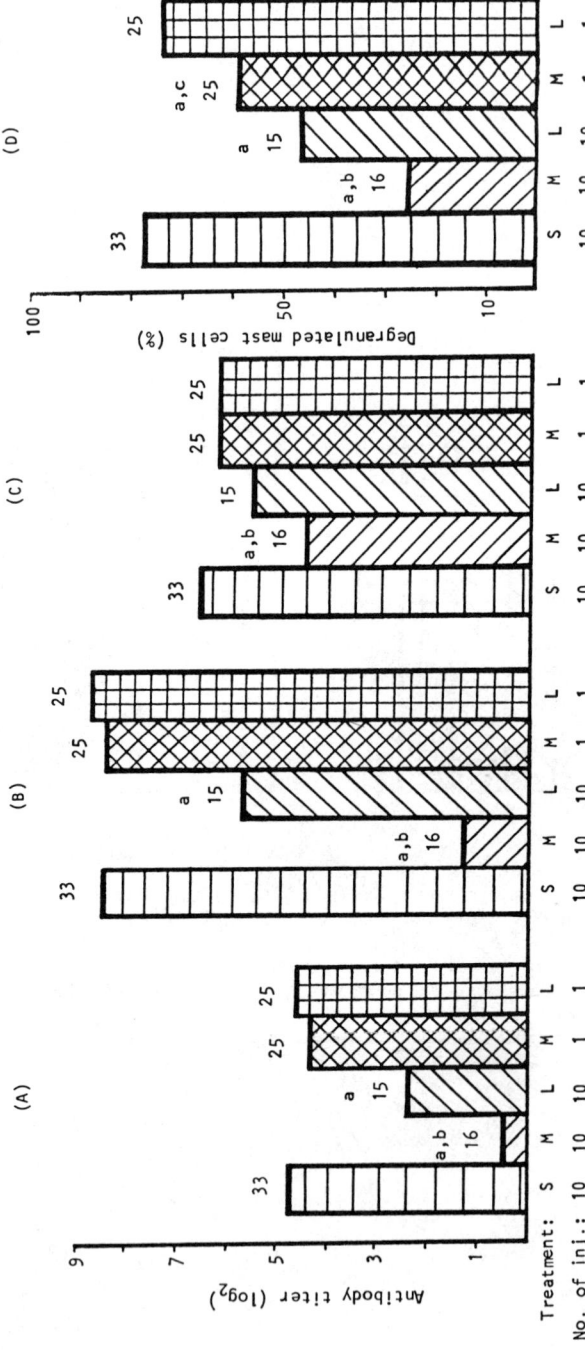

FIGURE 2. Serum passive cutaneous anaphylaxis (PCA) (A), ELISA (B), and IgG (C) antiovalbumin (OA) antibody titers, and mast cell degranulation (D) in sensitized rats treated with saline solution (S), and 4 mg/kg of body weight of Met-Enk (M) and Leu-Enk (L), and challenged with shocking dose of OA. *Figures above bars* indicate the number of animals in each group. Statistically significant differences: $^a p < 0.001$, 1 injection of Met-Enk, or 10 injections of Met-Enk or Leu-Enk vs saline solution; $^b p < 0.001$, 10 injections of Met-Enk vs 10 injections of Leu-Enk; $^c p < 0.01$, 1 injection of Met-Enk vs 1 injection of Leu-Enk.

Enk in particular, may bind directly to opioid receptors on mast cells[4] and thus inhibit the release of vasoactive substances involved in anaphylactic shock. Another possibility is that Met-Enk antagonizes physiologically the exacerbating activity of endogenous beta-endorphin[5] and thus exerts its antianaphylactic activity. These results suggest that the immunosuppressive activity of Met-Enk should be considered in the clinical prevention of systemic anaphylaxis.

## REFERENCES

1. JANKOVIĆ, B. D. & D. MARIĆ. 1986. Clin. Neuropharmacol. 9(Suppl. 4): 476-478.
2. JANKOVIĆ, B. D. & D. MARIĆ. 1987. Ann. N.Y. Acad. Sci. 496: 115-125.
3. JANKOVIĆ, B. D. & D. MARIĆ. 1987. Immunol. Lett. 15: 153-160.
4. CASALE, T. B., S. BOWMAN & M. KALINER. 1984. J. Allergy Clin. Immunol. 73: 775-781.
5. AMIR, S. & J. M. REE. 1985. Brain Res. 329: 329-333.

# Neurokinin-Induced Generation of Interleukin-1 in a Macrophage Cell Line

### EDWARD S. KIMBALL, FRANCIS J. PERSICO, AND JEFFREY L. VAUGHT

*Janssen Research Foundation*
*Spring House, Pennsylvania 19477*

Substance P is one of a number of neuropeptides responsible for the transmission of pain in afferent nerve fibers in the joint[1] and has also been indirectly implicated in the exacerbation of the arthritic state through a number of actions on different cell types. Substance P (SP) was recently demonstrated to activate synoviocytes to secrete $PGE_2$ and collagenase,[2] and it is also known to activate macrophages to secrete prostaglandins and active oxygen metabolites.[3] *In vivo,* substance P was shown to amplify experimental adjuvant arthritis in rats when injected intraarticularly.[4] Interleukin-1 (IL-1), a peptide hormone that is a product of activated macrophages and synoviocytes, has been implicated as a major mediator of the joint pathology that accompanies chronic arthritic disease. For example, IL-1 has a wide variety of biologic activities that are pertinent to arthritic disease, including fibroblast secretion of prostaglandins and collagenase, fibroblast proliferation, chondrocyte activation, and bone resorption. Additionally, IL-1 has been detected in synovial fluid from patients with rheumatoid arthritis. Because of the interesting parallels in some of the biologic activities of IL-1 and substance P, we were prompted to examine whether some of the arthritogenic properties of SP might be due to IL-1 induction.

The P388D1 mouse macrophage cell line was used as the source of IL-1. In the culture system employed, IL-1 inducer was provided in serum-free medium for 4 hours. After washing the cells, the cells were maintained in serum-free medium for an additional 18 hours. IL-1 activity in the supernatants was determined by their ability to induce IL-2 secretion by the LBRM/TG6 cell line. IL-2 was determined by increased proliferation of the IL-2-dependent T-cell line HT2.[5]

FIGURE 1 is a representative experiment showing a response to dilutions of P388D1 supernatant fluids from cultures treated with either SP, lipopolysaccharide (LPS), control medium, or the substance P antagonist D-Pro$^2$, D-Trp$^{7,9}$-SP (DPDT). Substance P (30 ng/ml) was capable of causing significantly increased levels of IL-1 secretion when compared with control medium (RPMI). SP-induced secretion was inhibitible by co-incubation with 100 ng/ml of DPDT. However, LPS-induced IL-1 secretion was not significantly affected by DPDT, suggesting that this may be an SP receptor-mediated process. DPDT itself was only a weak IL-1 inducer that did not elevate IL-1 secretion significantly above those levels seen with control medium. Other structurally related neurokinins that were examined for their ability to induce IL-1 secretion were the C-terminal SP-octapeptide $SP_{4-11}$ and neurokinins A and B (NK-A and NK-B). As shown in FIGURE 2, all three peptides were active in this system.

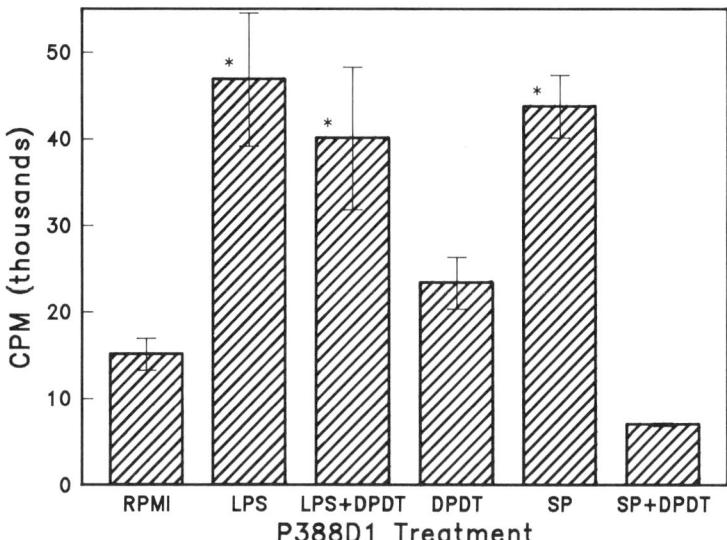

**FIGURE 1.** Substance P induction of IL-1 secretion. Response of LBRM/HT2 cells to culture supernatants (1:8 dilutions) from P388D1 cells stimulated with LPS (300 ng/ml), SP (30 ng/ml substance P), DPDT (100 ng/ml), SP + DPDT (30 ng/ml SP + 100 ng/ml DPDT), and LPS + DPDT (300 ng/ml LPS + 100 ng/ml DPDT) compared to unstimulated P388D1 controls (RPMI). Results are expressed as average counts per minute (cpm) ± SE of triplicate cultures. *Asterisks* indicate a significant difference ($p < 0.001$), using analysis of variance, from unstimulated cultures.

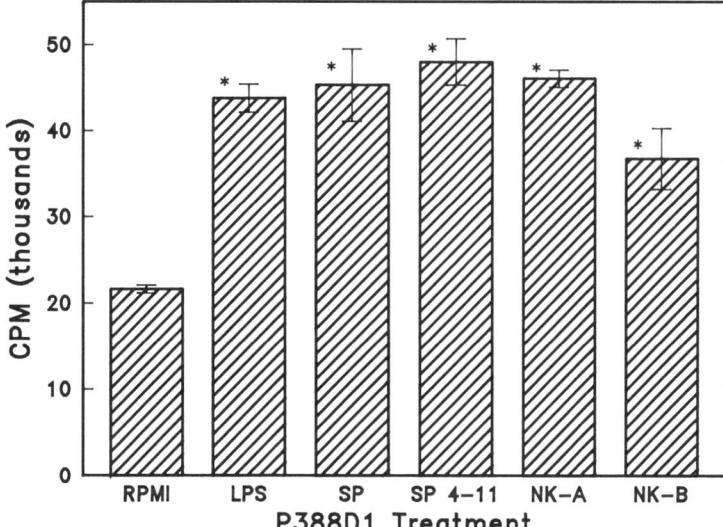

**FIGURE 2.** IL-1 induction by structural homologs of substance P. Response of LBRM/HT2 cells to culture supernatants (1:2 dilutions) from P388D1 cells stimulated with LPS (300 ng/ml), or various neuropeptides at 30 ng/ml. SP (substance P), $SP_{4-11}$ (C-terminal octapeptide of SP; supernatant was tested at a 1:8 dilution), NK-A (neurokinin A), and NK-B (neurokinin B) were compared with those in unstimulated P388D1 controls (RPMI). *Asterisks* indicate a significant difference ($p < 0.001$), using analysis of variance, from unstimulated cultures.

These results support the hypothesis that SP as well as other neurokinins may play a role in the generation and maintenance of the inflammatory condition in rheumatoid arthritis by promoting IL-1 production. The demonstration of neuropeptide activity on lymphoid cells further suggests that neurogenic stimulation of immunologic mechanisms may also play a significant role in other autoimmune neuropathies such as multiple sclerosis.

## REFERENCES

1. FOREMAN, J. C. & C. L. JORDAN. 1984. Trends Pharm. Sci. **5:** 116.
2. LOTZ, M., D. A. CARSON & J. H. VAUGHN. 1987. Science **235:** 893.
3. HARTUNG, H.-P., K. WOLTERS & K. V. TOYKA. 1986. J. Immunol. **136:** 3856.
4. LEVINE, J. D., et al. 1984. Science **226:** 547.
5. LARRICK, J. W., L. BRINDLEY & M. V. DOYLE. 1985. J. Immunol. Methods **79:** 39.

# Enkephalins Modulate *in Vivo* Immune Reactions Through Delta- and Mu-Opioid Receptors[a]

BRANISLAV D. JANKOVIĆ[b] AND DRAGAN MARIĆ

*Immunology Research Center*
*Vojvode Stepe 458*
*11221 Belgrade, Yugoslavia*

Earlier experiments, performed in rats and mice, demonstrated that opioid pentapeptides, methionine-enkephalin (Met-Enk) and leucine-enkephalin (Leu-Enk), modulate humoral and cellular immune responses *in vivo*.[1-4] However, the mode of action of enkephalins on immune reactions is still unclear. It is generally accepted that opioid peptides, including enkephalins, bind to mu-, delta-, and kappa-opioid receptors.[5-7] Consequently, the immunomodulatory action of Met-Enk and Leu-Enk may depend on these opioid receptors. To evaluate this possibility, two opioid receptor antagonists were employed in the present study: N,N-diallyl-Tyr-Aib-Aib-Phe-Leu (ICI 174864; Imperial Chemical Industry, England) and naloxone (NX; Sigma, USA). ICI 174864 is known as a highly selective antagonist for delta-receptors, whereas NX is specific for mu-receptors when used in low doses. However, a high dose of NX acts as a nonselective blocker of all types of opioid receptors. For this reason, both high and low doses of NX were used in the experiment.

Male BALB/c mice were given intraperitoneal injections of 0.5 mg/kg of ICI 174864; 0.5 or 5 mg/kg of NX; and 5 mg/kg of Met-Enk and Leu-Enk alone or in combination with ICI 174864 and NX. In the last case, an antagonist was administered every 12 hours and enkephalin every 24 hours (one injection of enkephalin between two injections of antagonist per day): 1 day before and 4 days after intraperitoneal immunization with $5 \times 10^8$ sheep red blood cells (SRBC). The dose of 5 mg/kg of enkephalin was previously shown to enhance the humoral immune response in mice.[8] Immunized controls were treated with antagonist or saline solution alone. Animals were sacrificed 4 days after challenge with SRBC and spleen cells used in direct plaque-forming cell (PFC) assay. Serum samples obtained on the day of sacrifice were tested for the presence of circulating anti-SRBC antibody by means of a microhemagglutination reaction.

As shown in TABLES 1 and 2, both Met-Enk and Leu-Enk enhanced the PFC response and hemagglutinin production when used without antagonists. However, ICI 174864 and NX, when used alone, suppressed humoral immune reactions, thus suggesting the involvement of mu- and delta-opioid receptors in humoral immune response. ICI 174864 applied in combination with enkephalins antagonized the

---

[a]This work was supported by the Republic of Serbia Research Fund, Belgrade, Yugoslavia, and Thymoorgan Pharmazie, Vienenburg, F.R.G.).

[b]To whom correspondence should be addressed.

TABLE 1. Antagonist Effect of ICI 174864 on Immunopotentiating Action of Met-Enk and Leu-Enk in Mice Immunized with SRBC and Tested for PFC Response and Serum Anti-SRBC Antibody Titer

| Treatment of Mice | Dose (mg/kg of body weight) | Humoral Immune Response (mean ± SD) | |
|---|---|---|---|
| | | No. of PFC/$10^6$ Cells | Antibody Titer ($\log_2$) |
| Saline | | 1,904 ± 150 | 5.9 ± 0.5 |
| ICI 174864 | 0.5 | 1,307 ± 112[a] | 5.4 ± 0.3[b] |
| Met-Enk | 5 | 2,505 ± 222[a,c,d] | 7.0 ± 0.3[a,c,d] |
| Met-Enk/ICI 174864 | 5/0.5 | 2,057 ± 142[b] | 6.3 ± 0.2[b] |
| Leu-Enk | 5 | 2,246 ± 205[a] | 6.6 ± 0.5[a] |
| Leu-Enk/ICI 174864 | 5/0.5 | 2,160 ± 161[a] | 6.5 ± 0.4[a] |

Statistically significant differences:
[a] $p < 0.001$ and [b] $p < 0.01$, Met-Enk; Leu-Enk; and/or ICI 174864 vs saline solution.
[c] $p < 0.001$, Met-Enk vs Met-Enk and ICI 174864.
[d] $p < 0.01$, Met-Enk vs Leu-Enk.

TABLE 2. Effect of NX on Immunopotentiating Action of Met-Enk and Leu-Enk in Mice Immunized with SRBC and Tested for PFC Response and Serum Anti-SRBC Antibody Production

| Treatment of Mice | Dose (mg/kg of body weight) | Humoral Immune Response (mean ± SD) | |
|---|---|---|---|
| | | No. of PFC/$10^6$ Cells | Antibody Titer ($\log_2$) |
| Saline | | 2,019 ± 180 | 6.0 ± 0.4 |
| NX | 0.5 | 1,670 ± 189[a,d,k] | 5.7 ± 0.3[b,d,k] |
| NX | 5 | 807 ± 123[a,l] | 4.6 ± 0.2[a,l] |
| Met-Enk | 5 | 2,666 ± 196[a,c,e] | 6.8 ± 0.4[a,c,e] |
| Met-Enk/NX | 5/0.5 | 2,599 ± 174[a,h] | 6.6 ± 0.5[a,i] |
| Met-Enk/NX | 5/5 | 1,973 ± 201 | 6.1 ± 0.5 |
| Leu-Enk | 5 | 2,318 ± 135[a,f,g] | 6.4 ± 0.3[a,f,g] |
| Leu-Enk/NX | 5/0.5 | 378 ± 83[a,j] | 3.7 ± 0.6[a,j] |
| Leu-Enk/NX | 5/5 | 105 ± 129[a] | 2.3 ± 0.3[a] |

Statistically significant differences:
[a] $p < 0.001$ and [b] $p < 0.01$, Met-Enk; Leu-Enk; and/or NX vs saline solution
[c] $p < 0.001$, Met-Enk vs Leu-Enk.
[d] $p < 0.001$, low dose of NX vs high dose of NX.
[e] $p < 0.001$, Met-Enk vs Met-Enk and high dose of NX.
[f] $p < 0.001$, Leu-Enk vs Leu-Enk and low dose of NX.
[g] $p < 0.001$, Leu-Enk vs Leu-Enk and high dose of NX.
[h] $p < 0.001$ and [i] $p < 0.01$, Met-Enk and low dose of NX vs Met-Enk and high dose of NX.
[j] $p < 0.001$, Leu-Enk and low dose of NX vs Leu-Enk and high dose of NX.
[k] $p < 0.001$, low dose of NX vs Leu-Enk and low dose of NX.
[l] $p < 0.001$, high dose of NX vs Leu-Enk and high dose of NX.

immunoenhancing activity of Met-Enk but not that of Leu-Enk (TABLE 1). Low doses (0.5 mg) of NX, however, prevented the immunopotentiating action of Leu-Enk but not that of Met-Enk (TABLE 2). These findings imply that in humoral immunity Met-Enk operates through delta-opioid receptors, whereas Leu-Enk acts primarily via mu-opioid receptors. Further experiments revealed that high doses (5 mg) of NX produced even a greater anti-Leu-Enk effect. However, this dose of NX also compromised to certain extent the immunoenhancing activity of Met-Enk, probably because NX, beside blocking mu-receptors, blocked also a number of delta-receptors.

These results suggest that both delta- and mu-opioid binding sites are involved in humoral immune reactions. Which of these two opioid receptors accounts more for the expression of immune reactions is a matter of conjecture. Because (a) 0.5 mg of ICI 174864, which blocks only delta-receptors, produced more pronounced immunosuppression than did an identical dose of NX, which blocks only mu-receptors, and because (b) Met-Enk, which binds to delta-receptors, exerted a stronger immunoenhancing effect than did Leu-Enk, which binds to mu-receptors preferentially, it may then be deduced that a larger portion of immune processes is realized through delta-receptors. This assumption seems to be substantiated by a recent demonstration that Met-Enk is a more potent modulator than Leu-Enk of the complex biochemical processes underlying anaphylactic shock in the rat.[4] Besides, the conformational states of enkephalins may partly account for the preferential binding of Met-Enk to delta-receptors and Leu-Enk to mu-receptors. It has been shown[9-11] that an enkephalin may occur in folded or extended form depending on the microenvironmental conditions, the folded form reacting with mu-receptors and the extended form preferring delta-receptors. At the present state of the art, the possibility that other opioid receptors and nonopioid receptors are involved in enkephalin-induced immunomodulation should also be taken into consideration.

## REFERENCES

1. JANKOVIĆ, B. D. & D. MARIĆ. 1986. Clin. Neuropharmacol. **9:** (Suppl. 4): 476-478.
2. JANKOVIĆ, B. D. & D. MARIĆ. 1987. Ann. N.Y. Acad. Sci. **496:** 115-125.
3. MARIĆ, D. & B. D. JANKOVIĆ. 1987. N.Y. Acad. Sci. **496:** 126-136.
4. JANKOVIĆ, B. D. & D. MARIĆ. 1987. Immunol. Lett. **15:** 153-160.
5. KOSTERLITZ, H. W., J. A. H. LORD, S. J. PATERSON & A. A. WATERFIELD. 1980. Br. J. Pharmacol. **68:** 333-342.
6. CHAILLET, P., A. COULAUD, M.-C. FOURNIER-ZALUSKI, G. GACEL, B. P. ROQUES & J. CONSTENTIN. 1983. Life Sci. **33** (Suppl. 1): 685-688.
7. UPTON, N., R. D. E. SEWELL & P. S. J. SPENCER. 1982. Eur. J. Pharmacol. **78:** 421-429.
8. MARIĆ, D. & B. D. JANKOVIĆ. 1987. Fed. Proc. **46:** 1446.
9. SOÓS, J., I. BERZÉTEI, S. BAJUSZ & A. Z. PONAI. 1980. Life Sci. **27:** 129-133.
10. MAIGRET, B., S. PREMILAT, M.-C. FOURNIER-ZALUSKI & B. P. ROQUES. 1981. Biochem. Biophys. Res. Commun. **99:** 267-274.
11. CAMERMAN, N., D. MASTROPAOLO, A. CAMERMAN & J. KARLE. 1983. J. Neurochem. **41:** (Suppl.): 598A.

# Opioid Receptors on Murine Splenocytes

## Possible Coupling to K⁺ Channels

### D. J. J. CARR, J. K. BUBIEN, W. T. WOODS, AND J. E. BLALOCK

*Department of Physiology and Biophysics*
*University of Alabama at Birmingham*
*University Station*
*Birmingham, Alabama 35294*

Opioid peptides appear to mediate numerous effects on both *in vitro* and *in vivo* parameters of immunity including antibody production[1] and the generation of cytotoxic T lymphocytes.[2] In addition, high affinity, stereospecific opiate binding sites have been identified on cells of the immune system.[3] These observations led us to investigate the biochemical nature of opiate-specific receptors on murine splenocytes. By *in situ* cross-linking $^{125}$I-$\beta$-endorphin to murine brain or splenocyte membranes in the presence or absence of unlabeled naloxone and subsequently subjecting the labeled membrane extracts to sodium dodecyl sulfate polyacrylamide gel electrophoresis and autoradiography of the resultant gel, we determined a major binding chain of the splenic opiate receptor to have an apparent molecular weight of 46 kd and a less prominent binding chain to have an apparent molecular weight of 31 kd (FIG. 1, lane D). The labeling is specific, because in the presence of excess unlabeled naloxone, no bands are apparent (FIG. 1, lane C). It would appear that the $\beta$-endorphin binding chains on splenocytes may represent a subset of those observed in brain tissue (compare lanes A and D in FIG. 1).

In addition to demonstrating opiate receptor-like molecules on murine splenocytes, we also investigated second messenger pathways that may be affected by opiate peptides. One such pathway, ion channels, has been associated with cell activation and function. Of the ionic channels studied in immunocytes, K⁺ channels were described as being involved in T-cell activation[4] and natural killer cell cytolytic activity.[5] These findings led us to propose that this is a major ionic conductance in cells of the immune system and worthy of inquiring whether the opiate receptor-ligand interaction influenced its gating. Therefore, we applied the patch clamp technique[6] to study ion channel responses to the opiate peptide, $\beta$-endorphin. We identified a similar voltage-gated potassium conductance in murine T cells as has been identified in human T cells (FIG. 2, Part A). To test the hypothesis that $\beta$-endorphin modulation of immune function may be at least partly mediated through this type of channel, we added $\beta$-endorphin ($7 \times 10^{-7}$ M) to the solution bathing T cells that were undergoing continuous single channel conductance measurements. After 10 minutes of exposure to extracellular $\beta$-endorphin, the channel openings ceased (FIG. 2, Part B). After a 5-minute exposure to the opiate receptor antagonist naloxone ($1 \times 10^{-4}$ M), unitary openings with characteristics similar to the previous ones were observed (FIG. 2, Part C). These results indicate that $\beta$-endorphin on immunocytes (T cells), as on neurons,[7] reduces membrane $K^+$ conductance presumably by decreasing potassium channel openings in an opiate-receptor-specific manner.

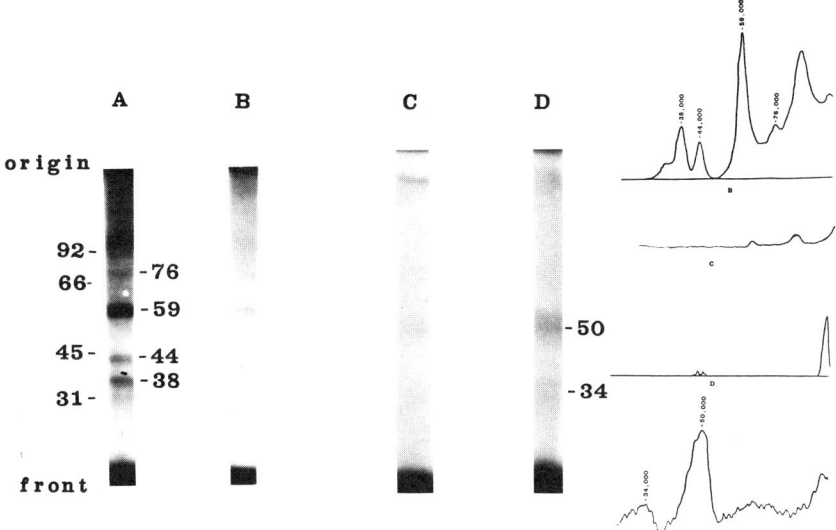

**FIGURE 1.** Autoradiographic analysis of $^{125}$I-$\beta$-endorphin cross-linked to mouse brain (lanes A and B) or spleen cells (lanes C and D). Membranes were prepared by homogenizing cells or tissue with a glass homogenizer (15-20 strokes) in 50 mM of $K_2HPO_4$ (pH 7.4) containing 1 mM of EDTA, 60 $\mu$g/ml of trasylol, 100 $\mu$g/ml of pepstatin, 100 $\mu$g/ml of leupeptin, and removing debris by centrifugation (100 $\times$ g, 5 minutes). Brain (250 $\mu$g) or spleen (1.25 mg) membranes were placed in 50 mM of $K_2HPO_4$ (pH 7.4) containing 50 $\mu$g/ml of bacitracin in a total volume of 1 ml. $^{125}$I-$\beta$-endorphin (Amersham) was added ($2.5 \times 10^{-9}$ M final concentration) in the presence or absence of unlabeled naloxone ($1 \times 10^{-4}$ M). After 1 hour of incubation at 25°C, excess ligand was removed (centrifugation, 800 $\times$ g), and membranes were washed twice in 50 mM of $K_2HPO_4$. Membranes were cross-linked using disuccinimidyl suberate (3 mM) on ice for 15 minutes before cross-linking was terminated with an equal volume (1 ml) of 0.1 M Tris-HCl, pH 7.4, 1 mM of EDTA. The labeled cross-linked membranes were subjected to SDS-polyacrylamide gel electrophoresis (11% acrylamide), and the resultant gels were dried and analyzed by autoradiography. Lane A is brain with $^{125}$I-$\beta$-endorphin. Lane B is lane A + naloxone. Lane D is spleen with $^{125}$I-$\beta$-endorphin. Lane C is lane D + naloxone. Densitometric analysis of each gel lane is shown to the right of the figure.

In conclusion, we have identified a splenic opiate-specific receptor composed of at least two binding chains. These polypeptides appear responsible for the recognition of ligands as well as the operation of certain ion channels, thus linking specific opiate receptor-ligand interactions with secondary messenger events. This further demonstrates the similarity in molecular responses to opiate peptides by immunocytes and neurons.

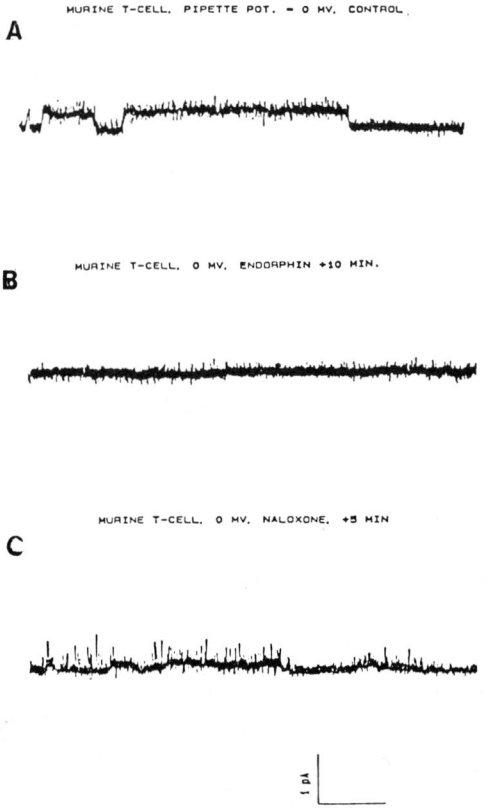

**FIGURE 2.** $\beta$-endorphin suppresses conductance in murine T cells, and the effect is partially naloxone-reversible. A patch of a prepared T-lymphocyte membrane was gigaohm sealed with a suction pipette containing 50 mM of $K^+$, 10 mM of $Na^+$, 0.004 mM of $Ca^{2+}$, 50 mM of gluconate, and 5 mM of Hepes, pH 7.0. The bathing solution was RPMI-1640 (2% fetal bovine serum) and the membrane was in the cell-attached configuration. Under the electrochemical $K^+$ gradient dictated by the pipette solution and the cytosol, outward currents were observed at 0 holding potential (Part A). After a 10-minute exposure of the cell to $\beta$-endorphin (7 $\times$ $10^{-7}$ M), all events ceased entirely (Part B). After this same cell was exposed to naloxone (1 $\times$ $10^{-4}$ M) for 5 minutes, partial reversal of the endorphin effect occurred (Part C). The effect of endorphin on T-cell channel conductance was observed in 10 of 13 cells recorded. The partial reversal by naloxone was observed in 2 of 5 cells recorded. By establishing current/voltage relations under different $K^+$ electrochemical gradients (i.e., using 50, 100, and 200 mM of $K^+$), we confirmed that the major conductance affected by $\beta$-endorphin was $K^+$, which appeared to be similar to $K^+$ channel conductances previously reported.[4]

## REFERENCES

1. JOHNSON, H. M., E. M. SMITH, B. A. TORRES & J. E. BLALOCK. 1982. Proc. Natl. Acad. Sci. USA **79**: 4171-4174.
2. CARR, D. J. J. & G. R. KLIMPEL. 1986. J. Neuroimmunol. **12**: 75-87.
3. LOPKER, A., L. G. ABOOD, W. HOSS & F. J. LIONETTI. 1980. Biochem. Pharmacol. **29**: 1361-1365.
4. DECOURSEY, T. E., K. G. CHANDY, S. GUPTA & M. D. CAHALAN. 1984. Nature **307**: 465-466.
5. SIDELL, N., L. C. SCHLICTER, S. C. WRIGHT, S. HAGIWARA & S. H. GOLUB. 1986. J. Immunol. **137**: 1650-1658.
6. NEHER, E. & B. SAKMANN. 1976. Nature **260**: 779-802.
7. CHANG, K. - J. 1984. *In* The Receptors, Vol. 1: 1-81. Academic Press, New York.

# Somatotropin and Prolactin Enhance Respiratory Burst Activity of Macrophages[a]

CARL K. EDWARDS, III,[b,c] JEANETTE M. SCHEPPER,[c] LIBBY M. YUNGER,[c] AND KEITH W. KELLEY [b]

[b] *Laboratory of Immunophysiology*
*University of Illinois*
*Urbana, Illinois 61801*

[c] *Research and Development Division*
*IMC Pitman-Moore Inc.*
*Terre Haute, Indiana 47808*

Macrophages elicited by injection of inflammatory agents or obtained from animals infected with intracellular parasites are primed so that they respond to phagocytosis of opsonized-zymosan (Op-Zym), with a marked increase in the respiratory burst NADPH oxidase system.[1] This capacity to increase the release of reactive oxygen metabolites, including superoxide anion ($O_2^-$), plays an important role in the enhanced microbicidal capacity of activated macrophages.[2] The possible neuroimmunomodulatory role of somatotropin (ST) and prolactin (PRL) in macrophage activation of mononuclear phagocytes *in vitro* has been addressed in our studies. Porcine peripheral blood monocyte-derived mononuclear phagocytes were obtained from healthy 10-week-old pigs and cultured overnight with increasing concentrations (1-1000 ng/ml) of pituitary-derived, native porcine prolactin (npPRL), native porcine ST (npST), or recombinant porcine ST (rpST). All three hormones at concentrations of 100 ng/ml and greater caused at least a tenfold increase in the production of $O_2^-$ (from 40 nmol of $O_2^-$/mg of protein per hour to > 700) after stimulation with Op-Zym. For comparison, mononuclear phagocytes that were exposed overnight to 10 EU/ml of lipopolysaccharide released 228 nmol $O_2^-$/mg of protein per hour. Concurrent incubation with specific antibodies to PRL and ST blocked more than 90% of the $O_2^-$ that was induced by their respective hormones. Experiments with porcine bronchoalveolar lung macrophages that were free of residual lymphocytes (> 98% α napthyl butyrate esterase positive) indicated that significantly higher amounts of $O_2^-$ (> 400 nmol $O_2^-$/mg of protein per hour) were released when either npST or rpST was included in the culture medium, and this effect was also blocked by a specific antibody to ST.

To date, gamma-interferon (IFN-γ) has been the most completely characterized substance known to be produced by mammalian cells that augments the production

---

[a]This work was supported in part by grants to K. W. K. from NIH AG06246-01, USDA 86-CRCR-;1-2003, and IMC Pitman-Moore, Inc. K-0503.

of reactive oxygen metabolites by macrophages. ST and PRL are synthesized by the adenohypophysis, and they may also be produced by activated lymphocytes.[3,4] Data in this report provide the first evidence that PRL and ST augment the production of $O_2^-$ by mononuclear phagocytes *in vitro*. Because macrophages are capable of exerting antimicrobial activities towards a wide range of intracellular pathogens *in vivo* through an enhanced respiratory burst, our current studies are focused on the *in vivo* effects of ST and PRL on other components of macrophage function and in animal disease models.

## REFERENCES

1. HAMILTON, T. A. & D. O. ADAMS. 1987. Immunol. Today **8**: 151.
2. ADAMS, D. O. & T. A. HAMILTON. 1984. Ann. Rev. Immunol. **2**: 283.
3. HIESTOOD, P. C., P. WLEKLER, R. NORDMAN, A. GRIEDER, & C. PERMMANGHAL. 1986. Proc. Natl. Acad. Sci. USA **83**: 1599.
4. MONTGOMERY, D. W., C. F. ZUKOSKI, G. N. SHAH, A. R. BUCKLEY, T. PACHOLCZYK, & O. H. RUSSELL. 1987. Biochem. Biophys. Res. Commun. **145**: 692.

# Effect of Sound Stress on the Migration of Prethymic Stem Cells[a]

CATHERINE E. BOMBERGER AND JACK L. HAAR

*Department of Anatomy*
*Medical College of Virginia*
*Richmond, Virginia 23298*

The thymus has been established as an essential organ for the normal development of immune function in young mammals. Recent evidence suggests that the thymus also plays an active role in the maintenance of the immune system through life.[1] To perform its role as a primary lymphoid organ, the thymus must attract extrinsic stem cells or prothymocytes. Precursor cells migrate from the bone marrow during the neonatal period throughout adulthood to carry out this function.[2,3]

A blind well assay system was developed to examine the "bone marrow-thymus axis" *in vitro*. It was used to demonstrate that a subset of murine bone marrow cells is capable of migrating through a Nuclepore membrane toward a supernatant derived from cultured newborn mouse thymuses. The migrated cells are enriched for a "null" cell population, that is, Thy 1 and surface immunoglobulin negative cells.[4] When injected into an irradiated host, these cells are capable of repopulating the thymus in a significantly higher percentage than do nonmigration-enriched bone marrow cells. This significant *in vivo* thymus homing suggests that selective migration to thymus supernatant enriches for a prethymic cell population.[5]

In the present study the effect of sound stress on the bone marrow-thymus axis was examined using the *in vitro* migration assay. Histologic sections and weights of thymus, spleen, and adrenal glands were also examined for alterations resulting from the sound stress.

Young adult female CBA/J mice were exposed to a 2-second, high intensity sound (110 db at 2900 Hz, variable interval of 1 minute) 2 hours daily for 5 days. Twenty-four hours later, the femurs and tibias were dissected from the animals; bone marrow cells were separated and suspended in media. *In vitro* migration assays were carried out using blind well chambers. Thymus supernatant from 3-day-old mice was used as the attractant in the bottom wells separated from the bone marrow cells in the top wells by Nuclepore membranes having 5-μm diameter pores. After 90 minutes of incubation, cells migrating to the bottom chambers were collected, counted, and compared to the number of migrated cells from the bone marrow of nonstressed mice. Migrations to Iscove's media alone were carried out simultaneously to calculate the nonspecific background migration.

The *in vitro* assay showed a significant decrease in the percentage of migration of bone marrow cells from experimental sound-stressed animals when compared with control nonstressed age-matched mice (TABLE 1). When thymus, spleen, and adrenal glands of the experimental animals were compared with those of the control animals, no significant changes in organ weights (TABLE 2) and no apparent histologic changes

[a]This study was supported by NIH grant 04384.

TABLE 1. *In Vitro* Migration Assay[a]

| Stress | | | Control | | |
|---|---|---|---|---|---|
| Supernatant | Media | Difference[b] | Supernatant | Media | Difference |
| 11.60 | 5.24 | 6.36 | 14.72 | 5.55 | 9.17 |
| 14.73 | 12.59 | 214 | 18.12 | 14.18 | 3.94 |
| 17.35 | 8.14 | 9.21 | 19.29 | 7.92 | 11.37 |
| 19.86 | 14.62 | 5.24 | 20.37 | 9.72 | 10.65 |
| 13.09 | 7.89 | 5.20 | 12.75 | 6.37 | 6.38 |
| 17.37 | 7.22 | 10.15 | 16.53 | 8.19 | 8.34 |
| 16.06 | 6.43 | 9.63 | 23.50 | 9.79 | 13.71 |
| 9.71 | 4.02 | 5.69 | 10.02 | 4.86 | 5.16 |
| | | (6.70) | | | (8.59) |

[a] % migration = no. cells migrated/$1 \times 10^6$ cells.
[b] Difference = supernatant-media. Using Student $t$ test, $p = 0.05$.

TABLE 2. Organ Weights (mg/g of mouse weight)[a]

| Organ | Stress | Control | Control/Stress Ratio |
|---|---|---|---|
| Thymus | 2.50 | 2.47 | .99 |
| Spleen | 3.21 | 3.04 | .95 |
| Adrenal | 0.494 | 0.494 | 1.00 |

[a] Values represent mean of 8 thymus and spleen weights and 6 adrenal weights.

were observed. These results suggest that the migration assay reflects alterations resulting from sound stress that occur before changes in the size and weight of lymphoid organs or adrenal glands are detectable.

Future studies will evaluate whether the production of prethymic stem cells is decreased in response to stress, or whether stem cell production remains unaltered while the capacity of these cells to migrate toward a thymus supernatant *in vitro* is affected.

## REFERENCES

1. SCOLLAY, R., J. SMITH & V. STAUFFER. 1986. Immunol. Rev. **91**: 129.
2. FORD, E. C., H. S. MICKLER, E. P. EVANS, J. G. GRAY & D. A. OGDEN. 1966. Ann. N.Y. Acad. Sci. **129**: 283.
3. ROSSE, C. 1981. *In* The Handbook of Cancer Immunology, Vol. 6. H. Waters, Ed.: 251. Garland STPM Press, New York.
4. HAAR, J. L. & F. LOOR. 1981. Thymus **3**: 187.
5. HAAR, J. L., W. M. GROGAN, J. D. POPP & J. K. TAUBENBERGER. 1987. Cell Tissue Kin. **20**: 227.

# Interaction of Endogenous Opioids and Developing T Lymphocytes

DELANE BAILEY, LEONOR GONZALES, AND
MARIE METLAY

*SUNY College at Old Westbury*
*Department of Biological Sciences*
*Old Westbury, New York 11568*

Data from several fields of study have established a definite link between the central nervous system (CNS) and the immune system. T lymphocytes were shown to possess receptors for the opioids; in addition, administration of the drugs alters the normal complement of these cells in the circulation.

To date the major emphasis of work in this field has centered on the interaction of circulating or mature T lymphocytes with the neural peptides. We were specifically interested in quantifying the endogenous levels of the opioids that are bound to receptors of thymocytes (developing T lymphocytes) and correlating these levels with specific subclasses of T lymphocytes. The neural peptides that were studied include beta-endorphin and (met)- and (leu)-enkephalin. All analyses employed thymus from normal, untreated, RF/J mice. The level(s) of both the typical T-cell markers and endogenous opioids bound to receptors was monitored by flow cytometry using a Becton Dickinson FACS Analyzer.

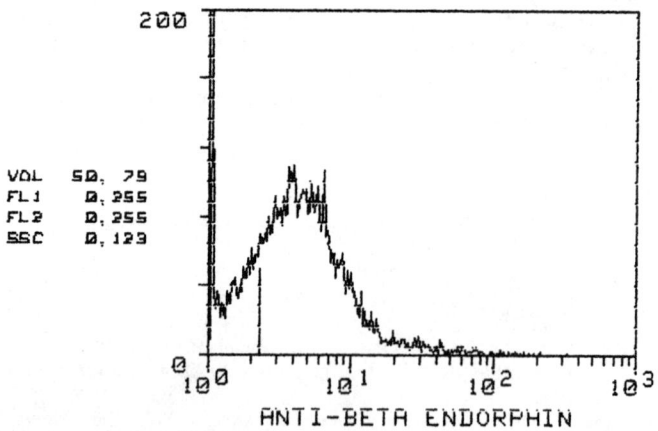

**FIGURE 1.** FACS histogram of thymocytes stained in a two-step process with rabbit antibody to beta-endorphin followed by FITC-conjugated antibody to rabbit. The $X$ axis is in fluorescent units and divisions on the $Y$ axis represent the number of cells.

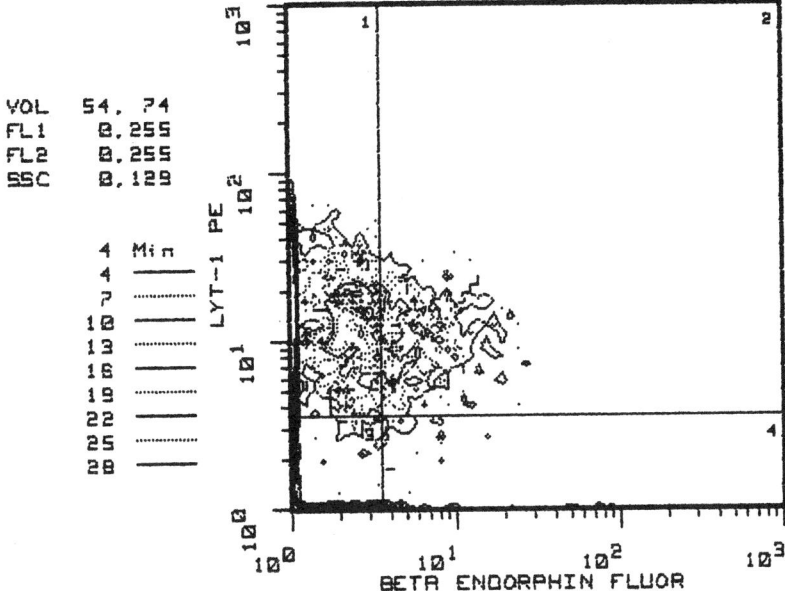

**FIGURE 2.** FACS contour graph of thymocytes stained with both fluoresceinated anti-beta-endorphin and phycoerythrein-conjugated anti-Lyt-1. The cells are scatter gated to include only lymphocytes in the analysis.

In normal untreated mice the detectable level of beta-endorphin bound to receptors on thymocytes was found to vary among individual mice, but was as high as 75%. FIGURE 1 depicts a representative histogram of the levels of antibody to beta-endorphin bound to thymocytes from a normal mouse. Negative cells (to the left of the marker) were defined as those cells whose fluorescence fell within the range observed for 95% of the background controls. In this histogram 70% of the cells stain positive for antibody to beta-endorphin. The variability that is observed in levels of bound opioid is not age related and in fact can be observed between litter mates. The measurable levels of (met)- and (leu)-enkephalins were always lower than that of beta-endorphin (data not shown).

To simultaneously monitor the level of T-cell markers expressed on the surface of the thymocytes and the amount of opioid bound to receptors on these thymocytes, two-color analyses were performed. FIGURE 2 is a contour graph that correlates the levels of antibody to Lyt-1 and beta-endorphin on the cell surface. Statistical analysis of this graph (data not shown) reveals that nearly all cells that have beta-endorphin bound to cell surface receptors are positive for the T-cell marker Lyt-1; however, 48% of the cells that are positive for Lyt-1 are not positive for beta-endorphin. This suggests that a specific subset of Lyt-1 positive cells may be positive for the opioids. This phenomenon is presently being investigated in this laboratory.

# Neuroendocrine Regulation of Immune Parameters

## Photoperiod Control of the Spleen in Syrian Hamsters

### GEORGE C. BRAINARD, MARCIA WATSON-WHITMEYER, ROBERT L. KNOBLER, AND FRED D. LUBLIN

*Department of Neurology*
*Jefferson Medical College*
*Philadelphia, Pennsylvania 19107*
*and*
*Department of Biology*
*School of Life and Health Sciences*
*University of Delaware*
*Newark, Delaware 19716*

A new approach for investigating the mechanism of neural regulation of immune function uses the interaction of photoperiodism with immune parameters.[1] Most species have evolved adaptations for seasonal fluctuations in temperature, day length, food availability, and rainfall. Hence, there are seasonal fluctuations in behavior, physiology, and morphology in nearly all mammals.[5] The primary environmental signal that controls seasonal physiology is the ambient photoperiod. Recently, it was shown that photoperiod triggers changes in reproductive status and selected parameters of the immune system. Hamsters exposed to artificial wintertime photoperiods (10 hours light and 14 hours dark; LD 10:14) had significantly higher spleen weights, splenic lymphocyte, and macrophage counts as compared to hamsters exposed to summertime photoperiods (LD 14:10). In contrast, photoperiod had no significant effect on thymus weight or antibody production.[2] The purpose of this study was to examine if the pineal gland mediates the effects of photoperiod on the immune system, because the pineal gland regulates photoperiod-reproductive responses.

Groups of adult Syrian hamsters were exposed to a long photoperiod (LD 14:10), a short photoperiod (LD 10:14), or a short photoperiod (LD 10:14) after pinealectomy. After 14 weeks of exposure, the animals were sacrificed and the testes, spleens, and thymus glands were weighed. Data were analyzed by one-way ANOVA and Student Newman-Keuls test.

Hamsters maintained in a long photoperiod had high testicular weights, whereas hamsters kept in a short photoperiod had low testes weights. Pinealectomized hamsters in a short photoperiod were reproductively active and had high testicular weights. Testicular weights of intact animals in a short photoperiod were significantly lower

($p$ <0.001) than those of the other two groups (FIG. 1). There were no significant differences in thymus weight among the three groups. The spleens of short photoperiod, intact animals were significantly heavier ($p$ <0.001) than the spleens of the other two groups (FIG. 2).

These data confirm earlier observations that photoperiod can modify spleen weight[1,4,6,7] and that the pineal gland mediates the photoperiod-induced change in spleen weight. The pineal gland mediates the effects of photoperiod in the reproductive axis by its hormone, melatonin, which signals other components of the reproductive axis about the external photoperiod.[5] The pineal gland may affect spleen weight and

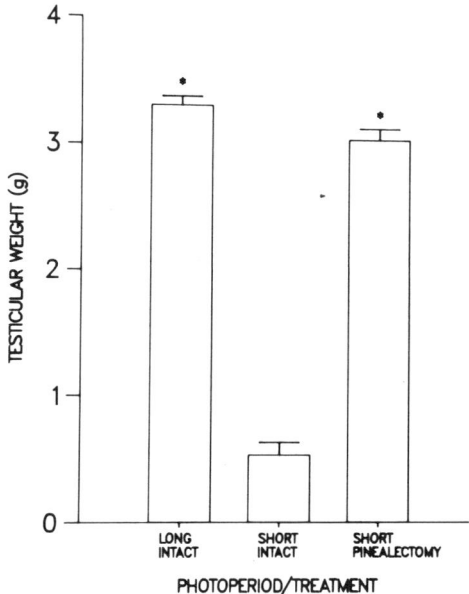

**FIGURE 1.** Mean ± standard error of the mean testicular weights of intact immunized male Syrian hamsters or pinealectomized animals in simulated winter (short) or summer (long) photoperiods for 14 weeks. The *asterisk* indicates $p$ <0.001 versus short-photoperiod intact animals.

other immune parameters by direct action of melatonin or indirectly by melatonin's action on the reproductive system. Male hamsters in short photoperiods have decreased prolactin and testosterone levels.[2,5] Sex steroids and pituitary hormones have been known to influence immune tissues.[3] The mechanism by which photoperiod influences the spleen remains to be clarified.

In conclusion, this report establishes that the pineal gland directly or indirectly mediates the effects of environmental photoperiod on the spleen. Photoperiodically sensitive mammals are an excellent model for clarifying the interactions of the neuroendocrine and immune system.

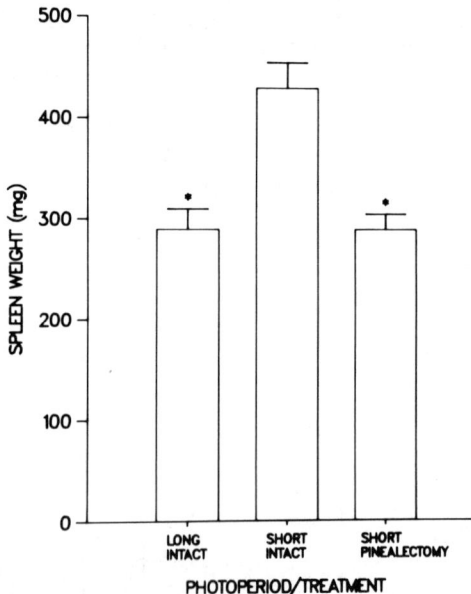

**FIGURE 2.** Mean ± standard error of the mean spleen weights of intact immunized male Syrian hamsters or pinealectomized animals in simulated winter (short) or summer (long) photoperiods for 14 weeks. The *asterisk* indicates $p < 0.001$ versus short-photoperiod intact animals.

## REFERENCES

1. BRAINARD, G. C., R. L. KNOBLER, P. L. PODOLIN, M. LAVASA & F. D. LUBLIN. 1987a. Life Sci. **40:** 1319-1326.
2. BRAINARD, G. C., M. K. VAUGHAN & R. J. REITER. 1987b. Endocrinology **119:** 648-654.
3. GROSSMAN, C. J. 1984. Endocrine Rev. **5:** 435-455.
4. HOFFMAN, R. A., K. DAVIDSON & K. STEINBERG. 1982. Growth **46:** 150-162.
5. REITER, R. J. 1980. Endocrinol. Rev. **1:** 109-131.
6. VAUGHAN, M. K., G. B. HUBBARD, T. H. CHAMPNEY, G. M. VAUGHAN, J. C. LITTLE & R. J. REITER. 1987. Am. J. Anat. **179:** 131-136.
7. VRIEND, J. & J. K. LAUBER. 1973. Nature **244:** 37-38.

# Sympathectomy Augments the Severity of Experimental Allergic Encephalomyelitis in Rats[a]

EWA CHELMICKA-SCHORR,[b,c,d,e] MARGARET CHECINSKI,[b,d] AND BARRY G. W. ARNASON [b,d]

[b]*Department of Neurology,* [c]*Pediatrics, and*
[d]*The Brain Research Institute*
*University of Chicago*
*Chicago, Illinois*

We previously showed that ablation of the peripheral sympathetic nervous system of adult (axotomy) or neonatal (sympathectomy) mice with 6-hydroxydopamine hydrobromide is followed by significant enhancement of antibody response by spleen cells to thymus-independent antigen, a decrease in the population of splenic B lymphocytes, an increase in the number of suppressor lymphocytes within the spleen, and an increase in the number of $\beta$-adrenergic receptors on spleen lymphocytes.[1-3] We now report on the influence of sympathectomy on the severity of allergic experimental encephalomyelitis (EAE) in Lewis rats.

Lewis rats were sympathectomized by injecting newborns with 6-hydroxydopamine (6OH-DA) intraperitoneally for 10 days at a dose of 150 $\mu g/g$ of body weight per day. 6OH-DA was dissolved in 0.9% NaCl containing 0.1 mg/ml of ascorbic acid as an antioxidant. Control mice were injected with 0.9% NaCl containing 0.1 mg/ml of ascorbic acid.

Six to 8-week-old sympathectomized or control rats were immunized with 20% guinea pig brain and spinal cord homogenate in complete Freund's adjuvant injected into foot pad (0.1, 0.05, or 0.03 cc). Four experiments were performed. Results were comparable and data have been pooled.

Clinical disease was assessed as 1+ mild paresis; 2+ paraparesis; 3+ tetraplegia and/or death. In two experiments, surviving animals were killed between 17 and 23 days after immunization and autopsied. Histology was read by one of us blindly, and histologic lesions were scored as follows: 0 if no lesion was seen, 1+ mild, 2+ moderate, and 3+ severe. Difference between groups was calculated using the Chi-square test. Animals sympathectomized at birth had more severe clinical disease than did controls. Thirty-three of 43 sympathectomized rats (76.7%) versus 14 of 32 controls (43.3%) developed severe (3+) clinical EAE. The difference is significant at $p$ value < 0.01. Severity of the histologic lesion did not differ between experimental and control animals (TABLE 1).

---

[a]This work was supported by a gift from the Lucille P. Markey Charitable-Trust to B.G.A. and NIH grant NINCDS to E.C.S., NS-18413.

[e]To whom all correspondence should be addressed.

The work presented here supports the hypothesis that interactions occur between the sympathetic nervous system (SNS) and immune system. There is compelling evidence that SNS modulated the immune response in living animals. The presence of SNS innervation has been documented in lymph nodes, spleen, thymus, and Peyer's patches.[4-6] It was also shown that lymphocytes possess $\beta$-adrenergic receptors and that adrenergic ligands affect lymphocyte stimulation.[7,8] EAE is a T-cell-mediated disease. Helper T cells most likely play a primary role in tissue destruction, but disease severity is also influenced by suppressor T cells. Because suppressor cells have more $\beta$-adrenergic receptor than helper cells, the augmented severity of EAE observed after sympathetic ablation could be a result of altered suppressor cell activity due to lack of adrenergic input.

TABLE 1. Effect of Sympathectomy on EAE in Rats

| Group | Clinical Disease[a,b] | | | | | Histologic Disease[c,d] | | | |
|---|---|---|---|---|---|---|---|---|---|
| | 0 | + | ++ | +++ | | 0 | + | ++ | +++ |
| Control | 3 | 1 | 14 | 14 | B | 1 | 8 | 5 | 0 |
| | | | | | SC | 0 | 4 | 6 | 4 |
| Sympathectomized | 0 | 5 | 5 | 33 | B | 5 | 8 | 6 | 3 |
| | | | | | SC | 3 | 7 | 7 | 5 |

Abbreviations: B = brain; SC = spinal cord.
[a] Four experiments (32 control and 43 sympathectomized animals).
[b] Difference significant at $p < 0.01$ (Chi-square method).
[c] Two experiments (14 control and 22 sympathectomized animals).
[d] Difference was not significant for brain and spinal cord.

## REFERENCES

1. MILES, K., J. QUINTANS, E. CHELMICKA-SCHORR & B. G. W. ARNASON. The sympathetic nervous system modulates antibody response to thymus-independent antigens. J. Neuroimmunol. 1981. **1:** 101.
2. MILES, K., S. ATWEH, G. OTTEN, B. G. W. ARNASON & E. CHELMICKA-SCHORR. 1984a. $\beta$-adrenergic receptors on splenic lymphocytes from axotomized mice. Int. J. Immunopharmacol. **6:** 171.
3. MILES, K., E. CHELMICKA-SCHORR, S. ATWEH, G. OTTEN & B. G. W. ARNASON. Sympathetic ablation alters lymphocyte membrane properties. 1985. J. Immunol. **6:** 135.
4. GIRON, L. T., K. A. CRUTCHER & J. N. DAVIS. 1980. Lymph nodes—a possible site for sympathetic neuronal regulation of immune responses. Ann. Neurol. **8:** 520-525.
5. REILLY, F. D., R. S. MCCUSKEY & H. A. MEINEKE. 1976. Studies of the hemopoietic microenvironment. VIII. Adrenergic and cholinergic innervation of the murine spleen. Anat. Rec. **105:** 100.
6. WILLIAMS, J. M., R. G. PETERSON, P. A. SHEA, J. F. SCHMEDTJE, D. C. BAUER & D. L. FELTEN. 1981. Sympathetic innervation of murine thymus and spleen: Evidence for a functional link between the nervous and immune systems. Brain. Res. Bull. **83:** 91.
7. HADDEN, J. W. 1975. Cyclic nucleotides in lymphocyte function. Ann. N. Y. Acad. Sci. **256:** 352-363.
8. WILLIAMS, L. T., R. SNYDERMAN & R. J. LEFKOWITZ. 1976. Identification of $\beta$-adrenergic receptors in human lymphocytes by $(-)$ $^3$H-alprenolol binding. J. Clin. Invest. **57:** 149-155.

WORKSHOP 16. AUTOIMMUNE MODELS OF DEMYELINATION

# Susceptibility to PLP-Induced EAE Is Regulated by Non-H-2 Genes[a]

VINCENT K. TUOHY,[b,c] RAYMOND A. SOBEL,[d,e] AND MARJORIE B. LEES[b,c]

[b]Department of Biochemistry
E. K. Shriver Center
Waltham, Massachusetts 02254

Departments of [c]Neurology and [d]Pathology
Harvard Medical School
Boston, Massachusetts 02115

[e]Department of Pathology
Massachusetts General Hospital
Boston, Massachusetts 02114

Genetic regulation of susceptibility to myelin basic protein (MBP)-induced experimental allergic encephalomyelitis (EAE) has been mapped to the I-region of the H-2 complex in the mouse,[1,2] whereas control of susceptibility to EAE induced with whole spinal cord homogenate appears to be polygenic involving the K-region of H-2[3] as well as non-H-2 linked factors.[4-6]

The purpose of this study was to determine the role of H-2 and non-H-2 genes in the control of susceptibility to PLP-induced EAE in mice. Our approach involved the determination of susceptibility in strains of mice representing the major nonrecombinant H-2 haplotypes and in substrains within a susceptible strain. Female mice received two subcutaneous abdominal injections 1 week apart of 200 $\mu$g bovine PLP and Freund's adjuvant supplemented with *Mycobacteria tuberculosis*.

All strains of mice tested developed EAE, but the clinical and histopathologic expression of the disease varied considerably among the different strains (TABLE 1). Fifteen of 17 SJL (H-2$^s$) mice developed acute EAE, as evidenced by clinical signs of tail and hind limb paralysis 16-31 days after immunization. The histologic profile of the mice correlated well with the clinical severity of the disease and consisted of parenchymal perivascular infiltrates of mononuclear and polymorphonuclear leukocytes with the most severe pathology generally in the spinal cord. Half the recovered mice exhibited a relapsing form of the disease. Nylon wool-enriched T cells from inguinal lymph nodes of diseased animals responded by $^3$H-thymidine incorporation to PLP but were unresponsive to rabbit, human, rat, mouse, and bovine MBP. Control animals showed no clinical or histologic disease, and their lymph node cells were unresponsive to PLP.

In contrast to the acute form of EAE observed in SJL (H-2$^s$) mice, the other strains tested showed a slowly progressive chronic form of the disease, requiring 7-21

---

[a]This work was supported by NIH grants NS 16945, NS 13649, HD 04147, and National Multiple Sclerosis Society Grant RG 1792-A.

TABLE 1. Susceptibility of Various Strains of Mice to PLP-Induced EAE

| Strain | H-2 | Mice with Clinical and Histologic EAE | Mice with Histologic EAE | Day of Disease Onset |
|---|---|---|---|---|
| SJL | s | 15/17 | 17/17 | 16-31 |
| BALB/c[a] | d | 4/10 | 8/10 | 30-88 |
| AKR | k | 4/9 | 5/9 | 49-122 |
| C57BL/6 | b | 3/10 | 4/10 | 117-147 |
| DBA/1 | q | 3/9 | 6/9 | 95-140 |

[a] BALB/cAnNCrlBR mice from Charles River Laboratories, Wilmington, Massachusetts.

weeks to develop. Both clinical and histologic disease was observed in 4 of 9 AKR (H-2$^k$), 4 of 10 BALB/cAnNCr1BR (H-2$^d$), 3 of 9 DBA/1 (H-2$^q$), and 3 of 10 C57BL/6 (H-2$^b$) mice. Several other strains with the $k$ haplotype, namely, CBA, C3H, C57BR/cd, and B10.BR, were similarly affected. Within six other substrains of BALB/c (H-2$^d$) mice tested (TABLE 2), the incidence of disease varied markedly from almost complete susceptibility (BALB/cPt) to total resistance (BALB/cWt and BALB/cORNL).

Although H-2 genes may play a role in determining the clinical and histologic expression of disease, these data indicate that the primary control of susceptibility to PLP-induced EAE is not H-2 determined. The varied clinical, histologic, and genetic factors involved in PLP-induced EAE in mice may be comparable to the expression of multiple sclerosis in humans.

TABLE 2. Susceptibility of BALB/c Substrains to PLP-Induced EAE

| BALB/c Substrain | Mice with Clinical and Histologic EAE | Mice with Histologic EAE | Day of Disease Onset |
|---|---|---|---|
| BALB/cPt[a] | 8/9 | 8/9 | 42-78 |
| BALB/cJ | 2/8 | 4/8 | 85-121 |
| BALB/Ka[b] | 2/9 | 2/9 | 110-140 |
| BALB/cByJ | 3/9 | 3/9 | 92-112 |
| BALB/cWt[a] | 0/9 | 0/9 | ... |
| BALB/cORNL[a] | 0/10 | 0/10 | ... |

[a] Supplied by Dr. Michael Potter, Laboratory of Genetics, NCI, NIH, Bethesda, Maryland.
[b] Supplied by the Department of Therapeutic Radiation, Division of Radiation Biology, Stanford University, Palo Alto, California.

## REFERENCES

1. FRITZ, R. B., M. J. SKEEN, C.-H. J. CHOU, M. GARCIA & I. K. EGOROV. 1985. J. Immunol. **134:** 2328.
2. PERRY, L. L. & M. E. BARZAGA. 1987. J. Immunol. **138:** 1434.
3. BERNARD, C. C. A. 1976. J. Immunogenet. **3:** 63.
4. LINTHICUM, D. S. & J. A. FRELINGER. 1982. J. Exp. Med. **155:** 31.
5. MONTGOMERY, I. N. & H. C. RAUCH. 1982. J. Immunol. **128:** 421.
6. KNOBLER, R. L., D. S. LINTHICUM & M. COHN. 1985. J. Neuroimmunol. **8:** 15.

# Oligodendrocyte Proliferation and Enhanced CNS Remyelination after Therapeutic Manipulation of Chronic Relapsing EAE[a]

## C. S. RAINE, R. HINTZEN, U. TRAUGOTT, AND G. R. W. MOORE

*Departments of Pathology (Neuropathology),
Neurology and Neuroscience
Albert Einstein College of Medicine
Bronx, New York 10461*

Previous works on autoimmune demyelination from these laboratories demonstrated that (a) combinations of myelin lipids and myelin basic protein (MBP) are required to effect demyelination and (b) when strain 13 guinea pigs with chronic relapsing experimental allergic encephalomyelitis (EAE) induced by whole spinal cord in adjuvant are treated with MBP combined with galactocerebroside (GC), clinical improvement and extensive remyelination of spinal cord lesions are observed.[1,2] Remyelinated lesions showed a decrease in inflammatory activity and widespread proliferation of oligodendrocytes. Similar but less extensive proliferation has been described in multiple sclerosis in the absence of intervention.[3] The present study examines different regions of the central nervous system (CNS) for this phenomenon during EAE after MBP/GC treatment with a view to elucidating the origin of the remyelinating cells.

In short-term (2-5 month) treated animals with EAE, there was a marked increase in the number of oligodendrocytes within remyelinated areas (FIG. 1). These cells were identified by morphologic (light and electron microscope) and immunocytochemical (anti-MBP, anti-GC, and anticarbonic anhydrase antisera and peroxidase labeling) criteria. Suggestive evidence was found for cells having been derived by mitotic division from surviving parenchymal oligodendrocytes and by differentiation from perivascular glial cell precursors. To support the latter was the observation of clustered oligodendrocytes within layers of perivascular astrocytes at the perimeter of white matter fascicles in optic nerve tissue, regions normally not populated by oligodendrocytes. Morphometric analysis of optic nerves from normal, treated, and untreated animals showed that the oligodendrocyte to astrocyte ratio was 1.64:1, 1.09:1, and 0.64:1, respectively. The decreased ratio in treated animals despite a significant increase in the number of oligodendrocytes was found to be a reflection of a persistent increase in fibrous astrocytes occurring during active disease. In some lesions, cells with the phenotype of fibrous astrocytes had the ultrastructural features

---

[a] This work was supported in part by HHS grants NS 08952 and NS 11920; and NMSS grants RG 1001-F-6 and 1634-A-1.

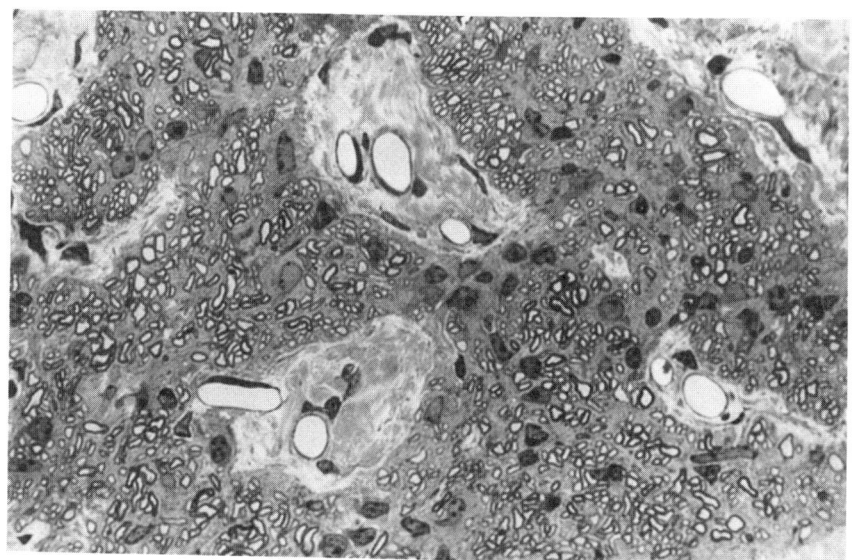

**FIGURE 1.** In this section of optic nerve from a strain 13 guinea pig with chronic relapsing EAE treated with myelin basic protein and galactocerebroside, note the widespread CNS remyelination evidenced by the many thinly myelinated fibers, the high number of glial cells, most of which are oligodendrocytes (darker nuclei with clumped heterochromatin), and fibrotic changes around blood vessels. Astrocytes (larger, paler nuclei) are also visible. Chronic relapsing EAE, 13.5 months after inoculation with spinal cord tissue in adjuvant, 6 months after treatment with MBP/GC. One micron epoxy section stained with toluidine blue. (Original magnification × 300.)

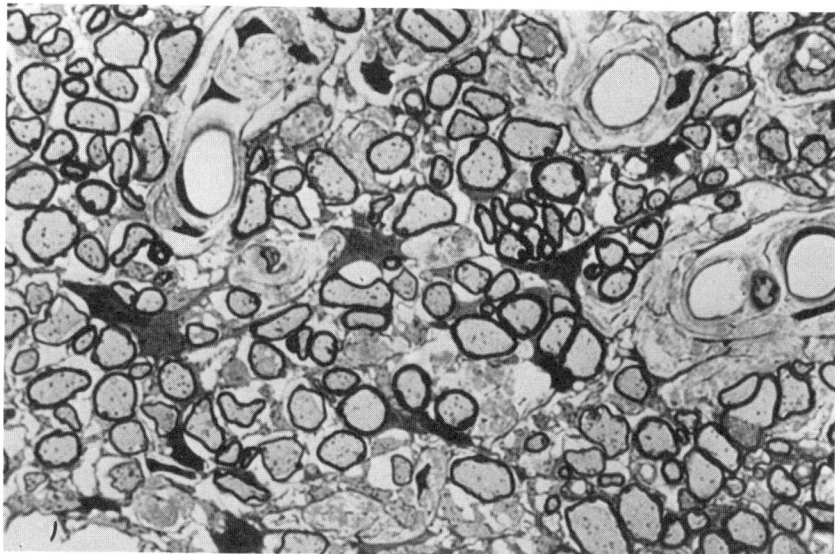

**FIGURE 2.** In a thinly remyelinated spinal cord lesion from an MBP/GC-treated animal, note the spider-like cells extending processes towards nerve fibers. By immunocytochemistry and ultrastructure, these cells possessed features of both astrocytes and oligodendrocytes. Extensive parenchymal collagen deposition and perivascular fibrosis are also evident. Chronic relapsing EAE 10 months after inoculation; 4.5 months after treatment. (Original magnification × 750.)

of both astrocytes and oligodendrocytes and appeared to be involved in myelination (FIG. 2).

The data suggest that cells ostensibly indistinguishable from fibrous astrocytes might under certain conditions differentiate into myelinating oligodendrocytes. We believe this reparatory process to be the result of the down-regulation of an MBP-specific T-cell response and the production of anti-GC antibodies that have a stimulatory effect upon oligodendrocytes.[4] A similar effect was observed in mice with Theiler's virus-induced encephalomyelitis that were either treated with MBP/GC directly or injected with hyperimmune antisera to white matter.[5,6] In this latter model also, antibody to GC was implicated in oligodendrocyte stimulation. The present approach may have relevance to the therapy of multiple sclerosis.

## REFERENCES

1. TRAUGOTT, U., S. H. STONE & C. S. RAINE. 1982. J. Neurol. Sci. **56:** 65-73.
2. RAINE, C. S. & U. TRAUGOTT. 1983. Lab. Invest. **48:** 275-284.
3. RAINE, C. S., L. C. SCHEINBERG & J. M. WALTZ. 1981. Lab. Invest. **45:** 534-546.
4. RAINE, C. S. 1984. Lab. Invest. **50:** 608-635.
5. LANG, W., M. RODRIGUEZ, V. A. LENNON & P. W. LAMPERT. 1984. Ann. N.Y. Acad. Sci. **436:** 98-102.
6. RODRIGUEZ, M., V. A. LENNON, E. N. BENVENISTE & J. E. MERRILL. 1987. J. Neuropathol. Exp. Neurol. **46:** 84-95.

# Effects of OX8+ Lymphocytes on *in Vitro* Lymphocyte Reactivity During Experimental Allergic Encephalomyelitis

D. M. ESSAYAN, J. A. COHEN, B. ZWEIMAN, AND
R. P. LISAK

*University of Pennsylvania
School of Medicine
Philadelphia, Pennsylvania*

It has been postulated that the usually self-limited course of acute experimental allergic encephalomyelitis (EAE) in the Lewis rat induced by sensitization to myelin basic protein (MBP) is due in major part to the effects of a suppressor T cell.[1,2] There is an increased frequency of OX8+ (putative suppressor) cells in the lymphoid cell accumulation in the CNS of such recovered rats.[3] To test the hypothesis that such OX8+ cells do modulate lymphocyte responses to MBP, we investigated the effects of OX8+ cells on the *in vitro* proliferative responses to MBP and a control (EAE-irrelevant) antigen of lymphocytes obtained during clinically manifest EAE.

## MATERIALS AND METHODS

Draining lymph node cells were obtained from Lewis rats with clinically manifest EAE 12 days after injection of 50 µg MBP and 1 LF tetanus toxoid (TT) in complete Freund's adjuvant (CFA) as previously reported by us.[4] Using monoclonal antibodies against rat lymphocyte subsets, cell aliquots were depleted by panning of: (a) only B (OX12+) cells; and (b) OX12+ and OX8+ cells. To replicate cultures containing 50,000 W3/25+ helper) cells and sufficient irradiated syngeneic thymocytes (as antigen presenters and feeder cells to make a total of 200,000 cells) were added: (a) MBP (30 µg/ml); (b) TT (2 Lfu/ml); and (c) diluent (negative control). Incorporation of treated thymidine was assessed 4 days later. Pokeweed-mitogen-induced secretion of anti-MBP and anti-TT antibodies was determined over 7 days by these cultured cells by ELISA, as reported previously by us.[5,6]

## RESULTS

Draining node cells previously depleted of OX8+ cells from 28 ± 4% to 3 ± 1% (TABLE 1) did not proliferate to either MBP or TT to a greater extent than did

TABLE 1. Phenotype Profiles in Day 12 Rat Lymph Node Cells

| Markers | Phenotype | OX12+ Cells Depleted | OX12+ and OX8+ Cells Depleted |
|---|---|---|---|
| 3W/25 | Helper T | 75 ± 2[a] | 94 ± 1 |
| OX8 | Suppressor/cytotoxic T | 28 ± 4 | 3 ± 1 |
| OX19 | Pan - T | 94 ± 1 | 97 ± 1 |
| OX12 | B | 3 ± 1 | 4 ± 1 |
| OKT$_4$ | Human CD$_4$ (neg. control) | 2 ± 1 | 1 ± 1 |

[a] Mean ± SEM percentage of cells expressing the particular phenotypic marker.

aliquots of the same cells not depleted of OX8+. This lack of difference was seen whether the degree of proliferation was estimated by a stimulation index or differences in mean counts per minute (cpm) between cultures with and without antigen (TABLE 2). Because there was considerable variation among animals in the degree of antigen-induced proliferation, a ratio of responses in OX8+-depleted and OX8+-nondepleted cells is shown in TABLE 2.

Following culture with pokeweed mitogen for 7 days, the OX8+-depleted and OX8+-nondepleted node cells from three animals secreted similar amounts of anti-MBP and anti-TT antibodies. There was little antibody secretion by cells cultured without pokeweed mitogen.

## DISCUSSION

These findings suggest that OX8+ cells do not inhibit antigen-induced proliferative responses or antibody secretion in node cells obtained during clinically manifest EAE.

TABLE 2. Comparison of the Proliferative Response to MBP or TT of OX8-Depleted Lymph Node Cells to That of Non-OX8-Depleted Cells[a]

| | Ratio of SI[b] Without OX8/With OX8 | | Ratio of Δ cpm[c] Without OX8[a]/With OX8 | |
|---|---|---|---|---|
| Animal | MBP | TT | MBP | TT |
| BT 6.128 | 0.4 | 1.4 | 0.6 | 2.1 |
| BT 6.139,40 | 1.5 | 1.0 | 1.1 | 0.7 |
| BT 6.155,57 | 0.6 | 0.7 | 0.7 | 0.8 |
| BT 6.158,60 | 0.6 | 1.0 | 0.7 | 1.1 |
| BT 6.161,63 | 1.2 | 1.7 | 0.6 | 0.9 |

[a] All aliquots were also depleted of B cells (OX12+) and contained added antigen-presenting cells.

[b] SI (stimulation index) = mean cpm in MBP-containing cultures/mean cpm in control cultures.

[c] Δ CPM = mean cpm in MBP-containing cultures minus mean cpm in control cultures.
SI without OX8 vs SI with OX8, $p = 0.3$.
Δ cpm without OX8 vs cpm with OX8, $p = 0.1$.

Studies of cells obtained at other time points are underway. It is possible that the OX8$^+$ cells found in the CNS during EAE may have suppressor activities not found in lymph node cells. Therefore, we will use our technique for isolating lymphocytes from the EAE-involved spinal cord[4] to investigate this possibility. Another possibility is that the suppressor cell activity in this setting is not concentrated in the OX8$^+$ cell subpopulation. Of course, the relation of any *in vitro* findings to the *in vivo* events leading to remission of acute EAE has to be resolved, with the possibility that other modulatory factors are involved.

## REFERENCES

1. ADDA, D. H., E. BERAUD & H. DEPIEDS. 1975. Eur. J. Immunol. **7:** 620.
2. WELCH, A. M., J. H. HOLDA & R. H. SWANBORG 1980. J. Immunol. **125:** 6.
3. HICKEY, W. F. & N. K. GONATAS. 1984. Cell Immunol. **85:** 284.
4. COHEN, J. A., D. M. ESSAYAN, B. ZWEIMAN & R. P. LISAK. 1987. Cell Immunol. **108:** 203.
5. ZWEIMAN, B., A. R. MOSKOVITZ, A. M. RASTAMI *et al.* 1982. J. Neuroimmunol. **2:** 331.
6. SANDBERG-WOLLHERM, M., B. ZWEIMAN, A. I. LEVINSON *et al.* 1986. J. Neuroimmunol. **11:** 205.

# Evidence for an Immunosuppressive Autoantibody in Experimental Allergic Encephalomyelitis

## IAIN A. M. MacPHEE AND DONALD W. MASON

*MRC Cellular Immunology Unit*
*Sir William Dunn School of Pathology*
*University of Oxford*
*Oxford OX1 3RE, England*

Lewis rats immunized with myelin basic protein (MBP) in complete Freund's adjuvant experience a single episode of paralysis and after recovery are refractory to further disease induction.[1] The processes bringing about this refractory state, which may be similar to those involved in the remissions observed in multiple sclerosis, are still poorly understood. Here we examine in EAE the possible role of an immunoregulatory autoantibody found in convalescent animals.

We consistently failed to adoptively transfer refractoriness to EAE with T lymphocytes, but serum from convalescent animals is a potent inhibitor of clinical signs (FIG. 1). This suppression is also seen when serum is transferred from animals immunized with whole brain homogenate in complete Freund's adjuvant.[2] Although

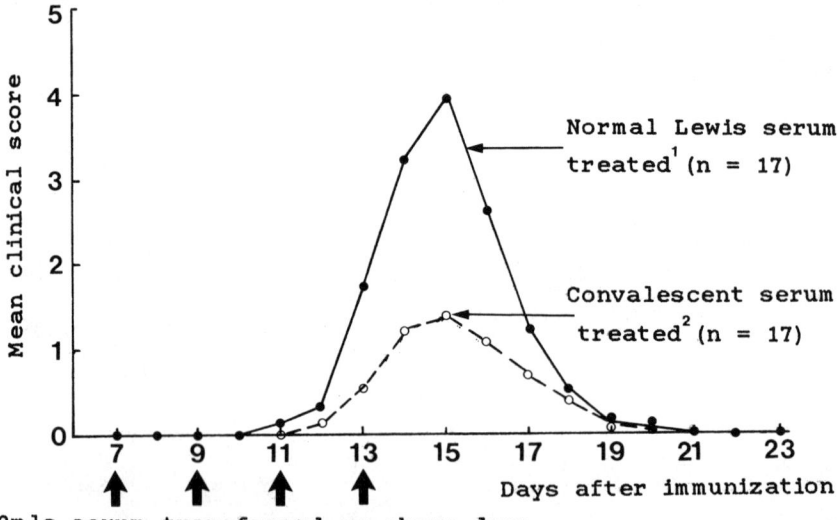

**FIGURE 1.** Suppression of experimental allergic encephalomyelitis by adoptive transfer of serum from convalescent animals. Data are pooled from four separate experiments using three different batches of serum. By Wilcoxon's rank sum test, $p$ 1 vs 2 <0.001.

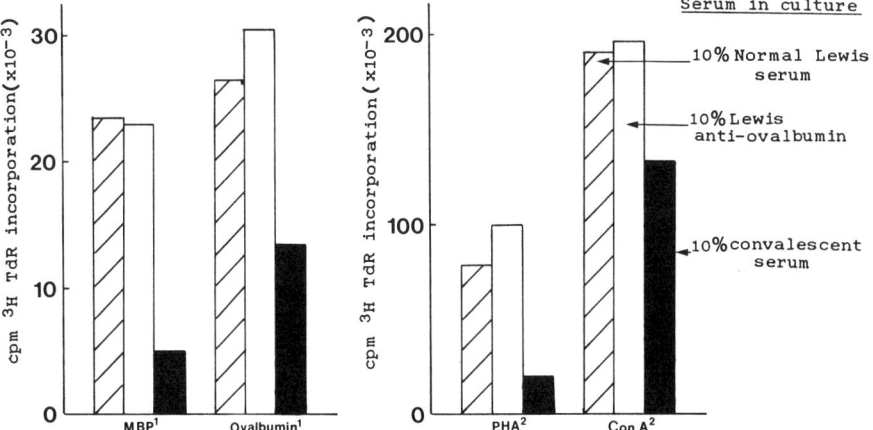

FIGURE 2. Serum from convalescent Lewis rats inhibits lymphocyte proliferation *in vitro*. These are data from one experiment that has been repeated at least twice with the same results. (1) Spleen cells from animals immunized with MBP or ovalbumin were cultured *in vitro* with the given antigen. (2) Normal Lewis spleen cells were cultured *in vitro* with the given lectin.

convalescent animals are not susceptible to reinduction of EAE with MBP in complete Freund's adjuvant, their spleens do contain memory cells that will adoptively transfer disease to naive recipients after culture with MBP.[1] We demonstrated that this is also the case in animals in which disease is completely prevented by adoptive transfer of convalescent serum. It follows that EAE in these animals, as with naturally convalescent animals, is inhibited by prevention of the activation of effector cells rather than their specific elimination.

Memory cell reactivation can be studied *in vitro* by culturing lymphocytes from primed animals with the specific antigen. Serum from convalescent animals substantially inhibits such responses to both MBP and ovalbumin (FIG. 2). These sera also inhibit T-lymphocyte activation by the mitogens phytohemagglutinin (PHA) and concanavalin A (Con A), demonstrating that this inhibitory activity is not exclusively specific for reactivation of cells by MBP. The inhibitory factor copurifies with immunoglobulin when isolated by ion exchange chromatography and gel filtration. However, the specificity of this putative immunosuppressive autoantibody is still not clear. Immunosuppressive autoantibodies have previously been shown to be present in serum from patients with AIDS,[3] leprosy,[4] and systemic lupus erythematosus.[5] The possibility that similar autoantibodies induce remissions in multiple sclerosis thus merits investigation.

## REFERENCES

1. SEDGWICK, J. D. & D. W. MASON. 1986. J. Neuroimmunol. **13:** 217-232.
2. PATERSON, P. Y. & S. M. HARWIN. 1963. J. Exp. Med. **117:** 755-774.
3. STRICKER, R. B., T. M. MCHUGH, D. J. MOODY, W. J. W. MORROW, D. P. STITES, M. A. SHUMAN & J. A. LEVY. 1987. Nature **327:** 710-712.
4. KERR, M. A., Y. M. HUSSEIN, R. C. POTTS, J. SWANSON BECK & M. M. SHERIFF. 1987. Immunology **61:** 117-123.
5. OKUDAIRA, K., R. P. SEARLES, J. S. GOODWIN & R. C. WILLIAMS, JR. 1982. J. Immunol. **129:** 582-586.

# Changes in T-Cell Subsets in Experimental Allergic Neuritis

T. YAMASHITA, T. NEGISHI, K. NOMURA,
T. HOSOKAWA, R. OHNO, AND K. HAMAGUCHI

*Department of Neurology*
*Saitama Medical School*
*Saitama 350-04, Japan*

There have been few reports on changes in T-cell subsets in experimental allergic neuritis (EAN), an animal model of Guillain-Barré syndrome.[1,2] In this study, changes in T-cell subsets in blood and spleen cells were investigated by means of flow cytometry during the course of EAN. Cellular reactivity to P2 protein (P2) and serum anti-P2

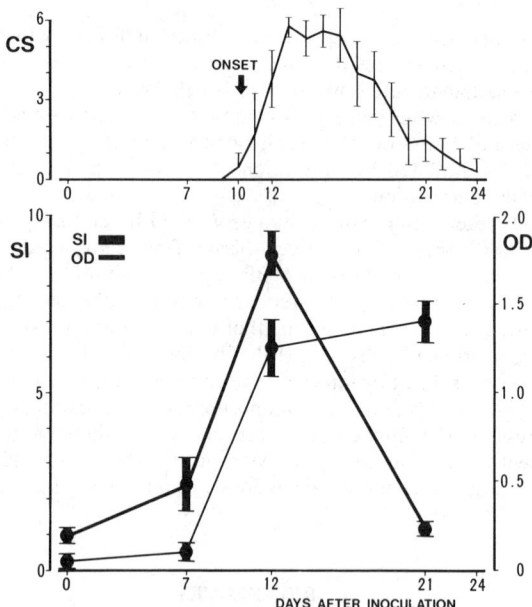

FIGURE 1. Clinical course of experimental allergic neuritis and immune responses to P2 protein. *Upper column* shows changes in mean values of clinical scores on the scale of Hughes *et al.*,[3] with slight modification. The mean time of onset was 10.5 days, and the clinical scores rapidly reached their maximum on day 14, continued to be high until day 16, and thereafter gradually declined. *Lower column* shows the results of the lymphocyte proliferation test and enzyme-linked immunosorbent assay in peripheral blood from another 15 animals sacrificed on days 7, 12, and 21 after immunization. *Vertical bars* indicate the mean ± 1 standard deviation. CS = clinical score; SI = stimulated index; OD = optical density at 405 nm.

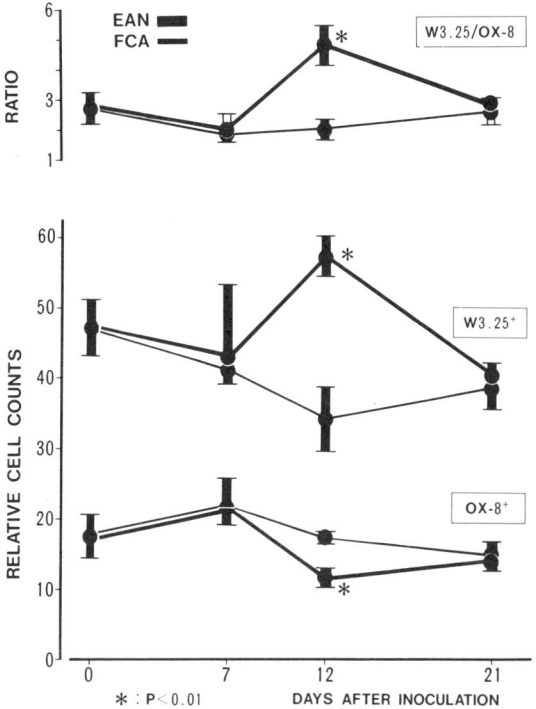

**FIGURE 2.** Changes in T-cell subsets in peripheral blood during experimental allergic neuritis (EAN) and adjuvant controls (CFA). T-cell subsets were analyzed by flow cytometry. After labeled cells were stained with a few drops of propidium iodide solution to detect the dead cells, $1 \times 10^4$ cells were analyzed using a fluorescent activated cell sorter (FACS440). *Vertical bars* indicate mean ± 1 standard deviation. *: $p < 0.01$ when compared with adjuvant controls.

antibody were also examined using the lymphocyte proliferation test and enzyme-linked immunosorbent assay, respectively.

For analysis of T-cell subsets, lymphocytes were stained using mouse monoclonal antibodies to surface antigens of T lymphocytes as the first antibody and FITC-labeled goat anti-mouse IgG(Fab')$_2$ serum as the second antibody.

Forty-six Lewis rats (male, 12-16 weeks old) were used in this study. Thirty rats were challenged with peripheral nerve myelin in complete Freund's adjuvant (CFA). Fifteen of these rats were observed daily for 24 days, and the severity of neurologic signs was scored on the scale by Hughes *et al.*[3] Another 15 rats with EAN were sacrificed on days 7, 12, and 21, and blood samples and spleen cells were obtained for flow cytometry, lymphocyte proliferation test, and enzyme-linked immunosorbent assay. As the adjuvant controls, nine Lewis rats were challenged with CFA alone. Normal control values for each test were obtained from seven untreated rats. Myelin fraction was prepared from bovine spinal roots by the method of Uyemura *et al.*,[4] and P2 was purified according to the method of Kitamura *et al.*[5]

Cellular hypersensitivity to P2, represented by the stimulation index, was first detected on day 7, was clearly manifested on day 12 (just after the clinical onset), and then returned to normal on day 21 (recovery period). However, antibody titer to P2, represented by optical density, became elevated from day 12 and remained high during the recovery period (FIG. 1).

When each parameter in T-cell subsets obtained from EAN was compared with those from adjuvant controls, a significantly higher value of W3.25$^+$ ($T_H$, $T_{inducer}$, $T_{DTH}$) and a lower value of OX-8$^+$ ($T_S$, CTL) were observed in EAN on day 12, with a resulting elevation in the W3.25:OX-8 ratio. These changes returned to their normal ranges on day 21. Similar findings were observed in spleen cells, and no significant fluctuations in W3.13$^+$ (pan-T) were found in blood and spleen cells (FIG. 2).

Changes in W3.25$^+$ could play an important role in the evolution of EAN as well as in recovery from it. Further studies on the subclasses of T-cell subsets will be needed to clarify the details of the immunoregulatory mechanism in the pathogenesis of EAN.

## REFERENCES

1. FEASBY, T. E. et al. 1984. J. Neuroimmunol. **6:** 209-214.
2. BROSNAN, J. V. et al. 1985. Brain **108:** 315-334.
3. HUGHES, R. A. C. et al. 1981. Ann. Neurol. **9**(suppl.): 125-133.
4. UYEMURA, K. et al. 1972. J. Neurochem. **19:** 2607-2614.
5. KITAMURA, K. et al. 1981. Biomed. Res. **2:** 347-363.

# Presence and Distribution of Nervous System-Associated Mast Cells That May Modulate Experimental Autoimmune Encephalomyelitis

## EDWARD L. ORR

*Department of Anatomy*
*Texas College of Osteopathic Medicine*
*Fort Worth, Texas 76107*

Experimental autoimmune (allergic) encephalomyelitis (EAE) is an animal model of multiple sclerosis (MS). Histologically, animals with EAE develop edema, inflammation, and demyelination of dorsal root ganglia, spinal roots, spinal cord, and brain.[1] In rodents, these histopathologic changes are accompanied by paresis or paralysis of the tail, hindlimbs, and forelimbs, urinary incontinence, and even death.[1] Similar histopathologic and clinical symptoms are seen in MS, justifying the use of EAE as a model for MS.[2]

Recently, we became interested in the possibility that mast cells, especially those closely associated with the brain, spinal cord, and other nearby tissues, may be important mediators of the edema and inflammation of EAE. Consequently, we determined the relative number and distribution of mast cells present on or near the surface of the central nervous system and CNS-related structures in SJL X BALB mice, as a prelude to evaluating the roles these cells may play in the development and expression of EAE.

## METHODS

Male $F_1$-hybrids of SJL/J X BALB/C mice were anesthetized with ether and decapitated. The calvarium with attached dura mater, brain, and spinal column were collected from each animal and fixed by immersion in neutral-buffered formalin for at least 2 days. The spinal columns were subsequently divided by midsagittal section, and the spinal cords, pia mater, and arachnoid were removed from the spinal canals. All tissues were then rinsed in tap water, stained by dipping the tissues 2-4 times in 0.5% toluidine blue, and rinsed again in two changes of tap water and one change in tap water acidified with a few drops of 1.0 M HCl. The tissues were then viewed and photographed using a dissecting microscope fitted for photomicroscopy. Under these conditions, mast cells stain pink to purple against a background of light to dark blue.

## RESULTS AND DISCUSSION

Numerous mast cells were found aligned along the sinuses, blood vessels, and nerves of the calvarial dura mater and in association with the blood vessels of the spinal periosteum and epidural surface of the spinal dura mater (not shown). Although the leptomeninges and surfaces of the spinal cord and most of the brain contained

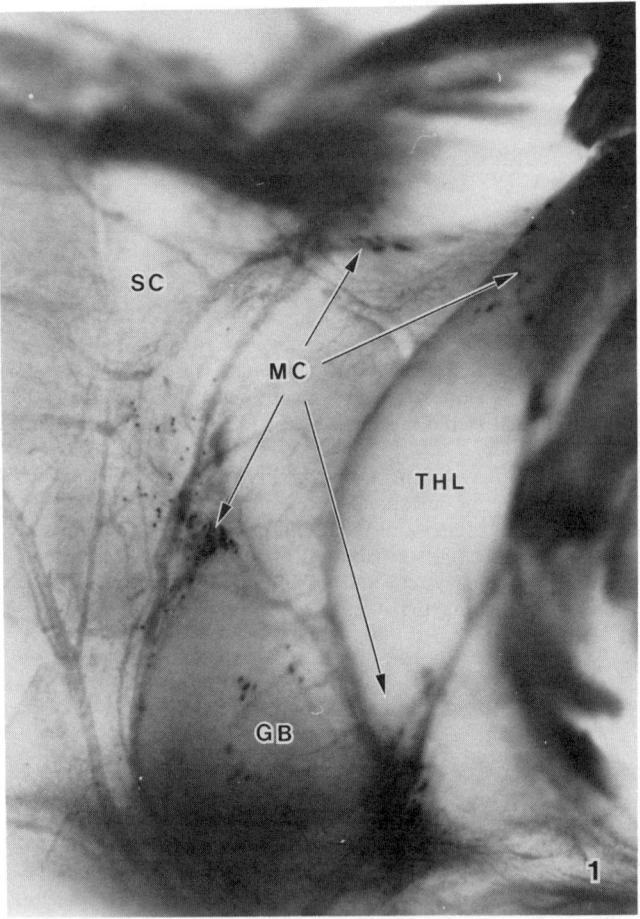

**FIGURE 1.** Mast cells (MC) in the velum interpositum of the mouse brain. The hippocampal formation has been removed to expose the velum interpositum which overlies the dorsal and lateral surfaces of the diencephalon and midbrain. The dissected brain was then stained with toluidine blue, and the dorsolateral surface of the diencephalon was photographed through a dissecting microscope. The dorsolateral surfaces of the right medial geniculate body (GB), thalamus (THL), and superior colliculus (SC) can be seen. (Original magnification × 40; reduced by 32%.)

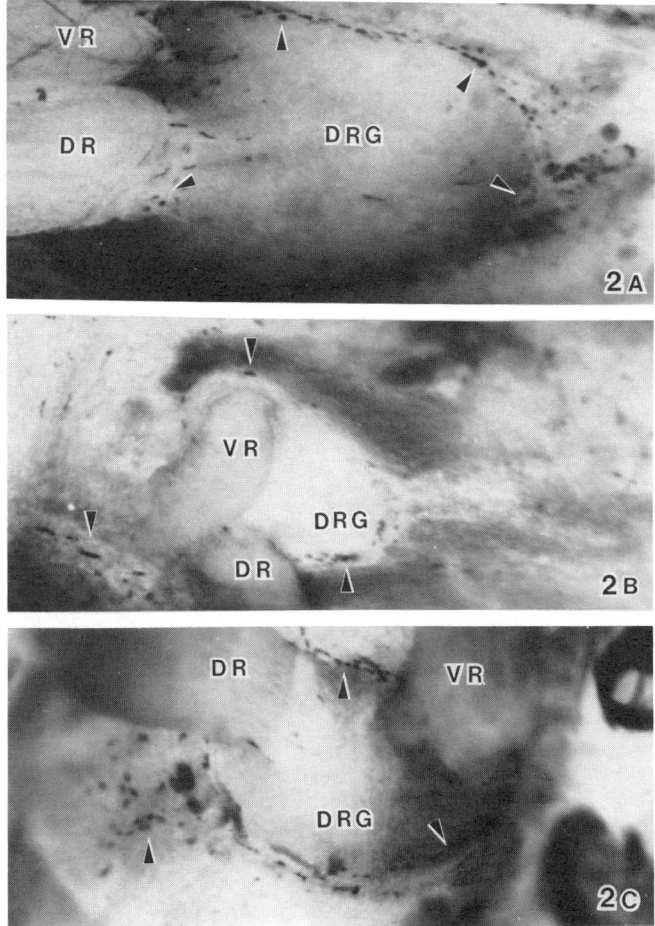

**FIGURE 2.** Periganglionic mast cells encircling the dorsal root ganglia (DRG) of the mouse. DRGs were exposed by dissection, stained with toluidine blue, and photographed *in situ* through a dissecting microscope. (**A**) Periganglionic mast cells (*arrows*) associated with a lumbar DRG; (**B**) periganglionic mast cells (*right arrows*) associated with a midthoracic DRG. Also seen are mast cells (*left arrow*) in the periosteum of the spinal canal; (**C**) Periganglionic (*right arrows*) and periosteal (*left arrow*) mast cells near a cervical DRG. DR = dorsal root; VR = ventral root. (Original magnification × 40; reduced by 69%.)

very few mast cells, variable numbers of mast cells were found in association with blood vessels supplying or draining certain regions of the brain. The largest number of mast cells were located along blood vessels that traverse the velum interpositum of the transverse fissure (FIG. 1). Thus, mast cells were numerous around the blood vessels that perfuse or drain the thalamus, corpora quadrigemini, hippocampal formation, and choroid plexi of the lateral and third ventricles. Large numbers of mast cells were also observed as periganglionic rings around dorsal root ganglia (DRGs) and on or within dorsal and ventral roots proximal to the DRGs. Moreover, the largest numbers of periganglionic and spinal root mast cells were associated with the lumbar DRGs (FIG. 2A), whereas the lowest numbers were present around the thoracic DRGs (FIG. 2B). Substantial numbers of mast cells were also present around most of the cervical DRGs (FIG. 2C).

These results demonstrate that nervous system-associated mast cells are regionally distributed in a manner consistent with the pattern of occurrence of the edema and inflammation of EAE.[1] Such a distribution supports our hypothesis that products of these cells released into or near blood vessels and/or the cerebrospinal fluid could control or modulate the edema and inflammation that occurs in EAE.

## REFERENCES

1. RAINE, C. S. 1985. *In* Handbook of Clinical Neurology, Vol. 3 (47). Demyelinating Diseases. J. C. Koeteier, Ed.: 429-466. Elsevier, Amsterdam.
2. ARNASON, B. G. W. 1983. *In* Neurologic Clinics, Vol. 1 (3). J. P. Antel, Ed. Saunders, Philadelphia: 765-782.

# Role of Mast Cells in Peripheral Nervous System Demyelination

DAVID JOHNSON, HOWARD L. WEINER, AND
PIERRETTE A. SEELDRAYERS

*Center for Neurologic Diseases*
*Brigham and Women's Hospital*
*Harvard Medical School*
*Boston, Massachusetts*

It was previously reported that degranulation of peripheral nerve mast cells is an early event in the development of experimental allergic neuritis (EAN).[1-3] We examined the possible consequences of this degranulation and ways in which it may be initiated.

Vasoactive amines released by degranulating mast cells have been implicated in the development of demyelination by contributing to increased permeability of blood vessels.[1-3] We examined the effects of another granule component, neutral protease, on PNS myelin. Rat serosal mast cells were degranulated with Compound 48/80, a standard mast cell secretagogue, and the supernatant was incubated with freshly prepared bovine PNS myelin. The proteases released on degranulation degraded 72 ± 1.7% of $P_0$ protein in 3 hours. As $P_0$ is the major PNS myelin protein, such extensive degradation may be expected to be associated with significant structural disruption.

As basic peptides can stimulate degranulation of mast cells,[4] we also examined the effects of the cationic myelin proteins $P_2$ and myelin basic protein (MBP) on isolated serosal mast cells. Degranulation was assayed by measuring the release of the granule enzyme $\beta$-hexosaminidase. Incubation of mast cells with either $P_2$ or MBP led to the release of approximately 50% of total mast cell $\beta$-hexosaminidase, which was comparable to the effect obtained with Compound 48/80 (TABLE 1). Myelin-

TABLE 1. Effect of Myelin Proteins on Mast Cell Degranulation

| Degranulating Agent | Percentage of $\beta$-Hexosaminidase Released |
|---|---|
| Control | 7.5 |
| 48/80 (1 µg/ml) | 48 |
| MBP (100 µg/ml) | 56 |
| $P_2$ (100 µg/ml) | 45.8 |

NOTE: Rat peritoneal mast cells ($2 \times 10^5$) were incubated for 20 minutes at 37°C with degranulating agents. Cells were centrifuged, and enzyme assays were performed on pellets and supernatants. Enzyme release is expressed as the percentage of combined total in pellet and supernatant.

induced degranulation is unlikely to be a primary cause of demyelination, but release of $P_2$ or MBP, or of their breakdown products, may be able to potentiate local mast cell degranulation.

To examine the primary causes of mast cell degranulation in EAN, the disease was induced in Lewis rats by immunization with bovine PNS myelin in complete Freund's adjuvant. Sera were tested for the presence of IgE antibodies against myelin components using the rat basophil leukemia line RBL-2H3, which bears similar high affinity IgE receptors to those on mast cells. Cross-linking of occupied IgE receptors of mast cells or basophils by the appropriate antigen causes degranulation. Cells were preincubated with sera from control or EAN animals and then with purified bovine $P_2$ protein, and degranulation was assayed by release of granule $\beta$-hexosaminidase. RBL incubated with both EAN sera and $P_2$ released significant amounts of granule enzyme (TABLE 2), suggesting that animals with EAN produce IgE antibodies against $P_2$. If IgE-mediated degranulation of PNS mast cells occurs *in vivo*, release of myelinolytic mast cell proteases and vasoactive amines could serve as a focus for inflammatory demyelination, as degranulating mast cells also release chemoattractants.

TABLE 2. IgE Antibodies in Experimental Allergic Neuritis (EAN)

| Condition | Percentage of $\beta$-Hexosaminidase Released |
|---|---|
| No serum | 17 |
| $P_2$ alone | 18.25 |
| $P_2$ and control serum | $15.1 \pm 1.2$ ($n = 3$) |
| $P_2$ and EAN serum | $37 \pm 4.4$ ($n = 3$) |

NOTE: Basophils ($1 \times 10^6$) were preincubated with 50 $\mu$l of serum or medium for 30 minutes at 30°C. They were washed once and then incubated with cytochalasin (2 $\mu$g/ml) and purified $P_2$ (20 $\mu$g/ml) for 30 minutes at 37°C. Cells were pelleted and supernatants assayed for release of $\beta$-hexosaminidase. Values are expressed as percentage of total value obtained by lysing cells with 1% Triton X-100.

## REFERENCES

1. POWELL, H. C., S. L. BRAHENY, R. R. MYERS, M. RODRIGUEZ & P. W. LAMPERT. 1983. Early changes in experimental allergic neuritis. Lab. Invest. **48:** 332-338.
2. BROSNAN, C. F. & F. A. TANSEY. 1984. Delayed onset of experimental allergic neuritis in rats treated with reserpine. J. Neuropathol. Exp. Neurol. **43:** 84-93.
3. BROSNAN, C. F., W. D. LYMAN, F. A. TANSEY & T. H. CARTER. 1985. Quantitation of mast cells in experimental allergic neuritis. J. Neuropathol. Exp. Neurol. **44:** 196-203.
4. DUFTON, M. J., R. J. CHERRY, J. W. COLEMAN & D. R. STANWORTH. 1984. The capacity of basic peptides to trigger exocytosis from mast cells correlates with their capacity to immobilize band 3 proteins in erythrocyte membranes. Biochem. J. **223:** 67-71.

# Resistance to Induction of Experimental Allergic Encephalomyelitis

## Role of Adjuvant Components and Antigen

T. BRENNER, R. MIZRACHI, AND O. ABRAMSKY

*Department of Neurology*
*Hadassah University Hospital and*
*Hebrew University-Hadassah Medical School*
*Jerusalem, Israel*

We previously demonstrated that pregnant rats immunized with encephalitogenic antigen transfer a transient resistance to induction of experimental allergic encephalomyelitis (EAE) in encephalitogen-challenged offspring.[1] The resistance to EAE induction is transferred during the whole lactating period, until weaning, and not during pregnancy. Through the milk, antimyelin basic protein (MBP) antibodies are transferred to the newborn animals. The degree of protection against EAE diminished with age and was correlated with anti-MBP antibody levels in the offspring sera. The present study was designed to investigate the effect of maternal immunization with adjuvant components, in the presence or absence of encephalitogenic antigen, on the susceptibility of offspring to induction of EAE. Outbred female rats (HUS) were immunized during the third week of pregnancy. After weaning, offspring of both sexes were sensitized with encephalitogenic material. Animals were bled from the tail vein before immunization and then at intervals of 1-2 weeks. (All serial tests were performed simultaneously.) For EAE induction, rats were sensitized with 50 mg of guinea pig spinal cord (GPSC) in complete Freund's adjuvant (CFA, Difco) supplemented with $10^{10}$ organisms of *Bordetella pertussis* vaccine (Rafa). Animals were examined daily for neurologic signs of EAE. The clinical and histologic signs were scored as described previously.[1] With solid-phase radioimmunoassay (RIA), antipertussis antibodies were determined on microtiter plates coated with $10^9$ *Bordetella pertussis* organisms. Bound serum antibodies were identified with $^{125}$I-goat anti-rat Ig (Amersham). Anti-MBP antibodies were determined also by solid-phase RIA as described previously.[2] The type of adjuvant and antigen used for immunization of pregnant rats affected the susceptibility of offspring to EAE induction. As shown in TABLE 1, 75% of challenged offspring born to nonimmunized mothers developed moderate or severe EAE. Of the challenged offspring born to CFA or GPSC immunized mothers, 80 and 40%, respectively, developed moderate EAE. However, none of the challenged offspring born to pertussis vaccine (PV), PV with CFA, or GPSC, PV, and CFA immunized mothers developed any signs of EAE. Antipertussis and anti-MBP antibodies were detected in the challenged mothers as well as in their nonimmunized offspring (TABLE 2).

TABLE 1. Effect of Maternal Immunization on Susceptibility of Offspring to Experimental Allergic Encephalomyelitis (EAE) Induction[a]

| | EAE Parameters | | |
|---|---|---|---|
| Immunization | Incidence of Disease in Immunized Offspring | Maximum Score | Duration of Disease (days) |
| None | 30/40 | 4.0 ± 0.5 | 4.6 ± 0.5 |
| GPSC + CFA + PV | 0/16[b] | 0 | 0 |
| CFA + PV | 0/13[b] | 0 | 0 |
| CFA | 16/20 | 2.5 ± 0.5[b] | 5.0 ± 0.9 |
| GPSC | 8/20[b] | 1.0 ± 1.0[b] | 2.7 ± 0.1[b] |
| PV | 0/21 | 0 | 0 |

[a] Female rats were immunized during the third week of pregnancy with: guinea pig spinal cord (GPSC), complete Freund's adjuvant (CFA), and pertussis vaccine (PV). The offspring were challenged with GPSC + CFA + PV after weaning.
[b] $p < 0.05$.

Circulating antipertussis and anti-MBP antibodies appeared 10-15 days after immunization in both control nonpregnant and pregnant rats. In the nonimmunized offspring born to an immunized mother, the antibodies were undetectable at delivery, but during lactation and in the period following, antipertussis and anti-MBP were high. These antibodies decreased gradually after weaning. The degree of protection

TABLE 2. Serum Levels of Antipertussis and Anti-MBP Antibodies in Relation to Maternal Immunization, Offspring Age, and Susceptibility to Induction of Experimental Allergic Encephalomyelitis (EAE)[a]

| Immunization | Antipertussis (1:000) | Anti-MBP (1:00) | Incidence of EAE |
|---|---|---|---|
| Control (not immunized) | 2,377 ± 46 | 543 ± 60 | — |
| Control EAE animals (30 days pi) | 9,884 ± 71[b] | 3,900 ± 350[b] | 25/30 |
| Animals immunized during pregnancy (30 days pi) | 9,074 ± 482[b] | 4,055 ± 500[b] | 20/25 |
| Offspring born to immunized mothers (at delivery) | 3,233 ± 430 | 711 ± 50 | — |
| Offspring born to immunized mothers (at weaning, 30 days of age) | 8,555 ± 366[b] | 3,655 ± 200[b] | 0/16[b] |
| Offspring born to immunized mothers (at 70 days of age) | 5,228 ± 503[b] | 1,750 ± 100[b] | 12/20[c] |

[a] Antipertussis and anti-MBP antibodies were determined by solid-phase radioimmunoassay. Results are mean counts per minute, bound ± SE (pi = postimmunization).
[b] $p < 0.05$.
[c] Mild disease.

against EAE diminished with age and was correlated with the level of antipertussis and anti-MBP antibodies in the offspring sera.

In conclusion, pregnant rats immunized during pregnancy with pertussis vaccine (PV), PV with GPSC in CFA, or PV with CFA transferred resistance to induction of EAE in encephalitogenic-challenged offspring. Immunization with GPSC alone imparted partial protection, whereas immunization with CFA did not protect the offspring against EAE induction. The degree of protection against EAE diminished with age and correlated with antipertussis and anti-MBP antibodies. We believe that such transfer of resistance and antibodies may serve as a model both for the study of milk-transmitted maternal immunocompetent factors as well as the mechanisms involved in producing resistance to EAE.

## REFERENCES

1. BRENNER, T., H. OVADIA, S. EVRON, R. MIZRACHI & O. ABRAMSKY. 1986. J. Neuroimmunol. **12:** 317-327.
2. BRENNER, T., R. P. LISAK, A. ROSTAMI, F. A. MCMORRIS & D. H. SILBERBERG. 1986. J. Neurochem. **46:** 54-60.

# Demyelination of the Peripheral Nervous System Causes Neurologic Signs in Myelin Basic Protein-Induced Experimental Allergic Encephalomyelitis

## Implications for the Etiology of Multiple Sclerosis[a]

MICHAEL P. PENDER

*Department of Medicine*
*University of Queensland*
*Clinical Sciences Building*
*Royal Brisbane Hospital*
*Brisbane, Queensland 4029, Australia*

Experimental allergic encephalomyelitis (EAE) is an autoimmune disease induced by inoculation with whole central nervous system (CNS) tissue, myelin basic protein (MBP), or myelin proteolipid protein. It is widely studied as a model of multiple sclerosis (MS), a human CNS demyelinating disease of unknown etiology. In MS, CNS demyelination is a major cause of neurologic signs. However, because of the reported absence of demyelination in some animals with neurologic signs of EAE, it has been suggested that the signs of EAE, especially acute EAE, are due not to demyelination but to other factors such as edema.[1,2] But these reported studies failed to use adequate histologic techniques to assess demyelination or to thoroughly examine the whole nervous system, particularly the lumbar, sacral, and coccygeal spinal cord and the peripheral nervous system (PNS), which is known to be involved in EAE. We recently showed in rabbits and rats with whole spinal cord-induced acute EAE that there is ample demyelination in the PNS and CNS to account for the neurologic signs.[3] I am reporting that, in MBP-induced acute EAE in the Lewis rat, the ventral and dorsal spinal roots are principal sites of demyelination, whereas the spinal cord and brain are only slightly demyelinated, although considerably inflamed.

MBP was prepared from guinea pig spinal cord (after removal of the spinal roots) by the method of Deibler *et al.*,[4] and its purity was ascertained by sodium dodecyl sulfate polyacrylamide gel electrophoresis. MBP in 0.9% saline solution was emulsified in an equal volume of incomplete Freund's adjuvant containing 4 mg/ml of *Myco-*

---

[a] This work was supported by the National Multiple Sclerosis Society of Australia.

*bacterium butyricum*. Male rats, 8-10 weeks old, received 0.1 ml of emulsion in a footpad of each hindfoot. The total dose of MBP was 50 μg per rat. Light and electron microscopic histologic studies were performed on rats with hindlimb weakness, as previously described.[3] These studies demonstrated inflammation and mild demyelination in the spinal cord and brainstem (FIG. 1). However, the principal sites of demyelination were the lumbar, sacral, and coccygeal ventral and dorsal spinal roots (FIG. 2). The vast majority of random 0.5-2 μm sections through individual spinal roots showed demyelination. Electrophysiologic studies indicated that this PNS demyelination is an important cause of the neurologic signs in these animals (Pender,

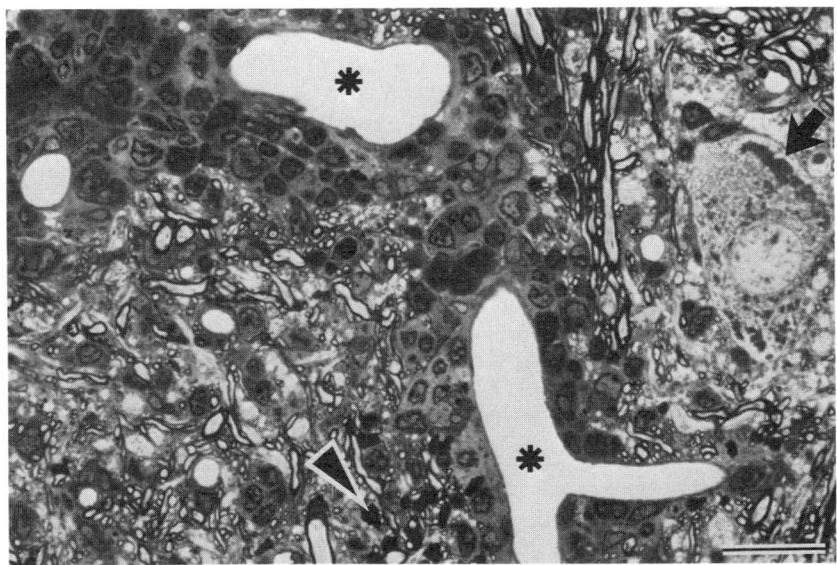

**FIGURE 1.** Transverse section through the ventral horn of the L5 spinal cord of a rat with severe hindlimb weakness due to MBP-induced acute EAE 2 days after the onset of tail weakness and on the day of onset of hindlimb weakness. There is marked perivascular cuffing with mononuclear cells (*asterisks* in vessels) and infiltration of these cells into the adjacent parenchyma. Extravasated erythrocytes are also present (*arrowhead*). The cell body of a motor neurone can be seen (*arrow*). Epok 812 section stained with toluidine blue. Bar = 25 μm.

in preparation). There was minimal involvement of the dorsal root ganglia and peripheral nerves.

Thus, in the Lewis rat, immunization with MBP results in a demyelinating polyradiculitis with little CNS demyelination. PNS demyelination is an important cause of the neurologic signs of acute MBP-EAE in these animals and is due to the close similarity, if not identity, of CNS MBP and PNS $P_1$ protein.[5] The predominance of spinal root demyelination over CNS demyelination may be due to a lesser blood-tissue barrier in the roots.[6] In contrast, it has recently been reported that T-cell lines and clones specific for MBP induce considerable CNS demyelination in irradiated nude mice.[7] Differences in the distribution of demyelination in rats and mice could be due to interspecies differences in the blood-nerve barrier, Ia antigen expression, or MBP concentration in the spinal roots or to differences in MBP epitopes in intact

CNS and PNS myelin. Sensitization to MBP may account for the PNS involvement in patients developing neurologic complications after inoculation with antirabies vaccine containing sheep brain.[8] Although MS may sometimes involve the PNS, the neurologic signs of MS are generally regarded as being due to CNS demyelination. If MBP is the target antigen in MS, the relevant epitope must be recognized in CNS but not in PNS myelin.

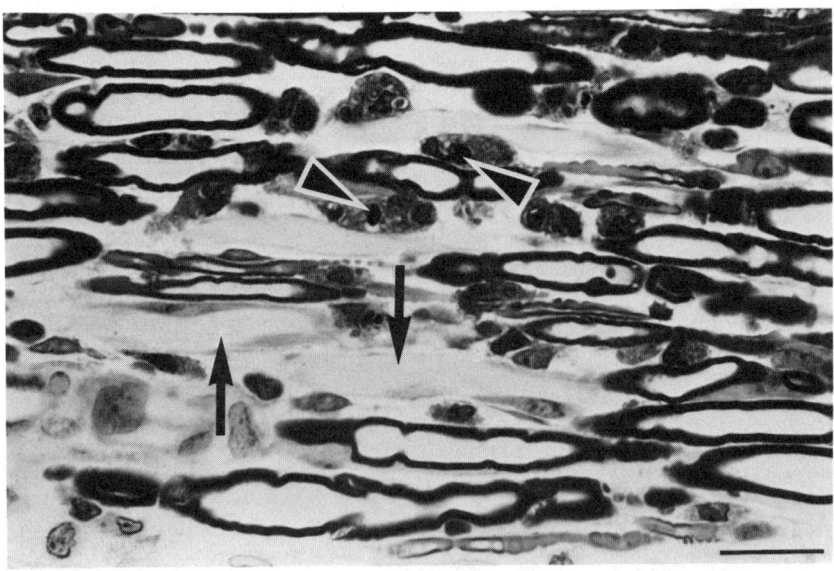

**FIGURE 2.** Longitudinal section through an S4 ventral root of a rat with MBP-induced acute EAE 3 days after the onset of tail weakness. Demyelinated axons are present (*arrows*). Mononuclear cells containing myelin debris (*arrowheads*) lie adjacent to some of the demyelinated axons. HistoResin (LKB Bromma) section stained with cresyl violet. Bar = 25 μm.

## REFERENCES

1. KERLERO DE ROSBO, N., C. C. A. BERNARD, R. D. SIMMONS & P. R. CARNEGIE. 1985. J. Neuroimmunol. **9:** 349-361.
2. SEDGWICK, J., S. BROSTOFF & D. MASON. 1987. J. Exp. Med. **165:** 1058-1075.
3. PENDER, M. P. 1987. J. Neuroimmunol. **15:** 11-24.
4. DEIBLER, G. E., R. E. MARTENSON & M. W. KIES. 1972. Prep. Biochem. **2:** 139-165.
5. GREENFIELD, S., S. BROSTOFF, E. H. EYLAR & P. MORELL. 1973. J. Neurochem. **20:** 1207-1216.
6. OLSSON, Y. 1968. Acta Neuropathol. (Berlin) **10:** 26-33.
7. TABIRA, T. & K. SAKAI. 1987. Lab. Invest. **56:** 518-525.
8. HEMACHUDHA, T., D. E. GRIFFIN, J. J. GIFFELS, R. T. JOHNSON, A. B. MOSER & P. PHANUPHAK. 1987. N. Engl. J. Med. **316:** 369-374.

# Genetic Regulation of Susceptibility and Severity of Demyelination[a]

ROBERT L. KNOBLER,[b,c] FRED D. LUBLIN,[b]
D. SCOTT LINTHICUM,[d] MEL COHN,[e] ROGER
D. MELVOLD,[f] HOWARD L. LIPTON,[f] BENJAMIN
A. TAYLOR,[g] AND WESLEY G. BEAMER[g]

[b]*Department of Neurology*
*Jefferson Medical College*
*Philadelphia, Pennsylvania*

[d]*Department of Pathology*
*University of Texas Health Sciences Center*
*Houston, Texas*

[e]*Developmental Biology Laboratory*
*The Salk Institute*
*La Jolla, California*

[f]*Departments of Microbiology-Immunology and Neurology*
*Northwestern University*
*Chicago, Illinois*

[g]*The Jackson Laboratory*
*Bar Harbor, Maine*

Susceptibility to virus-induced and autoimmune demyelinating central nervous system (CNS) diseases is genetically regulated. Three CNS diseases with similar histopathology, acute (A) and relapsing (R) experimental allergic encephalomyelitis (EAE),[1] and Theiler's murine encephalomyelitis virus (TMEV)-induced demyelination,[2] occur in SJL mice. BALB/c mice are resistant, but susceptible to mouse hepatitis virus type 4 (MHV-4)-induced demyelination, to which SJL mice are resistant.[1] The availability of nine recombinant-inbred (RI) strains, the CXJ series, provides a resource for unmasking BALB/c or SJL/J genes that may regulate the occurrence and severity of disease and recovery.

Each RI strain in a series contains a unique reassortment of genes derived from one progenitor or the other. For a useful RI series, the progenitors should differ in phenotype and genotype at a number of loci. Progressive inbreeding of F2 progeny eventually leads to distinct strains.[3] For any given allele, the strain distribution pattern (SDP) characterizes its source, from either progenitor, for each strain of the RI series.

---

[a] This work was supported by research grant RG 1722-A-3 from the National Multiple Sclerosis Society, TIDA K07-NS00961 from the NINCDS, and the Arthur L. Swim Foundation.

[c] Address for correspondence: Dr. Robert L. Knobler, 1025 Walnut Street, Philadelphia, PA 19107.

By comparing SDPs with mapped loci on each chromosome, genetic mapping can be accomplished.

Different CXJ RI strains, and thus different genes, showed susceptibility to each of these four demyelinating diseases (TABLE 1). Some were susceptible to all four models (CXJ 6 and 8), some only to both virus-induced diseases but neither autoimmune disease (CXJ 9), some to both autoimmune diseases but neither virus-induced disease (CXJ 1), and some to one but not the other form of autoimmune demyelination (CXJ 3). The responses to R-EAE were further refined with 14 SWXJ RI strains between R-EAE-resistant SWR and susceptible SJL/J. Three clinically different groups included high, middle, and low responders in regard to onset and severity (TABLE 2). Clinical recovery patterns provided further differentiation. For example, SWXJ 3 and 14 both developed R-EAE with early onset and frequent relapses, but SWXJ 3 retained deficits, whereas SWXJ 14 recovered better.

Previously, this approach showed that a single gene for MHV-4 susceptibility mapped to mouse chromosome 7,[4] and identified as coding the virus receptor. TMEV demyelination was closely linked to the beta chain of the mouse T-cell receptor by its SDP in CXJ mice.[2] The present studies demonstrate that MHV-4, TMEV, A-EAE, and R-EAE demyelinating diseases are under separate genetic regulation (TABLE 1). Even variability in the clinical course, such as that in R-EAE (TABLE 2), depends on host genetic makeup. RI strain profiles can thus be used to identify the number of genes and gene products, which influence the clinical severity of demyelination and the degree of recovery. Furthermore, because there are histocompatible RI strains that differ in susceptibility to the different models of experimental demyelination, these differences can be exploited in the bone marrow and brain transplant paradigms being used in our laboratory to further dissect the pathogenesis of the individual diseases. This may provide an experimental means for understanding the genetic basis of clinical variability in the multigenic human demyelinating disease, multiple sclerosis.

TABLE 1. Susceptibility to MHV (JHM Strain), TMEV, Acute and Relapsing EAE and Vasoactive Amines in CXJ Recombinant Inbred Strains of Mice

| Strain | H-2 | Virus Studies | | EAE Studies | | Histamine Sensitivity | |
|---|---|---|---|---|---|---|---|
| | | MHV | TMEV | Acute | Relapsing | Natural | Induced |
| CXJ 1 | d | Nil | Nil | + | + | + | + |
| CXJ 3 | d | Nil | + | Nil | + | + | + |
| CXJ 4 | s | + | + | + | ND | Nil | + |
| CXJ 6 | s | + | + | + | + | Nil | + |
| CXJ 8 | d | + | + | + | + | Nil | + |
| CXJ 9 | d | + | + | Nil | Nil | Nil | + |
| CXJ 10 | d | Nil | + | Nil | ND | Nil | + |
| CXJ 11 | d | + | Nil | + | ND | Nil | + |
| CXJ 15 | s | Nil | + | Nil | ND | Nil | + |
| BALB | d | + | Nil | Nil | Nil | Nil | Nil |
| SJL | s | Nil | + | + | + | + | + |

ND = not done.

TABLE 2. Strain Distribution Pattern for the Clinical Expression of Relapsing EAE in the SWXJ RI Series

| Strain | H-2 | Frequency Avg. No. of Relapses | Average Onset (mo.) | Severity Mild Moderate Severe |
|---|---|---|---|---|
| SWXJ 14 | s | 3 | 2 | Severe |
| SWXJ 11 | s | 3 | 6 | Mod-Severe |
| SWXJ 8 | s | 2 | 3 | Severe |
| SWXJ 3 | s | 3 | 2 | Severe |
| SJL | s | 2 | 6 | Moderate |
| SWXJ 12 | s | 2 | 9 | Mild-Mod |
| SWXJ 6 | s | 1 | 8 | Mild |
| SWXJ 2 | s | 2 | 9 | Mild |
| SWXJ 13 | q | 2 | 3 | Mild |
| SWXJ 10 | q | 1 | 9 | Mild |
| SWXJ 9 | q | 2 | 9 | Mild-Mod |
| SWXJ 5 | q | 1 | 10 | Mild-Mod |
| SWXJ 4 | q | 2 | 7 | Mild |
| SWXJ 1 | q | 2 | 6 | Mild-Mod |
| SWXJ 7 | q | 0 | 10 | Minimal |
| SWR | q | 0 | 10 | Minimal |

## REFERENCES

1. KNOBLER, R. L., D. S. LINTHICUM & M. COHN. 1985. Host genetic regulation of acute MHV-4 encephalomyelitis and acute experimental autoimmmune encephalomyelitis in CXJ (BALB/cKe × SJL/J) recombinant-inbred mice. J. Neuroimmunol. **8:** 15-28.
2. MELVOLD, R. W., D. M. JOKINEN, R. L. KNOBLER & H. L. LIPTON. 1987. Variations in genetic control of susceptibility to Theiler's murine encephalomyelitis virus (TMEV)-induced demyelinating disease. I. Differences between susceptible SJL/J and resistant BALB/c strains map near the T cell beta-chain constant gene on chromosome 6. J. Immunol. **138:** 1429-1433.
3. TAYLOR, B. A. 1981. Recombinant inbred mice. *In* Genetic Variants and Strains of the Laboratory Mouse. M. C. Green, Ed.: 397-407. Gustav Fischer Verlag, New York.
4. KNOBLER, R. L., B. A. TAYLOR, M. K. WOODELL, W. G. BEAMER & M. B. A. OLDSTONE. 1984. Host genetic control of mouse hepatitis virus type-4 (JHM strain) replication. II. The gene locus for susceptibility is linked to the *Svp-2* locus on murine chromosome 7. Exp. Clin. Immunogenet. **1:** 217-222.

# Adoptive Transfer Experimental Autoimmune Encephalomyelitis

## Evidence for Central Nerve and Spinal Root Dysfunction[a]

KURT HEININGER,[b,c] WALTER FIERZ,[d] BÄRBEL SCHÄFER,[b] HANS-PETER HARTUNG,[b] AND KLAUS V. TOYKA[b]

[b]Department of Neurology
University of Düsseldorf
Düsseldorf, West Germany

[d]Section of Clinical Immunology
Department of Internal Medicine
University of Zürich
Zürich, Switzerland

In adoptive transfer experimental autoimmune encephalomyelitis (AT-EAE), a myelin basic protein (MBP)-specific T-cell line mediates the disease in naive Lewis rats.[1] Although the immunopathology of the disease model has been studied extensively, the functional disorder of central and peripheral conduction has not been investigated.

In this study, injection of $5 \times 10^6$ line cells in 8-10-week-old female Lewis rats induced fulminant tetraplegia after a latent period of 4 days followed by death on day 5. Electrophysiologic testing[2] of central afferent conduction by somatosensory-evoked potentials revealed a profound slowing of conduction with delayed latencies of cervical and lumbar responses. In addition, the roots were affected, as shown by a variety of standard conduction studies (FIG. 1). Treatment with 4-aminopyridine, a potassium channel-blocking agent,[3] could partially reverse the slowing of conduction (FIG. 2). Because axonal potassium channels are exposed during paranodal demyelination, resulting in a delay or blockade of the nerve impulse, this pharmacologic finding is best explained by paranodal demyelination as an important pathogenic mechanism.

A lower cell dose ($10^6$ cells) induced only moderate clinical signs, with paraparesis paralleled by milder conduction slowing and conduction failure of central neurons and roots. The peripheral nerves distal to the spinal roots were free of electrophysiologic changes in the higher and lower cell dose animals.

[a]This work was supported by the Deutsche Forschungsgemeinschaft SFB 200/B5, the Hertie-Stiftung, and the Schweizerische Nationalfonds (Projekt-no. 3.998-0.86) (W. F.).

[c]ADDRESS: Neurolog. Klinik, Moorenstr. 5, 4000 Düsseldorf, Düsseldorf, FRG.

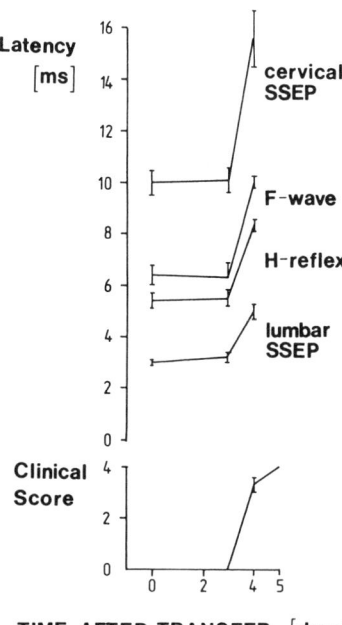

**FIGURE 1.** Time course of clinical signs and electrophysiologic findings in rats injected with $5 \times 10^6$ myelin basic protein-specific T cells (higher dose). Mean values of six recipient rats ($\pm$ SD) are given. *Top to bottom,* latencies of the C response, the first negative potential of the somatosensory-evoked potentials (SSEP) recorded at the C7 spinal level. F-wave latencies of the sciatic nerve on stimulation at the malleolus, H-reflex latencies of the sciatic nerve upon stimulation at the sciatic notch, and latencies of the S response of the lumbar SSEP recorded at the D13/L1 spinal level. The clinical status was scored using a 5-grade scale (0 = normal, 4 = death).

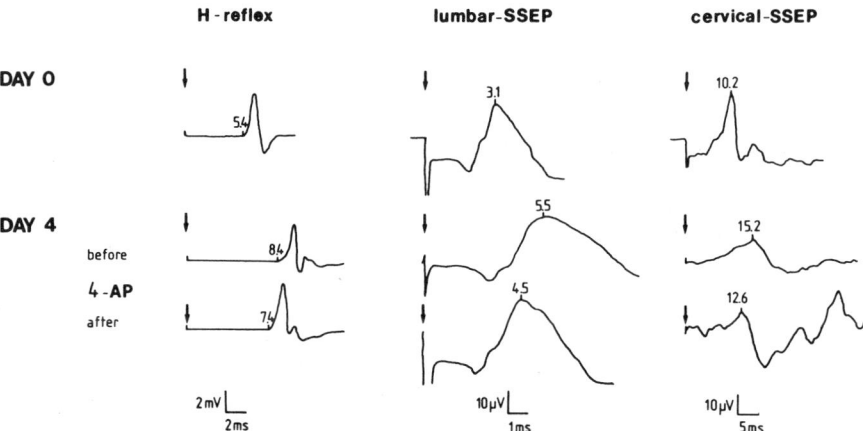

**FIGURE 2.** Effect of 4-aminopyridine (4-AP, 1 mg/kg intraperitoneally) in a rat injected with $5 \times 10^6$ myelin basic protein-specific T cells. Redrawn original recordings of H reflex, S response of lumbar SSEP, and C response of cervical SSEP on day 0 and on day 4 before and 15 minutes after injection of 4-AP. Note change in gain and time scale.

Light microscopy showed marked inflammation with perivascular and meningeal infiltration of lymphocytes and macrophages and only minor demyelination in the brain, spinal cord, and adjacent roots. The signs of inflammation were dose dependent, and the caudal parts of the spinal cord were more affected than the cranial parts. Longitudinal sections of the spinal cord specimen did not reveal any definite structural alterations at the paranodal myelin sheath. The peripheral nerves were free of pathologic changes in the high-dose and low-dose animals.

These findings indicate that (1) the nerve fiber dysfunction in AT-EAE is cell dose dependent in quality and quantity, (2) changes are suggestive of paranodal pathology, and (3) the peripheral nervous system distal to the spinal roots is spared.

### REFERENCES

1. BEN NUN, A., H. WEKERLE & I. R. COHEN. 1981. The rapid isolation of clonable antigen-specific T-lymphocyte lines capable of mediating autoimmune encephalomyelitis. Eur. I. Immunol. **11**: 195-198.
2. HEININGER, K., G. STOLL, C. LININGTON, K. V. TOYKA & H. WEKERLE. 1986. Conduction failure and nerve conduction slowing in EAN induced by $P_2$-specific T-cell lines. Ann. Neurol. **19**: 44-49.
3. SHERRATT, R. M., H. BOSTOCK & T. A. SEARS. 1980. Effects of 4-aminopyridine on normal and demyelinated mammalian nerve fibres. Nature **283**: 570-572.

# Index of Contributors

Abramsky, O., 729-731
Adams, D. S., 649-651
Alexander, E. L., 387-388
Allinquant, B., 286-289
Altman, A., 324-326
Alvord, E. C., Jr., 315-318, 581-584
Anderson, E., 440-441
Andersson, M., 624-627
Antel, J., 498-500
Arezzo, J. C., 571-572
Arnason, B. G. W., 4-12, 585-588, 707-708
Arnheim, N., 269-270
Audhya, T. K., 298-300
Avrameas, S., 290-292

Bach, J. F., 298-300, 504-505
Bach, M. A., 594-596
Baig, S., 277-281
Bailey, D., 702-703
Bambridge, L., 498-500
Barolat, G., 573-575
Bartels, J., 452-454
Basta, P., 255-257
Beamer, W. G., 735-737
Bellini, W. J., 352-353
Bergström, T., 624-627
Berrih-Aknin, S., 504-505, 506-507
Biberfeld, P., 293-297
Bigner, D. D., 64-77
Blalock, J. E., 694-697
Blancher, A., 290-292
Blomstrand, C., 624-627
Bodmer, S., 218-227, 437-439
Bomberger, C. E., 700-701
Bonifacio, E., 528-529
Borkowski, J., 652-653
Boulet, S., 498-500
Bourdette, D. N., 537-539
Brackenbury, R., 39-46
Brainard, G. C., 642-644, 704-706
Braun, D. G., 665-668
Brenner, T., 729-731
Brew, B., 162-175
Brosnan, C. F., 571-572
Brown, G. B., 452-454
Brown, M., 585-588
Brown, M. J., 445-448
Brun-Vezinet, F., 619-623
Bubien, J. K., 694-697
Budka, H., 630-633

Burks, J. S., 301-305
Burns, F., 576-577

Cadrobbi, P., 615-618
Calvelli, T. A., 628-629
Campbell, G. K., Jr., 578-580
Carbone, K. M., 661-662
Carlquist, M., 520-522
Carr, D. J. J., 694-697
Carter, J. L., 535-536
Casey, J. M., 611-614
Cashman, N., 498-500
Castro, E. E., 306-308
Checinski, M., 707-708
Chelmicka-Schoff, E., 707-708
Chieco-Bianchi, L., 615-618
Chofflon, M., 330-332
Christensson, B., 293-297
Ciulla, T. A., 271-276
Clanet, M., 290-292
Clark, E. A., 455-458, 581-584
Clatch, R. J., 674-677
Cobain, T. J., 372-373, 528-529
Cohen, J. A., 445-448, 715-717
Cohen-Kaminsky, S., 504-505, 506-507
Cohn, M., 735-737
Cohn, V. H., 269-270
Coleman, M., 602-604
Conti-Tronconi, B. M., 511-512
Cook, S. D., 533-534
Cragg, L., 498-500
Crane, M., 669-671
Cuzner, M. L., 501-503
Członkowska, A., 608-610

Dawkins, R. L., 372-373, 513-515, 528-529
Dawson, D. M., 535-536
Dawson, G., 433-436
Degos, J. D., 286-289
de Groot, C. J. A., 549-550
Deibler, G. E., 345-348
Demaine, A., 266-268
De Rossi, A., 615-618
de Silva, S., 176-186
Devare, S. G., 611-614
de Vellis, J., 324-326
Devereux, C., 533-534
Dhib-Jalbut, S., 645-648
Diamantstein, T., 563-565
Difiglia, C. J., 327-329

Dijkstra, C. D., 549-550
DiMartino, M. J., 578-580
D'Imperio, C., 573-575, 642-644
Doherty, P. C., 228-239
Doll, S. C., 678-680
Doolittle, T. H., 271-276
Dorries, R., 663-664
Dowling, P. C., 533-534
Doyon, B., 290-292
Drachman, D. B., 176-186
Duchala, C. S., 661-662
Dwyer, D. S., 452-454

Edwards, C. K., III, 698-699
Emerson, D., 602-604
Eng, H., 520-522
Essayan, D. M., 715-717

Fallis, R., 349-351
Fallis, R. J., 535-536
Fazakerley, J. K., 672-673
Felgenhauer, K., 378-380
Fields, K. L., 327-329
Fierz, W., 122-161, 563-565, 738-740
Fisher, M. C., 681-683
Fontana, A., 218-227, 437-439
Francavilla, E., 615-618
Frank, M. M., 387-388
Fredrikson, S., 282-285
Frei, K., 218-227, 437-439
Fuchs, S., 504-505
Fudenberg, H. H., 602-604
Fujii, N., 516-519
Fujii, Y., 530-532
Fujinami, R. S., 210-217
Fujino, R., 639-641
Funauchi, M., 636-638

Gallo, P., 615-618
Geller, H. M., 445-448
Gill, T. J., III, 493-494
Gin, W., 513-515
Goldowitz, D., 252-254
Goldstein, G., 298-300
Gonzales, L., 702-703
Govaerts, A., 286-289
Greene, M. I., 445-448
Griesmann, G. E., 516-519
Griffin, D. E., 491-492, 566-567
Griffiths, M. S., 528-529
Grimaldi, L. M. E., 611-614
Grimsley, G., 372-373
Groscurth, P., 218-227
Guilbert, B., 290-292
Gulcher, J. R., 333-336

Haar, J. L., 700-701

Hafler, D. A., 306-308, 330-332, 535-536, 557-559
Håkansson, C., 624-627
Hamaguchi, K., 376-377, 720-722
Hanna, N., 578-580
Happ, M. P., 576-577
Harms, H., 663-664
Hartung, H. P., 122-161, 427-429, 563-565, 738-740
Hashim, G., 337-339, 594-596
Hatanaka, M., 636-638
Hauser, S. L., 271-276, 301-305
Hawkins, B. R., 513-515
Hayashi, K., 551-553
Hayashi, T., 271-276, 301-305
Hayes, G. M., 501-503
Heber-Katz, E., 576-577
Heininger, K., 122-161, 427-429, 563-565, 738-740
Hemesath, T. J., 333-336
Henderson, C. E., 628-629
Hermodsson, S., 624-627
Hess, M., 269-270
Hintzen, R., 712-714
Hochkeppel, H. K., 665-668
Hofer, E., 437-439
Hoffman, S. A., 466
Hohlfeld, R., 511-512
Holmdahl, R., 560-562
Honda, Y., 106-114
Hoppe, F., 508-510
Hosokawa, T., 376-377, 720-722
Hruby, S., 581-584
Huang, Z.-X., 516-519

Ikebe, S.-i., 592-593
Ikeda, M., 639-641
Irie, H., 546-548
Ishigaki, Y., 551-553, 554-556
Itagaki, S., 319-323
Ito, H., 258-260

Jackevicius, S. L., 455-458, 581-584
Jacobson, S., 352-353, 645-648
Janković, B. D., 684-687, 691-693
Jerusalem, F., 378-380
Johnson, C. L., 352-353
Johnson, D., 727-728
Johnson, G. C., 649-651
Johnson, H. M., 324-326
Johnson, T. C., 678-680
Joiner, K. A., 387-388
Jones, R., 540-542
Jörnvall, H., 520-522
Joseph, J., 573-575
Jow, B., 523-524
Juji, T., 106-114

# INDEX OF CONTRIBUTORS

**K**ahn, C., 176-186
Kam-Hansen, S., 282-285
Karaszewski, J., 585-588
Kashkin, J. M., 628-629
Kastrukoff, L. F., 654-656
Kelley, K. W., 698-699
Khalili-Shirazi, A., 672-673
Kies, M. W., 345-348
Kim, B., 669-671
Kim, S. U., 654-656
Kimball, E. S., 681-683, 688-690
Kindt, T. J., 271-276
Kirchner, T., 508-510
Klareskog, L., 560-562
Klausner, R. D., 1-3
Knobler, R. L., 252-254, 324-326, 573-575, 642-644, 704-706, 735-737
Knogge, W., 530-532
Koetsier, J. C., 549-550
Kohriyama, T., 442-444
Koike, F., 343-344
Komiya, T., 554-556, 605-607
Korlak, J., 608-610
Koski, C. L., 387-388
Kouvelas, E., 290-292
Kress, Y., 628-629
Krolick, K. A., 340-342
Kuczyńska, A., 608-610
Kuncl, R. W., 176-186
Kunz, H. W., 493-494

**L**ambert, E. H., 516-519
Larsson, P., 560-562
Latov, N., 258-260, 442-444
Lau, A. S., 654-656
Lavi, E., 488-490
Lazzarin, A., 611-614
Lebon, P., 286-289, 309-311, 619-623
Lees, M. B., 709-711
Lefvert, A. K., 520-522, 525-527
Lennon, V. A., 516-519
Levinson, A. I., 115-121
Li, D., 597-601
Li, X., 576-577
Lindsley, M. D., 657-660
Lindstrom, J., 530-532
Link, H., 277-281
Linthicum, D. S., 735-737
Lipton, H., 652-653, 669-671
Lipton, H. L., 674-677, 735-737
Lisak, R. P., 115-121, 715-717
Litwak, M., 571-572
Long, E. O., 352-353
Löwhagen, G.-B., 624-627
Lublin, F. D., 252-254, 573-575, 642-644, 704-706, 735-737
Lund, R. D., 493-494

Luo, M., 652-653
Lyman, W. D., 628-629

**M**ackay, I. R., 372-373
MacPhee, I. A. M., 718-719
Mallat, M., 52-63
Marcus, S. G., 573-575
Marić, D., 684-687, 691-693
Marini, J., 252-254
Martin, R., 449-451
Maselli, R., 585-588
Maselli, R. A., 523-524
Mason, D. W., 718-719
Matell, G., 293-297
Matsiota, P., 290-292
Matsuki, K. 106-114
Matthaei, I., 549-550
Matsuda, S., 636-638
McCarron, R. M., 349-351
McCormick, D. J., 516-519
McFarland, H. F., 99-105, 352-353, 645-648
McFarlin, D. E., 349-351, 645-648
McGeer, E. G., 319-323
McGeer, P. L., 319-323
McGinnis, S., 442-444
McGuire, T. C., 649-651
McIntosh, K. R., 176-186
McKay, R., 47-51
McMorris, F. A., 381-383, 430-432
Mehra, R., 315-318
Mehta, P. D., 261-263
Melvold, R. D., 735-737
Mertens, H. G., 449-451
Meshul, C. K., 537-539
Metlay, M., 702-703
Meyermann, R., 463-465
Miller, S., 669-671
Miller, S. D., 674-677
Miner, L. L., 511-512
Mizrachi, R., 729-731
Moench, T. R., 491-492
Moore, G. R. W., 312-314, 712-714
Moore, P. M., 115-121
Morel, E., 298-300
Mori, F., 639-641
Morimoto, C., 306-308
Morimoto, K., 592-593
Moroni, M., 611-614
Mozell, R. L., 430-432
Mueller, H.-W., 461-462
Müller-Hermelink, H. K., 508-510
Murasko, D. M., 488-490
Murray, E. M., 488-490

**N**akajima, M., 636-638
Nakayasu, H., 546-548
Naohara, T., 106-114

Narayan, O., 661-662, 634-635
Nardelli, E., 91-92, 378-380
Narendran, A., 466
Negishi, T., 376-377, 720-722
Nelson, D. J., 523-524
Neumann, D., 504-505
Newsom-Davis, J., 25-38, 266-268
Nishiguchi, E., 636-638
Nishitani, H., 636-638, 639-641
Nomura, K., 376-377, 720-722
Noronha, A. B. C., 4-12
Northrup, B., 573-575
Nutter, D., 589-590

Offner, H., 337-339, 537-539, 540-542
Oger, J., 597-601
O'Gorman, M., 597-601
Ohno, R., 376-377, 720-722
Ohta, K., 636-638, 639-641
Ohta, M., 636-638, 639-641
Olsson, T., 277-281, 560-562
O'Neill, A., 333-336
Orav, J., 535-536
Orr, E. L., 723-726
Ortlauf, J., 449-451
Ota, K., 546-548
Owhashi, M., 576-577

Page, N., 459-460
Parish, C. R., 543-545
Paty, D. W., 597-601
Pender, M. P., 732-734
Perreault, M., 642-644
Perruisseau, G., 459-460
Pesce, M. A., 442-444
Persico, F. J., 688-690
Petersen, R., 315-318, 581-584
Pevear, D. C., 652-653
Phenix, P., 642-644
Pialoux, G., 619-623
Pinamaneni, S., 589-590
Polman, C. H., 549-550
Posner, J. B., 440-441
Price, R. W., 162-175
Prochiantz, A., 52-63

Raimond, F., 298-300
Raine, C. S., 312-314, 568-570, 571-572, 712-714
Rao, K., 493-494
Rascol, A., 290-292
Rashbaum, W. K., 628-629
Reboul, J., 619-623
Reder, A., 585-588
Reder, A. T., 4-12, 589-590
Reuben-Burnside, C. A., 345-348
Rey, M. A., 619-623

Richert, J. R., 345-348
Richman, D. P., 523-524
Robinson, M. A., 271-276
Rodriguez, M., 240-251, 657-660
Rohowsky-Kochan, C., 533-534
Roos, R. P., 611-614
Rose, L. M., 315-318, 455-458, 581-584
Rubinstein, A., 628-629
Rubinstein, L. J., 78-90
Ruzicka, E., 286-289
Ryberg, B., 384-386
Ryschkewitsch, C. F., 665-668

Safar, D., 506-507
Saida, K., 636-638
Saida, T., 636-638, 639-641
Samelson, L. E., 1-3
Sanders, M. E., 387-388
Saneto, R. P., 324-326
Sano, Y., 387-388
Sato, T., 551-553, 554-556, 592-593, 605-607
Satoh, J., 343-344
Schäfer, B., 122-161, 427-429, 563-565
Schafer, B., 738-740
Schalke, B., 508-510
Schepper, J. M., 698-699
Schluep, M., 378-380, 459-460
Schluesener, H. J., 264-265
Schroeder, C. E., 571-572
Schuller, E., 286-289, 619-623
Schwender, S., 663-664
Sears, D., 269-276
Seboun, E., 271-276
Seeldrayers, P. A., 727-728
Sekaly, R. P., 352-353
Selmaj, K., 568-570, 571-572
Sergott, R. C., 445-448
Shelton, D., 530-532
Shen, N., 576-577
Sherman, P., 255-257
Shin, M. L., 374-375, 381-383, 387-388
Shirazi, Y., 381-383
Siepl, C., 218-227, 437-439
Silberberg, D. H., 488-490, 495-497
Singh, V. K., 602-604
Sminia, T., 549-550
Smyka, W., 589-590
Sobel, R. A., 306-308, 709-711
Soffer, D., 665-668
Spielman, R. S., 269-270
Stanley, J., 566-567
Stazzone, L., 535-536
Steck, A. J., 91-92, 378-380, 459-460
Stefansson, K., 333-336
Steinhauer, E., 628-629
Sticht-Groh, V., 449-451
Stoll, G., 461-462

# INDEX OF CONTRIBUTORS

Stoner, G. L., 665-668
Streletz, L. J., 573-575
Strigård, K., 560-562
Sun, D., 463-465
Sundewall, A.-C., 525-527
Suzumura, A., 488-490, 495-497
Szuchet, S., 433-436

Tabira, T., 187-201, 343-344
Tago, H., 319-323
Takahashi, K., 546-548
Tami, J. A., 340-342
Tanaka, H., 546-548
Tarasewicz, D., 333-336
Tavolato, B., 615-618
Taylor, B. A., 735-737
ter Meulen, V., 202-209, 663-664
Thiemann, R. L., 657-660
Ting, J., 255-257
Tokunaga, K., 106-114
Tong-Lin, S., 551-553
Tournier-Lasserve, E., 594-596
Toyka, K. V., 122-161, 427-429, 511-512, 563-565, 738-740
Traugott, U., 309-311, 712-714
Troiano, R., 533-534
Tsuda, H., 554-556
Tuohy, V. K., 709-711
Tyor, W. R., 491-492
Tzartos, S., 508-510

Vandenbark, A. A., 337-339, 537-539, 540-542
Vandervegt, F. P., 452-454
Vanguri, P., 374-375
Vartanian, T., 433-436
Vaught, J. L., 688-690
Vernet-der-Garabedian, B., 298-300
Vrionis, F., 64-77

Waksman, B. H., 13-24
Walker, D. L., 665-668
Warner, N., 581-584
Watanabe, R., 663-664
Watson-Whitmeyer, M., 704-706
Webb, H. E., 672-673
Webster, H. deF., 665-668
Wege, H., 663-664
Weiner, H. L., 264-265, 306-308, 330-332, 535-536, 557-559, 727-728
Weiner, L. P., 269-270
Weiss, S. R., 488-490
Wekerle, H., 463-465, 508-510
Welsh, K., 266-268
Westarp, M. E., 566-567
Whitham, R. H., 537-539
Wikstrand, C. J., 64-77
Willcox, N., 266-268
Willenborg, D. O., 543-545
Willoughby, E., 597-601
Wolff, C. E., 578-580
Wong, V., 513-515
Woodroofe, M. N., 501-503
Woods, W. T., 694-697
Wrann, M., 437-439
Wucherpfennig, K. W., 264-265

Yamashita, T., 376-377, 720-722
Yu, R. K., 258-260, 442-444
Yu, Y. L., 513-515
Yuemura, K., 376-377
Yunger, L. M., 698-699

Zachau, A., 277-281
Zhang, W. J., 372-373, 513-515
Zimmer, M., 573-575
Zink, M. C., 634-635
Zito, G., 533-534
Z-Lu, C., 282-285
Zweiman, B., 115-121, 715-717